Lecture Notes of the Institute for Computer Sciences, Social Informatics and Telecommunications Engineering 714

The LNICST series publishes ICST's conferences, symposia and workshops.

LNICST reports state-of-the-art results in areas related to the scope of the Institute.

The type of material published includes

- Proceedings (published in time for the respective event)
- Other edited monographs (such as project reports or invited volumes)

LNICST topics span the following areas:

- General Computer Science
- E-Economy
- E-Medicine
- Knowledge Management
- Multimedia
- Operations, Management and Policy
- Social Informatics
- Systems

Hirokazu Tanaka · Matti Hämäläinen ·
Daisuke Anzai
Editors

Body Area Networks

20th EAI International Conference, BodyNets 2025
Okayama, Japan, December 2–4, 2025
Proceedings

Springer

Editors
Hirokazu Tanaka
Hiroshima City University
Hiroshima, Japan

Matti Hämäläinen
University of Oulu
Oulu, Finland

Daisuke Anzai
Osaka Metropolitan University
Osaka, Japan

ISSN 1867-8211 ISSN 1867-822X (electronic)
Lecture Notes of the Institute for Computer Sciences, Social Informatics and Telecommunications Engineering
ISBN 978-3-032-38656-4 ISBN 978-3-032-38657-1 (eBook)
https://doi.org/10.1007/978-3-032-38657-1

This Springer imprint is published by the registered company Springer Nature Switzerland AG
The registered company address is: Gewerbestrasse 11, 6330 Cham, Switzerland

Preface

We are delighted to introduce the proceedings of the 2025 European Alliance for Innovation (EAI) International Conference on Body Area Networks (Bodynets 2025), titled "Intelligent Edge Cloud for Dependable Globally Connected BAN," held in Okayama, Japan, from 2–4 December 2025. Bodynets 2025 provided an international forum for researchers, scientists, and practitioners from around the world to present and exchange ideas on the research, development, and deployment of smart body technologies and Body Area Networks.

The technical program of Bodynets 2025 consisted of 40 peer-reviewed papers, framed within a diverse range of tracks, each focusing on critical and emerging aspects of body area network technologies. These papers were selected from 97 submissions. Each submission was reviewed following a double-blind process with a minimum of 3 reviews per paper. The tracks included:

- **THz Sensing and Tissue Characterization for Body Area Networks**, focusing on terahertz and sub-terahertz time-domain spectroscopy for biological tissue characterization and its impact on communication performance in BAN and SmartBAN systems.
- **Sensing, Localization, and Motion Analysis in Body Area Networks**, exploring advanced sensing and localization techniques for body-centric systems, including 3D implant localization, magnetic-field-based positioning, and multimodal motion recognition.
- **Physical-Layer Techniques for Medical and Body-Centric Systems**, addressing physical-layer innovations such as secure biometric authentication, hybrid inductive–capacitive wireless power transfer for implants, biomedical system applications, and propagation modeling in challenging environments.
- **Advanced Sensing and Signal Processing for Health Monitoring**, covering non-contact vital sign monitoring, wearable ECG artifact removal, cognitive state and visual function assessment, and pressure-based health monitoring systems.
- **Clinical, Implantable, and Wearable Systems for Healthcare Applications**, focusing on the design and application of implantable, wearable, and networked systems for healthcare, including emergency care optimization, neurostimulation hardware, long-range monitoring platforms, personalized cardiovascular modeling, and performance-oriented wearables.
- **Molecular Communication and Bio-Inspired Networking Models**, exploring theoretical and computational advances in molecular and bio-inspired communications, including reaction–diffusion modeling, electrical-to-molecular interfaces, and collective behavior of bio-nanomachine clusters.
- **Body Area Networks and Wearable Systems for Reliable Health Monitoring**, addressing adaptive MAC protocols, UWB ranging in IEEE 802.15.6ma BANs, non-invasive IoT-based home monitoring, heatstroke detection, and physiological biofeedback methods.

- **Reliable and Interference-Resilient Wireless Networks for Healthcare**, focusing on reliability enhancement and interference robustness through reinforcement-learning-based WLAN optimization, advanced error control and HARQ schemes, and coexistence-aware UWB BAN communications.
- **Human-Centric Sensing, Haptics, and Data Standardization**, covering textile sensibility evaluation, virtual vital-sign sensing, haptics technology considerations, and standardized frameworks for sensor data distribution and heterogeneous media stream alignment.

In addition to the technical paper presentations, the conference featured a special panel session titled "Standardization Session on Wearable Technologies," fostering discussion on standardization challenges and future directions in wearable and body-centric systems.

The technical program was further enriched by three keynote speeches delivered by distinguished experts in the field:

- **Stefano Caputo**, Optical Wireless Communications for In- and On-Body Communications
- **Hiroyuki Shinoda**, Haptics with Body Area Networks: Improving Mental Health while Enhancing Human Ability
- **Shinichiro Haruyama**, Navigation System Utilizing Visible Light Communication (VLC) and Its Standardization – A Promising Application of Optical Wireless Communication Technology in Body Area Environments

We would like to express our sincere gratitude to the steering chairs and the organizing committee for their dedication and tireless efforts in making Bodynets 2025 a success. We also thank the members of the Technical Program Committee for their careful and professional review of the submitted papers. Finally, we extend our appreciation to all authors for contributing their high-quality research to the conference.

We believe that Bodynets 2025 offered a valuable forum for researchers, developers, and practitioners to exchange ideas and discuss scientific and technological advances in Body Area Network technologies. We hope that these proceedings will serve as a useful reference for the research community and for all those interested in this rapidly evolving field.

Hirokazu Tanaka
Matti Hämäläinen
Daisuke Anzai

Organization

Organizing Committee

General Chair

Hirokazu Tanaka	Hiroshima City University, Japan

General Co-chairs

Lorenzo Mucchi	University of Florence, Italy
Chika Sugimoto	Yokohama National University, Japan

TPC Chairs

Matti Hämäläinen	University of Oulu, Finland
Daisuke Anzai	Osaka Metropolitan University, Japan

Sponsorship and Exhibit Chair

Kai Ishida	Shonan Institute of Technology, Japan

Local Chair

Takahiro Ito	Hiroshima City University, Japan

Publicity and Social Media Chair

Marco Hernandez	University of Oulu, Finland

Publications Chair

Maurizio Magarini	Politecnico di Milano, Italy

Web Chair

Kento Takabayashi	Toyo University, Japan

Panels Chair

Jari Iinatti	University of Oulu, Finland

Tutorials Chairs

Manato Fujimoto	Osaka Metropolitan University, Japan

Technical Program Committee

Balasingham Ilangko	Oslo University Hospital, Norway
Dudley-McEvoy Sandra	London South Bank University, UK
Fujimoto Manato	Osaka Metropolitan University, Japan
Harjula Erkki	University of Oulu, Finland
Hernandez Marco	University of Oulu, Finland
Hyry Jaakko	Nagoya Institute of Technology, Japan
Iinatti Jari	University of Oulu, Finland
Ishida Kai	Shonan Institute of Technology, Japan
Ito Takahiro	Hiroshima City University, Japan
Katz Marcos	University of Oulu, Finland
Kumpuniemi Timo	University of Oulu, Finland
Magarini Maurizio	Politecnico di Milano, Italy
Mikhaylov Konstantin	University of Oulu, Finland
Mucchi Lorenzo	University of Florence, Italy
Nguyen Diep	University of Technology Sydney, Australia
Särestöniemi Mariella	University of Oulu, Finland
Sayrafian Kamran	National Institute of Standards and Technology, USA
Sugimoto Chika	Yokohama National University, Japan
Takabayashi Kento	Toyo University, Japan
Tanaka Hirokazu	Hiroshima City University, Japan
Taparussanagorn	Attaphongse Asian Institute of Technology, Thailand

Contents

Physical-Layer Techniques for Medical and Body-Centric Systems

Advanced Sensing and Signal Processing for Health Monitoring

Clinical, Implantable, and Wearable Systems for Healthcare Applications

Molecular Communication and Bio-Inspired Networking Models

Body Area Networks and Wearable Systems for Reliable Health Monitoring

Reliable and Interference-Resilient Wireless Networks for Healthcare

Human-Centric Sensing, Haptics, and Data Standardization

THz Sensing and Tissue Characterization

Study of TeraHertz Time Domain Spectroscopy for Tissue Characterization in Body Area Networks

Marco Hernandez(✉)

Center for Wireless Communications, University of Oulu, Oulu, Finland
Marco.Hernandez@oulu.fi

Abstract. TeraHertz time-domain spectroscopy (THz-TDS) systems have emerged as mature technologies with significant potential in several research fields, consumer electronics, industry, and medical applications. The paper presents an initial study on the use of THz technology on the human body and the potential impact of implants or a fusion center with THz wireless links on the body, both on- and in-body. This study intends to observe the THz absorption and refraction on [pork] skin samples to start building a simulation model to study SAR on human tissues.

Keywords: THz Time Domain Spectroscopy · THz tissue characterization · Body Area Networks

1 Introduction

The next generation of Body Area Networks (BAN) envisions incorporating a use case for Brain-Computer Interface (BCI) that necessitates a reduction in sensor form factor and an increase in aggregated data rate. Indeed, current electrodes implanted in the human brain can accommodate a plaque of 100 electrodes covering $3\,\text{cm}^2$ with a sampling rate of 1 kHz per electrode and a resolution of 14 bits. Consequently, the aggregated data rate for this set of electrodes is 1.4 Mb/s. If the intention is to cover a larger area of the brain, such as accommodating four arrays, it would require 56 Mb/s to handle the aggregated data rate. Hence, a future generation of BANs will require: a small form factor, high speed, and the possibility of implementing Wireless Power Transfer (WPT), as brain surgery cannot be performed frequently. That is why TeraHertz (THz) technology is a candidate, as Visual Light Communications (VLC) requires Line Of Sight (LOS), and acoustic devices are low-speed.

THz waves can be absorbed and emitted by substances. THz Time Domain Spectroscopy (THz-TDS) is an instrument that was initially conceived to determine the chemical composition of materials, but lately, it has expanded to a wide range of other applications.

This work is partially supported by 6G Flagship (Grant 369116) funded by the Research Council of Finland and Infotech Oulu via SEHU project.

H. Tanaka et al. (Eds.): BodyNets 2025, LNICST 714, pp. 3–15, 2026.
https://doi.org/10.1007/978-3-032-38657-1_1

The non-ionizing nature of THz radiation makes it possible to detect biological tissues non-invasively. Moreover, THz waves are part of the fingerprint spectrum (the electromagnetic absorption pattern by a substance is highly complex but unique to each substance's structure). However, the measurements with THz-TDS can be coupled with the penetration of THz waves into tissues to study SAR. Moreover, the relatively high-resolution THz-TDS can be used for imaging as well. The paper is divided into an overview of THz-TDS, uncertainties in the measurements, and an experiment with pork tissues with the TeraPulse 4000.

2 Overview of TeraHertz Time-Domain Spectroscopy

THz-TDS is a versatile, high-precision tool, offering detailed material characterization unmatched by many other techniques. The time-domain approach provides both amplitude and phase data, making it ideal for research and industrial quality control. THz-TDS consists of:

1. Femtosecond fiber laser: Generates ultra-short ($\backsim$100 fs) optical pulses.
2. THz Emitter: Downconverts laser pulses into THz radiation via a photoconductive antenna (PCA). When the fs laser hits the PCA, carriers are excited, producing THz pulses via transient current.
3. THz Detector: Measures the terahertz pulses after interaction with the sample via a PCA optimized for sensitivity or an electro-optic crystal.
4. Optical Delay Line: Adjusts the timing between the *pump* and *probe* beams for time-domain analysis.
5. Sample Chamber: Holds the material under test in the THz beam path.
6. Control & Analysis Software: Processes the acquired time-domain data into frequency-domain spectra.
7. Configurations: Transmission mode (THz pulses pass through the sample, and absorption and phase shifts are measured), Reflection mode (THz pulses reflect off the sample surface; used for opaque or thick materials), and Attenuated Total Reflection (ATR) mode (THz waves undergo total internal reflection in a prism, with an evanescent wave probing the sample).
8. Repetition Rate: $\backsim$80 MHz (standard for time-domain systems).
9. Average Power: $\backsim$10–50 mW (ensures stable THz generation).
10. Frequency Range: 0.1–4 THz.
11. Dynamic range: $>$70 dB (enables detection of weak signals).
12. Spectral Resolution: $<$1 GHz (depends on time-delay scan length).
13. Acquisition Speed: Milliseconds per scan.

THz-TDS is a technique used to measure material properties, such as the index of refraction and conductivity, as well as spectral absorption, among others. It is also used for imaging.

Typically, the THz pulse is generated via optical rectification in a crystal or Photo-Conductive Antenna (PCA). The THz pulse is then focused through a sample and subsequently detected in another crystal or PCA via free-space electro-optic detection. The measured signal is proportional to the Electric field of the pulse, such that the magnitude and phase are preserved, and the complex transmission coefficient can be extracted. From this, the full complex value of the sample material parameters can be extracted. A THz pulse is generated via optical rectification in a crystal (optical downconversion to a THz pulse). The THz pulse is then focused through a sample and subsequently detected in another crystal via free-space electro-optic detection. Figure 1 shows the schematic diagram of a THz–TDS system.

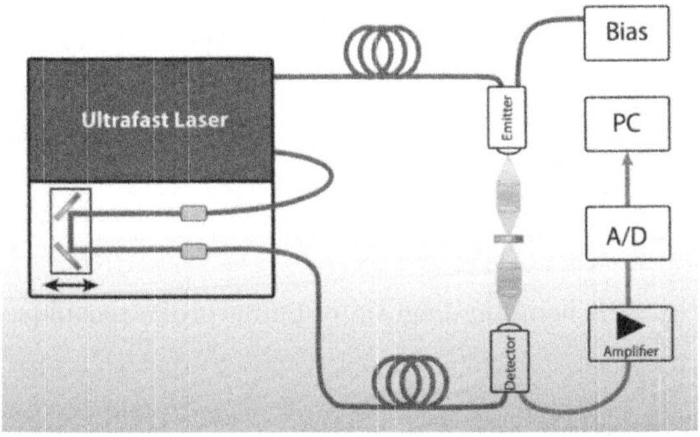

Fig. 1. Schematic diagram of a THz–TDS system.

A split of the original laser beam (the probe beam) arrives at the detector with a controlled time delay relative to the pump beam (pulse THz signal after downconversion). The detector detects the electric field of the pump THz pulse triggered by the probe THz pulse at each delay time. By scanning the delay, the entire electric field of the THz pulse is mapped as a function of time, or the time-domain signal.

This time-domain sampling detection is done using the pump-probe technique. It is a powerful experimental method used to investigate ultrafast events. The idea is to use two synchronized laser pulses. The pump pulse acts as the probing electric field that interacts with the sample. The probe pulse triggers the detector at a controlled delay time, such that the detector measures the result of the change of the probing electric field interacting with the sample, as illustrated in Fig. 2.

The data analysis & interpretation can be summarized as follows:

1. Time-Domain Waveform: Raw data shows the electric field of the THz pulse over time. The sample's interaction produces time delays (phase shifts) and amplitude changes (absorption).
2. Frequency-domain spectrum: The amplitude spectrum shows absorption features. The phase spectrum reveals refractive index changes.
3. Extracting material properties: Refractive Index (n) calculated from phase delay. Absorption Coefficient (α), derived from amplitude attenuation.
4. Dielectric function (ε): Obtained from n and α via the Kramers-Kronig relations.

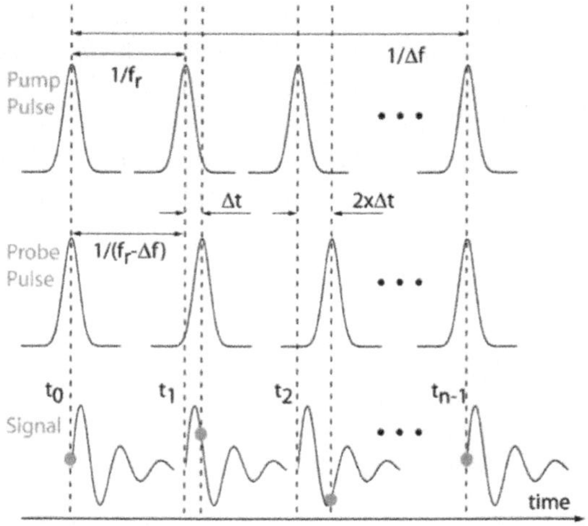

Fig. 2. Schematic diagram of pump-probe technique.

2.1 THz Transmission and Detection

The laser femtosecond pulse hits a biased GaAs/InGaAs substrate with nanoscale electrodes. Photons create electron-hole pairs in the semiconductor. The applied bias field accelerates carriers, producing a transient current that radiates THz waves.

The THz Electric field is proportional to the time derivative of the photocurrent density $J(t)$ as:

$$E(t) \propto \frac{dJ(t)}{dt} \tag{1}$$

The THz detection is based on Electro-Optic Sampling (EOS). The pump THz pulse and delayed probe pulse co-propagate in an electro-optic crystal (e.g., ZnTe), where the THz electric field induces birefringence (the difference in the index of refraction between two beams passing through a substance that has this property) in the crystal, modifying the probe's polarization. A Wollaston prism and photodiodes measure polarization rotation, reconstructing $E(t)$. The detected signal is given by

$$\triangle I \propto E(t)\, L\, r_{41}\, I_{probe} \tag{2}$$

where L is the crystal thickness, and r_{41} is the electro-optic coefficient ($\backsim$ 4 pm/V for ZnTe).

The optical time-delay line is a motorized stage adjusting the optical path length with <100 nm precision, where delay taps are typically $\backsim$ 300 ps (for 4 THz resolution). The optical path calculation for a delay τ is given by

$$\triangle L\, c\, \tau / n_{air} \tag{3}$$

where c is the speed of light, and $n_{air} \approx 1$.

Measurements are typically averaged to increase the SNR to greater than 70 dB, and the FFT uses a Hanning window to reduce spectral leakage. Water vapor absorption lines are subtracted using reference data.

3 Uncertainties in THz Time-Domain Spectroscopy Measurements

Calculating uncertainties in THz time-domain spectroscopy measurements involves analyzing errors from instrumental noise, sample alignment, environmental factors, and data processing. Major sources of uncertainty are as follows:

1. Instrumental Noise: Laser Power Fluctuations affect THz generation and detection stability. Quantification is done by measuring the THz amplitude variation over repeated scans.
2. Detector Noise: Shot noise, thermal Noise, electro-optic sampling (EOS), or photoconductive detection noise. Quantification is performed by recording the baseline noise (in the absence of a THz pulse) and calculating the RMS noise level.
3. Optical delay line positioning errors introduce mechanical jitter in the time-delay stage, affecting timing precision. Quantification is done by measuring stage repeatability (typically $< 0.1\ \mu$m, equivalent to $\backsim$ 0.3 fs timing error.
4. Thickness variation: Non-uniform samples introduce errors in refractive index (n) and absorption coefficient (α). Quantification is performed by measuring thickness at multiple points (using a micrometer or interferometry) and calculating the standard deviation.
5. Surface Roughness & Scattering: Scattering losses distort amplitude measurements. Quantification is done by using profilometry to measure surface roughness and apply correction models.
6. Misalignment Errors: Sample tilt or beam misalignment causes phase shifts. Quantification is done by measuring the angular dependence of the THz signal (e.g., $\pm 1^{o}$ tilt produces $\backsim$ 1% amplitude error).
7. Water vapor: Ambient water vapor absorbs THz at specific frequencies (e.g., 0.56, 0.75, 1.1 THz). Mitigation is done by purging with dry air, nitrogen, or subtracting the reference spectrum.
8. Temperature drifts: it affects laser stability and sample properties. Quantification is done by monitoring lab temperature and correlating it with signal drift.
9. Fourier transform issues: Window functions (Hanning, Blackman) introduce spectral leakage. Quantification by comparing FFT results with/without windowing.
10. Peak fitting errors: Errors in extracting $n(\omega)$ and $\alpha(\omega)$ from transmission/reflection models. Quantification is done by using Monte Carlo simulations to propagate noise through fitting algorithms.

Reducing uncertainties is given by

1. Improve SNR: Increase laser power (without damaging the emitter). Use longer averaging (e.g., 1000 scans).
2. Environmental control: Purge with dry air to minimize water vapor absorption. Stabilize lab temperature (± 0.1°C).
3. Calibration: Use reference samples (e.g., Si wafer) to validate system performance.
4. Advanced Fitting: Use machine learning or Bayesian inference for robust parameter extraction.

3.1 Transmission Amplitude Uncertainty

The dominant uncertainty in THz-TDS is often amplitude noise or transmission amplitude uncertainty, and is calculated as follows:

1. Measure the reference signal (without sample), acquire N repeated scans of the reference THz pulse, and compute the mean time-domain and standard deviation of the detected electric field (E_{ref}, σ_{ref}). Repeat the same for the measure sample signal: $(E_{samp}, \sigma_{samp})$.
2. The complex transmission is given by

$$\tilde{T}(\omega) = \frac{\tilde{E}_{samp}(\omega)}{\tilde{E}_{ref}(\omega)} \tag{4}$$

and uncertainty propagation is given by

$$\delta\tilde{T}(\omega) = \tilde{T}(\omega)\sqrt{\left(\frac{\sigma_{samp}(\omega)}{\tilde{E}_{samp}(\omega)}\right)^2 + \left(\frac{\sigma_{ref}(\omega)}{\tilde{E}_{ref}(\omega)}\right)^2} \tag{5}$$

3. The complex refractive index $\tilde{n} = n + ik$ is extracted from

$$\tilde{n}(\omega) = 1 + (c\omega/\delta d)\ln(\tilde{T}(\omega)) \tag{6}$$

where δd is the sample thickness measurement uncertainty.

3.2 Signal-to-Noise Ratio Calculation

The SNR quantifies the quality of THz-TDS data by comparing the signal power or amplitude to the noise floor. However, the SNR for THz-TDS has been conventionally defined by physics scientists as the ratio.

$$\text{SNR} = \frac{\mu}{\sigma} \tag{7}$$

where μ is the sample mean signal or expected value, and σ is the standard deviation of the noise or an estimate thereof. This definition is closely related to the sensitivity index (also known as the discriminability index or detectability index). The reason is that the "noise" is not only thermal noise as conventionally assumed in wireless communications, but also includes other uncertainties as mentioned in Sect. 3.

Thus, the discriminability or detectability of a signal depends on the separation and the spread of the noise-alone and signal-plus-noise probability distributions. Discriminability or detectability is improved by increasing the separation (a stronger signal) or by decreasing the spread (reducing noise). In either case, there is less overlap between the probabilities of occurrences. Describing how discriminable the signal is from the no-signal (or noise-alone) requires capturing the separation and the spread of their probability distributions. The most widely used measure is called d-prime ($d' = separation/spread$). Notice that d' is an estimate of the strength of the signal embedded in uncertainties. This value does not depend upon the criterion the subject is adopting. Still, it is a true measure of the internal response, and the reason Eq. 7 is used to quantify the SNR in THz-TDS. However, careful consideration must be given that the SNR and other desired parameters must be quantified from measurement data, and consequently, the use of statistical analysis is required.

This paper deals with two univariate distributions a (noise-alone) and b (signal-plus-noise) with the same standard deviation σ, such that d' is the separation between the means of the two distributions in units of the standard deviation given by

$$d' = \frac{|\mu_a - \mu_b|}{\sigma} \tag{8}$$

As we are dealing with measurement data, the analysis of data is done with statistical tools, in this case, estimation statistics. Here d' is a statistical effect size, which is a value measuring the strength of the relationship between two variables in a population, or a sample-based estimate of that quantity, as is our case.

Hence, assuming that the signal under test has two states (noise-alone and signal-plus-noise), separated by $\mu = \mu_a - \mu_b$, and that σ (the spread) does not change between the two states. If the signal data is known to be constant, then σ can be calculated using the standard deviation of the signal. If the signal data is not constant, then σ can be calculated from the data, where the signal is zero (or noise-alone).

Below is a step-by-step method to compute SNR for THz-TDS. The SNR is computed as follows:

1. Acquire the time-domain waveforms: Reference scan (no sample, just air), and "noise" scan (block THz beam or measure at a time delay where no THz pulse exists).
2. Measure the root-mean-square (RMS) of the received THz signal.

3. Measure the noise floor: Select a noise window (e.g., 10–20 ps after the pulse, where no THz signal is present) and compute RMS noise as:

$$E_{noise} = \sqrt{\frac{1}{N}\sum_{i=1}^{N}(E(t_i) - \langle E\rangle)^2} \tag{9}$$

where N is the number of points in the noise window, and $\langle E\rangle = 1/N\sum_{i=1}^{N} E(t_i)$ is the sample mean of noise level.
4. The SNR is given by

$$\text{SNR} = 20\,\text{Log}\left(\frac{E_{rms}}{E_{noise}}\right). \tag{10}$$

E_{noise} is a coarse estimate of the uncertainties of the THz data capture, including thermal noise, shot noise, thickness & alignment errors. Noise reduction can be accomplished by introducing a moving average filter, by smoothing high-frequency noise, analyzing multiple peaks for resonant samples, and averaging over multiple scans.

4 THz Pulse Propagation in Life-Form Tissues

Performing THz propagation studies on life-form tissues using the THz-TDS involves a careful experimental setup designed to capture both spectral absorption and temporal delay, revealing tissue-specific information such as hydration, structure, and pathological differences. Here's how to approach it: THz radiation is non-ionizing and interacts strongly with polar molecules, especially water, making it ideal for probing hydration content, collagen/fat differences. Cancerous vs. healthy tissue. THz-TDS instruments typically cannot penetrate deeply ($\backsim$ 0.1–2 mm) into tissue due to water absorption, so the reflection mode in the instrument is typically used. Indeed, the transmission mode is typically used for thin tissues (samples $\backsim$ 1 mm thick) due to high water absorption. The reflection mode is typically used for thicker tissues, like muscle, and it measures the reflected THz signal from the tissue surface (useful for in vivo or ex vivo measurements).

4.1 THz Propagation on Skin Pork Tissue

In a first approach to the characterization of human tissues, we conducted a measurement campaign to study the effect of THz radiation on samples of pork skin. The TeraPulse 4000 in Transmission Mode is used for the experiments. The instrument is covered with plastic to avoid contamination and purged with dry air as shown in Fig. 3.

Pork chops were cut with several thicknesses of pork skin, with fat, and with fat and muscle. Those were used as a proxy for human tissues. The pork's fat skin was cut as much as possible, but a more precise cutting instrument would be required.

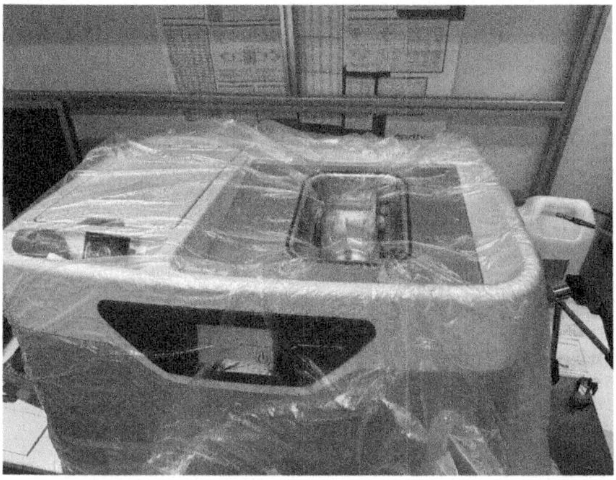

Fig. 3. The THz-TDS TeraPulse 4000.

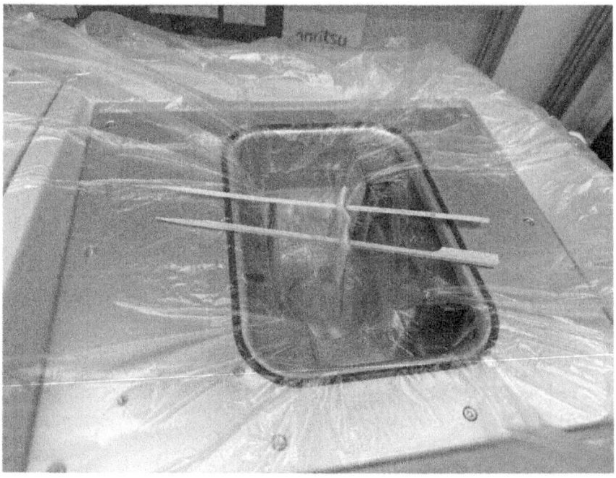

Fig. 4. Pork skin samples in TeraPulse 4000.

The samples were placed in wooden sticks as indicated in Fig. 4.

Although pork's skin may be a good approach to human skin, it must be considered that it is dead tissue with more fat than an average human and without capillary veins or blood flow. However, the impact on THz measurements is the main evaluation.

4.2 TeraPulse 4000

We performed a set of experiments with the TeraPulse 4000. The instrument records traces in the time domain. The time-domain waveform processing firstly removes the system response as indicated in Eq. 11.

$$T(\omega) = \frac{E_{sample}(\omega)}{E_{ref}(\omega)} \tag{11}$$

Apply a Hanning window to reduce spectral leakage. For transmission measurements, the refractive index is given by

$$n(\omega) = 1 + \frac{c\,\Delta\phi(\omega)}{\omega\, d} \tag{12}$$

where $\Delta\phi(\omega)$ is the phase difference, and d is the sample thickness.

The absorption coefficient is given by

$$\alpha(\omega) = -\frac{2}{d}\ln\left(\frac{|T(\omega)|(n(\omega+1))^2}{4n(\omega)}\right) \tag{13}$$

4.3 Experimental Results

We present some experimental results for a skin cut of 2 mm. Figure 5 is the THz pulse detected after passing through the sample. Figure 6 shows the reference THz pulse (no sample). Figure 7 and Fig. 8 show the corresponding spectrum.

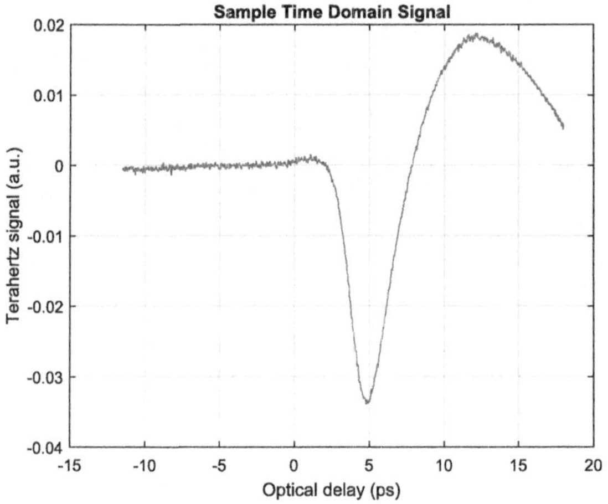

Fig. 5. Sample time-domain signal.

The refractive index and absorption coefficient spectra are calculated from the amplitude, phase spectra, and according to Eq. 12 and Eq. 13, respectively. The refractive index spectrum is shown in Fig. 9 and the absorption index spectrum is shown in Fig. 10.

The dynamic range of the measured absorption spectrum is based on the SNR consideration. However, the SNR is based on a coarse estimation of noise. In a future study, the different sources of noise will be characterized more precisely.

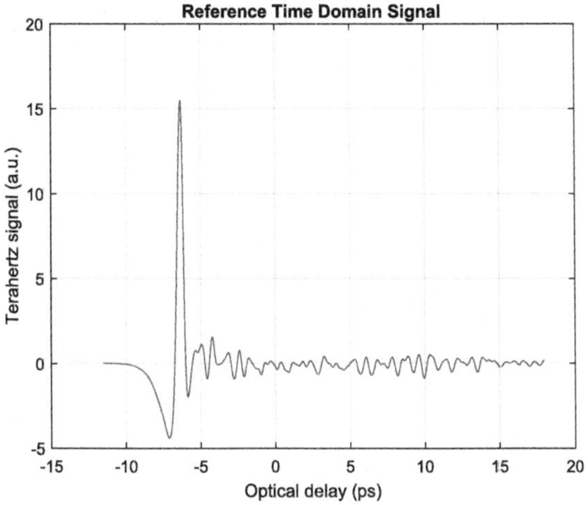

Fig. 6. Reference time-domain signal.

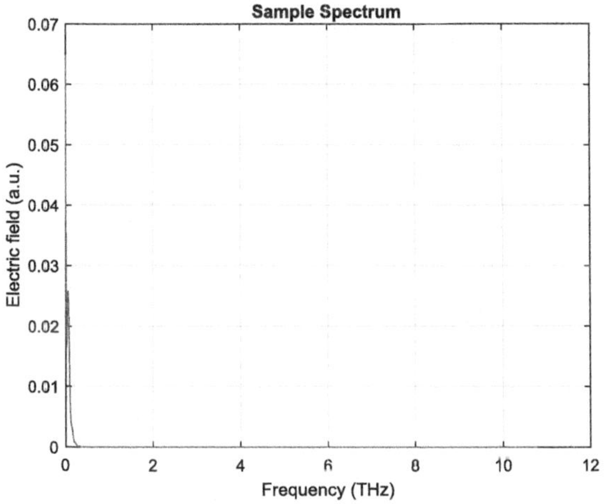

Fig. 7. Sample spectrum.

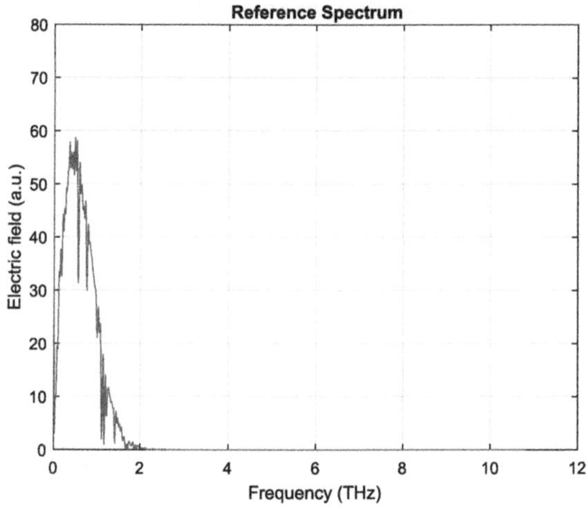

Fig. 8. Reference spectrum.

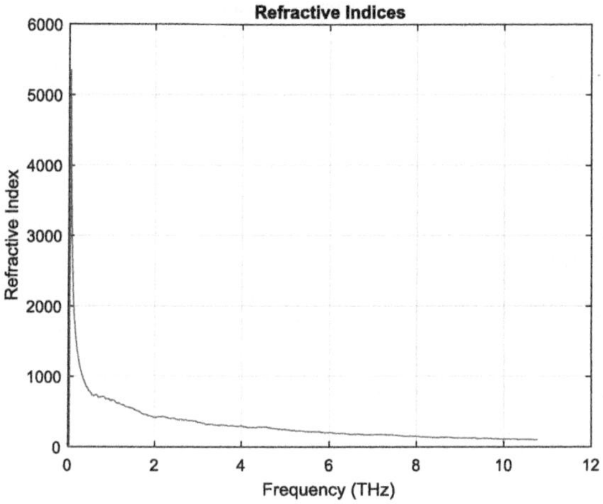

Fig. 9. Refractive index.

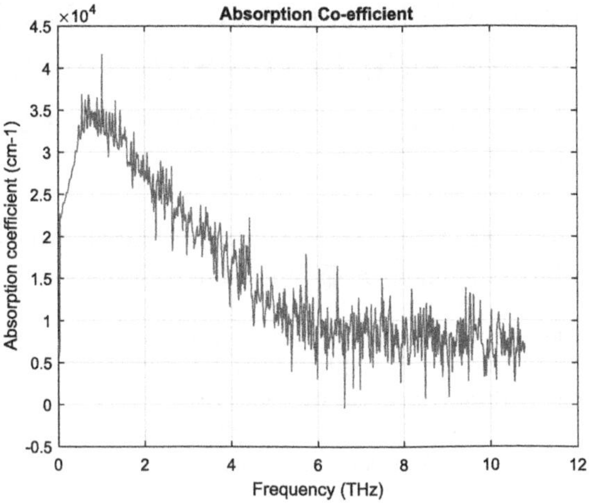

Fig. 10. Absorption index.

5 Conclusions

As described above, the absorption coefficient spectrum is measured by directing a beam of THz radiation to the sample and detecting the intensity of the radiation that passes through it. The transmitted energy can be used to calculate the absorption coefficient spectrum. As shown in Fig. 10, there is a significant absorption around 1 THz, and variable otherwise. The absorption coefficients depend on varying concentrations of collagen and water molecules in the samples.

All in all, there is an indication that THz-TDS can detect changes in the spatial structure of the skin and, in general, other tissues, as it is possible to detect, differentiate, and identify specific skin or tissue structures, such as glands, capillaries, and others, which enables medical imaging. Future research work is to validate and specify an electromagnetic simulation model that can be used to study SAR, WPT, and the impact of THz radiation on biological cells.

References

1. Son, J.K. (ed.): Terahertz Biomedical Science & Technology. CRC Press, Boca Raton (2014)
2. Nikitkina, A.I., et al.: Terahertz radiation and the skin: a review. J. Biomed. Optics **26**(4) (2021)
3. Neu, J., et al.: Tutorial: an introduction to terahertz time domain spectroscopy. J. Appl. Phys. **124**, 231101 (2018)
4. TeraView Ltd. TeraPulse 4000 User's Guide, Cambridge (2019)

Layered Dielectric Characterization of Human Skin in the Sub-Terahertz and Terahertz Frequency Ranges

Silvia Mura[1(✉)], Elisabetta Marini[1], Maurizio Magarini[1], Matti Hämäläinen[2], and Marco Hernandez[2]

[1] Department of Electronics, Information and Bioengineering, Politecnico di Milano, Milan, Italy
{silvia.mura,elisabetta.marini,maurizio.magarini}@polimi.it
[2] University of Oulu, Oulu, Finland
matti.hamalainen@oulu.fi

Abstract. Sub-terahertz (sub-THz) and terahertz (THz) radiation offer unique opportunities for non-invasive diagnostics and imaging due to their sensitivity to water content and molecular dynamics in biological tissues. In this work, a comprehensive dielectric model of human skin and its cellular constituents is developed across these frequency ranges. The model combines multi-Debye relaxation theory with effective medium formulations to account for intracellular water dynamics and macromolecular relaxation processes. Key cellular parameters, including water content, protein and lipid fractions, and ionic conductivity, are integrated from experimentally validated sources. The proposed framework enables realistic predictions of frequency-dependent permittivity for different skin layers and cell types, providing a physically interpretable description of sub-THz and THz tissue interactions. This approach establishes a foundation for the design and optimization of next-generation diagnostic and imaging techniques operating in these frequency bands.

Keywords: Terahertz Radiation · Millimeter-wave · Dielectric Modeling · Multi-Debye Relaxation · Human Skin · Cellular Permittivity

1 Introduction

The interaction between sub-terahertz (sub-THz) and terahertz (THz) radiation with biological tissues has gained increased attention for diagnostics, imaging, and sensing applications [1,2]. In these frequency ranges, electromagnetic waves couple to vibrational and rotational modes, revealing intermolecular forces and collective molecular dynamics. This sensitivity is especially relevant in water-rich biological media, where sub-THz and THz waves enable non-ionizing, non-

H. Tanaka et al. (Eds.): BodyNets 2025, LNICST 714, pp. 16–31, 2026.
https://doi.org/10.1007/978-3-032-38657-1_2

destructive probing of tissue hydration and cellular water content. While sub-THz radiation penetrates deeper due to lower absorption, THz waves offer higher spectral resolution, making the two ranges complementary in biomedical contexts.

At the molecular level, weak interactions such as hydrogen bonds and van der Waals forces govern biomolecular structure and functions [3,4]. The sub-THz and THz window ($0.1 - 10\,\text{THz}$) coincides with many rotational and vibrational molecular modes, granting access to molecular and collective motions beyond the reach of infrared spectroscopy [4]. In aqueous environments, these frequencies are particularly sensitive to hydrogen-bond dynamics, providing insights into the organization and fluctuations of biomolecular systems, because water is the predominant constituent of biological tissue. Consequently, spectroscopy in the sub-THz and THz domains has emerged as a powerful approach to investigate the structural organization and functional dynamics of biomolecular systems [5].

Propagation in biological tissues depends mainly on water absorption, given their 60–80% water content [6,7]. Scattering also contributes, arising from the structural heterogeneity of tissues, while reflections at interfaces with different refractive indices provide imaging contrast, for instance in distinguishing malignant from healthy tissue [6,7]. Dispersion further modulates wave propagation, influencing time-domain spectroscopy results [7].

Modeling sub-THz and THz propagation in tissue often rely on frequency-dependent complex permittivity $\varepsilon(\omega) = \varepsilon'(\omega) - j\varepsilon''(\omega)$, with the imaginary part accounting for absorption. Advanced approaches employ numerical simulations or finite element methods in COMSOL to capture realistic geometries, dielectric heterogeneity, and scattering effects [8,9].

Skin is a key focus for sub-THz and THz studies, being the body's outermost layer and a target for cancer detection [10,11], non-invasive imaging [12], and body-centric communications [13]. Its layered structure—epidermis, dermis, and hypodermis—shows distinct dielectric properties linked to hydration, macromolecular content, and lipid composition [14]. Therefore, realistic modeling of propagation in these frequency ranges therefore requires a multi-layer description of skin that accounts for its anatomical and cellular heterogeneity.

The dielectric response of biological cells in these ranges is commonly modeled using Debye-type relaxation. This formalism describes the frequency-dependent complex permittivity as the result of dipolar relaxation processes, which are especially relevant for polar species, such as water, proteins, and lipids [15]. Multi-Debye formulations account for multiple relaxation processes: the parameters can be tuned according to water content, protein and lipid composition, and ionic conductivity, offering a physically interpretable framework for predicting cellular dielectric properties and constructing realistic tissue-level models. Linking water dynamics and macromolecular contributions to overall permittivity is thus fundamental to advancing sub-THz and THz sensing and imaging in biomedical applications.

In this work, we propose a comprehensive dielectric model of human skin and its cellular constituents across the sub-THz and THz frequency ranges. The framework integrates multi-Debye relaxation theory with effective medium formulations to describe intracellular water and macromolecular inclusions, yielding realistic frequency-dependent permittivity predictions validated against experimental data.

The paper is organized as follows. Section 2 describes the multilayer skin model and the considered cellular constituents. Section 3 details the dielectric computation framework. In Sect. 4, we analyze intra-body wave propagation. Section 5 describes the voxel-based simulation framework used to model realistic skin tissue scenarios.

2 Skin Model and Cells

Human skin is a complex, multilayered organ whose structural and compositional heterogeneity strongly influences its electromagnetic behavior in the millimeter-wave, sub-THz, and THz frequency ranges [16–18]. It is composed of multiple layers with distinct water content, protein and lipid composition, and cellular organization, leading to depth-dependent variations in dielectric properties. Understanding these variations is crucial for accurate modeling of sub-THz and THz propagation and for reliable interpretation of imaging and sensing data.

The overall dielectric response of skin arises from the combined contributions of cellular and extracellular components, including water, proteins, lipids, and ionic species [2,19]. In this context, only cellular structures whose dimensions are comparable to the wavelengths or penetration depths of sub-THz and THz radiation are expected to significantly interact with the electromagnetic field, contributing to scattering and absorption phenomena. Modeling the skin as a multilayer system, as illustrated in Fig. 1, enables the representation of these heterogeneous effects on the macroscopic dielectric response. This framework provides a physically grounded basis for simulating sub-THz and THz tissue interactions and for predicting layer-specific electromagnetic contrasts.

2.1 Epidermis

The epidermis is the outermost skin layer and the primary interface with the external environment. Its thickness can reach up to 600 μm, and comprises five tightly interconnected strata. Lacking blood vessels, it depends on diffusion from the underlying dermis for nutrient and waste exchange. Functionally, it provides mechanical protection, prevents water loss, and supports immune defense [20–22]. The epidermis is primarily composed of specialized cell types [23]. The **keratinocytes**, the predominant cell population (90–95%), form the structural scaffold and produce keratin. Originating in the basal layer, they migrate outward through progressive differentiation stages that maintain tissue homeostasis: the *basal keratinocytes* in the stratum basale, are proliferative cells responsible for continuous renewal; the *spinous keratinocytes* in the stratum spinosum, provide mechanical strength; and the *granular keratinocytes* in the stratum granulosum,

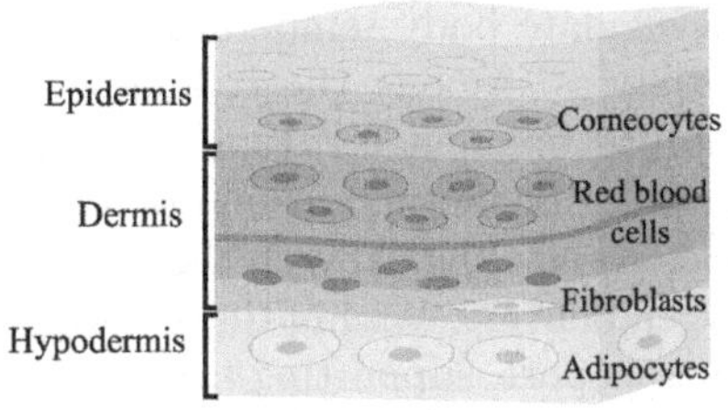

Fig. 1. Schematic representation of skin layers and some cell types.

accumulate keratohyalin and lipids before terminal differentiation. The **corneocytes** are the terminally differentiated keratinocytes, and are flattened, enucleated cells embedded in a lipid matrix, forming a robust barrier to mechanical stress and water loss. The **melanocytes**, located in the basal layer,produce melanin to protect against ultraviolet radiation. And the **Langerhans cells**, dendritic immune cells within the suprabasal layers, act as antigen-presenting cells, linking cutaneous and systemic immunity. The coordinated activity of these cell types enables the epidermis to function as a dynamic, multifunctional barrier that provides protection, pigmentation, sensory interface, and immunological defense.

2.2 Dermis

The dermis is the intermediate skin layer, composed mainly of fibrous connective tissue rich in collagen and elastin, which provide mechanical strength and elasticity [24]. It can be divided into two main regions and performs key functions, including maintaining tensile integrity, supporting blood circulation, enabling oxygen and nutrient exchange, and contributing to immune defense [25]. A dense capillary network within the dermis ensures continuous exchange of oxygen and metabolites between blood and tissue. The primary cellular component, the **fibroblasts**, synthesize collagen, elastin, and other extracellular matrix proteins, maintaining the dermis's structural and mechanical properties. The endothelial cells line the capillaries, regulating the transport of gases and solutes, while **red blood cells** within these vessels are essential for oxygen delivery and thermoregulation [24]. From an electromagnetic perspective, fibroblasts and red blood cells are particularly relevant, as their dimensions and water content fall within the interaction regime of sub-THz and THz radiation. These features make them major contributors to scattering and absorption, thus influencing the overall dielectric behavior of the dermal tissue.

2.3 Hypodermis

The hypodermis is the deepest skin layer, mainly composed of adipose and connective tissues that provide structural support, cushioning, and energy storage [26]. Its key functions include storing triglycerides for metabolic energy, minimizing heat loss to regulate body temperature, and protecting underlying organs from mechanical stress. Among the cellular components of this layer, the **adipocytes** are the predominant cell type, storing energy in the form of triglycerides and contributing to thermal insulation and mechanical protection. A dense network of blood vessels runs between the dermis and hypodermis, facilitating nutrient and oxygen delivery. Within these vessels, **red blood cells** play a critical role in oxygen transport, supporting tissue metabolism and homeostasis. Overall, the hypodermis functions as a flexible, energy-rich, and protective layer that supports the upper skin strata while contributing to thermoregulation, mechanical stability, and vascular integration.

2.4 Extracellular Matrix

The extracellular matrix (ECM) is a complex network of macromolecules that provides structural and biochemical support to cells, maintaining tissue integrity, strength, and intercellular signaling. In the skin, it plays a key role in preserving architecture, elasticity, and hydration through water-binding components that regulate viscoelasticity and permeability [27–29]. ECM composition and organization vary across skin layers, reflecting their distinct structural and physiological functions. In the *epidermis*, the ECM is confined mainly to the basement membrane, composed of collagen type IV, laminin, and proteoglycans that support cell adhesion and hydration. The *dermis* is ECM-rich, dominated by collagen I and III and elastin within a hydrated matrix of proteoglycans and glycosaminoglycans that retain bound water. The *hypodermis*, in contrast, contains a looser ECM forming connective septa around adipose lobules, with collagen and elastin fibers interspersed with proteoglycans that provide mechanical support and local water retention around lipid-rich adipocytes. These structural variations govern the mechanical, hydraulic, and dielectric behavior of each skin layer, establishing the ECM as a key determinant of the tissue's physical and electromagnetic properties across its full depth [30].

3 Computational Modeling of Cellular Permittivity in the Sub-THz-to-THz Band

In this study, the complex permittivity of human cells and their surrounding ECM is evaluated over 100 GHz–1 THz, where dielectric behavior is dominated by water dynamics and protein/lipid relaxation. The model combines a multi-Debye relaxation framework with Maxwell–Garnett effective medium theory, treating cells as heterogeneous mixtures of water, proteins, and lipids within the ECM.

The multi-Debye model captures the multi-scale dynamics of cellular water and macromolecules in the Sub-THz/THz range. Since ions cannot follow the applied field above 100 GHz, ionic conductivity is neglected. The complex permittivity of each component (water, proteins, and lipids) is expressed as [31]:

$$\varepsilon^*(\omega) = \varepsilon_\infty + \frac{\Delta\varepsilon_\alpha}{1 + j\omega\tau_\alpha} + \frac{\Delta\varepsilon_\beta}{1 + j\omega\tau_\beta} + + \frac{\Delta\varepsilon_\gamma}{1 + j\omega\tau_\gamma}, \quad (1)$$

where ε_∞ is the high-frequency permittivity, and $\Delta\varepsilon_{\alpha,\beta,\gamma}$ and $\tau_{\alpha,\beta,\gamma}$ are the strengths and characteristic times of the three dominant relaxation processes [32,33]. The *α-relaxation* arises from collective structural rearrangements in the hydration network [32], the *β-relaxation* corresponds to more localized motions at higher frequencies [33,34], and the *γ-relaxation* represents ultrafast motions [33]. Proteins exhibit all three processes with a dominant α contribution, while lipids mainly show β- and γ-relaxations [31].

Once the permittivity of each cellular component is defined, the effective permittivity of the whole cell, modeled as a water-based medium containing dispersed protein and lipid inclusions, is estimated using the Maxwell–Garnett effective medium theory [34]:

$$\tilde{\epsilon}(\omega) = \epsilon_{\text{host}}(\omega) + 3\epsilon_{\text{host}}(\omega)\frac{\sum_{n=1}^{N}\phi_n\frac{\epsilon_n-\epsilon_{\text{host}}}{\epsilon_n+2\varepsilon_{\text{host}}}}{1-\sum_{n=1}^{N}\phi_n\frac{\epsilon_n-\epsilon_{\text{host}}}{\epsilon_n+2\varepsilon_{\text{host}}}}, \tag{2}$$

where ϵ_{host} and ϵ_n are the permittivity of the water (i.e. intracellular liquid) and of the cellular inclusions, respectively, and $\phi_n = \frac{m_n}{m_{\text{total}}}$ is the volumetric fraction of each inclusion based on its mass fraction m_n with respect to the entire composite structure, m_{total}. Finally, the complex refractive index of the composite system is obtained as

$$n(\omega) = \sqrt{\tilde{\epsilon}(\omega)} = n'(\omega) - jn''(\omega). \tag{3}$$

It has a real part, governing the phase velocity, and an imaginary part, describing absorption [35,36]. This approach provides the frequency-dependent optical properties for each cell type and the ECM [31–33].

3.1 Cell Types and Properties

We consider the main epidermal and dermal cell types, as well as blood and connective tissue cells. Each cell is modeled as a composite structure, with water as the host medium and proteins and lipids as dispersed inclusions. Table 1 lists the Debye relaxation parameters, while Table 2 reports component concentrations in the considered skin cells [31–34,37,38].

Table 1. Debye relaxation parameters of water, proteins, and lipids (100 GHz–1 THz, 37 °C) [31–34]

Component	ε_∞	$\Delta\varepsilon_\alpha$	$\Delta\varepsilon_\beta$	$\Delta\varepsilon_\gamma$	τ_α (ps)	τ_β (ps)	τ_γ (ps)
Water	1.8	78	–	–	8.3	–	–
Proteins	2.0–2.5	10–50	1–5	0.5–2.0	1–100	0.1–10	0.01–0.1
Lipids	2.0–2.2	≈ 0	1–3	0.2–1.0	–	0.1–1.0	0.01–0.05

Table 2. Protein and lipid mass fractions and derived parameters for different skin cell types [37,38].

Cell Type	Water (%)	Protein (%)	Lipid (%)
Corneocytes	10–15	70–80	10–15
Granular Keratinocytes	70–75	20–25	3–5
Spinous Keratinocytes	75–80	15–20	2–3
Basal Keratinocytes	75–80	15–20	2–3
Langerhans Cells	70–75	20–25	3–5
Melanocytes	75–80	15–20	2–3
Red Blood Cells	65–70	28–32	1–2
Fibroblasts	75–80	15–20	2–3
Adipocytes	10–20	5–10	70–85

Water exhibits a dominant α-relaxation at 8.3 ps, reflecting collective dipolar reorientation. Proteins display multiple relaxation modes with broader time distributions, including side-chain (β) and localized (γ) motions, while lipids contribute at shorter timescales due to restricted headgroup and tail mobility. Most skin components are smaller than 0.1 mm, making them much smaller than typical THz wavelengths. Therefore, scattering is negligible and the cell can be treated as an effective homogeneous dielectric inclusion. However, larger structures can induce THz wave scattering, which must be considered in both experimental measurements and modeling [39].

By combining Debye parameters with the volumetric fractions of cellular constituents in (2), the complex permittivity of each skin cell type is obtained and used to derive the corresponding frequency-dependent refractive index.

3.2 Extracellular Matrix Composition and Dielectric Properties

The ECM exhibits distinct biochemical and structural compositions across the epidermis, dermis, and hypodermis, which collectively determine the dielectric response of the tissue [29,30]. In the *epidermis*, water accounts for 65–70% of the total mass, proteins (mainly collagen IV, laminin, and fibronectin) for 25–30%, and lipids for 5%, primarily in the stratum corneum. The *dermis* is similarly hydrated, containing 65–75% water, 20–30% proteins (mainly collagen I/III and elastin), and a negligible lipid fraction (2%). In the *hypodermis*, the composition shifts toward adipose tissue with 20–30% water, 5–10% proteins, and 60–75% lipids stored in adipocytes [28].

These compositional differences govern the dielectric behavior of each skin layer by influencing polarization and absorption, dominated by water in the epidermis and dermis, and by lipids in the hypodermis. The effective permittivity of the ECM in each layer is computed using (2), modeling it as a water-based medium with layer-dependent inclusion fractional volume, providing a comprehensive description of the skin's electromagnetic behavior [34].

4 Intrabody Wave Propagation Losses

Understanding the dielectric properties of cells and the extracellular matrix is essential for accurate modeling of sub-THz and THz wave propagation in biological tissues. The total path loss within the human body arises from three frequency-dependent components: spreading, molecular absorption, and scattering losses. The overall attenuation factor is expressed as in [31]:

$$L_{\text{tot}}(f) = L_{\text{spr}}(f) \times L_{\text{abs}}(f) \times L_{\text{sca}}(f), \tag{4}$$

where L_{spr} accounts for spherical wavefront spreading, L_{abs} represents molecular absorption losses, and L_{sca} denotes attenuation due to scattering processes.

4.1 Spreading Loss

Electromagnetic waves in biological tissues experience spreading losses, modeled as

$$L_{\text{spr}} = D\left(\frac{\lambda_g}{4\pi d}\right)^2, \tag{5}$$

where $\lambda_g = \lambda/n'$ is the wavelength in the medium, d the propagation distance, and D the transmitting antenna directivity. The refractive index is defined as $n = n' - jn'' = \sqrt{\tilde{\varepsilon}}$, where $\tilde{\varepsilon}$ is the complex permittivity of both cells and ECM, obtained from (2).

4.2 Molecular Absorption Loss

Molecular absorption arises from the interaction of THz waves with tissue constituents at their characteristic resonant frequencies [40]. It is modeled using the Beer–Lambert law [41]:

$$L_{\text{abs}} = e^{-\mu_{\text{abs}} d}, \tag{6}$$

where μ_{abs} is the molecular absorption coefficient, given by $\mu_{\text{abs}} = 4\pi n''/\lambda_g$ [42].

4.3 Scattering Loss

Light scattering in the skin originates from its microscopic heterogeneity and is evaluated *cell by cell*. Rayleigh scattering applies to particles smaller than the wavelength, while Mie theory describes larger structures such as red blood cells or adipocytes [4]. The scattering loss is expressed as

$$L_{\text{sca}} = e^{-(\mu_{\text{sca}}^{\text{small}} + \mu_{\text{sca}}^{\text{large}})d}, \tag{7}$$

where $\mu_{\text{sca}}^{\text{small}}$ and $\mu_{\text{sca}}^{\text{large}}$ are the scattering coefficients for small and large particles, respectively, accounting for tissue heterogeneity and avoiding the effective medium approximation [43].

For large particles, part of the incident energy is reflected while the rest is refracted. The total energy removed from the beam, the extinction has efficiency [44].

$$Q_{\text{ext}} = 2 - \frac{4}{p}\sin p + \frac{4}{p^2}(1 - \cos p), \qquad Q_{\text{sca}}^{\text{large}} = Q_{\text{ext}} - Q_{\text{abs}}. \tag{8}$$

where $p = 4\pi r(n-1)/\lambda = 2(n-1)\psi$ represents the phase delay through the particle center, and $\psi = 2\pi r/\lambda_g$ is the dimensionless size parameter. The scattering coefficient for large particles is then computed as $\mu_{\text{sca}}^{\text{large}} = \rho_{\text{large}} Q_{\text{sca}}^{\text{large}} \sigma_g$, where $\sigma_g = \pi r^2$ is the geometric cross section of a sphere given the radius r and ρ_{large} is the particle number density, which can be written in terms of the volume fraction.

For particles much smaller than the wavelength, the local electric field induces an oscillating dipole, leading to *Rayleigh scattering* [4]. The scattering efficiency of small spherical absorbing particles is given by [31].

$$Q_{\text{sca}}^{\text{small}} = \frac{8}{3}\psi^4 \text{Re}\left(\frac{n^2-1}{n^2+2}\right)^2, \tag{9}$$

In this case, the scattering coefficient for small particles is $\mu_{\text{sca}}^{\text{small}} = \rho_{\text{small}} Q_{\text{sca}}^{\text{small}} \sigma_g$.

Overall, attenuation in biological tissues is highly frequency-dependent, arising from the combined effects of spreading, molecular absorption, and scattering across multiple spatial scales.

5 Simulation Framework

Human skin tissue is simulated using a MATLAB-based voxelized framework. The tissue is discretized with voxels of size $dx = 0.01$ mm (10 μm) over a lateral extent of $X = Y = 0.1$ mm and depth $Z = 5.0$ mm. Cells are modeled as spheres with layer-specific diameters and concentrations. Table 3 summarizes the cell concentrations ρ, diameters d, and an average z-intervals Z_{layer} corresponding to their natural layer positions. The number of cells per layer is limited by literature-reported concentrations, while ECM concentration is determined from the remaining volume not occupied by cells.

Table 3. Cell Parameters in the Skin Model [45,46]

Cell Type	ρ [cells/mm^3]	d [µm]	Z_{layer} [µm]
Corneocytes	1.0×10^7	23	0–20
Granular Keratinocytes	0.8×10^6	15	20–50
Spinous Keratinocytes	0.7×10^6	15	50–120
Melanocytes	2.0×10^4	14	50–120
Basal Cells	1.0×10^6	8	120–130
Langerhans Cells	3.0×10^4	10	50–120
Merkel Cells	1.0×10^3	10	50–120
Fibroblasts	5.0×10^4	20	130–3000 (Dermis)
Red Blood Cells	6.0×10^5	8	Capillaries/Arterioles
Adipocytes	1.0×10^5	80	3000+ (Hypodermis)

5.1 Statistical Skin Scenario Definition

In the simulation, cells are modeled as spheres within their respective tissue layer volumes (V_{layer}). Each cell's position, $\mathbf{p} = [x, y, z]^{\mathrm{T}}$, is assigned via a *disc Poisson process*, which ensures a minimum center-to-center distance equal to the sum of the radii of any two cells:

$$\mathcal{P} = \left\{ \mathbf{p}_i \in V_{\text{layer}} \,\middle|\, \|\mathbf{p}_i - \mathbf{p}_j\| \geq \frac{d_i}{2} + \frac{d_j}{2},\ \forall j \neq i \right\}. \tag{10}$$

This defines a spatial probability distribution for the center of each cell in V_{layer}.

Vessels are represented as line segments inside the V_{layer} and with centers and orientations sampled from such a *line Poisson process*. It distributes lines or line segments in space according to a homogeneous Poisson point process over a parameter space defining position and orientation [47]. Lateral coordinates (x_v, y_v) of each vessel center are drawn from a homogeneous 2D Poisson point process over the layer plane, while the vertical coordinate z_v spans the layer thickness. Each segment is aligned along the vessel axis, with length determined by vessel type. Formally, the set of vessel center positions is

$$\mathcal{L} = \left\{ \mathbf{p}_v = (x_v, y_v, z_v) \in V_{\text{layer}},\ v = 1, \ldots, N_{\text{vessels}} \right\}, \tag{11}$$

where N_{vessels} is the total number of vessels of a given type. This approach produces a spatially homogeneous, statistically independent distribution of vessel centers in the lateral plane, while allowing control over vessel density, orientation, and length. Anatomical constraints are incorporated: dermal capillaries are confined to the upper layer near the epidermal–dermal interface, reflecting the dense superficial microvasculature, whereas vessels in the hypodermis span the full layer depth, consistent with the more uniform distribution of larger arterioles and venules.

Red blood cells are then randomly distributed within the vessels using a *disc Poisson process*, consistent with the vessel geometry and avoiding overlap.

Figure 2a shows a representative realization of cell placement in the epidermis, while Figs. 2b and 2c depict the corresponding distributions in the dermis and hypodermis, respectively.

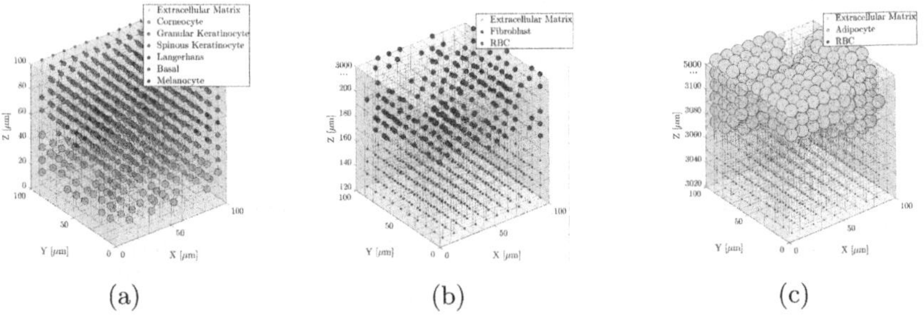

Fig. 2. Voxel-based 3D representation of skin with randomly distributed spherical cells, scaled by diameter, in (a) epidermis, (b) dermis, and (c) hypodermis.

6 Numerical Results

This section quantitatively analyzes THz propagation in multilayer skin models, highlighting frequency-dependent attenuation, absorption, and scattering at 100 GHz and 1 THz. Figures 3a–b show the relative contributions of attenuation mechanisms from Sect. 4 at 100 GHz and 1 THz. The skin's heterogeneous structure produces frequency-dependent losses. Spreading loss (L_{spr}) dominates, reflecting its reliance on the effective wavelength, contributing 35 dB over 5 mm at 100 GHz and 40 dB at 1 THz. Absorption loss (L_{abs}) is smaller at 100 GHz (8 dB) but rises to 15 dB at 1 THz due to stronger molecular absorption by water and biomolecules. These results highlight the importance of frequency selection in sub-THz and THz biomedical applications: higher frequencies enhance interactions with tissue water and molecular resonances, markedly affecting propagation.

Scattering (L_{sca}) remains minor at both frequencies but shows clear frequency dependence. At 100 GHz, wavelengths are much larger than cells, producing low, uniform Rayleigh scattering. At 1 THz, wavelengths approach cellular scales, shifting toward Mie scattering with stronger layer-specific effects. Total path loss sums spreading, absorption, and scattering, reaching 45 dB over 5 mm at 100 GHz and 65 dB at 1 THz, reflecting greater sensitivity of higher frequencies to tissue losses.

Tissue-specific absorption is shown in Figs. 4, with frequency-dependent trends reflecting each skin layer's composition. At 100 GHz, the epidermis shows a high absorption peak near 700–800 m^{-1} reflecting its high water content and strong dielectric losses, the dermis peaks around 200–300 m^{-1} from its collagen–water mix, and the hypodermis exhibits a broader, bimodal distribution ($\sim$ 100 and 350 m^{-1}) reflecting its adipose/connective tissue heterogeneity. At 1 THz, distributions shift higher, indicating increased losses due to enhanced dipolar relaxation of water molecules and stronger frequency-dependent coupling. The epidermis peaks sharply near 900 m^{-1}, the dermis centers around 500 m^{-1}, and the hypodermis ranges from 400–700 m^{-1}, showing moderate absorption. These results highlight how skin absorption depends on frequency and tissue composition: water-rich layers dominate, while lipid-rich hypodermis shows weaker, more variable absorption. Such probabilistic characterization is crucial for realistic THz propagation models accounting for tissue heterogeneity.

Tissue-specific scattering properties are shown in Fig. 5, where the probability distributions of the scattering coefficient (μ_{sca}) reflect structural rather than compositional differences of each layer. At 100 GHz, all layers exhibit

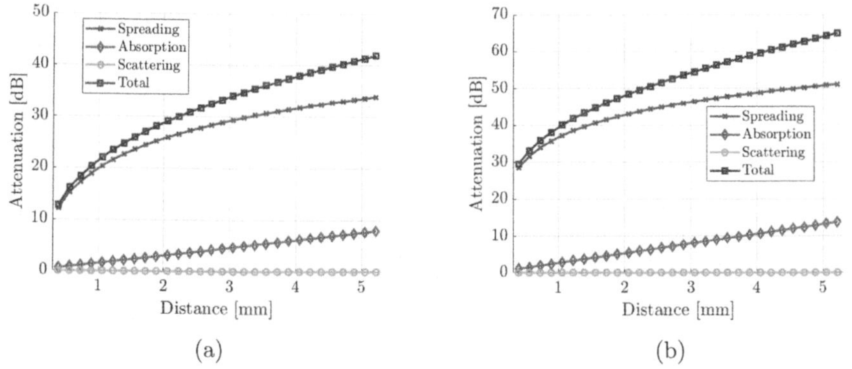

Fig. 3. Attenuation due to spreading, absorption, scattering, and the total vs distance, for (a) f = 100 GHz and (b) f = 1 THz.

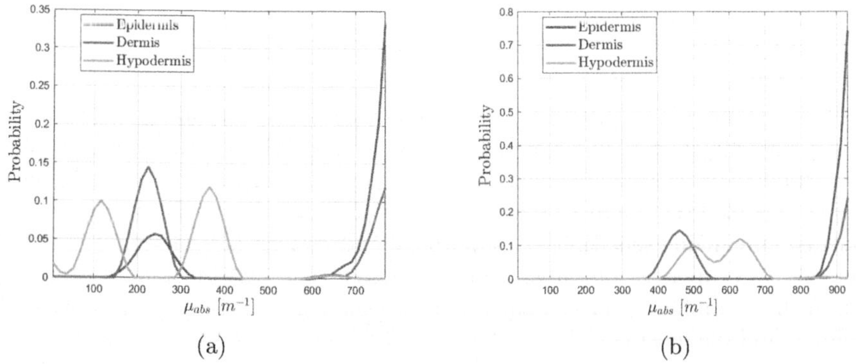

Fig. 4. Absorption coefficient probability density function for (a) f = 100 GHz and (b) f = 1 THz.

extremely low scattering, with sharp peaks near $2 \cdot 10^{-5}$ μm^{-1}. The epidermis and dermis show nearly identical distributions with probability densities above 0.45, indicating minimal Rayleigh scattering from cells and collagen fibers ($\lambda \approx 3$ mm $\gg$ 1–100 μm scatterers dimension). The hypodermis shows a similar trend with a slightly broader tail up to $2 \cdot 10^{-4}$ μm^{-1} due to larger adipocytes. At 1 THz, distributions broaden as Mie scattering emerges ($\lambda \approx 300$ μm), with epidermis and dermis developing extended tails up to 0.25–0.35 μm^{-1} at low probabilities ($\sim$ 0.01–0.02). The hypodermis shows a pronounced bimodal distribution with peaks near 0 and 0.01–0.35 μm^{-1}, reflecting its heterogeneous adipocyte content. Overall, scattering remains a secondary loss mechanism compared to absorption, even at THz frequencies.

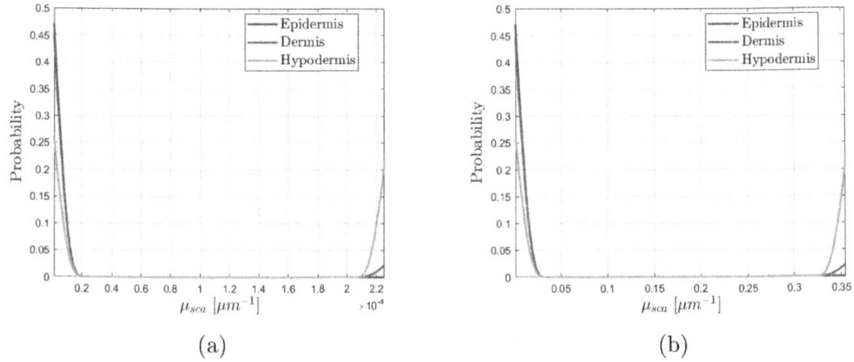

Fig. 5. Scattering coefficient for (a) $f = 100$ GHz and (b) $f = 1$ THz.

These results show that scattering becomes more relevant at higher frequencies, where cellular and subcellular heterogeneities interact more effectively with the electromagnetic field. However, the persistent dominance of low-scattering probabilities across all layers indicates that spreading, followed by absorption remain the primary attenuation mechanisms in skin tissue throughout the sub-THz and THz regimes.

This numerical analysis provides a quantitative understanding of THz interaction with multilayer skin. Lower frequencies (100 GHz) exhibit lower attenuation and deeper penetration, suitable for probing deeper tissues. Instead, higher frequencies (1 THz) increase absorption but offer better spatial resolution and contrast, enhancing sensitivity to superficial and structural variations. The complementary properties of these regimes suggest that hybrid or dual-frequency approaches, combined with adaptive power management, could improve THz imaging and diagnostics.

7 Conclusion

This work presents a comprehensive dielectric modeling framework for human skin in the sub-THz and THz ranges. By combining multi-Debye relaxation with effective medium theory, the model captures frequency-dependent permittivity of cellular constituents and the extracellular matrix across the epidermis, dermis, and hypodermis. Physiologically realistic parameters, including water content, protein and lipid fractions, and cellular heterogeneity, enable a physically interpretable description of tissue dielectric properties. Numerical simulations using a voxel-based statistical skin model reveal the distinct contributions of spreading, molecular absorption, and scattering to wave attenuation. At lower sub-THz frequencies, spreading dominates, allowing deeper penetration, while at higher THz frequencies, absorption and scattering increase, improving tissue contrast and layer differentiation.

Overall, this study provides a physically grounded framework for predicting electromagnetic interactions in skin, offering practical insights for designing and optimizing next-generation sub-THz and THz imaging and sensing systems.

References

1. Fischer, B.M., et al.: Far-infrared vibrational modes of dna components studied by terahertz time-domain spectroscopy. Phys. Med. Biol. **47**(21), 3807–3814 (2005)
2. Pickwell, E., Wallace, V.P.: Biomedical applications of terahertz technology. J. Phys. D Appl. Phys. **39**(17), R301–R310 (2006)
3. Wang, Y., et al.: The nano-bio interactions of nanomedicines: understanding the biochemical driving forces and redox reactions. Accounts Chem. Res. **52**(6), 1507–1518 (2019)
4. Cherkasova, O.P., et al.: Cellular effects of terahertz waves. J. Biomed. Opt. **26**(9), 090902 (2021)
5. Lee, Y.K., et al.: Frontier of terahertz spectroscopy: unveiling its potential in biochemical applications. BioChip J. **19**(3), 424–443 (2025)
6. Xu, K., Arbab, M.H.: Terahertz polarimetric imaging of biological tissues: Monte carlo modeling of signal contrast mechanisms due to mie scattering. Biomed. Optics Express **15**(4), 2328–2342 (2024)
7. Vilagosh, Z., et al.: Characterisation of biological materials at thz frequencies by attenuated total reflection. lard. Appl. Sci. **10**(23), 8692 (2020)
8. Mahdy, S., Hamdy, O.: Thz radiation distribution for the identification of infiltrating ductal carcinoma in human breast model: a computational study. Optical Quant. Electron. **56**(5), 831 (2024)
9. Yanina, I.Y., et al.: Measurement and modeling of the optical properties of adipose tissue in the terahertz range: aspects of disease diagnosis. Diagnostics **12**(10), 2395 (2022)
10. Woodward, R.M., et al.: Terahertz pulse imaging of ex vivo basal cell carcinoma. J. Invest. Dermatol. **120**(1), 72–78 (2003)
11. Ferdous, A.H.M.I., et al.: Innovative refractive index sensor utilizing terahertz spectrum for early cancer detection: a photonic crystal fiber approach. Cell Biochem. Biophys. **83**(1), 489–505 (2025)

12. D'Arco, A., et al.: Thz pulsed imaging in biomedical applications. Condens. Matter **5**(2), 25 (2020)
13. Ashworth, P.C., et al.: Terahertz pulsed spectroscopy of freshly excised human breast cancer. Optics Exp. **17**(15), 12444–12454 (2009)
14. Hanson, S.G., et al.: Dielectric properties of human skin measured in vivo in the frequency range 0.5–20 ghz. Bioelectromagnetics (2015)
15. Pickwell, E., et al.: Simulation of terahertz pulse propagation in biological systems. Appl. Phys. Lett. **84**(12), 2190–2192 (2004)
16. Yang, K., et al.: Permittivity characterization of human skin based on a quasi-optical system at sub-thz. arXiv preprint arXiv:2405.11863 (2024)
17. Yang, K., et al.: Human skin permittivity characterization for mobile handset evaluation at sub-thz. arXiv preprint arXiv:2405.06106 (2024)
18. Zhang, Y., et al.: Terahertz probe for real-time in vivo skin hydration evaluation. Adv. Photonics Nexus (2024)
19. Gabriel, S., et al.: The dielectric properties of biological tissues: III. Parametric models for the dielectric spectrum of tissues. Phys. Med. Biol. **41**(11), 2271–2293 (1996)
20. Fluhr, J., et al.: Epidermal barrier function in dry, flaky and sensitive skin: a narrative review. J. Eur. Acad. Dermatol. Venereol. **38**(5), 812–820 (2024)
21. Tang, X., et al.: Epidermal stem cells: skin surveillance and clinical perspective. J. Translat. Med. **22**(1), 779 (2024)
22. Hofmann, E., et al.: Modelling the complexity of human skin in vitro. Biomedicines **11**(3), 794 (2023)
23. Baker, P., et al.: Skin barrier function: the interplay of physical, chemical, and immunologic properties. Cells **12**(23), 2745 (2023)
24. Brown, T.M., Krishnamurthy, K.: Histology, Dermis. StatPearls Publishing (2022)
25. Lee, S., et al.: Resilience of dermis resident macrophages to inflammatory settings. Nat. Commun. **56**(10), 2105–2112 (2024)
26. Hirsch, J., et al.: Structure and function of the human hypodermis: insights from histology and imaging. J. Anatomy (2023)
27. Bosman, F.T., Stamenkovic, I.: Functional structure and composition of the extracellular matrix. J. Pathol. J. Pathol. Soc. Great Britain Ireland **200**(4), 423–428 (2003)
28. Karamanos, N.K., et al.: A guide to the composition and functions of the extracellular matrix. FEBS J. **288**(24), 6850–6912 (2021)
29. Watt, F.M., Fujiwara, H.: Cell-extracellular matrix interactions in normal and diseased skin. In: Cold Spring Harbor Perspectives in Biology (2011)
30. Krieg, T., Aumailley, M.: The extracellular matrix of the dermis: flexible structures with dynamic functions. Exp. Dermatol. (2011)
31. Elayan, H., et al.: Terahertz channel model and link budget analysis for intrabody nanoscale communication. IEEE Trans. NanoBiosci. (2017)
32. Gabriel, C.: Dielectric properties of biological materials. Bioeng. Biophys. Aspects Electromagn. Fields (2018)
33. Wolf, M., et al.: Relaxation dynamics of a protein solution investigated by dielectric spectroscopy. Biochimica et Biophysica Acta (BBA)-Proteins Proteomics (2012)
34. Tannino, M., Mangini, F., Dinia, L., Frezza, F.: A heuristic model to evaluate the dielectric properties of human tissues at microwave band based on water and solid content. J. Eng. Appl. Sci. **70**(1), 1–22 (2023). https://doi.org/10.1186/s44147-023-00187-8
35. Calvo-de la Rosa, J., et al.: Terahertz permittivity of pressed zno and cuo powder in polyethylene pellets: effect of porosity. IEEE Trans. Terahertz Sci. Technol. (2021)

36. Jepsen, P.U.: Phase retrieval in terahertz time-domain measurements: a "how to" tutorial. J. Infrared Millimeter Terahertz Waves (2019)
37. Madison, K.C.: Barrier function of the skin: "la raison d'etre" of the epidermis. J. Invest. Dermatol. **121**(2), 231–241 (2003)
38. Van Smeden, J., et al.: The important role of stratum corneum lipids for the cutaneous barrier function. Biochimica et Biophysica Acta (BBA)-Molec. Cell Biol. Lipids (2014)
39. Nikitkina, A.I., et al.: Terahertz radiation and the skin: a review. J. Biomed. Optics (2021)
40. Saxena, S., et al.: Limitations of effective medium models for tissue phantoms in the thz frequency range. Sci. Rep. (2024)
41. Shi, W., et al.: Quantitative detection of thz-atr spectra of aqueous samples under strong-field terahertz wave. iScience (2022)
42. Elayan, H., et al.: Multi-layer intrabody terahertz wave propagation model for nanobiosensing applications. Nano Commun. Netw. (2017)
43. Cheong, W., et al.: A review of the optical properties of biological tissues. IEEE J. Quant. Electron. (1990)
44. van de Hulst, H.: Light Scattering by Small Particles. Dover Publications (1981)
45. Nikitkina, A.I., et al.: Terahertz radiation and the skin: a review. J. Biomed. Optics (2021)
46. Graham, H.K., Eckersley, A., Ozols, M., Mellody, K.T., Sherratt, M.J.: Human skin: composition, structure and visualisation methods. In: Limbert, G. (ed.) Skin Biophysics. SMTEB, vol. 22, pp. 1–18. Springer, Cham (2019). https://doi.org/10.1007/978-3-030-13279-8_1
47. Kingman, J.F.C.: Poisson Processes. Clarendon Press (1992)

Experimental Characterization of Biological Tissue Dielectric Properties Through THz Time-Domain Spectroscopy

Elisabetta Marini[1(✉)], Silvia Mura[1], Marco Hernandez[2], Matti Hämäläinen[2], and Maurizio Magarini[1]

[1] Department of Electronics, Information and Bioengineering, Politecnico di Milano, Milan, Italy
{elisabetta.marini,silvia.mura,maurizio.magarini}@polimi.it
[2] University of Oulu, Oulu, Finland
{marco.hernandez,matti.hamalainen}@oulu.fi

Abstract. Terahertz (THz) radiation provides a non-ionizing, highly sensitive probe of the dielectric properties of biological tissues. In this study, we present a comprehensive experimental characterization of dielectric properties using pork skin tissue, a widely used surrogate for human tissue, as a biological sample. Measurements are conducted employing THz time-domain spectroscopy in the 0.1–11 THz frequency range with photoconductive antennas for both signal generation and detection. Frequency-dependent refractive indices, absorption, and complex permittivity are extracted from transmitted time-domain signals. Our results confirm strong absorption and low transmittance at low THz frequencies due to water content, while highlighting frequency-dependent dispersion and narrowband transmission features at higher frequencies. This work provides one of the first extended-frequency datasets of biological tissue dielectric properties, supporting realistic channel modeling for the design and development of intra-body nanosensor networks in the THz band.

Keywords: Terahertz · Time-domain spectroscopy · Photoconductive antennas · Biological tissue characterization · Dielectric properties

1 Introduction

The integration of nanoscale devices within the human body has the potential to radically transform modern medicine. By enabling continuous physiological monitoring, targeted therapies, and seamless interaction with biological systems, these nanosystems pave the way for personalized healthcare, early disease detection, and advanced biomedical interfaces [1]. The vision of intra-body wireless

H. Tanaka et al. (Eds.): BodyNets 2025, LNICST 714, pp. 32–46, 2026.
https://doi.org/10.1007/978-3-032-38657-1_3

nanosensor networks (WNSNs) encompasses numerous devices capable of sensing, processing, and communicating biomedical information in real time, thus supporting applications as diverse as precision drug delivery, neural interfacing for brain–machine interfaces (BMIs), and monitoring of chronic diseases [2,3].

A key enabler of this vision is intra-body communication (IBC), defined as the reliable and efficient exchange of information among nanoscale devices and between nanosensors and external gateways. Communication requirements are stringent: high data rates are needed for neural data acquisition, ultra-low latency is essential for closed-loop biomedical control, and power consumption must stay very low for safe, sustainable operation. These challenges have driven research into novel communication paradigms for the intra-body medium [2].

Several technological approaches have been proposed to realize intra-body communication (IBC). Molecular communication (MC), exploiting controlled release and detection of molecules, offers excellent biocompatibility and minimal energy consumption [3,4]. However, the stochastic nature of molecular diffusion causes high latency and limited data rates, restricting its use to delay-tolerant applications such as long-term monitoring or drug delivery. Ultrasonic communication provides improved propagation in tissues and potentially higher data rates. Yet, challenges such as device miniaturization, high power requirements, and limited integration with nanoscale architectures remain significant [2,3].

Electromagnetic (EM) communication is another promising solution, benefiting from decades of wireless technology progress. Different frequency bands have contrasting trade-offs: low frequencies (kHz–MHz) penetrate deeply but offer limited data rates; RF and microwave bands provide higher bandwidths, but tissue absorption reduces range; communication at millimeter waves offers wide bandwidths, yet strong attenuation in water-rich tissues severely limits practical range [3]. These constraints have motivated the search for even higher-frequency bands that could combine wide bandwidth with sufficient tissue penetration.

In this context, the terahertz (THz) band (0.1–10 THz) emerges as a particularly compelling candidate for IBC. THz radiation provides ultra-wide bandwidths for very high data rates and low latency, while remaining non-ionizing and biologically safer than X rays or other high-energy radiation. Recent advances demonstrate the feasibility of nanoscale transceivers resonating at THz frequencies, bridging the gap between miniaturization and communication performance [5–7]. These developments position the THz band as a central enabler for intra-body wireless nanosensor networks (WNSNs).

Despite these advantages, challenges remain. Biological tissues, rich in water, strongly absorb THz radiation, causing significant signal attenuation [8]. Tissue heterogeneity leads to complex scattering and dispersion [9]. Careful power management, thermal control, and optimized device placement are needed for safe and reliable operation. Accurate channel modeling that includes absorption, scattering, and dispersion is therefore essential [6,8,10]. Notably, studies on THz propagation in tissues often focus on narrower frequency ranges, such as 0.1–3.5 THz [11] or higher bands up to 20 THz [12], using techniques like frequency-domain spectroscopy or THz imaging.

Considering these limitations, it is clear that more comprehensive experimental data across the full THz range are needed for intra-body communication. To address this, the present work investigates THz propagation in porcine skin, a widely used surrogate for human tissue because of its structural and dielectric similarities. By employing THz time-domain spectroscopy (TDS) with photoconductive antenna (PCA) instrumentation, key dielectric parameters, including refractive index, absorption coefficient, and dielectric constant, are extracted across 0.1 to 10 THz. These parameters provide realistic inputs for channel modeling and highlight trade offs between achievable bandwidth and penetration depth in intra-body environments.

The paper is organized as follows. Section 2 presents the system model. Section 3 covers THz propagation in tissues, Sect. 4 describes the experimental setup, and Sect. 5 reports the results. Finally, Sect. 6 concludes the paper.

2 System Model

The interactions of THz radiation with cells and molecules in biological tissues are studied using TDS with PCAs for broadband generation and detection. Figure 1 shows the system workflow, providing a schematic of the experimental THz time-domain chain for biological tissue applications.

2.1 Photoconductive Antenna (PCA)

A PCA is typically fabricated on a semiconductor substrate, such as GaAs or InGaAs, with two metallic electrodes separated by a narrow gap of width d. The semiconductor has a valence band (VB) and a conduction band (CB), separated by an energy gap E_G. At equilibrium, electrons populate the VB, ensuring charge neutrality. When illuminated by a femtosecond laser pulse with photon energy exceeding E_G, electrons are excited into the CB, generating electron–hole pairs.

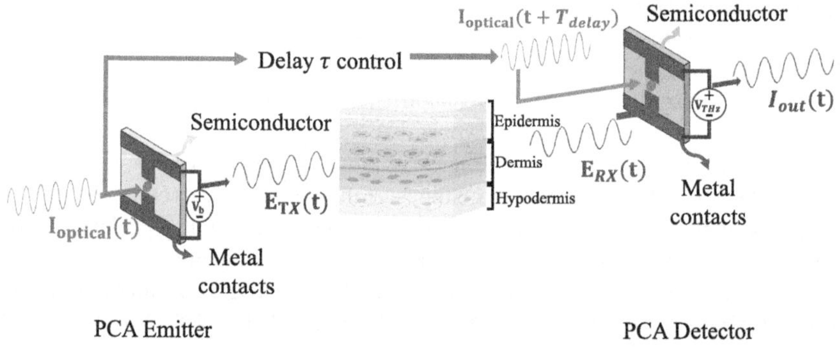

Fig. 1. Figurative diagram of the THz time-domain spectroscopy system for tissue analysis. The THz pulse, generated and detected using PCAs, interacts with the tissue, and the response is processed to reconstruct the waveform.

Under an external bias, these carriers accelerate, producing a transient photocurrent that generates THz radiation [13,14]. The emitted THz field, $E_{TX}(t)$, can be modeled as the emitter response, $h_{emitter}(t)$, to the optical excitation combined with the bias voltage. In detection, a delay τ is introduced to the optical path, allowing the transmitted THz pulse, $E_{RX}(t)$, to interact with the detector PCA, described by $h_{detector}(t)$, enabling time-domain sampling of the waveform.

Pulse characteristics depend on semiconductor parameters such as carrier lifetime, mobility, and saturation velocity, as well as optical pulse duration and bias field. Electrode geometry (e.g., dipole, bow-tie, or interdigitated structures) further influences the radiation pattern and efficiency, providing spectral tunability for specific applications.

2.2 THz Signal Generation

The PCA converts ultra-fast optical pulses into electromagnetic radiation in the THz domain, and its behavior is modeled by the temporal response $h_{emitter}(t)$. When the PCA operates as an emitter, a static bias voltage, $V_b = 10\,\mathrm{V}$, is applied across the electrodes, establishing a static electric field in the gap region E_{bias}. A laser pulse of duration $\tau_{pulse} = 10 - 100\,\mathrm{fs}$, typically delivered by a pulsed $Ti : sapphire$ laser at a wavelength of $\lambda = 800$ nm, irradiates a GaAs substrate of thickness $L = 0.1\,\mathrm{mm}$ across a gap of $d = 5\,\mu\mathrm{m}$ between the two metal contacts. The optical excitation has an average power P_{avg} of a few hundred mW, and a repetition frequency $f_r = 80\,\mathrm{MHz}$ [15].

The photons of the focused femtosecond laser carry an energy $E_{laser} = hf$, where $f = \frac{c}{\lambda}$ is the optical frequency determined by the speed of light c and the wavelength λ. This photon energy exceeds the semiconductor band gap E_G, thereby generating electronhole pairs. These carriers are accelerated by the static field, producing a transient photocurrent $I_p(t)$. The carrier density $n(t)$ follows dynamics that can be modeled as [16–18]

$$\frac{dn(t)}{dt} = G(t) - \frac{n(t)}{\tau_c}, \tag{1}$$

where $G(t)$ is the carrier generation rate and τ_c the carrier recombination lifetime. The average carrier density $\overline{n}$ can be estimated from the number of photons absorbed in the active volume of the device. Specifically, it can be expressed as

$$\overline{n} \simeq \frac{N_p}{V_A}, \tag{2}$$

where V_A is the active volume and N_p the number of photons per pulse, reported in [19] as

$$N_p = \frac{E_{\text{pulse}}}{h\nu} = \frac{P_{\text{avg}}/f_r}{hc/\lambda} \simeq 10^8, \tag{3}$$

with h denoting Planck's constant. The induced photocurrent can then be written as [19,20]

$$I_p(t) = A\,E_{bias}\,q\,\mu\,n(t) \simeq 10^{-2}\,A, \tag{4}$$

where A is the beam-illuminated area, q the elementary charge, and μ the mobility.

The THz radiation field emitted in the far field is proportional to the temporal derivative of the photocurrent [18–20]:

$$E_{\mathrm{TX}}(t) \propto \frac{dI_p(t)}{dt}. \tag{5}$$

Considering the femtosecond pulse duration, and taking into account the geometry of the PCA and propagation to the far-field, the corresponding radiated field is on the order of

$$E_{\mathrm{TX}}(t) \simeq 10^4 - 10^6\, V/m. \tag{6}$$

These relations link the optical excitation, material properties, and antenna geometry to the amplitude and temporal profile of the emitted THz waveform.

2.3 THz Signal Detection

When a PCA operates as a detector of THz radiation, its response, $h_{detector}(t)$, converts the incident THz pulse from the sample, $E_{RX}(t)$, into a photocurrent $I_{\mathrm{det}}(t)$ that carries information about the sample properties. In a PCA detector, a delayed portion of the same femtosecond laser pulse generates electron–hole pairs in the semiconductor. The incident THz field $E_{\mathrm{RX}}(t)$ accelerates these carriers, producing a time-dependent photocurrent $I_{\mathrm{det}}(t)$ proportional to the THz signal. This photocurrent can be expressed as [21]

$$I_{det}(t) = g_d(t) \cdot V_{\mathrm{THz}}(t), \tag{7}$$

where $g_d(t)$ is the time-dependent photoconductance determined by the optical gating pulse and the carrier lifetime, and $V_{\mathrm{THz}}(t)$ is the voltage induced across the antenna gap by the incident THz radiation. The induced voltage $V_{\mathrm{THz}}(t)$ is proportional to the incident THz field, with the proportionality set by the effective antenna length L_{eff} [21], yielding

$$V_{\mathrm{THz}}(t) = L_{\mathrm{eff}} \cdot E_{\mathrm{RX}}(t). \tag{8}$$

Therefore, the output photocurrent as a function of the optical delay T_{delay}, which represents the relative temporal delay between the pump and probe optical pulses, can be written as [18–20]

$$I_{\mathrm{out}}(t) \propto E_{\mathrm{RX}}(t + T_{delay}). \tag{9}$$

The delay T_{delay} is a controlled, constant parameter for each acquisition point, independent of the detection channel. This preserves both the magnitude and phase of the THz radiation transmitted or reflected by the sample, enabling extraction of its complex transmission (or reflection) coefficient. The detected current is then amplified and processed by the readout electronics. By scanning the optical delay, the complete temporal waveform of $E_{\mathrm{RX}}(t)$ is reconstructed. A Fourier transform provides the spectral amplitude and phase, from which material parameters such as refractive index, absorption coefficient, and dielectric constant are derived to characterize the tissue response to THz radiation.

2.4 System Operation for Intra-body Analysis

The intra-body PCA-based THz system operates by sequentially generating, propagating, and detecting pulses to analyze biological tissues. The emitted pulse travels through tissue, experiencing absorption, dispersion, and scattering due to the tissue's dielectric properties. Tissue effectively modulates both the amplitude and phase of the transmitted or reflected waveform. The recorded signal encodes absorption and phase delay induced by the tissue, enabling quantitative and qualitative analysis of intra-body propagation. Temporal propagation within the biological tissue can be modeled as

$$E_{\mathrm{RX}}(t) = E_{\mathrm{TX}}(t) * h_{\mathrm{tissue}}(t), \tag{10}$$

where $*$ is the convolution operation and $h_{\mathrm{tissue}}(t)$ is the time-dependent tissue channel response accounting for absorption, dispersion, and scattering, quantified with the tissue's complex permittivity ϵ.

Figure 2 details the three main stages of the considered system and the corresponding operations for each block:

1. **THz signal generation**: The THz radiation is generated by the PCA, whose response to the incoming optical radiation is described by the impulse response $h_{emitter}(t)$.
2. **Biological tissue response**: The tissue interacts with the incident electromagnetic field $E_{TX}(t)$, resulting in $E_{RX}(t)$. This interaction can be described by the tissue channel response $h_{tissue(t)}$, which depends on the tissue's absorption coefficient and dielectric properties [22];
3. **THz signal detection**: as the resulting radiation $E_{RX}(t)$ is carrying the information on tissue properties, it is converted in an electric measurable quantity from which it is possible to extract the dielectric parameters.

3 Terahertz Propagation in Biological Tissues

The propagation of THz radiation in biological tissues is determined by their complex dielectric properties, which govern energy storage, dissipation, and attenuation. The THz range (0.1–10 THz) is highly sensitive to water content and molecular vibrations, making it an effective probe for soft tissues, hydration, and cellular organization [22]. At the molecular level, biological function depends on weak interactions, such as hydrogen bonds and Van der Waals forces, which shape biomolecular assembly and tissue structure [23,24]. The energy of THz photons (0.4–40 meV) overlaps with rotational, vibrational, and collective molecular modes [24], revealing dynamics often inaccessible to higher-energy techniques like infrared spectroscopy. Understanding the dielectric response in this range is crucial, linking molecular dynamics to macroscopic electromagnetic behavior and defining absorption, dispersion, and propagation.

When radiation propagates through a material of thickness d, the resulting outgoing intensity follows Beer–Lambert's law [25]:

$$|E_{RX}(\omega)| = |E_{TX}(\omega)|e^{-\alpha(\omega)d}, \tag{11}$$

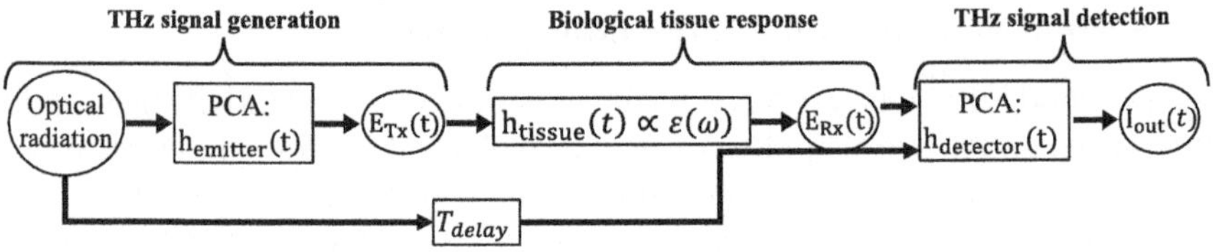

Fig. 2. Stages of the proposed framework. The experiment comprises three main steps: signal generation, tissue interaction, and signal detection.

where $\alpha(\omega)$ is the absorption coefficient. Experimental characterization is commonly performed using THz time-domain spectroscopy (THz-TDS), which enables direct measurement of the complex transmission coefficient [11]:

$$T(\omega) = \frac{E_{\mathrm{RX}}(\omega)}{E_{\mathrm{TX}}(\omega)}. \tag{12}$$

From the transmittance, tissue parameters can be extracted, as they depend on the magnitude of $T(\omega)$ and on the phase difference $\phi(\omega) = \arg\left(\frac{E_{RX}(\omega)}{E_{TX}(\omega)}\right)$ [11, 26,27]. The absorption coefficient $\alpha(\omega)$ and the refractive index $n(\omega)$ are obtained as

$$\alpha(\omega) \approx -\frac{1}{d}\ln\left(\frac{|E_{RX}(\omega)|}{|E_{TX}(\omega)|}\right), \quad n(\omega) = 1 + \frac{c\,\phi(\omega)}{\omega d}. \tag{13}$$

The extinction coefficient $k(\omega)$, which quantifies the material's electromagnetic losses, is expressed as

$$k(\omega) = \frac{c\,\alpha(\omega)}{2\,\omega}. \tag{14}$$

Using $n(\omega)$ and $k(\omega)$, the complex permittivity is obtained through

$$\tilde{\varepsilon}_r(\omega) = [n(\omega) - ik(\omega)]^2 = \varepsilon_r'(\omega) - i\varepsilon_r''(\omega), \tag{15}$$

where $\varepsilon_r'(\omega)$ represents the real part, the dielectric constant, representing the material's ability to store energy, and and $\varepsilon_r''(\omega)$ represents the imaginary component, the dielectric loss, quantifying energy dissipation through absorption and relaxation mechanisms. This is possible thanks to the direct dependence of the absorption coefficient $\alpha(\omega)$ and the refractive index $n(\omega)$ on the amount of the transmitted radiation with respect to the received amount.

The dielectric response of tissues is strongly influenced by water content, temperature, and molecular composition. For water-rich soft tissues, empirical relationships link static permittivity ε_s, high-frequency permittivity ε_∞, and relaxation time τ to the water mass fraction W_c:

$$\varepsilon_s = a_1 + b_1 W_c, \quad \varepsilon_\infty = a_2 + b_2 W_c, \quad \tau = a_3 + b_3 W_c, \tag{16}$$

where a_1, a_2, a_3 represent the baseline values for a dry or low-water-content medium, while b_1, b_2, b_3 describe the rate of variation of each parameter with the water mass fraction W_c. Finally, the frequency-dependent dielectric function can be modeled using a generalized Debye relaxation to account for both bulk and bound water contributions [28]:

$$\tilde{\varepsilon}_r(\omega) = \varepsilon_\infty + \sum_{j=1}^{N} \frac{\Delta\varepsilon_j}{1 + i\omega\tau_j}, \tag{17}$$

where $\Delta\varepsilon_j = \varepsilon_{sj} - \varepsilon_{\infty j}$ and τ_j represent the relaxation strength and relaxation time of the jth process, respectively.

Accurate characterization of the THz channel in biological tissues, through the determination of the real and imaginary parts of the relative permittivity, $\varepsilon_r'(\omega)$ and $\varepsilon_r''(\omega)$, as well as the refractive index $n(\omega)$, extinction coefficient $k(\omega)$, and absorption coefficient $\alpha(\omega)$, is essential. It enables reliable interpretation of THz imaging contrast, quantitative evaluation of tissue hydration, and understanding of molecular interactions involving water and proteins. Such knowledge is crucial for designing biocompatible THz systems with minimal energy deposition and signal loss in biological media. From these considerations, it emerges that these systems are particularly well suited for investigating multilayered biological tissues, as the analysis of both transmission and reflection allows the extraction of relevant parameters, including microstructural composition. This capability makes PCA-based THz spectroscopy a powerful, non-invasive tool for dermatological research.

4 Experimental Framework

This study presents a detailed investigation of the electromagnetic properties of pork skin using the TeraPulse 4000 THz-TDS system. The measurement campaign aimed to characterize the tissue's dielectric properties, refractive index, and absorption behavior in the 0.01–11 THz range, with the emitted pulse centered at 0.5 THz. The TeraPulse 4000 operated in transmission mode, generating femtosecond laser pulses centered at 800 nm with a spectral resolution of 1 GHz. The average optical power was 800 mW at an 80 MHz repetition rate. The THz beam was focused to a 3 mm spot with a pulse duration of 100 fs. Biological samples were positioned between the emitter and detector to maintain a constant optical path. The main system specifications are summarized in Table 1. Pork skin can be selected as a representative model for human skin due to its comparable anatomical structure and physiological properties, making it a suitable proxy for biomedical investigations in imaging, spectroscopy, and therapeutic applications. The observed THz pulse reflects the dispersive behavior associated with the frequency-dependent dielectric response of the skin. Comparison between the measured parameters of pork skin and reported values for human skin [29] shows close agreement, confirming its relevance as a surrogate tissue in THz studies. As summarized in Table 2, the quantitative similarity between pork and human skin parameters, with only minor deviations due to hydration and thickness differences, further supports the use of pork skin as a reliable biological analog in THz dielectric characterization.

Table 1. TeraPulse 4000 system specifications

Parameter	Value
Frequency range	0.01–11 THz
Spectral resolution	1 GHz
Dynamic range	>90 dB
Laser wavelength	800 nm
Pulse duration	100 fs
Repetition rate	80 MHz
Average power	800 mW
Beam diameter	3 mm

In our experiments, fresh pork skin samples were collected post-mortem and stored at 4°C to preserve their native properties. Preparation involved removing the subcutaneous fat layer and trimming the tissue to $5 \times 7\,\text{cm}^2$ with a thickness of about 2–3 mm, depending on fat nonuniformity. Measurements were performed immediately to prevent dehydration. The samples were mounted on wooden sticks inside the chamber, which was covered with a thin plastic layer to prevent contamination, as shown in Fig. 3.

Both reference and sample time-domain signals were then recorded over a 30 ps window with 0.1 ps resolution. Averaging over 1000 scans was performed to improve the signal-to-noise ratio. The complex transmission coefficient $\hat{T}(\omega)$ was obtained by Fourier transforming the time-domain signals, enabling extraction of the amplitude and phase of the transmitted pulse. From these, the frequency-dependent complex refractive index, $\hat{n}(\omega) - i\hat{\kappa}(\omega)$, was retrieved. The real part $\hat{n}(\omega)$ described the phase velocity, while the imaginary part $\hat{\kappa}(\omega)$ represented absorption losses through $\hat{\alpha}(\omega) = 2\omega\hat{\kappa}(\omega)/c$.

The reported spectra may include minor uncertainties affecting the absolute magnitudes shown. These can arise from internal scaling or normalization by the instrument, as well as practical factors such as sample thickness, alignment, or phase processing. Small variations may occur when comparing data across studies due to differences in calibration, data processing, or experimental conditions (e.g., temperature, hydration, or humidity). Nevertheless, the spectra provide a consistent and reliable reference for analyzing the dielectric properties

Table 2. Comparison between measured parameters of pork skin and literature values for human skin at [0–2]THz frequency range

Parameter	Pork skin [30,31]	Human skin [29,32,33]
Absorption	30–200 cm^{-1}	70–300
Refractive Index	1.7–2.4	1.5–2.6
Dielectric Constant (Real part)	2–3	2–4

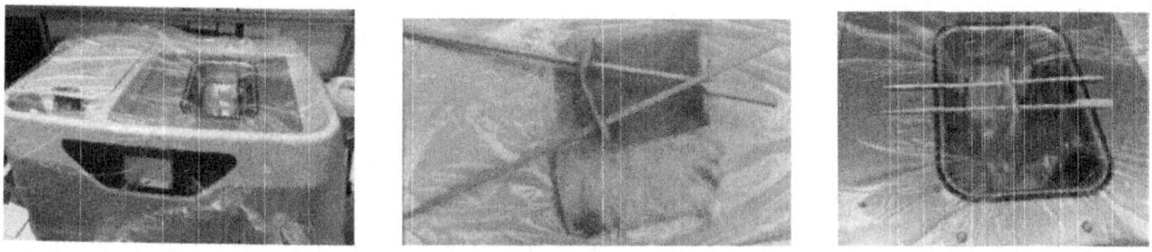

(a) (b) (c)

Fig. 3. Experiment setup overview. a) The instrumentation was covered with plastic to avoid contamination. b) Skin samples were hooked up to wooden sticks. c) Skin samples in the instrument chamber to perform the experiments,

of hydrated biological tissues. The following section discusses the measurements in terms of transmittance, absorption coefficient, and dielectric constant.

5 Numerical Results

This section presents and discusses the numerical results for THz wave propagation through a layer of pig skin. The investigated frequency range extends from 0.01 to 11 THz, with the most relevant part zoomed to 2 THz in Figs. 4–6, where the main dielectric relaxation processes occur. The electromagnetic response in this band is largely governed by tissue water content, affecting transmission, absorption, and dispersion.

Figure 4 presents the transmittance spectrum. Over most of the frequency band, transmission remains near zero due to strong absorption, with narrow peaks observed around 6–7 THz and smaller features between 7 and 9 THz. These narrowband spikes may originate from resonance effects such as Fabry–Pérot multi-reflections [11] and from internal interference effects or from vibrational resonances of molecular constituents such as collagen and lipids [34]. In

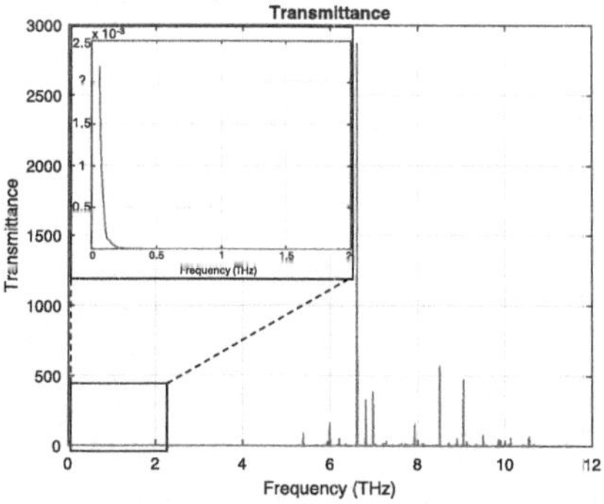

Fig. 4. Measured transmittance in the [0–12] THz range. A zoomed figure shows the behavior near the incident radiation frequency.

fact, in this range, absorption is less dominated by dipolar relaxation of free water and more influenced by specific vibrational modes of bound water and structural proteins, leading to weak, narrowband variations in the transmittance spectrum. The inset up to 2 THz highlights the most physically relevant region, where transmittance rapidly decreases with increasing frequency as a result of the strong absorption of THz waves by the high water content of the tissue [35–37].

From the transmittance spectrum, we extract the absorption coefficient $\hat{\alpha}(\omega)$, shown in Fig. 5(a). The absorption first increases up to about 1 THz and then decreases with frequency. The strong low-frequency absorption (0–1 THz) reflects tissue hydration, as water molecules induce significant dielectric losses due to dipole relaxation [35–37], confirming that hydration dominates the THz response of pig skin at low frequencies. The rapid oscillations may arise from intrinsic vibrational or rotational modes, numerical artifacts, or frequency-dependent scattering by tissue heterogeneities, such as adipose cells and collagen bundles [34]. Beyond 2 THz, the absorption coefficient decreases further, indicating reduced dielectric losses as the response shifts from collective water relaxation to localized vibrational absorption. This trend aligns with previous studies on porcine and human skin, where absorption decays at higher THz frequencies, reflecting the transition from relaxation- to resonance-dominated behavior [29–34].

Similarly, from transmittance we can also retrieve the refractive index $\hat{n}(\omega)$, shown in Fig. 5(b). At very low frequencies, $\hat{n}$ reaches large values, then decreases steeply within the first 0.5 THz and gradually levels off at higher frequencies. When focusing on the 0.01–2 THz region, it is evident that the refractive index decreases monotonically with frequency: despite the abnormal high values due to internal normalization, the trend is consistent with previously reported results on water and biological tissues [32]. Above 2 THz, the refractive index tends to stabilize toward lower values, approaching the asymptotic limit typical of bound

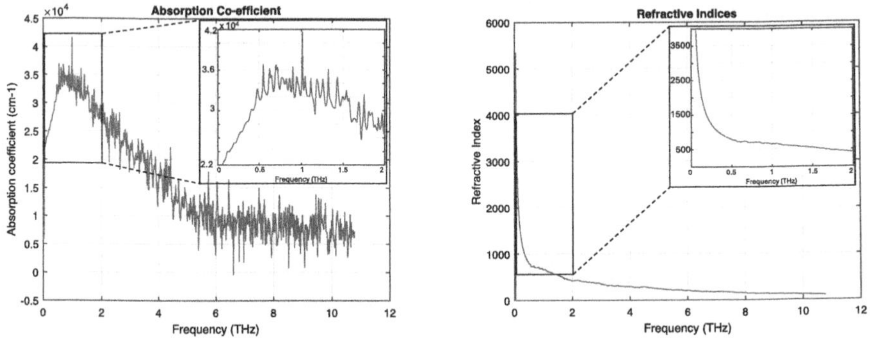

(a) (b)

Fig. 5. a) Absorption coefficient of pig skin in the 0–12 THz range. b) refractive index of pig skin in the 0–12 THz range. A zoomed figure shows the behavior in a closed range around the frequency of the incident radiation.

water and macromolecular media [34]. This plateau reflects the saturation of dispersive effects as the dipolar relaxation contribution vanishes, and the phase velocity becomes weakly frequency-dependent in the vibrational regime.

Overall, the results confirm that at low THz frequencies pig skin exhibits strong absorption and low transmittance, mainly due to its high water content. This behavior is consistent with the trends of $\hat{\alpha}(\omega)$ and $\hat{n}(\omega)$ for water predicted by the Debye model [32], highlighting the dominant role of hydration. From an application perspective, the results indicate that the upper part of the THz spectrum may be more favorable for imaging or sensing through biological tissues, as absorption decreases with frequency. Since THz radiation is strongly absorbed by liquid water, imaging applications can exploit the differences in water content between healthy and pathological tissues: for example, normal human skin typically contains about 70–72% free water, while many cancers contain 82–85% [38]. From these trends, we can anticipate the behavior of the complex dielectric constant $\varepsilon(\omega) = \varepsilon' - j\varepsilon''$. In particular, the results are consistent with a Debye-type dielectric dispersion, where molecular dipoles (primarily water) can follow the oscillating electric field at low frequencies, but fail to respond fast enough at higher THz frequencies [32].

As shown in Fig. 6, at low frequencies $\hat{\varepsilon}'$ reaches very large values, reflecting the strong tissue polarizability, while $\hat{\varepsilon}''$ is strongly negative, indicating significant absorption. As frequency increases toward the THz range (1–2 THz), $\hat{\varepsilon}'$ decreases and $\hat{\varepsilon}''$ rises toward zero, showing reduced absorption. Both $\hat{\varepsilon}'$ and $\hat{\varepsilon}''$ eventually stabilize at lower values. This trend aligns with the results for $\hat{\alpha}(\omega)$ and $\hat{n}(\omega)$, since $\hat{\varepsilon}''$ is directly related to the absorption coefficient and $\hat{\varepsilon}'$ to the refractive index. In the high-frequency region, both reach nearly constant values, indicating a steady-state dielectric response dominated by bound water and structural vibrations rather than collective dipole relaxation [34]. This flattening of the permittivity spectra marks the transition from the Debye relaxation domain to the vibrational absorption domain above a few terahertz.

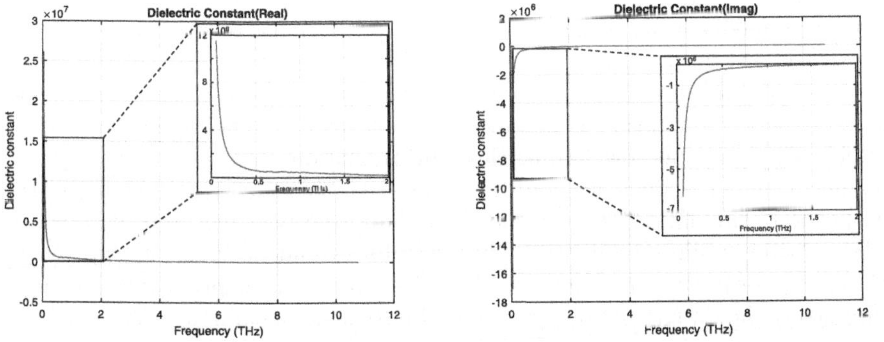

(a) (b)

Fig. 6. Real (a) and imaginary (b) parts of the dielectric constant. A zoomed view shows the behavior near the incident radiation frequency.

Furthermore, it is important to relate the dielectric response of porcine skin to the size of its structural components with respect to the THz wavelength. The main constituents, including keratinocytes, melanocytes, adipose cells, fibroblasts, and collagen fibers, have dimensions from a few to several tens of micrometers. Consequently, the observed spectral behavior primarily arises from the collective dielectric response of water and macromolecules rather than from scattering at cellular boundaries. This dimensional relationship explains why, in the 0 to 2 THz range, absorption and dispersion are dominated by Debye-type relaxation of free and bound water, while specific structural resonances become relevant only at higher frequencies. When the wavelength approaches the size of microstructures such as collagen bundles, local scattering and vibrational resonances can contribute to overall attenuation and dispersion [34].

In summary, the numerical results highlight the strong influence of water content on the THz response of pig skin, with high absorption and refractive index at low frequencies and reduced absorption at higher frequencies. The trends in $\hat{\alpha}(\omega)$, $\hat{n}(\omega)$, and $\hat{\varepsilon}(\omega)$ follow Debye-type behavior, confirming that hydration dominates the lower THz range. At higher frequencies, absorption and refractive index gradually decrease and stabilize, marking a transition to a less lossy yet dispersive regime. Despite low transmittance, frequency-dependent attenuation and phase delay provide a consistent description of wave propagation through hydrated skin. These parameters define key features of the THz channel, suggesting that selecting the operating frequency can optimize penetration and contrast, forming a basis for an analytical channel model capturing both dispersive and lossy characteristics relevant for intra-body communication and sensing.

6 Conclusions

This work presented an experimental characterization and modeling of porcine skin in the 0.01–11 THz range using PCA-based THz time-domain spectroscopy. The measured refractive index, absorption coefficient, and complex permittivity demonstrated that hydrated biological tissues behave as highly attenuating and dispersive media, with dielectric properties predominantly governed by water-related relaxation processes.

By mapping these frequency-dependent properties to a channel framework, a first experimental THz channel model was developed. The model captures the strong absorption at low frequencies, the transition to a less lossy dispersive regime at higher frequencies, and the associated phase delays, which are critical for accurate simulation of intra-body THz links and near-field sensing scenarios where local coupling dominates. These results extend previous studies by providing a quantitative, frequency-resolved description of the propagation channel, supporting the design and optimization of next-generation nanoscale biomedical devices operating in the sub-THz and THz bands.

Acknowledgment. The work of E. Marini, S. Mura, and M. Magarini was supported by the Institute of Information & communications Technology Planning & Evaluation (IITP) grant funded by the Korea government (MSIT)(No.RS-202400508465).

References

1. Ghorbian, M., Ghobaei-Arani, M., Babaei, M.R., Ghorbian, S.: Nanotechnology and nanosensors in personalized healthcare: a comprehensive review. Sens. Bio-Sens. Res. **47**, 100740 (2025)
2. Naranjo-Hernández, D., et al.: Past results, present trends, and future challenges in intrabody communication. Wirel. Commun. Mob. Comput. **2018**(1), 9026847 (2018)
3. Vizziello, A., Magarini, M., Savazzi, P., Galluccio, L.: Intra-body communications for nervous system applications: current technologies and future directions. Comput. Netw. **227**, 109718 (2023)
4. Anjum, M., Wang, H.: Molecular communication for wireless body area networks. In: Encyclopedia of Wireless Networks, pp. 1–5. Springer, Heidelberg (2019). https://doi.org/10.1007/978-3-319-32903-1_152-1
5. Hanson, G.W.: Fundamental transmitting properties of carbon nanotube antennas. IEEE Trans. Antennas Propag. **53**(11), 3426–3435 (2005)
6. Jornet, J.M., Akyildiz, I.F.: Fundamentals of electromagnetic nanonetworks in the Terahertz band. Found. Trends Netw. **7**(2–3), 77–233 (2013)
7. Jornet, J.M., Akyildiz, I.F.: Channel capacity of electromagnetic nanonetworks in the Terahertz band. In: Proceedings of IEEE ICC, pp. 1–6 (2010)
8. Guo, H., Johari, P., Jornet, J.M., Sun, Z.: Intra-body optical channel modeling for in vivo wireless nanosensor networks. IEEE Trans. Nanobiosci. **15**(1), 41–52 (2015)
9. Kucheryavenko, A., et al.: Terahertz-wave scattering in tissues: examining the limits of the applicability of effective-medium theory. Phys. Rev. Appl. **20**(5), 054050 (2023)
10. Jornet, J.M., Akyildiz, I.F.: Channel modeling and capacity analysis for electromagnetic nanonetworks in the Terahertz band. IEEE Trans. Wirel. Commun. **10**(10), 3211–3221 (2011)
11. Peretti, R., et al.: THz-TDS time-trace analysis for the extraction of material and metamaterial parameters. IEEE Trans. Terahertz Sci. Technol. **9**(2), 136–149 (2018)
12. Hale, P., et al.: 20 THz broadband generation using semi-insulating GaAs interdigitated photoconductive antennas. Opt. Express **22**, 26358–26364 (2014)
13. El-Ghazaly, S., Joshi, R., Grondin, R.: Electromagnetic and transport considerations in subpicosecond photoconductive switch modeling. IEEE Trans. Microw. Theory Techn. **38**(5), 629–637 (2002)
14. Khiabani, N., Huang, Y., Shen, Y.-C., Boyes, S.: Theoretical modeling of a photoconductive antenna in a terahertz pulsed system. IEEE Trans. Antennas Propag. **61**(4), 1538–1546 (2013)
15. Pawar, A.Y., Sonawane, D.D., Erande, K.B., Derle, D.V.: Terahertz technology and its applications. Drug Invent. Today **5**, 157–163 (2013)
16. Wilson, N., Aarnio, H., Österbacka, R.: Comparing the loss of charge carrier generation with the loss of V OC at low temperatures in organic bulk-heterojunction blends. Phys. Scr. **98**(11), 115985 (2023)
17. Qin, J., Liu, X.-K., Yin, C., Gao, F.: Carrier dynamics and evaluation of lasing actions in halide perovskites. Trends Chem. **3**(1), 34–46 (2021)
18. Piao, Z.S., Tani, M., Sakai, K.: Carrier dynamics and THz generation in biased semiconductors. J. Commun. Res. Lab. **46**(3), 263–269 (1999)

19. Wahlstrand, J.K., Heilweil, E.J.: Contactless THz-based bulk semiconductor mobility measurements using two-photon excitation. Opt. Express **26**(23), 29848–29853 (2018)
20. Castro-Camus, E., Lloyd-Hughes, J., Johnston, M.B.: Three-dimensional carrier-dynamics simulation of Terahertz emission from photoconductive switches. Phys. Rev. B **71**(19), 195301 (2005)
21. Burford, N.M., El-Shenawee, M.O.: Review of Terahertz photoconductive antenna technology. Opt. Eng. **56**(1), 010901 (2017)
22. Pickwell, E., Wallace, V.P.: Biomedical applications of Terahertz technology. J. Phys. D Appl. Phys. **39**(17), R301 (2006)
23. Wang, Y., Cai, R., Chen, C.: The nano-bio interactions of nanomedicines: understanding the biochemical driving forces and redox reactions. Acc. Chem. Res. **52**(6), 1507–1518 (2019)
24. Cherkasova, O.P., et al.: Cellular effects of Terahertz waves. J. Biomed. Opt. **26**(9), 090902 (2021)
25. Shi, W., Li, C., Wang, H., Wang, Z., Yang, L.: Quantitative detection of THz-ATR spectra of aqueous samples under strong-field Terahertz wave. iScience **26**(1), 105871 (2023)
26. de la Rosa, C., et al.: Terahertz permittivity of pressed ZnO and CuO powder in polyethylene pellets: effect of porosity. IEEE Trans. Terahertz Sci. Technol. **11**(4), 402–407 (2021)
27. Jepsen, P.U.: Phase retrieval in Terahertz time-domain measurements: a "how to" tutorial. J. Infrared Millim. Terahertz Waves **40**, 395–411 (2019)
28. Elayan, H., Shubair, R.M., Jornet, J.M., Johari, P.: Terahertz channel model and link budget analysis for intrabody nanoscale communication. IEEE Trans. Nanobiosci. **16**(6), 491–503 (2017)
29. Sullivan, T.P., Eaglstein, W.H., Davis, S.C., Mertz, P.: The pig as a model for human wound healing. Wound Repair Regen. **9**(2), 66–76 (2001)
30. He, M., Azad, A.K., Ye, S., Zhang, W.: Far-infrared signature of animal tissues characterized by terahertz time-domain spectroscopy. Opt. Commun. **259**(1), 389–392 (2006)
31. Helminiak, J., et al.: Temperature dependence of the dielectric function of dehydrated biological samples in the THz band. Biomed. Opt. Express **14**(4), 1472–1479 (2023)
32. Peralta, X.G., et al.: Terahertz spectroscopy of human skin tissue models with different melanin content. Biomed. Opt. Express **10**, 2942–2955 (2019)
33. Piro, G., Bia, P., Boggia, G., Caratelli, D., Grieco, L., Mescia, L.: Terahertz electromagnetic field propagation in human tissues: a study on communication capabilities. Nano Commun. Netw. **10**, 51–59 (2016)
34. Nikitkina, A.I., et al.: Terahertz radiation and the skin: a review. J. Biomed. Opt. **26**(4), 043005 (2021)
35. Jepsen, P.U., Cooke, D.G., Koch, M.: Terahertz spectroscopy and imaging-modern techniques and applications. Laser Photon. Rev. **5**(1), 124–166 (2011)
36. Arikawa, T., Nagai, M., Tanaka, K.: Characterizing hydration state in solution using Terahertz time-domain attenuated total reflection spectroscopy. Chem. Phys. Lett. **457**(1–3), 12–17 (2008)
37. Saxena, S., et al.: Limitations of effective medium models for tissue phantoms in the THz frequency range. Sci. Rep. **14**(1), 22968 (2024)
38. Vilagosh, Z., et al.: Characterisation of biological materials at THz frequencies by attenuated total reflection: lard. Appl. Sci. **10**(23), 8692 (2020)

Performance of Data Channel Migration Procedure for SmartBAN

Hirokazu Tanaka(✉) and Takahiro Ito

Hiroshima City University, Hiroshima 731-3194, Japan
hitanaka@hiroshima-cu.ac.jp

Abstract. Research and development of healthcare IoT, such as health management using wearable sensors, has been actively progressing. The development of these healthcare IoT is supported by the progress of wireless networks and Body Area Network (BAN) technology that enables flexible connections of wearable sensors placed near the human body is a typical example.

In this study, SmartBAN on which is a BAN standard specified by International Electrotechnical Commission (IEC) and European Telecommunications Standards Institute (ETSI) is focused and its coexistence characteristics are evaluated. SmartBAN features a mechanism to change to another channel when channel quality is degraded due to interference. Since SmartBAN usually has multiple nodes connected to one HUB for communication, if the channel condition is not good, it takes time for all nodes to complete the transition to a new channel. As a basic performance analysis, we evaluate the time required for SmartBAN to change channels through simulation.

Keywords: Body Area Network · SmartBAN · Channel migration

1 Introduction

Active Assisted Living (AAL) has emerged as a significant application area of healthcare IoT [1–3]. AAL aims to support the independence of elderly individuals and those with age-related disabilities by employing Information and Communications Technologies (ICT). With the global trend of aging populations, including in Japan, the demand for AAL services is expected to continue growing.

A typical AAL service includes a monitoring service and support for independent living that utilizes vital, environmental, and location information collected by wearable and environmental sensors. Such services are expected to stimulate new business opportunities in device development, system integration, and service provision.

The growing demand for AAL services using wearable sensors has promoted the development of wearable devices with embedded vital sensors. This progress is supported by technological advances that have miniaturized sensors, facilitated their integration into devices, and enabled wireless networking through IoT technologies. Consequently, wearable sensors are widely used in healthcare, not only in clinical settings but also in daily life, for health monitoring and elderly care.

H. Tanaka et al. (Eds.): BodyNets 2025, LNICST 714, pp. 47–53, 2026.
https://doi.org/10.1007/978-3-032-38657-1_4

One of key enabling technologies for healthcare IoT is the Body Area Network (BAN) [4, 5], which connects wearable sensors around the human body. A BAN typically consists of nodes that transmit sensor data and a hub that collects data from the nodes via wireless communication. Among various BAN standards, SmartBAN that was standardized by IEC and ETSI is widely recognized [6–9].

SmartBAN defines four primary technical requirements: low power consumption, optimized QoS control, timely connectivity, and coexistence with other wireless devices. Among these, coexistence with other wireless devices is particularly important because SmartBAN operates in the 2.4 GHz ISM band, where Wi-Fi, Bluetooth, ZigBee etc. also operate. Interference from these systems, as well as other SmartBAN devices on the same channel, may cause the degradation of communication quality and errors. To cope with this, SmartBAN defines a protocol for channel migration when channel quality falls below a defined threshold. However, since SmartBAN HUB typically connects multiple nodes, the migration procedure will take longer until all nodes are ready for channel change. This may also reduce the quality of AAL service.

In this study, we evaluate, through simulation, the time required for SmartBAN channel changing in a BAN with multiple nodes and discuss its impact on AAL services.

2 Overview of SmartBAN System

2.1 System Concept

SmartBAN is a BAN standard that is defined for meeting the following four technical requirements. An overview of them is shown below.

(1) Lower power consumption

It specifies a MAC that is simpler than other MAC protocols such as IEEE802.15.6 [10]. Furthermore, the MAC specification allows for lower power consumption on the sensor node side by concentrating the load balance between the hub and the nodes on the hub as much as possible.

(2) Optimal control of QoS

A mechanism that allows the QoS level of the upper layer to be transmitted to the PHY layer is introduced. This mechanism allows flexible QoS settings and data transmission according to the QoS level by increasing the number of QoS levels.

(3) Timely connection

It is designed to shorten the initial connection time. Furthermore, it can send emergency signals, making it suitable for medical and healthcare services.

(4) Coexistence of BANs

As users wearing wearable sensors connected by BAN move around, BANs that use the same frequency may come close to each other. In that case, these BANs may cause interference. This is because even if a user confirms an empty channel and sets a BAN when connecting for the first time, as the user moves, other users who have established the same channel will approach. Therefore, SmartBAN supports a mechanism that allows you to understand the status of nearby BANs, the approach of BANs, etc., and take steps to change channels as necessary. This mechanism is also used to change channels when there is strong interference from other systems using the same frequency band, such as WiFi or Bluetooth.

SmartBAN solves these technical requirements by creating two types of channel configurations, consisting of a Control channel (C-ch) and a Data channel (D-ch), and by devising the definition of the D-ch frame format. SmartBAN uses 40 channels with a channel width of 2 MHz in the 2.4 GHz band. Of the 40 channels, 3 are C-ch and the rest are D-ch. C-ch broadcasts the HUB address, slot length, data channel number, etc., and D-ch performs data transmission and reception between the HUB and the Node. The HUB sends out beacons for both channels. Figure 1 shows the configuration of C-beacon and D-beacon. A Node that attempts to connect to a HUB receives the C-beacon and obtains information necessary for initial connection and data communication with the HUB, such as information on the D-ch used by the HUB. D-ch performs initial connection processing of Nodes and sends and receives data to and from the HUB. D-ch manages the D-ch beacon interval (hereinafter called Inter-Beacon Interval: IBI) by dividing it into three periods: Scheduled Access period (SAP), Control & Management period (CMP), and Inactive period (IAP). Here, SAP employs the TDMA method and CMP employs the Slotted Aloha method. Additionally, it is possible to set four levels of QoS parameters for the D-ch frame.

2.2 Data Channel Migration Protocol

When a D-ch migration is required, the HUB will notify the D-ch migration timing and new D-ch number using the D-beacon's Channel Mitigation Info. Channel Migration Info consists of Change Timing, which indicates the timing of D-ch migration, and Channel Number, which indicates the destination D-ch number. Normally operating Nodes change channels at the same timing as the HUB based on the information in

Channel Mitigation Info. While this D-ch migration process is being performed, the D- beacon sets the Channel Migration Indicator to '1' to indicate that the D-ch migration instruction is coming from the HUB. From the start of D-ch migration until changing to a new D-ch number, the C-beacon sets Interference Mitigation to '1' to notify that interference mitigation procedures are being executed.

Figures 2 shows an example where SmartBAN with three nodes connected to a HUB performs a channel migration procedure based on the channel migration information of D-beacon.

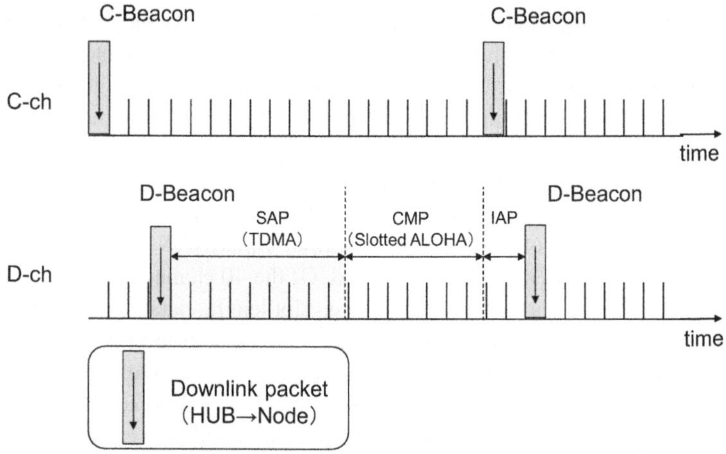

Fig. 1. Control and data channel structure in SmartBAN system

3 Performance Evaluation

3.1 Simulation Conditions

If multiple nodes are connected to a HUB, all nodes must be able to correctly receive the D-Beacon during the channel migration period, correctly read the Channel Migration Info, and migrate to the designated D-ch at the designated timing. If there is a node that cannot read the channel changing timing or the destination channel number, the BAN cannot properly complete the channel migration process. In this simulation evaluation, we will consider what the Change Timing value should be set in order to ensure that all Nodes can correctly receive D-Beacon's Channel Migration Info during the channel migration period and change to a new D-ch at the timing indicated by the HUB.

Table 1 shows the simulation conditions.

Table 1. Simulation Parameters

Parameter	Value/Condition
Number of Nodes	1, 3, 5,10, 16
D-Beacon length	320 bits
Change Timing	Max. 256 IBIs
Channel Model	AWGN channel

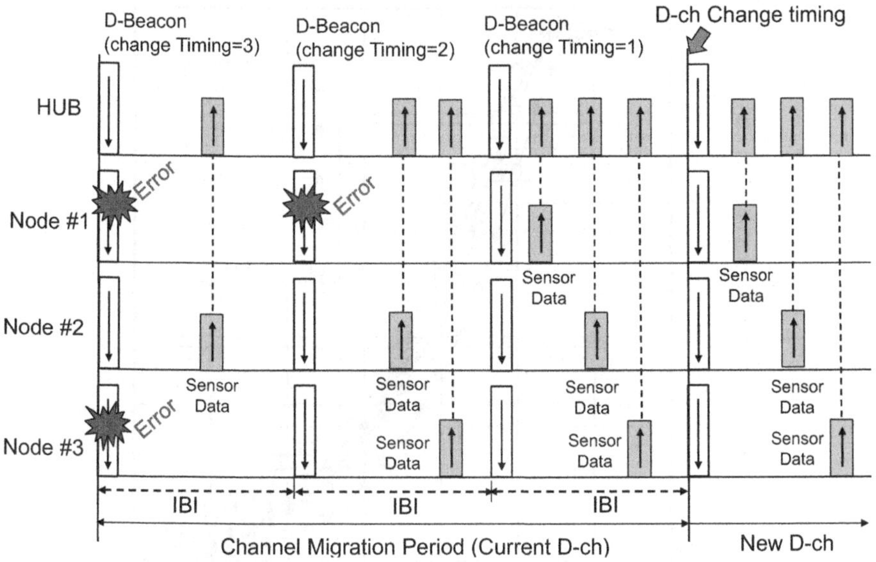

Fig. 2. An example of Data channel migration

3.2 Simulation Results

Figure 3 shows the simulation results. In Fig. 3, the horizontal axis shows Eb/N0 and the vertical axis shows the average number of IBIs required for channel migration. The curbs are shown when the number of nodes connected to HUB is 1, 3, 5, 10, and 16. As you can see from this figure, the more nodes connected to one HUB, the more number of IBI are required in order for all nodes to be able to chnage channels at the indicated timing. This shows that the larger the number of nodes connected to the HUB, the larger the Change Timing value needs to be. However, since there is less difference in performance characteristics when the number of Nodes is 10 or more, it is possible to set the Change Timing value to a value that does not make much of a difference. Also, it can be seen that in a region where Eb/N0 is approximately higher than 7 dB, Change Timing can be set to about 3IBIs.

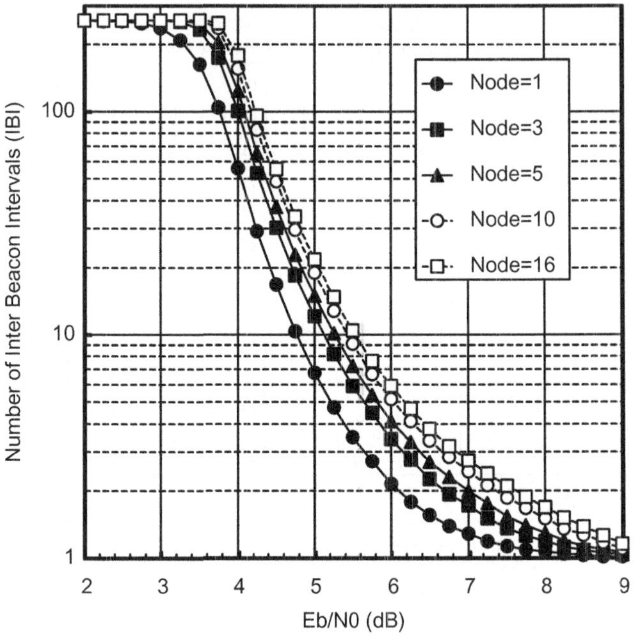

Fig. 3. Average number of IBI required until all nodes receive Channel Mitigation Info correctly and can perform Channel migration

4 Conclusion

In this study, we evaluated and investigated the performance of channel migration procedure in SmartBAN. We evaluated by simulation that the average number of IBIs required until all nodes connected to the HUB receive Channel Migration Info correctly and are able to perform channel migration. It has become quantitatively clear that the larger the number of nodes connected to the HUB, the larger the D-Beacon Change Timing value needs to be.

Acknowledgement. This research and development work was supported by the MIC/FORWARD # JPMI250830001.

References

1. Alowaydhah, S., Weerasekara, I., Walmsley, S., Keir, S., Marquez, J.: Perceived physical activity levels and objective measures: a mixed-methods study of residents aged 65 and above in assisted living homes in Australia. Wiley J. Aging Res. **2024**, 9688105 (2024)
2. Cicirelli, G., Marani, R., Petitti, A., Milella, A., D'orazio, T.: Ambient assisted living: a review of technologies, methodologies and future perspectives for healthy aging of population. Sensors. **21**(10), 3549 (2021)

3. Qian, K., Zhang, Z., Yamamoto, Y., Schuller, B.W.: Artificial intelligence internet of things for the elderly: from assisted living to health-care monitoring. IEEE Signal Process. Mag. **38**(4), 78–88 (2021)
4. Singh, S., Prasad, D.: Wireless body area network (WBAN): a review of schemes and protocols. Elsevier materials today: proceedings. **49**(Part 8), 3488–3496 (2022)
5. Mohanty, R.K., Sahoo, S.P., Kabat, M.R.: Sustainable remote patient monitoring in wireless body area network with multi-hop routing and scheduling: a four-fold objective based optimization approach. Springer Wireless Netw. **29**, 2337–2351 (2023)
6. IEC 63203-801-1: Wearable electronic devices and technologies - Part 801-1: Smart body area network (SmartBAN) - Enhanced ultra-low power physical layer, ED1, Nov. 2022
7. IEC 63203-801-2: Wearable electronic devices and technologies - Part 801-2: Smart body area network (SmartBAN) - Low complexity medium access control (MAC) for SmartBAN, ED1, Nov. 2022
8. ETSI TS 103 325, Smart Body Area Network (SmartBAN); Low Complexity Medium Access Control (MAC) for SmartBAN, version 1.1.1, Apr. 2015
9. ETSI TS 103 326: Smart Body Area Network (SmartBAN); Enhanced Ultra-Low Power Physical Layer, version 1.1.1, Apr. 2015
10. IEEE Std 802.15.6-2012 - IEEE Standard for Local and metropolitan area networks - Part 15.6: Wireless Body Area Networks

Sensing, Localization, and Motion Analysis in Body Area Networks

Evaluation of 3-Dimensional In-Body Device Localization Using Machine Learning Algorithms with Reduced Training Data

Taiki Egusa[1], Takumi Kobayashi[1], Jaakko Hyry[1], Manato Fujimoto[1,2](✉), Shingo Ata[1], and Daisuke Anzai[1]

[1] Osaka Metropolitan University, Osaka, Osaka 558-8585, Japan
manato@omu.ac.jp

[2] RIKEN Center for Advanced Intelligence Project AIP, Chuo-ku, Tokyo 103-0027, Japan

Abstract. Recently, active research has been conducted on the development of in-body cybernetic avatars (in-body CA) that can perform actions and operations on behalf of humans within the body with the aim of achieving a society with health longevity outcomes. These avatars are composed of various implantable devices, and it is important to acquire detailed information in vivo to localize device positions. We present a device localization method based on magnetic fields and evaluate the position estimation accuracy of the various machine learning algorithms using a bioequivalent liquid phantom that simulates the human body, to identify which algorithms are suitable for position estimations of in-body devices. In addition, since collecting training data is time-consuming, we also evaluate the relationship between the amount of training data and estimation accuracy, to reduce the required data volume while maintaining an acceptable level of error.

Keywords: Cybernetic Avatars · In-body Localization · Machine Learning

1 Introduction

Over the past few years, significant progress has been made in the development of in-body cybernetic avatars (in-body CA)[1] aimed at achieving a society with increased health longevity. An in-body CA refers to a system that enables safe and reliable remote control from outside the body, allowing for the monitoring of condition in vivo within organs and the gastrointestinal tract, as well as

This work was supported in part by JST Moonshot R&D Grant Number JPMJMS2214-06 and Grant-in-Aid for Scientific Research (KAKENHI) Grant Number JP24K00885.

[1] In-body Cybernetic Avatars, https://in-body-ca.org/index.html.

H. Tanaka et al. (Eds.): BodyNets 2025, LNICST 714, pp. 57–73, 2026.
https://doi.org/10.1007/978-3-032-38657-1_5

the interaction between the body and the external environment. This concept is realized through various implantable devices, which operate at millimeter, micro, and nano scales, and perform functions such as measuring internal body temperature and pH, delivering localized medication, and for removing tumors. Efforts to structure both temporal and spatial internal environmental information based on the data obtained from these devices are also considered. If applied to health monitoring, this approach could enable new methods for managing health and performing diagnostics from home. To this end, this study focuses on the 3-dimensional localization of in-body CA devices as a foundation for structuring spatiotemporal information within the body.

Conventional localization methods for in-body devices have utilized radio wave characteristics. Although millimeter-level accuracy has been achieved in previous studies using methods based on Received Signal Strength Indicator (RSSI) [1] and Time of Arrival (TOA) [2], these methods are significantly affected by the dielectric properties and conductivity of biological tissues. As a result, it is difficult to reproduce the same level of accuracy under actual measurement conditions due to individual differences in tissue composition and patient variability. In this study, we focus on a localization approach based on magnetic fields, because the relative permeability of human tissues is approximately one, and magnetic fields interact minimally with body media [8]. Furthermore, by using magnetoquasistatic fields, which exhibit characteristics of static fields, we aim to enable both wireless communication and device localization within the body. Specifically, localization is performed by measuring the magnetic fields emitted when the in-body device transmits information, using small sensors placed outside the body.

In general, it is difficult to construct mathematical models in complex radio environments or with fluctuating antenna patterns. In such cases, machine learning has been utilized to represent these environments in a learned feature space for localization. The same applies to in-body localization, where complex interference caused by body tissues and changes in antenna patterns due to device movement, make the environment difficult to model. Therefore, machine learning-based approaches have been explored for this task. However, comprehensive evaluations of the applicability of various machine learning algorithms to the in-body devices localization task remain limited. We study the feasibility of applying various traditional machine learning algorithms to this issue.

While machine learning offers advantages for modeling complex systems, it also requires a large amount of training data, the acquisition of which is time-consuming in real-world settings. To address this issue, we investigate the relationship between the amount of training data and estimation accuracy under a given acceptable error, to reduce the data requirement while maintaining good performance.

Accordingly, our contributions are summarized as follows:

1. Proposal of a localization method for in-body devices using magnetoquasistatic fields

2. Exploration of traditional machine learning algorithms for this localization task
3. Investigation into reducing the volume of training data required for machine learning

The rest of this paper is organized as follows: In Sect. 2, we summarize related studies that address the estimation of device location and clarify the position of the present study within the existing body of research. Section 3 describes our machine learning-based method for in-body devices localization utilizing quasi-static magnetic fields, while Sect. 4 details the hardware configuration of the implantable device and magnetic field measurement system employed in this study. Section 5 discusses the investigation into suitable machine learning algorithms for the in-body devices localization task, as well as the evaluation of methods for reducing the amount of training data. Section 6 elaborates on the tuning of the machine learning models. In Sect. 7, we present and analyze the results obtained from the evaluations described in Sect. 5. Finally, Sect. 8 provides the conclusion of this study.

2 Related Work

Nowadays, with the growing emphasis on achieving a society of healthy longevity, there has been active development of in-body CA, which can operate within the human body in place of a person or be remotely controlled from outside the body. Among the essential technologies required for such systems, in-body localization techniques for implantable devices have attracted increasing research attention. Related studies by Zeising et al. [8] and Saransh et al. [7] have proposed localization methods that utilize magnetic field generation machines such as coils placed outside the body. In these studies, magnetic field gradients generated by highly efficient planar electromagnetic coils installed externally are measured using magnetic field sensors embedded in implantable devices. The position of the device is then estimated based on the measured magnetic field intensity. The gradients generated by a static magnetic field are designed to monotonically decrease with distance in each of the three spatial dimensions (x, y, and z), enabling unique localization of the implantable device by measuring the magnetic field at its location. This approach also has the advantage of being robust to the device's rotational orientation within the body. However, it requires embedding magnetic field sensors in implantable devices and it depends on a large-scale external magnetic field generation system composed of planar coils with a diameter of approximately 60 cm, which compromises portability and limits applicability in general-use environments.

Additionally, related studies by Sasaki et al. [5,6] have proposed a localization method in which temporally alternating magnetic signals emitted by a target device are captured by receivers positioned in the surrounding environment. The location of the device is then estimated based on the measured signals. These studies specifically target indoor wireless device localization, using magnetic signals transmitted from the device and received by multiple receivers placed

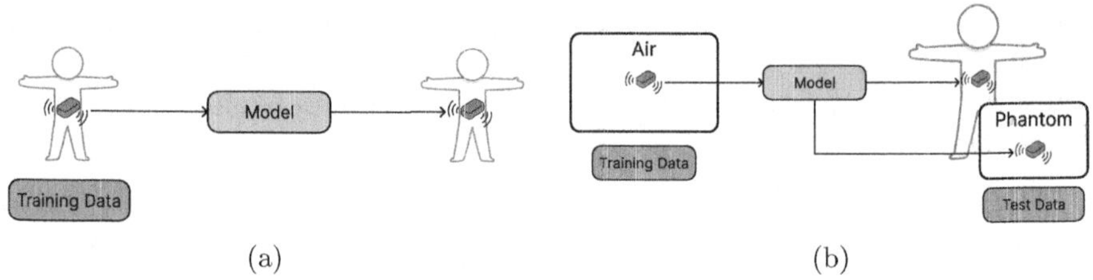

Fig. 1. Conceptual illustration: (a) Traditional method: Machine learning algorithms are trained in the body environment, (b) Our proposed method: Machine learning algorithms are trained in air and make predictions in the body environment.

indoors. The received signal strengths are used to estimate the transmitting location of the device and the estimation is performed using machine learning methods based on the nearest neighbor approach. However, these related works do not address the challenges of in-body localization, as they do not consider the effects of biological tissues on the propagation characteristics of magnetic signals or their impact on localization accuracy. Furthermore, they did not explore how localization accuracy might change when applying machine learning algorithms in addition to the nearest-neighbor approach.

When considering the previous issues, the present study contributes novelty by establishing a localization method that leverages magnetoquasistatic fields to minimize biological interference and by quantitatively evaluating the impact of the biological presence or absence on the performance of various machine learning algorithms used for localization.

3 Traditional Machine Learning-Based In-Body Device Localization Method Using Magnetoquasistatic Fields

This section describes the proposed localization method for in-body devices based on machine learning utilizing magnetoquasistatic fields. Conventional machine learning-based spatial localization methods generally assume that both the training and test data are obtained under identical or similar environmental conditions, and it is necessary to obtain the training data in advance within the environment where localization is to be performed. However, in the context of in-body devices localization, collecting training data for each individual is impractical, given the intended real-world application scenarios. Furthermore, individual anatomical differences may significantly degrade localization accuracy. Also, conventional localization methods require the acquisition of ground truth positional data within the target space to construct training datasets. However, obtaining accurate ground truth positional information inside the human body is extremely challenging in practice. To address these limitations, we propose a methodology, illustrated in Fig. 1, in which the machine learning model is trained using data acquired in air and subsequently evaluated using data collected in a biological tissue-equivalent liquid phantom. Ideally, the model would be trained on data obtained under actual in vivo conditions (as shown in Fig. 1(a)), however, since constructing individual models for each patient is not feasible, this study adopts an alternative approach (as shown in Fig. 1(b)), in which models trained on air-based data are evaluated in a phantom environment that simulates biological properties.

4 Hardware Configuration for In-Body Localization Based on Magnetoquasistatic Fields

Here we describe the hardware configuration used for in-body localization based on magnetoquasistatic fields. We aim to estimate the localization of an implantable device by utilizing the magnetic field generated during the transmission of information from within the body to the outside. Accordingly, the target signal source is assumed to be an alternating magnetic field, and the system is supposed to operate within a frequency range where the near-field component is dominant.

Figure 2(a) and Fig. 2(b) show overviews of the magnetic field generator and the measurement system used in the experiments, respectively. As shown in Fig. 2(a), the magnetic field source is a swallowable device that emits an alternating magnetic field at 10 kHz and is powered by a compact button cell battery. The magnetic field emitted from this source is measured at multiple external locations using the measurement system shown in Fig. 2(b), and the acquired magnetic field data is used for localization.

The measurement system uses four 3-axis magnetic field sensor modules that detect the magnetic signals emitted by the source to provide datasets for position estimation. Each 3-axis sensor module consists of three magneto-impedance (MI) sensors [3,4] corresponding to the x, y, and z axes, allowing for high-sensitivity detection of magnetic field strengths in all three directions at four different locations, using a total of twelve MI sensors.

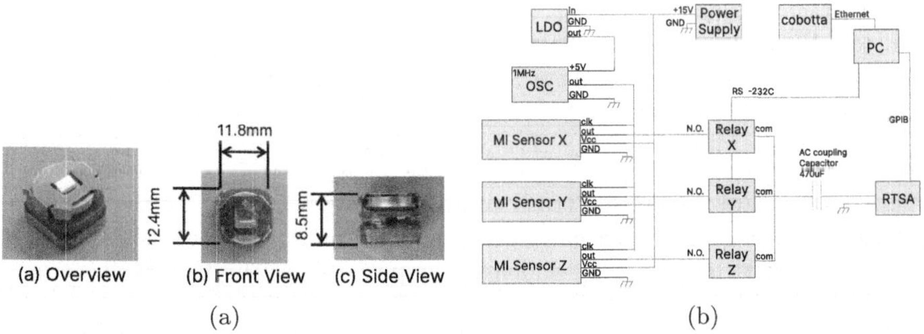

(a) (b)

Fig. 2. Overview of the magnetic field generation and measurement system: (a) Swallowable device emitting alternating magnetic field, (b) Block diagram of the 3-axis measurement system (1 of 4 locations).

Magnetic signals from these twelve MI sensors are selectively routed through a relay circuit to a real-time spectrum analyzer (RTSA) (RSA3308B, Tektronix), where their signal strengths are measured. To measure the received magnetic field strength at various spatial coordinates, the magnetic source is moved along the x, y, and z axes using a robotic arm (Cobotta, DENSO WAVE Inc.), enabling automated acquisition of measurements from all twelve sensors at each spatial coordinate.

Currently, the measurement system requires approximately 4 s to obtain the signal strength from one of the twelve MI sensors due to the limitations of the spectrum analyzer, the averaging signal, and the switching relay. Consequently, a full cycle of measurements across all twelve sensors takes around 48 s. If the magnetic source is moved to 20 different points along each of the x, y, and z axes, a complete scan involves 48×20^3 seconds, which corresponds to more than four days of continuous measurement. Furthermore, reducing the measurement interval increases the total time cubically. Although acquiring training data at finer intervals is expected to enhance localization accuracy, such prolonged measurement durations pose practical challenges. Therefore, in this study, we also investigate the effect of measurement interval on localization accuracy, identify the minimum interval required to achieve the desired accuracy, and explore machine learning algorithms that can suppress accuracy degradation even when data are sparsely sampled.

5 Experimental Method

We investigated both the applicability of traditional machine learning algorithms for estimating the localization of in-body devices and the possibility of reducing the required amount of training data. This chapter provides a detailed description of the proposed experimental methodology.

5.1 Evaluation Metrics

The machine learning algorithms are trained to minimize the error between the true coordinates and the predicted ones. For each data point, the prediction error is calculated using the Mean Squared Error (MSE), as defined below:

$$\mathrm{MSE}_i = \sqrt{(x_i - \hat{x}_i)^2 + (y_i - \hat{y}_i)^2 + (z_i - \hat{z}_i)^2}\,, \tag{1}$$

where x_i, y_i, z_i are the ground truth coordinates, and $\hat{x}_i, \hat{y}_i, \hat{z}_i$ are the predicted ones. The overall prediction accuracy of the algorithm is evaluated using the Root Mean Squared Error (RMSE), which is computed from the Euclidean error of each point:

$$\mathrm{RMSE} = \sqrt{\frac{1}{n}\sum_{i=1}^{n} \mathrm{MSE}_i^2}\,, \tag{2}$$

Table 1. List of the 45 machine learning algorithms used in this study

Machine Learning Models		
CCA	MLPRegressor	QuantileRegressor
SVR	SGDRegressor	ExtraTreeRegressor
Lars	PLSCanonical	ExtraTreesRegressor
Lasso	ElasticNetCV	MultiTaskElasticNet
Ridge	ARDRegression	KNeighborsRegressor
NuSVR	BayesianRidge	MultiTaskElasticNetCV
LarsCV	MultiTaskLasso	DecisionTreeRegressor
RidgeCV	DummyRegressor	RandomForestRegressor
LassoCV	PLSRegression	GaussianProcessRegressor
LassoLars	RANSACRegressor	OrthogonalMatchingPursuit
LinearSVR	TweedieRegressor	GradientBoostingRegressor
ElasticNet	LinearRegression	TransformedTargetRegressor
KernelRidge	MultiTaskLassoCV	PassiveAggressiveRegressor
LassoLarsCV	AdaBoostRegressor	OrthogonalMatchingPursuitCV
LassoLarsIC	TheilSenRegressor	HistGradientBoostingRegressor

where n denotes the number of data points. A smaller RMSE indicates higher prediction accuracy. Furthermore, we evaluate the Error Rate by setting a tolerance value and using the following formula:

$$\text{Error Rate} = \frac{1}{n}\sum_{i=1}^{n} \mathbb{I}(\text{MSE}_i > \text{tolerance}) \tag{3}$$

Here, $\mathbb{I}(\cdot)$ denotes the indicator function. In this study, the tolerance is set to 10 mm, and a lower Error Rate is considered to indicate higher algorithm accuracy.

5.2 Exploration of Traditional Machine Learning Algorithms

One of the limitations identified in related research is the insufficient exploration of a wide range of machine learning models. To address this, we perform a comprehensive evaluation of various machine learning algorithms for in-body devices localization tasks. Table 1 presents the list of the 45 algorithms examined and evaluated in this study. All algorithms are implemented using the scikit-learn library and applied to regression problems.

First, the prediction performance of each algorithm listed in Table 1 is evaluated without any hyperparameter tuning. This is because performing a complete hyperparameter search for all algorithms would require significant computational resources and time. Next, for the algorithms that show lower RMSE values, we search for the best hyperparameter to further improve performance. The performance of models trained with different sets of hyperparameters is then evaluated, and the best model is selected as the final model for the proposed system.

5.3 Reduction of Training Data

In machine learning-based localization methods, one major challenge is the time consuming nature of data acquisition for training purposes. Therefore, we analyze the minimum amount of training data required to achieve sufficient prediction accuracy with the selected algorithm. Specifically, we evaluate the degradation in localized performance as the training data is uniformly reduced. Let $\mathbb{D}$ be the original training dataset, and $\mathbb{D}_s$ be the subset obtained by uniform sampling. The size of $\mathbb{D}_s$ is defined using a constant sparsity ratio SR as follows:

$$|\mathbb{D}_s| = SR \cdot |\mathbb{D}|, \tag{4}$$

where $|\mathbb{D}_s|$ and $|\mathbb{D}|$ represent the number of data points in the sampled and original datasets, respectively, and SR denotes the sparsity ratio.

For the performance evaluation, we define acceptable prediction accuracy as either RMSE less than 10 mm or Error Rate under 10% with a tolerance of 10 mm. We then search for the minimum SR that satisfies this criterion.

6 Tuning of Machine Learning Models

This section describes hyperparameter tuning (hereafter referred to simply as "tuning") conducted during the exploration of suitable traditional machine learning algorithms for the task of in-body devices localization and the reduction of training data. Here, hyperparameters refer to parameters that are specified at the time of model construction and are used to control the behavior of the machine learning algorithms.

We utilize Ray Tune to perform 250 sampling iterations per model for the algorithm exploration task, and 100 sampling iterations for the data reduction task. The sampling process is guided by the Tree-structured Parzen Estimator (TPE) implemented in Optuna[2]. The corresponding search spaces are shown in Tables 2, 3, 4, 5 and 6. In the tables, values in parentheses denote the data type, and those in square brackets indicate the search range. "Localization" refers to the hyperparameter space used when exploring traditional machine learning algorithms fitting to the in-body devices localization task. In contrast, "Data Reduction" indicates the hyperparameter space used during data reduction.

[2] OPTUNA, optuna.samplers.TPESampler, https://optuna.readthedocs.io/en/stable/reference/samplers/generated/optuna.samplers.TPESampler.html.

7 Experimental Evaluation of the Proposed Method

This section presents an experimental evaluation of the proposed method. We conducted a comprehensive analysis using traditional machine learning algorithms provided by the Python-based machine learning library, scikit-learn. The experimental environment used in the evaluation is summarized in Table 7.

Table 2. Search Space for the Random Forest Regressor

Hyperparameter	Localization	Data Reduction
n_estimators (int)	[10, 1000]	[10, 1000]
criterion	squared_error absolute_error friedman_mse	squared_error absolute_error
max_depth (int)	[1, 25]	[5, 25]
min_samples_split (int)	[2, 10]	[2, 10]
min_samples_leaf (int)	[1, 10]	[1, 10]
min_weight_fraction_leaf (float)	[0.0, 0.5]	[0.0, 0.1]

Table 3. Search Space for the Extra Trees Regressor

Hyperparameter	Localization	Data Reduction
criterion	squared_error absolute_error friedman_mse	squared_error absolute_error
n_estimators (int)	[10, 1000]	[100, 1000]
max_depth (int)	[1, 25]	[1, 25]
min_samples_split (int)	[2, 10]	[2, 10]
min_samples_leaf (int)	[1, 10]	[1, 10]
min_weight_fraction_leaf (float)	[0.0, 0.5]	[0.0, 0.1]

Table 4. Search Space for the Gradient Boosting Regressor

Hyperparameter	Localization	Data Reduction
loss	squared_error absolute_error huber quantile	squared_error absolute_error huber quantile
learning_rate (float)	$[10^{-5}, 1.0]$	$[10^{-3}, 1.0]$
n_estimators (int)	[10, 1000]	[100, 1000]
subsample (float)	$[10^{-3}, 1.0]$	[0.1, 1.0]
criterion	friedman_mse squared_error	friedman_mse squared_error
min_samples_split (int)	[2, 100]	[2, 100]
min_samples_leaf (int)	[1, 100]	[1, 100]
min_weight_fraction_leaf (float)	[0.0, 0.5]	[0.0, 0.5]
max_depth (int)	[1, 25]	[1, 25]

Furthermore, using the experimental setup described in Sect. 4, we collect data points in two distinct environments: in the air and in the tissue equivalent liquid phantom. For the air condition, data points are sampled at 20 mm intervals within a 200 mm × 200 mm × 100 mm space. For the phantom condition, 100 random data points are collected within the same space. The distribution of these data points is illustrated in Fig. 3.

Table 5. Search Space for the Hist Gradient Boosting Regressor

Hyperparameter	Localization	Data Reduction
loss	squared_error absolute_error	squared_error absolute_error
learning_rate (float)	$[10^{-5}, 1.0]$	$[10^{-3}, 1.0]$
max_iter (int)	[10, 1000]	[10, 1000]
max_leaf_nodes (int)	[1, 100]	[2, 100]
max_depth (int)	[1, 25]	[1, 25]
min_samples_leaf (int)	[1, 25]	[1, 25]
l2_regularization (float)	[0.0, 1.0]	[0.0, 1.0]
max_features (float)	[0.0, 1.0]	[0.0, 1.0]
max_bins (int)	[2, 255]	[2, 255]

Table 6. Search Space for the k-Nearest Neighbors Regressor

Hyperparameter	Localization	Data Reduction
n_neighbors (int)	[1, 100]	[1, 12]
weights	uniform distance	uniform
algorithm	auto ball_tree kd_tree brute	auto ball_tree kd_tree brute
leaf_size (int)	[1, 100]	[1, 100]
p (int)	[1, 2]	1

Table 7. Experimental Environment

Hardware/Software	Specification/Version
CPU	AMD EPYC 9274F 24-Core Processor
Memory	768 GB
OS	Ubuntu 22.04 LTS
Python	3.10
scikit-learn	1.6.1
Ray Tune	2.43.0
Optuna	4.2.1

7.1 Exploration of Traditional Machine Learning Algorithms

Initially, each machine learning algorithm is trained and evaluated using its default parameters as provided by scikit-learn in order to identify promising candidates for the in-body devices localization task. The evaluation results are shown in Fig. 4, and among them, the following five algorithms, highlighted in orange, demonstrated particularly favorable performance: Extra Trees Regressor, Random Forest Regressor, Hist Gradient Boosting Regressor, k-Nearest Neighbors Regressor, and Gradient Boosting Regressor.

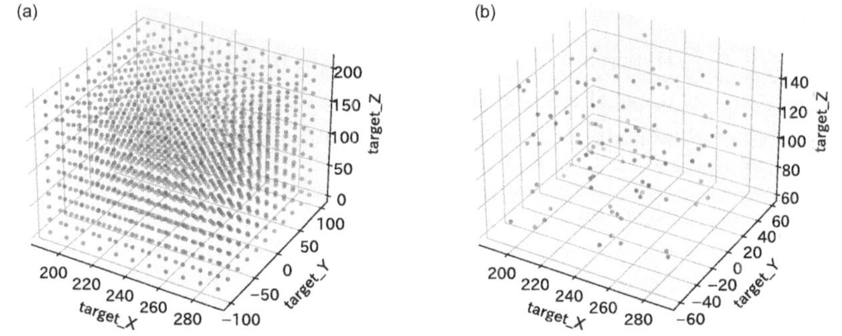

Fig. 3. The experimental space: (a) training data in the air and (b) test data in the tissue equivalent liquid phantom.

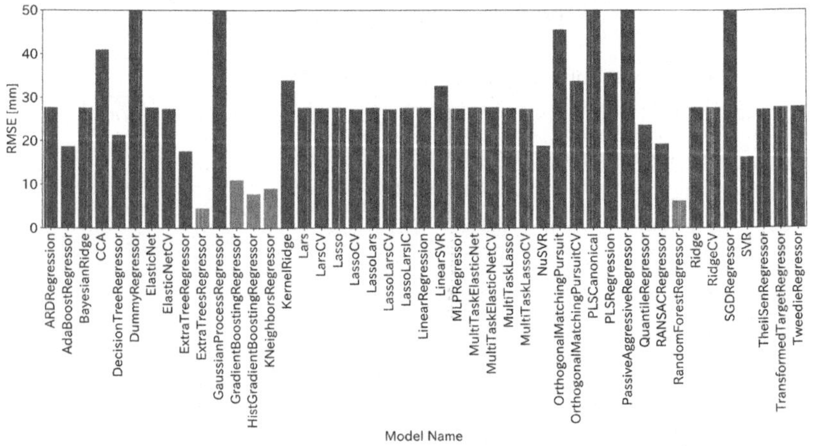

Fig. 4. RMSE of each algorithm using default parameters (under 50mm).

The RMSE values for each of the above models are as follows: Extra Trees Regressor: 4.4918 mm; Random Forest Regressor: 6.1819 mm; Hist Gradient Boosting Regressor: 7.7542 mm; k-Nearest Neighbors Regressor: 9.0465 mm; Gradient Boosting Regressor: 10.987 mm.

Subsequently, tuning is conducted for the five identified algorithms. Figure 5 presents the performance of each model using the top five hyperparameter combinations that achieved the best results. As can be seen, the Extra Trees Regressor exhibited the best overall performance, achieving a minimum RMSE of 4.68401 mm after tuning. The corresponding hyperparameters are summarized in Table 8.

These results suggest that ensemble-based algorithms, known for their high generalization capabilities, are well-suited for the in-body devices localization task. Moreover, tuning resulted in a notable performance improvement in the k-Nearest Neighbors Regressor, showing a significant enhancement in its perfor-

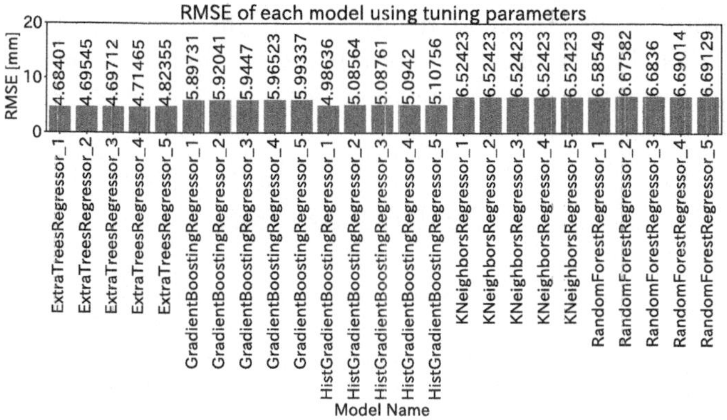

Fig. 5. Comparison of RMSE after hyperparameter tuning for each model.

Table 8. Best hyperparameter configuration for the model with the lowest RMSE

Hyperparameter	Value
criterion	squared_error
max_depth	21
min_samples_leaf	3
min_samples_split	8
min_weight_fraction_leaf	0.00013572654459646934
n_estimators	956

mance. Conversely, the Extra Trees Regressor demonstrated minimal variation before and after tuning, indicating that it can achieve high performance even with a relatively low number of tuning iterations. Finally, we analyze the error distribution of the best-performing model.

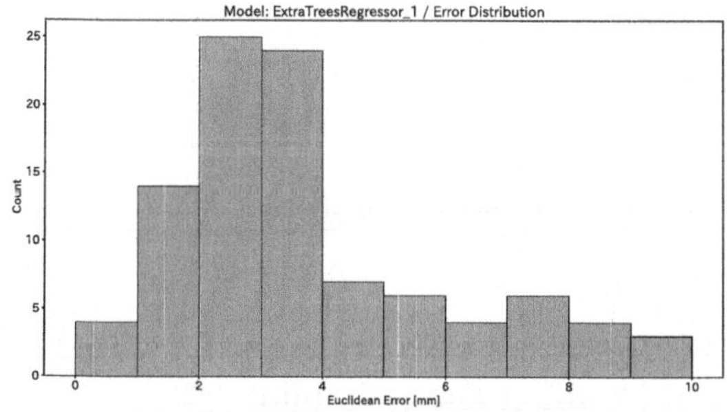

Fig. 6. Error distribution of the Extra Trees Regressor with the best-performing hyperparameters.

As shown in Fig. 6, the most frequent error falls within the 2 mm to 3 mm range. Additionally, the majority of errors are distributed within the 1 mm to 4 mm range, suggesting that the proposed method can achieve high localization accuracy for most data points.

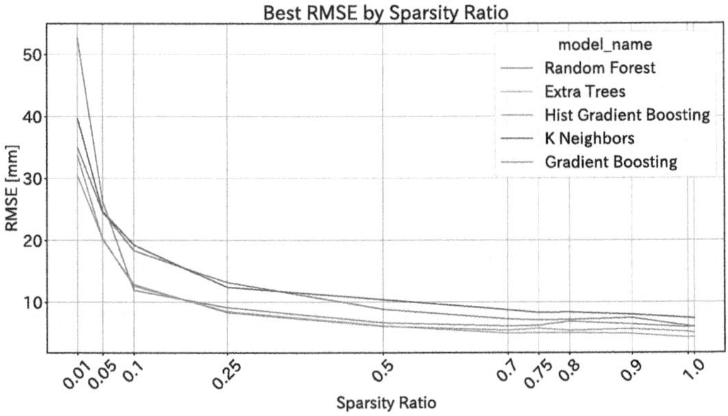

Fig. 7. RMSE transition for the amount of training data.

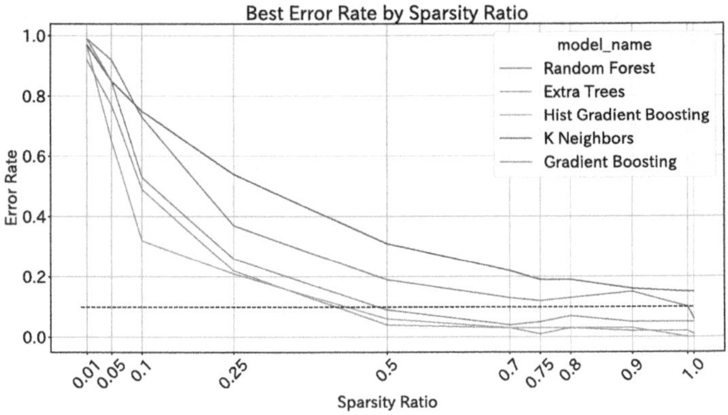

Fig. 8. Error rate transition for the amount of training data.

7.2 Reduction of Training Data Amount

We further investigate the extent to which the amount of training data can be reduced without significantly degrading performance. In this study, the sparsity ratio SR, defined in (4), is set to the following values: 0.01, 0.05, 0.1, 0.25, 0.5,

0.7, 0.75, 0.80, 0.90, 0.99, and 1.0. The estimation accuracy is evaluated for each case and the results are shown in Fig. 7 and 8, and it can be observed that the inference accuracy consistently decreases across all models when the amount of training data is reduced. Regarding the degree of accuracy degradation, the decline is relatively moderate when the sampling rate (SR) is greater than or equal to 0.5. This suggests that, beyond a certain amount of training data, the benefit of simply increasing the dataset size saturates, and alternative approaches other than mere data augmentation should be considered to further improve inference accuracy. In addition, since the accuracy deteriorates sharply when SR decreases from 0.25 to 0.01, it is expected that data augmentation methods could effectively improve inference performance in this range.

According to the results in Fig. 7, the minimum data amount required for the best-performing model to meet the RMSE criterion (set at 10 mm in this study) corresponds to $SR = 0.25$. This means that the training data amount can be reduced by 75% without violating the RMSE threshold. Similarly, based on Fig. 8, the minimum data volume required to satisfy the error rate criterion (set at 10%) is $SR = 0.5$, indicating a potential reduction of 50%. Furthermore, since RMSE is more sensitive to extreme errors compared to Error Rate, it can be inferred that the dataset includes relatively few instances of severely mispredicted data points and instead exhibits a broad distribution of moderate errors. This characteristic is also confirmed by Fig. 9 and 10.

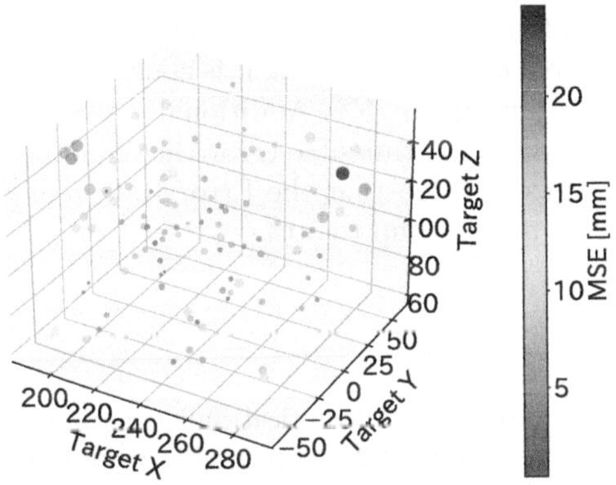

Fig. 9. Three dimensional plot of inference errors by Extra Trees for the data with $SR = 0.25$.

Finally, from Fig. 7 and 8, it can be seen that Extra Trees and Hist Gradient Boosting achieve the best performance across a wide range of data sizes, indicating that they are among the most suitable models for the in vivo device localization task. In particular, Extra Trees introduces greater randomness compared to Random Forest, and this property appears to have contributed to stronger suppression of overfitting under conditions where the number of training samples is limited.

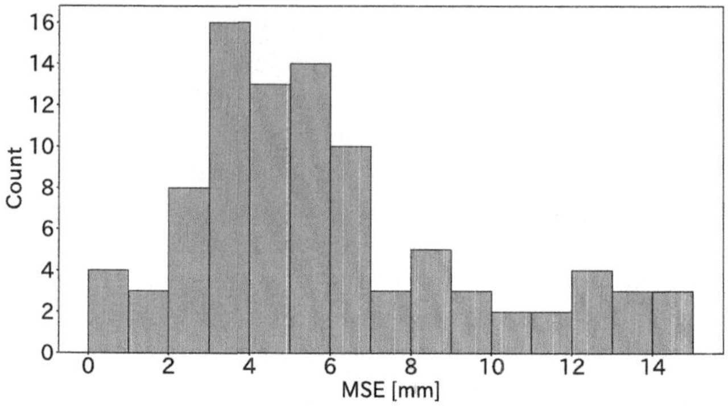

Fig. 10. Distribution of inference errors by Extra Trees for the data with $SR = 0.25$.

8 Conclusion

This study investigated a machine learning-based localization method utilizing magnetic fields and explored machine learning algorithms with an analysis of inference accuracy under constraints on the quantity of training data. The evaluation showed that ensemble algorithms such as Extra Trees, Random Forest, Hist Gradient Boosting, and Gradient Boosting, as well as the k-Nearest Neighbor, exhibited good performance. Furthermore, when examining the impact of reducing the amount of training data. Under the condition that the root mean square error (RMSE) remains below 10 mm, it is considered feasible to reduce the volume of training data by up to 75%. Additionally, we evaluated performance using the Error Rate under a permissible error threshold of 10 mm. The results suggest that, under the condition that the Error Rate remains below 10%, the training data can be reduced by up to 50%.

References

1. Anzai, D., Kato, T., Wang, J.: Theoretical and experimental analyses on location/channel parameters estimation for implantable medical devices. Electron. Lett. **53**(20), 1350–1352 (2017)
2. Ito, T., Anzai, D., Wang, J.: Novel joint toa/rssi-based wce location tracking method without prior knowledge of biological human body tissues. In: 2014 36th Annual International Conference of the IEEE Engineering in Medicine and Biology Society, pp. 6993–6996 (2014). https://doi.org/10.1109/EMBC.2014.6945237
3. Mohri, K., Honkura, Y.: Amorphous wire and CMOS IC based magneto-impedance sensors - origin, topics, and future. Sens. Lett. **5**, 267–270 (2007)
4. Panina, L.V., Mohri, K.: Magneto-impedance effect in amorphous wires. Appl. Phys. Lett. **65**(9), 1189–1191 (1994)
5. Sasaki, A.i., Ohta, E.: Magnetic-field-based position sensing using machine learning. IEEE Sens. J. **20**(13), 7292–7302 (2020). https://doi.org/10.1109/JSEN.2020.2979071

6. Sasaki, A., Ohta, E.: Improvement of prediction accuracy of magnetic field-based positioning with a high-isolation relay circuit. In: 5th International Workshop on Photonics applied to Electromagnetic Measurement (PEM2023), pp. 51–54 (2023)
7. Sharma, S., Ramadi, K.B., Poole, N.H., et al.: Location-aware ingestible microdevices for wireless monitoring of gastrointestinal dynamics. Nat. Electron. **6**(3), 242–256 (2023)
8. Zeising, S., Thalmayer, A.S., Lübke, M., Fischer, G., Kirchner, J.: Localization of passively guided capsule endoscopes–a review. IEEE Sens. J. **22**(21), 20138–20155 (2022). https://doi.org/10.1109/JSEN.2022.3205721

Performance Evaluation on Multiple Implantable Device Localization Based on Magnetic Fields

Riko Takano[1(✉)], Jaakko Hyry[2], Takumi Kobayashi[2], and Daisuke Anzai[2]

[1] Graduate School of Engineering, Nagoya Institute of Technology, Gokiso-cho, Showa-ku, Nagoya, Aichi 466-8555, Japan
r.takano.368@stn.nitech.ac.jp

[2] Graduate School of Informatics, Osaka Metropolitan University, 1-1, Gakuen-cho, Naka-ku, Sakai, Osaka 599-8531, Japan
{jaakko,kobayashi.takumi,d.anzai}@omu.ac.jp

Abstract. In recent years, technologies for acquiring and controlling information inside the body through implantable devices have gained significant attention and are expected to find applications in the medical and healthcare fields. To realize such technology, it is essential to accurately determine the spatial position of the implant in real time. In this study, we propose a position estimation method that utilizes the time-varying magnetic field generated by the implant during transmission. Given that the human body has a specific magnetic permeability of approximately 1, interference from magnetic fields is minimal. We measure the magnetic fields using multiple sensors placed outside the body and estimate the implant's position based on the distribution of these magnetic fields. For position estimation, we employ magnetic field distribution data acquired in air as training data, employing a position fingerprinting method that compares these values with real-time measurements. To address situations where multiple implants are present simultaneously, we introduce CDMA communication technology and applied direct spread modulation using different M-sequences for the transmission signals. Simulation results indicate that the root mean square error (RMSE) of the position estimation is as low as 2.9 mm, even with two transmitters operating at the same time, which demonstrates the effectiveness of the proposed method.

Keywords: Body area network (BAN) · implantable devices · magnetic field

This work was supported in part by JST Moonshot R&D Grant Number JPMJMS2214-06 and JSPS KAKENHI Grant Number JP21H01325.

H. Tanaka et al. (Eds.): BodyNets 2025, LNICST 714, pp. 74–80, 2026.
https://doi.org/10.1007/978-3-032-38657-1_6

1 Introduction

Recent developments in, in vivo cybernetic avatars have gained significant attention. This technology allows for the monitoring of internal bodily information, such as body temperature and pH levels within organs, and facilitates interactions within the body through remote external control. Notably, the ability to observe and control the internal environment via implantable devices is expected to lead to innovative applications in the medical and health fields. For viable real-world applications, it is crucial to develop a system capable of determining the spatial position and condition of the implantable device in real time and with high accuracy. One promising method for position estimation involves using magnetic fields [3]. The advantage of this approach is that the specific permeability of the human body is approximately 1, resulting in minimal interaction with living tissue. Traditionally, a method utilizing a three-dimensional static magnetic field generated by highly efficient planar electromagnetic coils installed externally has been employed [1]. However, this method requires careful consideration of the influence of geomagnetic fields [5].

In this study, we propose a position estimation method that leverages the time-varying magnetic field generated by the implant device during information transmission. Furthermore, we anticipate that in the future, multiple implantable devices coexist in the body, much like digital tablets. To address this, we suggest a position fingerprinting method that uses magnetic field strength distributions as training data and incorporates Code Division Multiple Access (CDMA) to enable simultaneous and highly accurate position estimation of multiple implantable devices.

2 Principle of Localization Based on Magnetic Fields

In this study, we measure the magnetic field generated by an implantable device within the human body as it transmits information. This measurement is conducted using multiple magnetic field sensors located outside the body, and the results are used to estimate the device's position. One advantage of using magnetic fields for position estimation is that the electromagnetic interaction with the human body is minimal, as the specific magnetic permeability of the human body is approximately 1. However, as the communication distance increases relative to the wavelength, the influence of the electric field becomes significant and is more affected by the human body. To address this, we propose a method for position estimation in the near field, where the interaction with the human body is small. This method utilizes a machine learning algorithm based on magnetic field data collected in advance in the air.

2.1 Localization Based on Machine Learning Algorithms

In this study, a k-nearest neighbor (k-NN) algorithm (k = 1) was employed for fingerprint-based localization. The training data consisted of magnetic field strength measurements collected at 1,331 grid points in air, each corresponding to a unique transmitter position. To enhance spatial resolution, spline interpolation was applied to the measured magnetic field data. The Euclidean distance between real-time measurements and pre-measured fingerprints was used as a similarity metric. The localization performance was verified through simulation by comparing the estimated transmitter positions with the true ones, using the root mean square error (RMSE) as the evaluation criterion. Position fingerprinting is an algorithm used to estimate the location of a target by comparing real-time measurements with previously recorded data [2]. This process involves two main phases: the training phase and the testing phase. During the training phase, measurements of magnetic field strengths are collected as position fingerprints. These fingerprints are determined by the spatial relationship between the transmitting implant device and the receiving magnetic field sensor, resulting in the creation of a two-dimensional magnetic field intensity map. In the testing phase, the location of the transmitter is estimated by comparing real-time observation data with the magnetic field strength map generated in the training phase. Figure 1 illustrates this process. Although having more pre-measured data can enhance the accuracy of position estimation, it is often impractical to collect a large amount of magnetic field data in advance. Therefore, interpolation techniques were applied to the collected data to generate a more detailed representation of the magnetic-field distribution.

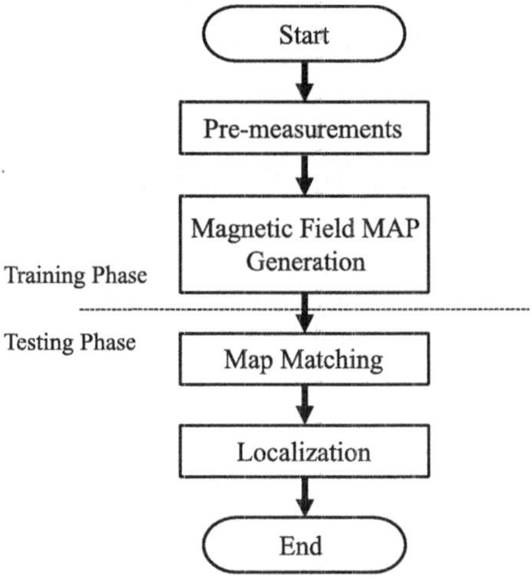

Fig. 1. Flowchart of Localization.

2.2 Signal Separation Using CDMA

A spread spectrum communication method refers to a technique in which a signal, originally occupying a narrow bandwidth for transmission, is transformed into one with a wider frequency bandwidth through additional processing. In this study, we employed a Direct-Sequence Spread Spectrum (DSSS) method, a specific type of spread spectrum communication technique, for signal separation. In this method, the frequency band of the signal is expanded by multiplying the original narrow-band modulated signal with a spreading code, which is typically a pseudo-random binary sequence. The equation that represents spread spectrum modulation is as follows:

$$S_{SS}(t) = S_{org}(t) \times S_{PN}(t) \tag{1}$$

On the receiving end, the process of restoring the original signal $S_{org}(t)$ from the spread signal $S_{SS}(t)$ is known as spread spectrum demodulation (or reverse spread). This demodulation can be accomplished by multiplying the received signal by the same spreading code used during transmission, maintaining the same phase. This relies on the property that $S_{PN}(t) \times S_{PN}(t) = 1$, and it can be expressed as follows:

$$S_{SS}(t) \times S_{PN}(t) = S_{org}(t) \times S_{PN}(t) \times S_{PN}(t) = S_{org}(t) \tag{2}$$

In this study, the M-sequence from the typical binary pseudo-noise (PN) series was utilized as the spreading code. This modulation and demodulation process enables CDMA communication, allowing multiple users to simultaneously use the same frequency band [4].

3 Computer Simulation Environment

Assuming a situation where two transmitters are present in the body, the micro loop antenna shown in Fig. 2 was used as the transmitter. The transmitter frequency was set to 11.3 MHz for use in actual measurements. The amplitude of the signal from the second transmitter was adjusted to match that of the first transmitter. Pre-measured data acquired in air based on the fingerprinting method was used as training data. Although the training data were obtained in air, this assumption is theoretically valid because the human body has a relative magnetic permeability of approximately one. Therefore, in the near-field region where the quasi-static magnetic component is dominant, the magnetic field distribution around the transmitting antenna is scarcely affected by the dielectric or conductive properties of the surrounding biological tissue. In contrast, the electric field component may vary depending on the medium properties; however, its influence is negligible under the operating frequency and geometry considered in this study. Consequently, the magnetic-field distribution measured in air can reasonably approximate that inside the human body, and it is valid to use the air-based data as training data for position estimation. The two transmitters were randomly placed in a space simulating the human body. The transmitted signals were spread using 31-bit M-sequences, each different from the other, to generate a direct spread signal. The estimated range was 200 mm × 200 mm. The signals from the two transmitters were added together to form the received signal, which was measured by the receiver. After reception, the same spreading code used for transmission was multiplied in phase, and correlation processing was performed. The peak of the correlation value obtained at this time was used as the test data. As electrical constants for the space simulating the human body, the conductivity $\sigma = 0.414$ S/m and dielectric constant $\varepsilon_r = 104$ were used. Finally, the acquired test data were compared with the training data to estimate the transmitter position using the nearest neighbor method. For comparison, we also simulated the case where the second transmitter was removed under similar conditions.

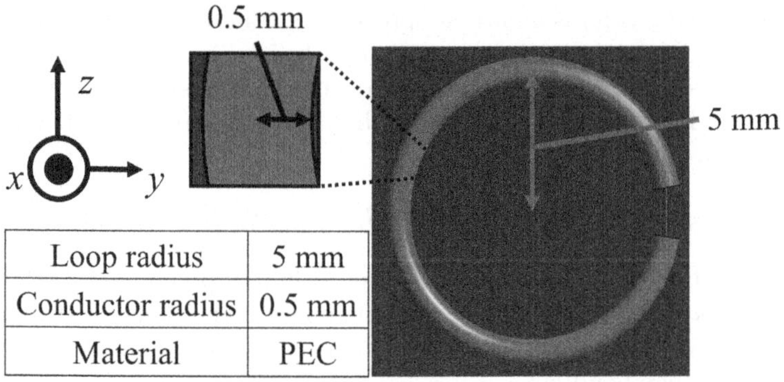

Fig. 2. Micro Loop Antenna.

4 Simulation Results

The estimation results for the case with one transmitter are shown in Fig. 3. In this scenario, the root mean square error (RMSE) was 2.1 mm, and 437 out of a total of 441 points were estimated correctly. Figure 4 displays the estimation results for the case with two transmitters. It illustrates the location of the first transmitter along with the estimation error at that location. The RMSE for this case was 2.9 mm, with 428 of the total 441 points being estimated accurately. While the accuracy of position estimation decreased with the addition of the second transmitter compared to the single transmitter case, it still demonstrated that accurate estimation is feasible. One potential reason for the reduced accuracy is that if the second transmitter is positioned very close to the line joining the first transmitter and the receiver, the interference from the second signal can be more pronounced. To enhance the accuracy of position estimation further, it may be beneficial to select training data appropriately based on the distance between the transmitter and the receiver.

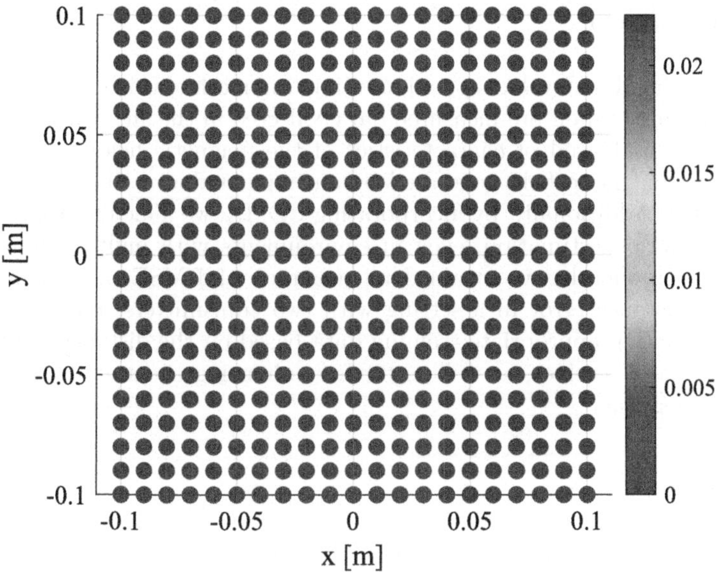

Fig. 3. Localization with one transmitter.

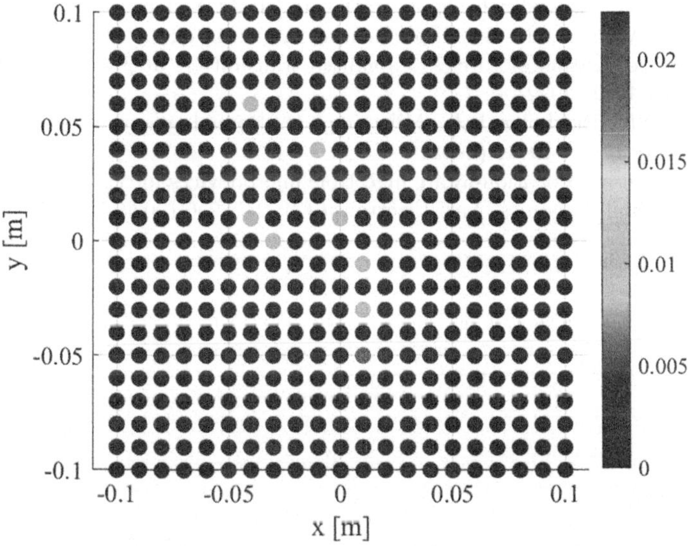

Fig. 4. Localization with two transmitters.

5 Conclusion

This study aimed to develop a position estimation method using a machine learning algorithm based on pre-measured data collected in the air, which is available inside body in the aid of characteristics of the magnetic fields.. This method utilized the magnetic field generated by an implant device during information transmission. Additionally, by incorporating CDMA, we aimed to achieve highly accurate position estimation, even in environments with multiple implantable devices. Consequently, we attained an accuracy of RMSE = 2.9 mm for the estimated distance error in a setting with two transmitters. Future work will focus on selecting appropriate training data based on the distance between the transmitter and receiver, as well as further enhancing accuracy by eliminating interference signals.

References

1. Li, J., Esteban-Fernández de Ávila, B., Gao, W., Zhang, L., Wang, J.: Micro/nanorobots for biomedicine: delivery, surgery, sensing, and detoxification. Sci. Rob. **2**(4), eaam6431 (2017)
2. Pu, Y.C., You, P.C.: Indoor positioning system based on ble location fingerprinting with classification approach. Appl. Math. Model. **62**, 654–663 (2018)
3. Salchak, Y.A., et al.: In-vivo experimental validation of the attenuation path loss model for localization of wireless implanted transmitters at 2.45 ghz. IEEE Access **10**, 84894–84912 (2022)
4. Schilling, D.L., Pickholtz, R.L., Milstein, L.B.: Spread spectrum goes commercial. IEEE Spect. **27**(8), 40–41 (2002)
5. Sharma, S., et al.: Location-aware ingestible microdevices for wireless monitoring of gastrointestinal dynamics. Nat. Electron. **6**(3), 242–256 (2023)

A Preliminary Study on Personalized 6-DoF Scapular Motion Recognition Using a Single-Device, Single-Site Optical MMG Array

Takashi Arai[1(✉)], Tomo Akamine[1], and Emi Tamaki[2]

[1] University of the Ryukyus, Nishihara, Okinawa, Japan
[2] H2L, Inc., Tokyo, Japan
{e225767,k248586}@ie.u-ryukyu.ac.jp

Abstract. This study investigates high-accuracy recognition of six degrees of freedom scapular motion for immersive VR flight with minimal user burden. Substantial inter-individual variability was quantified by contrasting a cross-subject model (40.33% mean accuracy) with a person-specific model (99.33%), revealing a large performance gap. Building on this, this study shows that a minimal configuration - a single optical mechanomyography (MMG) array at a serratus anterior-targeted window - achieves 97.33% accuracy with person-specific evaluation (10 trials per action). Learning-curve analysis further indicated that only 4–5 trials per action were sufficient to reach approximately 95% accuracy, supporting a short and practical calibration protocol. Early fusion of inertial measurement unit (IMU) features provided a consistent incremental gain of +1.67% points, improving accuracy to 99.00%. Accuracy was the primary evaluation metric because classes were balanced. These findings support a practical guideline: adopt "single optical MMG + personalization" as the default, and add IMU features only when needed. This work reports an engineering proof of concept focused on sensor placement and recognition; subjective outcomes such as embodiment and user experience are out of scope. Beyond the motivating VR flight scenario, the same minimal, personalized pipeline may extend to shoulder–scapular control in rehabilitation and sports, though such applications require dedicated validation.

Keywords: Scapular kinematics · Shoulder · Scapular motion recognition · Optical mechanomyography (MMG) array · Personalized modeling · Single-device single-site interface · IMU early fusion · Wearable sensing

1 Introduction

This study is ultimately motivated by immersive flight scenarios in VR, where users control virtual wings through scapular motion. Such imagery—common

H. Tanaka et al. (Eds.): BodyNets 2025, LNICST 714, pp. 81–99, 2026.
https://doi.org/10.1007/978-3-032-38657-1_7

in animation and games—guides the exploration of scapular kinematics as a compact and expressive input channel.

As an overview, Fig. 1 summarizes the single-device, single-site pipeline and the three placement windows (LS/MT/SA) used throughout the paper. Six Degrees of Freedom, 6-DoF, denotes six clinically established scapular actions, elevation, depression, protraction, retraction, upward rotation, downward rotation, defined per Prometheus Atlas [1]. We examine three *placement windows* for a single 14-channel optical MMG array, LS, levator scapulae targeted, MT, middle trapezius targeted, SA, serratus anterior targeted. Throughout, LS, MT, SA refer to windows, not single muscle isolation.

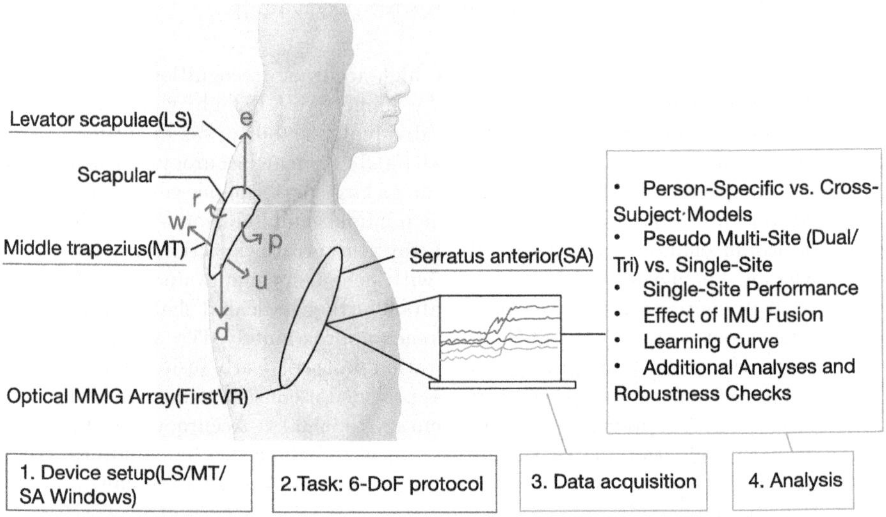

Fig. 1. System overview of the single-site pipeline. A single wearable device with a 14-channel optical MMG array (default placement: serratus anterior; alternative windows LS/MT illustrated) provides trial-wise features; a short person-specific calibration (4–5 trials per action) yields a personalized classifier predicting 6-DoF scapular actions *(abbreviations e, d, p, r, u, w appear in the figure; see Sect.* 2.3 *for operational definitions).* For clarity, the three windows are shown simultaneously; recording used one device sequentially (LS→MT→SA).

1.1 Background

The long-term goal is an immersive body-augmentation experience in which scapular movements could provide expressive control of virtual systems. Here, 6-DoF denotes the six clinically established scapular actions—elevation, depression, protraction, retraction, upward rotation, and downward rotation—defined according to the anatomical convention in the *Prometheus Atlas of Anatomy, 3rd*

Edition: General Anatomy and Musculoskeletal System [1]. If these actions can be reliably recognized, they could in principle be mapped to higher-level functions such as steering or posture control in extended reality. In this study, however, the focus is on establishing a low-burden and accurate sensing pipeline using a single-device, single-site optical MMG array (FirstVR) [2]. Embodied VR flying interfaces have also been explored, from demo-oriented systems such as Birdly [3] to research prototypes with empirical evaluation like Perch to Fly [16], as well as locomotion interfaces [4]. These contributions highlight that reliable recognition is critical, since misrecognition risks degrading users' sense of agency and presence. Guided by this observation, this study focuses on a *single-device, single-site* configuration to minimize burden while retaining accuracy. A 14-channel optical mechanomyography (MMG) array is attached to one anatomical *placement window* at a time—defaulting to a serratus anterior–targeted (SA) window, with levator scapulae–targeted (LS) and middle trapezius–targeted (MT) windows as alternatives. The term "single" therefore refers to both a single wearable device and a single attachment site per session (sequentially evaluated across LS/MT/SA). While VR flight motivates the design, the pipeline targets general shoulder–scapular interaction and is intended to be applicable to low-burden monitoring and input in rehabilitation and sports contexts.

1.2 Related Work

Approaches to shoulder and scapular sensing can be grouped by what they measure. Kinematics-focused methods estimate joint angles using magneto-inertial sensors placed on the thorax, scapula, and upper arm; multi-IMU protocols for scapulohumeral rhythm are well established [5] and remain a reference point in more recent surveys of scapular monitoring [6]. Sensor placement continues to be examined as it can affect tracking fidelity [7].

A second line measures skin-surface deformation as the result of motion. Bend sensors on the back have been explored for interface design [8], depth cameras have been used to capture scapular dyskinesis [9], and tape-like fiber-optic strain sensors have been reported for monitoring body motion [10]. Sato et al. demonstrated feasibility for rotational motion interfaces using bend sensors under clothing, though their system was limited to scapular abduction–adduction and required careful sensor positioning. Ibara et al. employed depth cameras to assess scapular dyskinesis in a non-contact manner, suitable for clinical observation but sensitive to lighting, occlusion, and inadequate for rapid or fine-grained motion. Ito et al. reported fiber-optic strain sensors for monitoring macroscopic skin strain, but these sensors are indirect with respect to muscle activity, require delicate handling, and involve higher cost.

A third family targets muscle activity as the cause of motion. Surface EMG (sEMG) is common; for example, multi-site classifiers have achieved high accuracies for shoulder movements using multiple channels [11]. While strong in performance, sEMG is highly sensitive to electrode placement: even small shifts can cause substantial degradation, and perspiration artifacts can alter skin–electrode impedance, reducing stability during prolonged use [12,14]. These factors limit robustness outside controlled laboratory conditions.

In contrast, the present study employs a single optical MMG array at one anatomical window (default SA), capturing muscle deformation signals that precede skeletal pose. Through short person-specific calibration and a person-specific classifier, our single-device configuration achieved 99.00% accuracy across six scapular motions when MMG signals were fused with IMU features at the SA-targeted window (Table 4), demonstrating that high performance can be realized with substantially reduced setup burden. This improvement from 97.33% (MMG only) to 99.00% (MMG+IMU) is consistent with prior reports that combining MMG and IMU enhances motion estimation in other contexts [15].

1.3 Research Objective

The objective of this study is to establish a low-burden and high-accuracy input foundation that enables immersive, embodied wing control in VR by accurately sensing scapular motion—a deep musculoskeletal action—through a compact configuration.

This idea was originally inspired by depictions in animation and fictional media, where wings extend from the scapular region and are animated in conjunction with emotional or intentional shoulder movements. These expressive metaphors suggest that scapular motion may serve as an intuitive, body-grounded input channel for virtual flight.

Interestingly, this fictional imagery aligns with fundamental biomechanical principles. In flying animals such as birds and bats, the scapula plays a crucial role in connecting the torso and forelimbs, supporting both postural control and wing propulsion. Its anatomical orientation and mobility enable a wide range of shoulder motion, particularly during the upward phase of flapping flight. These functional roles reinforce the feasibility of using scapular motion as a meaningful input modality in humans.

Despite this potential, practical sensing of scapular motion remains limited. Prior methods such as multi-site inertial sensors or multi-channel sEMG systems often require cumbersome setup and are sensitive to placement errors, making them less suitable for personalized or prolonged use. To address these limitations, this study explores whether a single-device configuration, combined with brief person-specific calibration, can deliver the fidelity needed for embodied control.

Furthermore, in interactive contexts where agency and presence are critical, recognition accuracy must be sufficiently high to avoid noticeable misclassifications. Prior studies in prosthetic control indicate that accuracy below 95% can negatively impact reliability and user trust [17]. Based on this insight, we adopt 95% within-subject classification accuracy as a practical threshold for reliable operation.

1.4 Research Goals

To achieve the above objective, the following five goals were defined and addressed in this study:

- **G1.** Develop a machine learning classifier capable of recognizing six degrees of scapular motion—elevation, depression, protraction, retraction, upward rotation, and downward rotation—using an optical MMG sensor array.
- **G2.** Compare classification performance across three sensor placement windows (levator scapulae, middle trapezius, and serratus anterior) to determine the optimal single-site configuration.
- **G3.** Evaluate the impact of person-specific modeling versus cross-subject generalization to quantify inter-individual variability and model transferability.
- **G4.** Examine the performance ceiling of the minimal single-MMG setup and assess the effect of early feature fusion with IMU data on classification accuracy.
- **G5.** Analyze the relationship between the number of calibration trials and recognition performance using learning curves.

All five goals were achieved in this study, and the corresponding methods and results are detailed in Sect. 2 and beyond.

2 Method

2.1 Participants

Five healthy male adults participated in the study (mean age 22.8 ± 1.1 years; mean height 167.2 ± 3.8 cm; mean body mass 57.0 ± 8.1 kg). Four were right-handed and one was left-handed; measurements were taken from the right shoulder for all participants. All participants received a full explanation of the study aims and procedures and provided written informed consent. Each participant confirmed no prior history of shoulder conditions that could affect joint function.

2.2 Apparatus and Sensor Placement

A single FirstVR wearable device integrating a 14-channel optical MMG sensor array and an IMU (3-axis accelerometer with orientation represented as a quaternion w, x, y, z) was used. The sampling rate for both MMG and IMU was 26–29 Hz. To examine window-specific performance with a minimal setup, the device was sequentially mounted on three placement windows on the right side of the body: an LS-targeted window (near the levator scapulae/superomedial scapular region), an MT-targeted window (between the scapular line and the paravertebral line, near the medial border of the scapula at the scapular spine level), and an SA-targeted window (mid-axillary line over the serratus anterior digitations). Because the device footprint spans several centimeters and anatomy varies across individuals, the LS-targeted window generally covered the levator scapulae together with upper and middle trapezius fibers, while the

MT-targeted window covered middle and lower trapezius fibers. Throughout the study, LS-targeted, MT-targeted, and SA-targeted denote placement windows rather than exclusive isolation of a single muscle. Functionally, the LS-targeted window reflects activity related to scapular elevation and downward return of an elevated arm. The MT-targeted window corresponds to scapular retraction and downward rotation. The SA-targeted window reflects scapular protraction and upward rotation of the glenoid cavity. These functional associations were considered when selecting the three representative placement windows. Landmarks were based on palpable bony references: the LS-targeted window was centered near the superior angle of the scapula along the line toward the cervical spine; the MT-targeted window was placed midway between the scapular spine and the thoracic midline at the T3–T6 level; and the SA-targeted window was placed on the mid-axillary line, approximately over the third to seventh ribs. In all placements, the device was fixed with medical tape and aligned perpendicular to the predominant local muscle-fiber orientation. Participants maintained a neutral standing posture during calibration and recording. For reproducibility, Fig. 2 illustrates the approximate sensor placement windows (LS/MT/SA) together with anatomical landmarks.

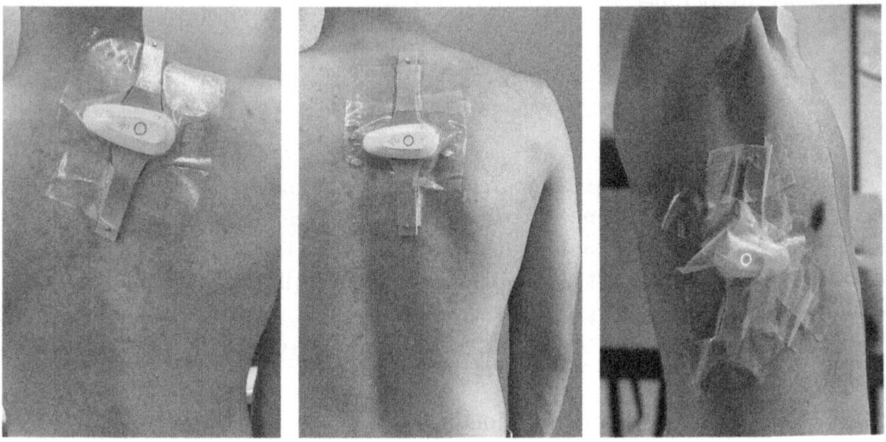

(a) LS-targeted window (b) MT-targeted window (c) SA-targeted window

Fig. 2. Representative photographs of sensor placement windows (LS/MT/SA) with anatomical landmarks for reproducibility.

2.3 Experimental Protocol

Before data collection, participants were prepared to execute the six scapular actions by (1) watching a standard demonstration video and (2) receiving a verbal explanation and live demonstration from the experimenter. Participants practiced each action several times; recording began once movement form was stable.

All measurements were conducted in a standing posture and initiated by a verbal cue. Each of the six scapular actions (elevation, depression, retraction, protraction, upward rotation, downward rotation) was performed in 10 trials. This number was selected to balance participant burden with sufficient data volume for person-specific modeling, LOGO validation, and learning-curve analysis (see Fig. 4).

Each trial lasted 9 s and followed the sequence: 3 s of initial rest → 3 s of transition to the target posture → 3 s of static hold at the target posture. This fixed timing structure was designed to capture both the dynamic onset and the quasi-static maintenance of each action, while ensuring temporal consistency across trials. In particular, the static hold phase enabled stable feature extraction from MMG and IMU signals. Although this duration slightly increased per-session recording time, it contributed to clean segmentation, reduced noise, and reproducible trial alignment—factors that supported the high accuracy observed in within-subject classification.

Sessions were run separately for the three targeted placement windows in a fixed order (levator scapulae, middle trapezius, serratus anterior). Rest intervals were approximately 10 s between trials, 5 min between actions, and at least 10 min between sessions.

Operational definitions of the six actions were as follows:

- Elevation (e): from a relaxed posture with the arms at the sides, shrug the shoulder.
- Depression (d): from a shrugged posture, actively lower the scapula back to the neutral resting position at the side.
- Protraction (p): from a starting posture with a closed fist at shoulder height and the elbow flexed to about 90°, thrust the fist straight forward as in a punch by extending the elbow, keeping the forearm in neutral rotation (thumb side up).
- Retraction (r): from a relaxed posture, draw the scapula toward the spine ("pinch" the shoulder blades).
- Upward rotation (u): from a relaxed posture, raise the straight arm vertically overhead.
- Downward rotation (w): from the overhead position, keep the elbow extended and sweep the arm backward and downward behind the body toward the contralateral posterior hip.

2.4 Data Processing and Feature Extraction

Raw MMG (14 channels) and IMU streams (3 axis acceleration and quaternion w, x, y, z) were segmented into 9 s trials following the protocol (3 s rest → 3 s transition → 3 s hold). For each trial, a single-window summary (no sliding windows) was used. Minor trial-to-trial variability in sampling rate (26–29 Hz) was not resampled; the single-window statistical features are insensitive to this small variation.

Feature Extraction. For every MMG channel, four statistics (mean, standard deviation, maximum, minimum) were computed and concatenated, yielding 56 features per device (14×4). When IMU early fusion was enabled, the same four statistics were computed for the seven IMU signals (3 accelerometer axes and 4 quaternion components) and concatenated to the MMG vector, adding 28 features (7×4).

Single-/Multi-site Composition. Single-site features were extracted per placement window. Dual- and tri-site features were formed by concatenating per-trial feature vectors across sites after aligning by participant, action, and trial index (1–10); only trials available at all specified sites were retained. Dual/tri-site conditions are based on offline concatenation of non-simultaneous recordings and are used to estimate the upper bound obtainable from increased channel count.

Learning Matrices and Labels. Per trial, one feature vector was stacked to form the feature matrix X. The corresponding action labels y (six classes: elevation, depression, protraction, retraction, upward rotation, downward rotation) and subject IDs were prepared with matching dimensions; labels were integer-encoded prior to training. No scaling or normalization was applied.

2.5 Experimental Design and Evaluation Metrics

Three conditions constructed from sequential recordings via offline concatenation of non-simultaneous trials (pseudo multi-site) were compared:

- Single-site: one device at each targeted placement window (LS-targeted/MT-targeted/SA-targeted).
- Dual-site pairs: any two of the three sites (three combinations), with per-trial feature vectors concatenated across the selected sites.
- Tri-site triplet: all three sites concatenated.

Concatenation aligned trials by the same subject, action, and trial index (1–10); only trials available at all required sites were retained. No temporal correlations from simultaneous recording were used.

Analyses. (i) Single-site comparison among the three targeted windows (person-specific models).
(ii) Pseudo multi-site comparison: the extent to which dual/tri-site concatenation outperforms single-site (person-specific models).
(iii) Progressive extension (MMG + IMU): starting from the best single-site configuration (selected automatically by the script), improvement when IMU features are concatenated.
(iv) Practicality (learning curves): for the best single-site configuration, the number of training trials per action was varied from 1 to 9 to estimate person-specific accuracy; in each test fold, n training trials were randomly sampled from the 9 available trials.

Classifier and Metrics. A `RandomForestClassifier` (`n_estimators`=100, `n_jobs`=−1, `random_state`=42) was used as the primary classifier due to its robustness to overfitting, tolerance to unscaled feature dimensions, and strong performance in prior studies involving biosignal classification [18]. In a within-study comparison (Table 5), RandomForest achieved the highest mean accuracy (97.33%) and lowest standard deviation (1.33% points), outperforming SVM (RBF kernel) and LightGBM. This suggests both effectiveness and consistency in person-specific settings.

Accuracy was adopted as the primary evaluation metric because the dataset is strictly class-balanced (six actions × 10 trials × 5 participants), and the application context involves trial-level classification where per-action correctness directly impacts user experience. While alternative metrics such as macro-F1 are recommended under class imbalance, accuracy is widely accepted and interpretable in balanced, multi-class tasks [19].

Validation Protocol. Person-specific models used Leave-One-Group-Out (LOGO), where the group was the trial index shared across all six actions; each fold held out one trial index for testing (across actions) and trained on the remaining trials. For dual/tri-site conditions, all sites corresponding to the held-out trial index were excluded together to prevent leakage. Cross-subject generalized models used Leave-One-Person-Out (LOSO): one participant was held out for testing while the remaining participants were used for training; class labels were integer-encoded prior to training.

Statistical Analysis. This study set $\alpha = 0.05$ and, unless otherwise noted, used two-sided tests. Accuracies were computed per participant and per condition. A *practical equivalence* margin for accuracy was prespecified at ±2.5 percentage points.

For paired comparisons (e.g., SA vs. SA+IMU), the **exact sign test** (ties excluded) was employed to avoid distributional assumptions under small sample size and to evaluate consistency of improvement direction. Ninety-five percent confidence intervals for mean paired differences were computed via participant-cluster bootstrapping (10,000 resamples).

Note. Dual/tri-site results are based on offline concatenation of non-simultaneous recordings and are not strictly equivalent to simultaneous multi-device acquisition; they serve as an upper-bound estimate of the benefit from increased channel count and to assess the viability of the minimal single-site configuration.

3 Results

3.1 Data Overview

A total of 900 trials (10 trials × 6 actions × 3 placement sites × 5 participants) were collected. No trials were missing; all 900 were valid (100% yield). Both

MMG and IMU streams operated at 26–29 Hz. The primary evaluation metric was accuracy (%), with confusion matrices used as supplementary analyses when appropriate. Because the dataset is class-balanced (equal numbers per action: 6 actions × 10 trials), macro-F1 was not reported in this study.

3.2 Person-Specific vs. Cross-Subject Models

The impact of inter-individual variability was quantified in the tri-site configuration (pseudo multi-site, concatenated LS+MT+SA). The person-specific model (within-subject cross-validation, LOGO) achieved a very high and stable mean accuracy of 99.33% ± 0.82% ($n = 5$). By contrast, the cross-subject model (between-subject cross-validation, LOSO) dropped to 40.33% ± 18.12% ($n = 5$) (Table 1). Although 40.33% is well above chance (16.67% for six balanced classes), it is far from adequate for high-fidelity, presence-preserving interaction. The $\approx$ 59 percentage-point gap and the large variability of the cross-subject model (SD = 18.12%) quantitatively underscore the severity of inter-individual differences and the necessity of person-specific optimization.

Table 1. Accuracy of person-specific and cross-subject models (participant-wise mean ± SD).

Model type	Mean accuracy (%)
Person-specific (LOGO)	99.33 ± 0.82
Cross-subject (LOSO)	40.33 ± 18.12

3.3 Pseudo Multi-site (Dual/Tri) vs. Single-Site

The benefit of increasing the number of devices was estimated using pseudo multi-site configurations constructed by offline concatenation of non-simultaneous recordings *(Table 2)*. The tri-site configuration (pseudo multi-site, concatenated LS+MT+SA) achieved a mean accuracy of 99.33% ± 0.82%, while the best dual-site pair (MT+SA) reached 99.00% ± 1.33%. As summarized in Table 2, compared to the best single-site configuration (SA-only: 97.33%), the average improvement from adding devices was limited to about +1–2 percentage points, suggesting that the SA-only configuration offers an excellent balance between accuracy and simplicity.

3.4 Single-Site Performance

Person-specific accuracy across the three single-site placements was compared to identify a minimal configuration. Mean accuracies (participant-wise mean ± SD) were SA-targeted 97.33%±1.33%, MT-targeted 96.67%±3.16%, and LS-targeted

Table 2. Accuracies (%) for pseudo multi-site vs. single-site configurations (participant-wise, LOGO). LS = levator scapulae–targeted; MT = middle trapezius–targeted; SA = serratus anterior–targeted.

Subject	Tri-site (LS+MT+SA)	MT+SA	MT-only	SA-only	LS+MT	LS+SA	LS-only
Sub-A	98.33	100.00	100.00	98.33	100.00	98.33	91.67
Sub-B	98.33	96.67	91.67	95.00	95.00	96.67	95.00
Sub-C	100.00	98.33	95.00	96.67	96.67	96.67	86.67
Sub-D	100.00	100.00	96.67	98.33	100.00	100.00	98.33
Sub-E	100.00	100.00	100.00	98.33	100.00	100.00	91.67
Mean	99.33	99.00	96.67	97.33	98.33	98.33	92.67
SD	0.82	1.33	3.16	1.33	2.11	1.49	3.89

92.67% ± 3.89% (Table 3). SA-targeted thus achieved the highest accuracy with the smallest variability, making it the most promising single-device option.

To further examine residual errors, participant-averaged confusion matrices are shown in Fig. 3(a)–(c). LS exhibited concentrated confusions between neighboring classes, MT showed more dispersed errors, and SA produced the sparsest off-diagonal entries. Adding IMU features at SA (Fig. 3d) reduced the few remaining off-diagonals, consistent with the summary in Table 3.

Table 3. Single-site accuracy (person-specific LOGO), reported as participant-wise mean ± SD.

Placement (single-site)	Mean accuracy (%)
LS-targeted window (levator scapulae)	92.67 ± 3.89
MT-targeted window (middle trapezius)	96.67 ± 3.16
SA-targeted window (serratus anterior)	97.33 ± 1.33

3.5 Effect of IMU Fusion

As visualized in Fig. 3(c) → (d), early fusion at SA reduces the already sparse off-diagonals to only rare neighbor-class flips, aligning with the +1.67 pp mean improvement in Table 4. Focusing on the recommended default configuration (single-site, SA-targeted), accuracy increased consistently by +1.67 percentage points for every participant, improving the mean from 97.33% to 99.00% (Table 4). Given $10 \times 6 = 60$ trials per person, this corresponds to one previously incorrect trial becoming correct. A 95% confidence interval for the mean difference, estimated via participant-cluster bootstrap (B=10,000), was [1.66, 1.67], which lies within the prespecified practical-equivalence margin (±2.5 pp). A two-sided sign test yielded $p = 0.0625$ ($n = 5$).

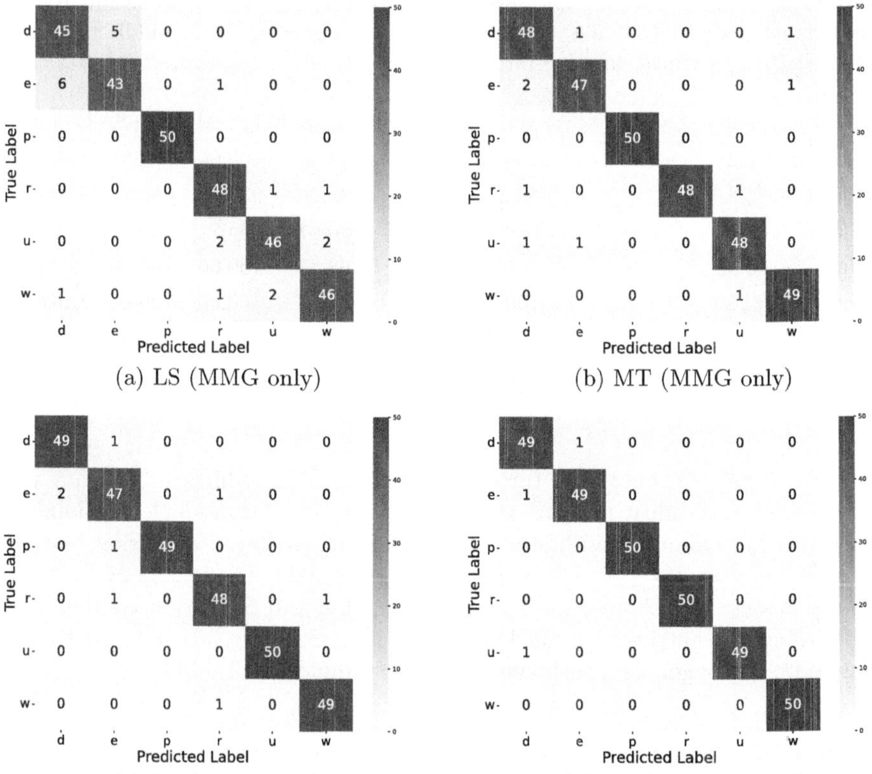

(a) LS (MMG only) (b) MT (MMG only)

(c) SA (MMG only) (d) SA (MMG + IMU)

Fig. 3. Participant-averaged confusion matrices (row-normalized; class order e, d, p, r, u, w). (a)–(c): single-site, MMG-only at LS/MT/SA. (d): SA with early fusion of IMU features. At LS (a), errors concentrate in the neighboring pair $e \leftrightarrow d$; at MT (b), errors are more dispersed; at SA (c), off-diagonals are the sparsest. Adding IMU (d) further suppresses residual off-diagonals at SA, leaving only rare flips between neighboring classes.

Table 4. Per-subject accuracy with and without IMU (single-site, SA-targeted). Values are in %. Δ is the absolute difference in percentage points.

Subject	MMG only	MMG + IMU	Δ (pp)
Sub-A	98.33	100.00	+1.67
Sub-B	98.33	100.00	+1.67
Sub-C	95.00	96.67	+1.67
Sub-D	96.67	98.33	+1.67
Sub-E	98.33	100.00	+1.67
Mean	97.33	99.00	+1.67
SD (across participants)	1.49	1.49	0.00

3.6 Learning Curve

Practicality was assessed via a learning-curve analysis for the SA-targeted single-site configuration as a function of the number of training trials per action (Fig. 4). With only one training trial per action, the mean (participant-wise) accuracy reached 81.33%; increasing to five trials raised accuracy to 96.67%, approaching the nine-trial performance (97.33%). These results suggest that a short calibration of about 4–5 trials per action is sufficient to achieve practically useful accuracy. This analysis used person-specific LOGO with random subsampling of n out of the nine trials per action in each fold. Models were trained on MMG features only; IMU features were not included. As visible in Fig. 4, accuracy rises steeply from $n = 1$ to $n = 4$–5 trials per action and then plateaus, while the error bars shrink, indicating reduced between-participant variability. This elbow around $n \approx 4$–5 empirically justifies a short calibration before deployment.

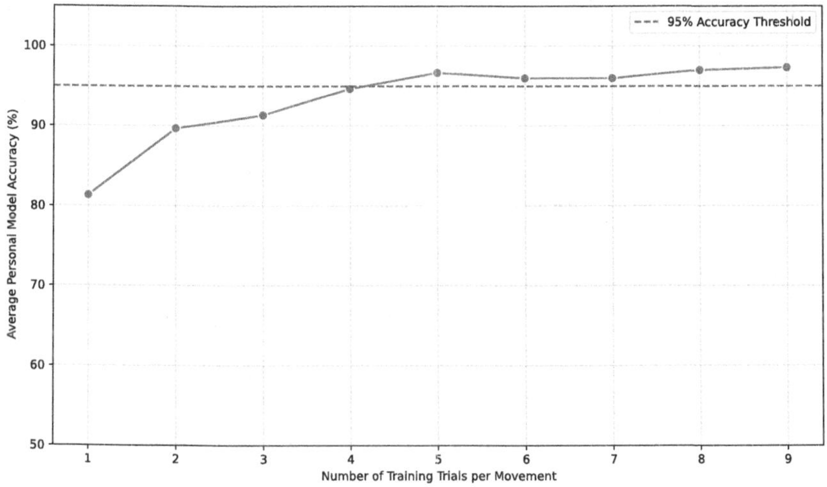

Fig. 4. Learning curve for the SA-targeted single-site configuration. Mean accuracy (participant-wise) vs. number of training trials per action. A clear elbow appears at 4–5 trials, after which gains plateau and variability (error bars) decreases, supporting a short calibration protocol.

3.7 Additional Analyses and Robustness Checks

Experimental Conditions. Two aspects of the experimental setup were examined.

Fixed session order. All participants followed the same session order (LS → MT → SA). Session-wise mean accuracies increased monotonically (Spearman's $\rho = 1.00$, $n = 3$), but participant-level distributions substantially overlapped;

given the small n and limited power, a decisive order effect is unlikely to have driven the main findings.

Feature scaling. For the SA-only configuration, applying z-score normalization yielded the same accuracy as the no-scaling setting (mean difference 0.00 percentage points), indicating that scaling had negligible impact in this task.

Model Robustness. Robustness was tested along two axes.

Classifier Sensitivity. To assess dependence on the learning algorithm, the SA-only analysis was repeated with models of different principles. LightGBM achieved 95.00% (SD 2.11), while an SVM with an RBF kernel reached 79.33% (SD 13.89). The RandomForest baseline remained highest at 97.33% (SD 1.33), indicating that high accuracy is not unique to a single algorithm, though tree-based models performed best under minimal tuning (Table 5).

Random-Seed Robustness. For the SA-only RandomForest, re-running training with five different random seeds yielded highly consistent results (across-seed SD of mean accuracy = 0.27 percentage points), indicating strong reproducibility.

Table 5. Classifier sensitivity analysis (SA-only; person-specific LOGO). Values are participant-wise mean and SD (%).

Classifier	Mean accuracy (%)	SD (%)
RandomForest	97.33	1.33
SVM (RBF kernel)	79.33	13.89
LightGBM	95.00	2.11

Statistical Comparison Across Configurations. *Per-subject stability.* In the SA-only configuration, all participants achieved $\geq$ 95.00% accuracy (see the "MMG only" column of Table 4); this indicates high and stable performance across users. *Practical equivalence: SA-only vs. MT+SA.* To assess whether adding a second device yields a practically meaningful gain, SA-only was compared with the best dual-site pair (MT+SA). As shown in Table 6, the per-subject improvement was consistently +1.67 percentage points (pp), yielding a mean difference of +1.67 pp. This lies within the pre-specified practical-equivalence margin of $\pm$2.50 pp (Methods), supporting the interpretation that MT+SA is *practically equivalent* to SA-only in this setting (formal TOST not performed).

Table 6. Per-subject accuracy (%) for SA-only vs. MT+SA (person-specific LOGO). Δ is MT+SA minus SA-only in percentage points.

Subject	SA-only	MT+SA	Δ (pp)
Sub-A	98.33	100.00	+1.67
Sub-B	95.00	96.67	+1.67
Sub-C	96.67	98.33	+1.67
Sub-D	98.33	100.00	+1.67
Sub-E	98.33	100.00	+1.67
Mean	97.33	99.00	+1.67
SD	1.33	1.33	0.00

4 Discussion

4.1 Summary and Implications

This study evaluated a minimal configuration for 6-DoF scapular motion recognition and found that a single optical MMG device placed over a serratus anterior–targeted window, combined with a person-specific model, achieves high accuracy while keeping user burden low. In the main experiment, the single-device personalized classifier reached 97.33% mean accuracy (six classes, LOGO). Together with the large gap observed between cross-subject and person-specific models in a separate contrast (40.33% vs. 99.33%), these results indicate that personalization is essential for presence-preserving control and that a one-size-fits-all model is unlikely to suffice for this task. The serratus anterior–targeted placement performed best among single-site configurations. A plausible interpretation is that the serratus anterior is both a prime mover for protraction and upward rotation and a stabilizer across actions, yielding class-separable MMG patterns; anatomically, its broad rib-digitations also suit spatial sampling with a 14-channel array. These are regarded as hypotheses rather than causal claims; strictly simultaneous comparisons and direct SNR assessments (e.g., ultrasound or thin-film sEMG) are natural next steps to test them. Adding IMU features via early fusion produced a small but consistent improvement (+1.67 percentage points on average, from 97.33% to 99.00%), corresponding to roughly one additional correct trial per participant in the 60-trial setting. A two-sided sign test yielded $p = 0.0625$ ($n = 5$), and the gain lay within a pre-specified practical-equivalence margin (±2.5 percentage points). Thus, in the present setting IMU plays an auxiliary role—useful for incremental stabilization or when specific confusions matter for interaction design, but not a replacement for the single-MMG baseline. Error analyses showed few misclassifications, concentrated between neighboring or kinematically adjacent classes (e.g., elevation vs. depression; upward vs. downward rotation). For interactive systems, such patterns argue for semantically safe mappings (assigning confusable pairs to low-risk functions) and lightweight temporal smoothing (e.g., short majority vote or hysteresis) to suppress transient errors without harming responsiveness. Practically, these findings support a deployment strategy that defaults to a single device over the serratus anterior with a short person-specific calibration (about 4–5 trials per action to approach 95% accuracy), and that adds IMU only when higher stability or application-specific safeguards are required. These conclusions mirror the patterns in Fig. 3: neighbor pairs ($e \leftrightarrow d$, $u \leftrightarrow w$) dominate the few residual errors, and the learning-curve elbow in Fig. 4 motivates a 4–5-trial calibration.

4.2 Prospective Applications

The motivating vision for this work is immersive flight. If six scapular actions can be detected with high fidelity, they can in principle be mapped to the control of a virtual wing's angle of attack, thrust, and flight attitude (roll, pitch, yaw). This would enable users to steer wings directly with their shoulders and back, extending prior embodied flying systems [3,16] with a physiology-grounded control space. Beyond flight, the same pipeline could support other domains where scapular function is central. In rehabilitation, standardized calibration could allow therapists to set per-action tolerance bands and monitor progress during unsupervised home training. In overhead sports, scapular activation checks could provide readiness scores or asymmetry alerts during practice. In workplace ergonomics, prolonged protraction–elevation bias could be detected and corrected through micro-break guidance. These broader scenarios remain prospective, but they illustrate how a single-device, single-site setup could support both expressive XR input and low-burden functional monitoring.

4.3 Limitations and Future Work

This proof-of-concept exhibits several limitations and corresponding next steps. Generalizability is limited by a small, homogeneous cohort ($n = 5$, young healthy males; right shoulder only). To establish external validity and capture inter-individual variability at scale, future work should expand to a larger, sex-balanced cohort, include both shoulders, and recruit clinical populations such as patients with scapular dyskinesis or post-operative conditions.

The present analysis was performed offline using 9 s single-window summaries. To evaluate real-time feasibility, streaming with short sliding windows (e.g., 200–500 ms) must be implemented to quantify end-to-end latency, explore accuracy–latency trade-offs, and assess false activation rates under online smoothing. Moreover, robustness to attachment repeatability and day-to-day drift remains untested, as the device was taped and evaluated within a single session only. Future studies should characterize the effects of re-attachment perturbations (translation/rotation) and cross-day drift, while developing practical countermeasures such as calibration warm-starts with only 1–2 trials and drift detection methods based on control-chart thresholds.

Another limitation arises from pseudo multi-site concatenation, as dual- and tri-site results were derived from non-simultaneous recordings. Hardware-synchronized, simultaneous multi-device acquisition will be necessary to obtain unbiased estimates of multi-site benefit. In addition, the experimental design used a fixed order of sensor placement (LS → MT → SA), leaving the possibility of residual sequence effects; counterbalanced or randomized orders are therefore needed in future studies.

With respect to evaluation metrics, accuracy was used as the primary measure because classes were balanced. However, complementary measures such as macro-F1, per-class cost-sensitive metrics, AUROC, and interaction-centric indices including stability and hysteresis-induced delay will be required to better reflect deployment needs. The protocol also focused on quasi-static postures; validation during dynamic phases and ballistic tasks, ideally with higher-rate streaming where supported, is necessary to determine task-general accuracy and to test whether IMU fusion yields greater benefits.

Finally, usability and adherence were not addressed. Future work should evaluate setup time, comfort, and long-session fatigue, as well as adherence and session completion rates. In rehabilitation contexts, therapist-supervised calibration workflows and remote review methods must be explored, while in XR scenarios, subjective outcomes such as embodiment and presence should be incorporated into evaluation.

5 Conclusion

This study set out to establish a low-burden and high-accuracy foundation for recognizing scapular motion as an embodied input modality, particularly for immersive applications such as VR flight control. To this end, five research goals were defined and systematically addressed: classifier development (G1), sensor placement comparison (G2), modeling personalization (G3), multimodal fusion (G4), and calibration protocol analysis (G5).

All five goals were successfully achieved. A person-specific classifier using a single-site optical MMG array placed over the serratus anterior achieved a mean accuracy of 97.33% under LOGO validation across six balanced classes. When inertial features were added via early feature fusion, the mean accuracy increased to 99.00%, representing a consistent gain of +1.67 percentage points across all participants. Among the three sensor placements, the serratus anterior consistently yielded the highest performance. Person-specific models substantially outperformed cross-subject generalization (99.33% vs. 40.33%), underscoring the importance of personalization. Learning-curve analysis indicated that only 4–5 calibration trials per action were sufficient to approach the 95% target accuracy, suggesting that high performance can be achieved with minimal user effort.

These results demonstrate that high-fidelity scapular motion recognition is feasible using a single-device, single-site configuration with short calibration, offering a practical pathway toward embodied, low-burden interfaces. At the same time, the present work remains preliminary. Generalizability is limited by the small and homogeneous sample (n=5, single session), pseudo multi-site analysis, and offline-only evaluation. Future work will address these limitations through real-time streaming, cross-day robustness testing, larger and more diverse cohorts including clinical populations, and integration with user-facing elements such as visual feedback, embodiment assessment, and long-term usability.

References

1. Schuenke, M., Schulte, E., Schumacher, U.: Prometheus: Atlas of Anatomy, Vol. 1: General Anatomy and Musculoskeletal System, 3rd edn. Thieme Medical Publishers, Stuttgart (2016). ISBN 9781626237186
2. Tamaki, E., Hosono, S., Iwasaki, K.: FirstVR: a muscle deformation sensors array device to detect finger gestures and noise reduction case. In: Proceedings of ICECC 2019, pp. 21–24. ACM (2019). https://doi.org/10.1145/3324033.3324041
3. Rheiner, M.: Birdly: an attempt to fly. In: ACM SIGGRAPH 2014 Emerging Technologies (Extended Abstract). ACM, Vancouver (2014). https://doi.org/10.1145/2614066.2614101
4. Bektaş, K., et al.: The systematic evaluation of an embodied control interface for virtual reality. PLOS ONE **16**(12), e0259977 (2021). https://doi.org/10.1371/journal.pone.0259977 virtual reality. PLOS ONE **16**(12), e0259977 (2021). https://doi.org/10.1371/journal.pone.0259977
5. Cutti, A.G., Giovanardi, A., Rocchi, L., Davalli, A., Sacchetti, R.: Ambulatory measurement of shoulder and elbow kinematics through inertial and magnetic sensors. Med. Biol. Eng. Comput. **46**(2), 169–178 (2008). https://doi.org/10.1007/s11517-007-0296-5
6. Antonacci, C., Longo, U.G., Nazarian, A., Schena, E., Carnevale, A.: Monitoring scapular kinematics through wearable magneto-inertial measurement units: state of the art and new frontiers. Sensors **23**(15), 6940 (2023). https://doi.org/10.3390/s23156940
7. Friesen, K.B., Sigurdson, A., Lang, A.E.: Comparison of scapular kinematics from optical motion capture and inertial measurement units during a work-related and functional task protocol. Med. Biol. Eng. Comput. **61**, 1521–1531 (2023). https://doi.org/10.1007/s11517-023-02794-2
8. Sato, M., Horikoshi, T.: Proposal of an interface device using scapular movement. In: Proceedings of the 29th Annual Conference of the Virtual Reality Society of Japan (1B1-01) (2024). https://conference.vrsj.org/ac2024/program/doc/1B1-01.pdf. (in Japanese)
9. Ibara, T., Yasukawa, M., Karashima, R., Fujita, K.: Establishment of scapular dyskinesis detection method using a depth sensor. Descente Sports Sci. **44**, 156–163 (2023). https://doi.org/10.57488/descente.44.0_156. (in Japanese)
10. Ito, M., Koyama, Y., Nishiyama, M., Yanagisawa, E., Hayashi, M., Watanabe, K.: Nursing movement monitoring system utilizing hetero-core fiber optic sensors embedded in medical thin films. IEEJ Trans. Sensors Micromach. **138**(12), 525–532 (2018). https://doi.org/10.1541/ieejsmas.138.525 (in Japanese)
11. Gini, G., Mazzon, L., Pontiggia, S., Belluco, P.: A classifier of shoulder movements for a wearable EMG-based device. J. Med. Rob. Res. **2**(02), 1740003 (2017). https://doi.org/10.1142/S2424905X17400037
12. Abdoli-Eramaki, M., Damecour, C., Christenson, J., Stevenson, J.: The effect of perspiration on the sEMG amplitude and power spectrum. J. Electromyogr. Kinesiol. **22**(6), 908–913 (2012). https://doi.org/10.1016/j.jelekin.2012.04.009

13. Rivela, D., Scannella, A., Pavan, E.E., Frigo, C.A., Belluco, P., Gini, G.: Processing of surface EMG through pattern recognition techniques aimed at classifying shoulder joint movements. In: Proceedings of the 37th Annual International Conference of the IEEE Engineering in Medicine and Biology Society (EMBC), pp. 2107–2110 (2015). https://doi.org/10.1109/EMBC.2015.7318804
14. Sanford, J., Patterson, R., Popa, D.O.: Concurrent surface electromyography and force myography classification during times of prosthetic socket shift and user fatigue. J. Rehabil. Assist. Technol. Eng. **4**, 1–13 (2017). https://doi.org/10.1177/2055668317708731
15. Miyake, S., Miyake, T.: Force estimation of five fingers using infrared optical sensors and an imu and its application to analysis of sports motion. IEEE Sensors J. **25**(6), 10122–10133 (2025). https://doi.org/10.1109/JSEN.2025.3528649
16. Zhang, Y., Riecke, B.E., Schiphorst, T., Neustaedter, C.: Perch to fly: embodied virtual reality flying locomotion with a flexible perching stance. In: Proceedings of DIS 2019, pp. 253–264. ACM (2019). https://doi.org/10.1145/3322276.3322357
17. Perry, B.N., et al.: Virtual integration environment as an advanced prosthetic limb training platform. Front. Neurol. **9**, 785 (2018). https://doi.org/10.3389/fneur.2018.00785
18. Kadavath, M.R.K., Nasor, M., Imran, A.: Enhanced hand gesture recognition with surface electromyogram and machine learning. Sensors **24**(16), 5231 (2024). https://doi.org/10.3390/s24165231
19. Farhadpour, S., Warner, T.A., Maxwell, A.E.: Selecting and interpreting multiclass loss and accuracy assessment metrics for classifications with class imbalance: guidance and best practices. Remote Sens. **16**(3), 533 (2024). https://doi.org/10.3390/rs16030533

A Comparative Study of Sensing Modalities for Classifying Active and Passive Motion

Haruki Higa[1(✉)], Momoko Oshiro[1], Satoshi Shimabukuro[1,2], Tomo Akamine[1], and Emi Tamaki[1,3]

[1] University of the Ryukyus, Okinawa, Japan
k248578@ie.u-ryukyu.ac.jp
[2] Okinawa Rehabilitation Welfare College, Okinawa, Japan
[3] H2L Inc., Tokyo, Japan

Abstract. Proprioceptive input and output for computers hold strong potential in gaming and rehabilitation. Active and passive movements differ fundamentally and yield distinct interactions. In this study, fourteen right-handed adults performed elbow flexion and extension under active and passive conditions. Data were recorded from agonist muscles using Surface Electromyography (sEMG) and Optical Myography (OMG). Clips were classified with Random Forest and Support Vector Machine. Across classifiers, sEMG showed consistently higher accuracy than OMG in our sample. Subject-specific (personal) training also performed better than cross-subject (overall) evaluation. These findings indicate that sEMG is preferable for classifying active and passive states from agonist sensing, especially with few channels.

Keywords: Proprioception · Active and Passive Movement · Surface Electromyography · Optical Myography · Movement Classification · Machine Learning

1 Introduction

1.1 Background

Proprioception comprises senses of position, movement, and effort. Internal state estimation is formed from inputs delivered by receptors in muscles, tendons, and joints [1]. Proprioception underpins motor control [2] and supports rehabilitation

This work was supported by Council for Science, Technology and Innovation, "Cross-ministerial Strategic Innovation Promotion Program (SIP), Development of foundational technologies and rules for expansion of the virtual economy" (JPJ012495). (funding agency: NEDO).

H. Tanaka et al. (Eds.): BodyNets 2025, LNICST 714, pp. 100–115, 2026.
https://doi.org/10.1007/978-3-032-38657-1_8

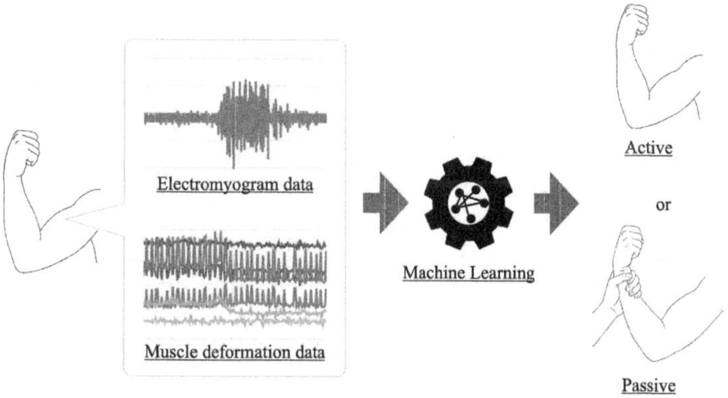

Fig. 1. Electromyogram (sEMG) and muscle deformation (OMG) data are each processed independently by machine learning to classify movements as Active or Passive.

and sports domains [3]. It also underlies input–output design in human–computer interaction (HCI) [4,5]. Proprioception is directly linked to enhancing presence in virtual reality (VR) [5] and to objective assessment in rehabilitation [6]. Even under identical kinematics, the generative origin—volitional (active) or externally generated (passive)—alters the match between predicted and actual sensory feedback via efference copy [7]. Misclassifying passive motion as active reduces sense of agency in VR [8] and increases variability in clinical evaluations [9]. Therefore, layering generative-origin classification on proprioceptive state estimation is essential for consistent VR experiences and objective clinical metrics. However, optimal sensors and methods for classifying these movements have not yet been identified.

1.2 Related Work and Research Gap

Recent advances in wearable sensing have enabled objective and quantitative assessment of muscle activity and deformation [10]. Surface electromyography (sEMG) [11] and Optical Myography (OMG), an optical muscle-deformation sensing modality [12], are widely used to evaluate muscle activity as biosignals [13]. sEMG records electrical potentials generated by skeletal muscle fibers during movement, particularly in superficial muscles [14]. It has been used to detect activation timing, to relate activation magnitude to produced force, and to index muscle fatigue [15]. sEMG is widely applied in rehabilitation [13] and HCI [10]. Howell et al. (1985) showed that sEMG activity during active eccentric contraction in healthy arms is markedly higher than during passive extension [16]. This clear difference suggests that sEMG amplitude can serve as an effective indicator for classifying movement modality.

OMG detects skin and muscle shape changes accompanying contraction as variations in reflected near-infrared light intensity from emitters and receivers [12,17]. Miyake et al. (2025) reported that OMG-based deformation can be converted to grip force, indicating correlation between deformation and force [18]. Internal muscle displacement manifests as skin-surface deformation through soft tissues, linking the two physiologically [19]. Cho et al. (2021) measured upper-arm skin deformation during passive and active movement using a flexible distance-sensor array and found significantly greater deformation in the biceps during active movement than passive movement [20].

Prior studies typically used a single device to observe differences between active and passive movements [16,20]. Few studies have directly compared sEMG and OMG for this specific classification task. As a result, a clear head-to-head comparison of sEMG and OMG under an identical task with an aligned analysis protocol remains limited, the relative effectiveness of commonly used feature families across modalities has not been systematically assessed, and the difference between inter-subject (Overall) and intra-subject (Personal) evaluation scopes remains insufficiently characterized. This work addresses these gaps by comparing sEMG and OMG on the same task with aligned feature/classification/evaluation protocols and by reporting performance in both Overall and Personal scopes.

Based on these prior findings [16,18,20], we test two hypotheses in this work: first, that sEMG amplitude during active movement is greater than during passive movement [16]; and second, that OMG-derived deformation during active movement is greater than during passive movement [18,20].

1.3 Objectives and Contributions

Objective. This study aims to determine whether sEMG or OMG is better suited to classify active and passive movements of the elbow joint. To achieve this objective, two machine-learning classifiers were employed: Random Forest (RF) and Support Vector Machine (SVM, RBF kernel; hereafter RBF-SVM) [21]. Classification accuracy was compared and evaluated. Figure 1 illustrates the overall sensing-to-classification pipeline and task framing.

Contributions. First, the study contributes to objectifying and standardizing movement assessment in rehabilitation. Accurate detection of transitions to active movement enables interventions aligned with recovery stage and may improve training efficacy. Second, the study provides foundational knowledge for identifying users' active engagement in HCI. By comparing the accuracy of OMG—whose practical advantages include ease of donning—with sEMG, guidance is provided for selecting the optimal sensor for specific applications.

2 Methodology

2.1 Participants

Fourteen healthy young adults participated (9 males, 5 females; mean age = 22.0±2.3 years; range 18–27 years). All participants were confirmed right-handed by a prescreening questionnaire. The absence of right-arm muscular fatigue and a good mental state were confirmed before testing.

Table 1 summarizes participant characteristics. Values are mean ± standard deviation. n denotes the number of participants.

Table 1. Participant characteristics. Values are mean ± standard deviation for age, height, and body mass. Data are reported separately for male (n=9) and female (n=5) participants, as well as for all participants combined (Overall, n=14).

Parameter	Male (n=9)	Female (n=5)	Overall (n=14)
Age (years)	21.3 ± 1.9	23.2 ± 2.6	22.0 ± 2.3
Height (cm)	168.1 ± 6.7	158.4 ± 7.7	164.3 ± 8.0
Weight (kg)	62.1 ± 12.0	52.6 ± 7.8	58.5 ± 11.1

Written informed consent was obtained after a detailed explanation of the study.

2.2 Apparatus

sEMG was measured using the TS-MYO device (Trunk Solution Inc.) [22]. This wireless sensor detected surface myoelectric signals and transmitted data via Bluetooth Low Energy (BLE) to a dedicated application. The sensor incorporated dry electrodes in a rectangular housing (37 × 27 × 12 mm; 10 g). Signals acquired by TS-MYO were amplified through an A/D converter and sampled at 1 kHz with 12-bit resolution. Figure 2 shows the TS-MYO device used for sEMG acquisition.

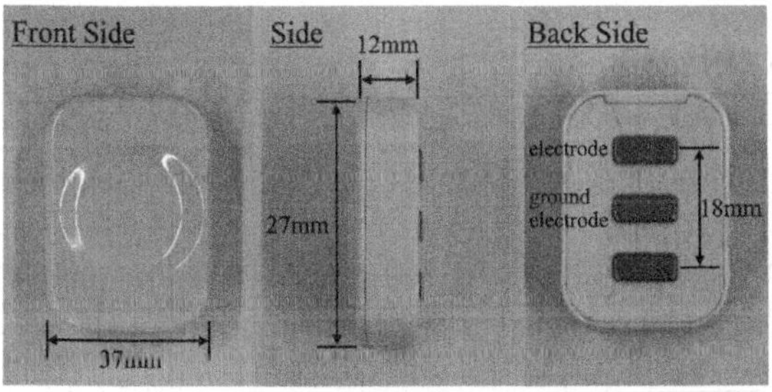

Fig. 2. TS-MYO device for sEMG acquisition. Two measuring electrodes and one ground electrode (18 mm spacing) are arranged on the back to detect surface myoelectric signals. The device uses dry electrodes and transmits data wirelessly via BLE.

Muscle deformation was recorded with the FirstVR (H2L Inc.), an optical-myography–based sensor array comprising 14 near-infrared emitter–receiver pairs [12], sampled at 27 Hz. Muscle contraction was quantified from reflected near-infrared light [18]. The device includes an onboard inertial measurement unit (IMU). To improve optical coupling to the skin, the cover material was changed from silicone to urethane foam. Data were transmitted to a PC via BLE. Figure 3 illustrates the FirstVR optical myography array and its IMU data streams.

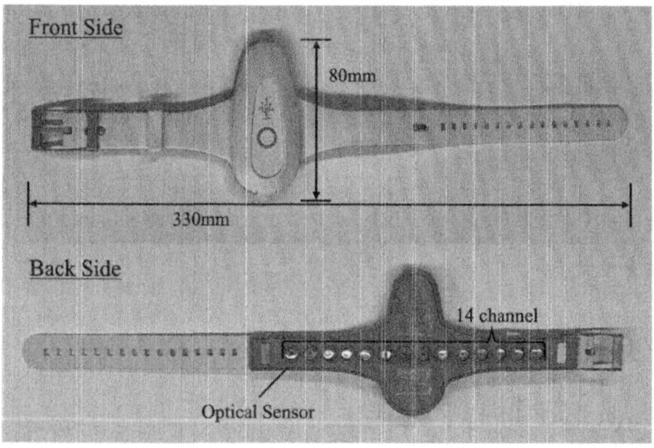

Fig. 3. FirstVR device for OMG and inertial sensing. A 14-channel infrared sensor array reads skin-reflected light to noninvasively measure muscle deformation associated with contraction. The device also integrates an IMU streaming 3-axis acceleration and orientation quaternions (27 Hz), which is used to compute a motion score and to define the analysis window. Data are transmitted to a PC via BLE.

The experimental setup consisted of TS-MYO (Trunk Solution Inc.), FirstVR (H2L Inc.), an iPad, and two personal computers.

2.3 Electrode Placement

Electrodes were placed on the triceps brachii (lateral head) for extension tasks and on the biceps brachii for flexion tasks. To reduce skin impedance, sites were wiped with alcohol swabs and allowed to dry before placement [15]. Placement followed the SENIAM guidelines [23]. Electrodes were aligned with muscle-fiber orientation [15]. Figure 4 depicts the electrode placement sites for the biceps and triceps. Figure 5 shows TS-MYO placement on the biceps and triceps. Figure 6 shows FirstVR placement on the biceps and triceps used during the tasks.

2.4 Movement Tasks

Subsequently, elbow movements were performed to a metronome at 60 beats per minute under the following conditions.

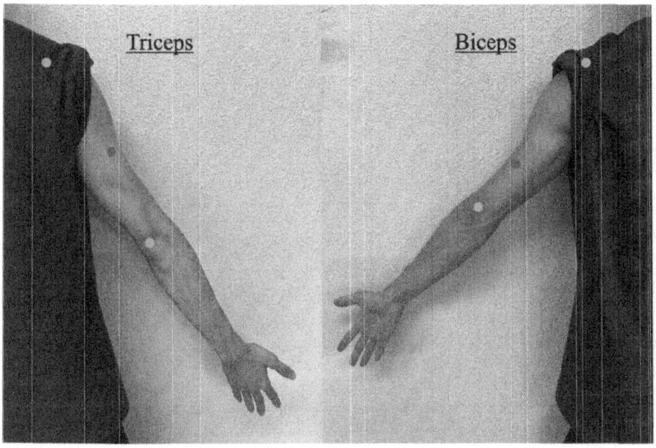

Fig. 4. Electrode placement sites. Triceps brachii (lateral head): two fingerbreadths lateral from the midpoint of the line connecting the posterior acromial ridge and the cubital fossa. Biceps brachii: on the line connecting the medial acromion and the cubital fossa, at one-third of the distance from the cubital fossa.

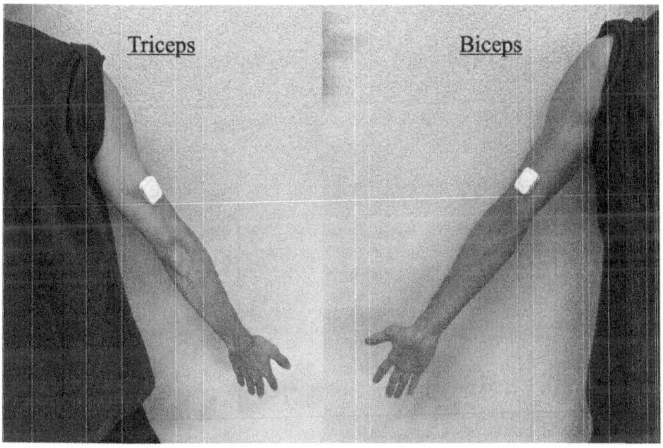

Fig. 5. TS-MYO placement on the triceps and biceps.

Triceps Brachii: Active movement: the elbow was voluntarily extended from 90° to 180°. Passive movement: the experimenter supported the arm and moved it along the same trajectory as active movement.

Biceps Brachii: Active movement: the elbow was voluntarily flexed from 0° to 90°. Passive movement: the experimenter supported the arm and moved it along the same trajectory as active movement.

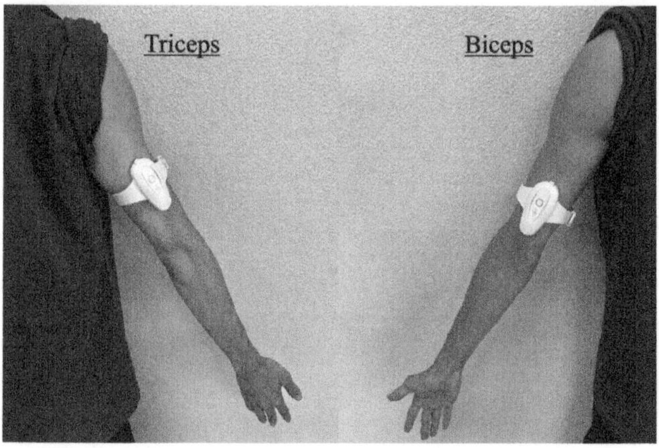

Fig. 6. FirstVR placement on the biceps and triceps.

Figure 7 illustrates active sequences (triceps: flexion → extension; biceps: extension → flexion).

Figure 8 illustrates passive sequences (triceps: flexion → extension; biceps: extension → flexion).

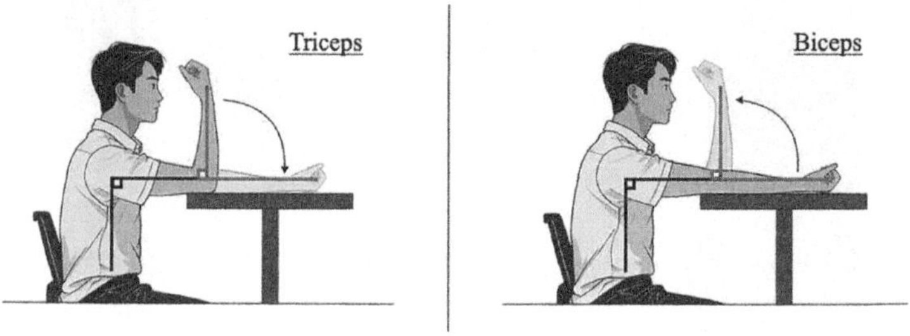

Fig. 7. Active movements. (Left) Triceps, from flexion to extension. (Right) Biceps, from extension to flexion.

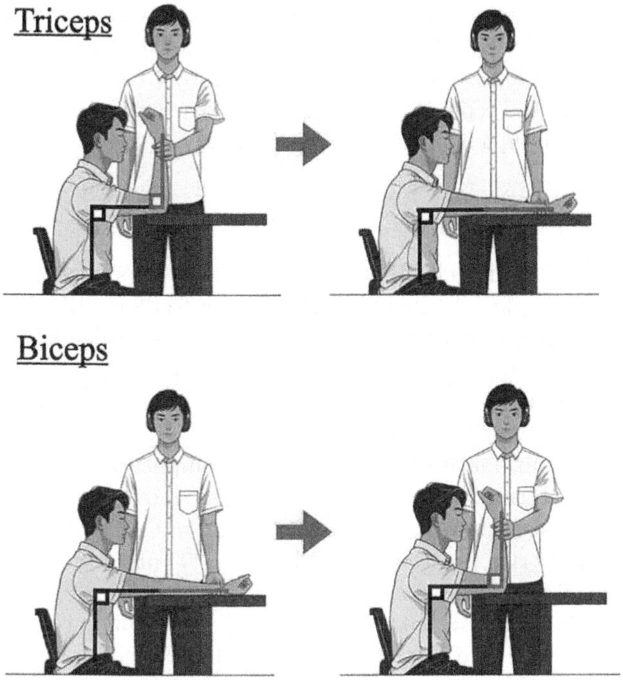

Fig. 8. Passive movements. Triceps: from flexion to extension. Biceps: from extension to flexion.

3 Analysis Methods

The objective was to determine whether sEMG or OMG is better suited to classify active and passive movements of the triceps and biceps. Classification performance for both sensors was compared using RF and RBF-SVM.

3.1 sEMG Preprocessing

sEMG was sampled at 1,000 Hz to satisfy Nyquist for the upper cutoff 450 Hz while retaining millisecond-level onset timing; this rate balances fidelity and data volume for surface EMG. First, a 20–450 Hz band-pass filter [24] and 60/120/180 Hz notch filters [25] were sequentially applied to isolate movement-related bands and suppress power-line noise. Next, signals were full-wave rectified. Muscle-activation envelopes were smoothed by computing a 50 ms root-mean-square (RMS) window [24]. Movement segments were identified manually by synchronizing with video [26]. To include anticipatory feedforward EMG up to ~200 ms before onset and to exceed the earliest emergence of feedback components (~130 ms post-onset) reported in prior work, while also accommodating filter/RMS edge transients and small segmentation jitter, we appended ±200 ms margins before and after each segment, yielding fixed-length clips of 2,400 samples (200 + 2,000 + 200) [27]. Because the RMS window lowers the effective bandwidth, we downsampled by bin-averaging ("binning") to match the OMG time base: the 2.4 s clip was represented as 66 samples (6 + 54 + 6; see OMG below), hereafter len66. Subsequent machine-learning analyses used len66 as input.

3.2 OMG Preprocessing

OMG was recorded with FirstVR at a fixed 27 Hz. A 2.0 s movement core therefore contains 54 samples. To include anticipatory feedforward activity and the earliest feedback while buffering endpoint effects, we appended ±200 ms margins ($\approx$ 5.4 frames/side, rounded to 6) as described in prior work [27], yielding fixed-length clips of 66 samples (6 pre + 54 core + 6 post), hereafter len66, which also aligns the temporal basis with sEMG.

Intervals were automatically extracted by computing the angular-velocity norm ω_t from quaternion differences (after short moving-average smoothing) and defining task onset and task offset from this IMU-derived timing cue [13].

The detected interval was then expanded by ±200 ms on both sides to obtain the common len66 representation.

Raw muscle-deformation data were smoothed by applying a centered (zero-phase) moving average to each optical channel [13]. Based on a sensitivity analysis, we selected a window width of $w = 19$ (at 27 Hz, $\sim$ 0.70 s) as the best trade-off between noise suppression and shape fidelity and fixed this setting for all data.

For baseline correction, we first smoothed the calibration trial and then computed a robust median over its central 90 frames. This participant×musclespecific value was used as a constant offset and subtracted from all clips of the same participant×muscle, thereby zero-centering each channel [28]. Because the agonist region overlapped channels 5–10, the OMG analysis used the group mean of channels 5–10 [28].

3.3 Classification

Each clip was classified into two classes (active, passive) using an RF and an RBF-SVM.

Four time-domain features of Hudgins et al. (Hudgins4: Zero Crossings(ZC), Slope Sign Changes(SSC), Mean Absolute Value(MAV), Waveform Length(WL)) [29] and eight basic statistics (Basic8: minimum, maximum, median, mode, mean, range, variance, standard deviation) were extracted. Feature definitions were kept consistent across sensors.

We used a robust noise-adaptive threshold based on the median absolute deviation (MAD), where MAD is defined as the median of $|x - \text{median}(x)|$ for a resting segment of each participant and channel.

For sEMG, ZC/SSC were computed per window from zero-mean, unrectified, unsmoothed signals using a MAD-based threshold; MAV, WL, and Basic8 were computed from the 50-sample RMSsmoothed signal. For OMG, ZC/SSC were computed from baseline-corrected, unsmoothed signals; MAV, WL, and Basic8 from baseline-corrected and smoothed signals.

Definitions and thresholding. Let a window of length $N = 66$ (the entire len66 clip) be given. For ZC/SSC, let $\tilde{x}_t$ be the zero-mean signal (sEMG: raw unrectified after per-window mean removal; OMG: baseline-corrected, unsmoothed after mean removal). A robust per-participant×muscle threshold is

$$\tau \;=\; 3 \times \mathrm{MAD}(x_{\mathrm{rest}}),$$

with the rest segment defined differently by modality: for sEMG, x_{rest} is computed from the same window's zero-mean signal (i.e., $\mathrm{MAD}(\tilde{x}_t)$ over N=66); for OMG, x_{rest} is taken from the central 90 frames of the calibration trial for the same participant×muscle ($\approx$ 3.3 s at 27 Hz).

Zero crossings (ZC) count sign changes between adjacent samples that exceed the threshold [29]:

$$\mathrm{ZC} = \sum_{t=1}^{N-1} \mathbf{1}\left[\tilde{x}_t\tilde{x}_{t+1} < 0 \;\wedge\; \left|\tilde{x}_{t+1} - \tilde{x}_t\right| > \tau\right].$$

Slope sign changes (SSC) count sign changes of the first difference over three samples, requiring a threshold exceedance [29]:

$$\mathrm{SSC} = \sum_{t=1}^{N-2} \mathbf{1}\Big[(\tilde{x}_{t+1} - \tilde{x}_t)(\tilde{x}_{t+2} - \tilde{x}_{t+1}) < 0 \wedge \\ \big(|\tilde{x}_{t+1} - \tilde{x}_t| > \tau \;\vee\; |\tilde{x}_{t+2} - \tilde{x}_{t+1}| > \tau\big)\Big].$$

For amplitude/variation features, let y_t be the feature-extraction signal in the window (sEMG: 50-sample RMSsmoothed envelope; OMG: baseline-corrected and smoothed with a centered moving average (MA) of window size w=19) [29]:

$$\mathrm{MAV} = \frac{1}{N}\sum_{t=1}^{N} \left|y_t\right|.$$

Waveform length (WL) (insensitive to constant offsets after baseline correction) [29]:

$$\mathrm{WL} = \sum_{t=1}^{N-1} \left|y_{t+1} - y_t\right|.$$

Training and evaluation. Out-of-fold (OOF) prediction was employed. For overall performance, GroupKFold grouped by participant ID to avoid intersubject leakage; for personal performance, StratifiedKFold per participant produced OOF predictions. Zero-mean centering and MAD-based thresholds τ were estimated within each training fold and applied to validation folds to prevent leakage. Metrics were accuracy, specificity (true negative rate, TNR), precision, recall (true positive rate, TPR), and F1; the primary index was the subject-macro mean. Classifier hyperparameters were shared and fixed across all conditions.

4 Results

4.1 RF

Across all conditions, personal outperforms overall (Tables 2–3). The gain is larger with OMG, indicating reduced within-subject variability. For sEMG, Table 2 shows that under overall the triceps favors Basic8, whereas the biceps is marginally better with Hudgins4. Switching to personal preserves this ranking while uniformly lifting scores. F1 moves in parallel with accuracy: Basic8 remains superior for the triceps, and differences for the biceps are small. Specificity and recall remain balanced, suggesting that accuracy differences reflect corresponding changes in false positives and false negatives. For OMG, Table 3 shows that personal greatly exceeds overall. Under overall, Basic8 is highest for both muscles, with F1 showing the same order. In personal, recall improves markedly, reducing missed active movements and raising composite indices. In summary, with RF, personal is consistently superior for both sEMG and OMG; Basic8 generally performs best, except for sEMG biceps under overall, where Hudgins4 slightly leads.

Table 2. Binary classification performance (OOF) with RF on sEMG. Values are subject-macro means. Best per muscle in bold.

Muscle	Feature	Scope	Accuracy	Specificity	Precision	Recall	F1
Triceps	Hudgins4	overall	0.600	0.643	0.703	0.557	0.601
	Hudgins4	personal	0.886	0.843	0.868	0.929	0.895
	Basic8	overall	0.707	0.700	0.753	0.714	0.728
	Basic8	**personal**	**0.929**	**0.900**	**0.919**	**0.957**	**0.936**
Biceps	Hudgins4	overall	0.650	0.714	0.781	0.586	0.626
	Hudgins4	**personal**	**0.964**	**0.971**	**0.971**	**0.957**	**0.964**
	Basic8	overall	0.607	0.571	0.633	0.643	0.769
	Basic8	personal	0.943	0.971	0.968	0.914	0.938

4.2 RBF-SVM

RBF-SVM also shows personal consistently surpassing overall (Tables 4–5). For sEMG, Table 4 shows that under overall both biceps and triceps are highest with Basic8, and F1 follows the same ordering. Switching to personal further improves both muscles while preserving the ranking. For OMG, Table 5 shows that overall performance is lower than sEMG, yet personal reliably improves results. From the overall stage, Basic8 is highest for both muscles, with F1 aligned. In personal, recall increases, suggesting a clearer active–passive boundary within individuals. Overall, personal remains advantageous for RBF-SVM, Basic8 generally ranks highest, and sEMG outperforms OMG; however, OMG reaches practical levels under personal.

Table 3. Binary classification performance (OOF) with RF on OMG. Values are subject-macro means. Best per muscle in bold.

Muscle	Feature	Scope	Accuracy	Specificity	Precision	Recall	F1
Triceps	Hudgins4	overall	0.564	0.600	0.594	0.529	0.580
	Hudgins4	personal	0.793	0.814	0.806	0.771	0.788
	Basic8	overall	0.586	0.671	0.650	0.500	0.592
	Basic8	**personal**	**0.871**	**0.886**	**0.882**	**0.857**	**0.870**
Biceps	Hudgins4	overall	0.429	0.443	0.373	0.414	0.472
	Hudgins4	personal	0.750	0.743	0.747	0.757	0.752
	Basic8	overall	0.464	0.557	0.434	0.371	0.551
	Basic8	**personal**	**0.914**	**0.914**	**0.914**	**0.914**	**0.914**

Table 4. Binary classification performance (OOF) with RBF-SVM on sEMG. Values are subject-macro means. Best per muscle in bold

Muscle	Feature	Scope	Accuracy	Specificity	Precision	Recall	F1
Triceps	Hudgins4	overall	0.614	0.700	0.732	0.529	0.585
	Hudgins4	personal	0.829	0.800	0.819	0.857	0.835
	Basic8	overall	0.736	0.757	0.825	0.714	0.751
	Basic8	**personal**	**0.879**	**0.871**	**0.877**	**0.886**	**0.880**
Biceps	Hudgins4	overall	0.550	0.629	0.625	0.471	0.588
	Hudgins4	personal	0.900	0.929	0.929	0.871	0.897
	Basic8	overall	0.600	0.729	0.701	0.471	0.667
	Basic8	**personal**	**0.971**	**0.986**	**0.982**	**0.957**	**0.968**

Table 5. Binary classification performance (OOF) with RBF-SVM on OMG. Values are subject-macro means. Best per muscle in bold.

Muscle	Feature	Scope	Accuracy	Specificity	Precision	Recall	F1
Triceps	Hudgins4	overall	0.564	0.557	0.610	0.571	0.557
	Hudgins4	personal	0.686	0.714	0.697	0.657	0.677
	Basic8	overall	0.607	0.671	0.657	0.543	0.707
	Basic8	**personal**	**0.814**	**0.814**	**0.814**	**0.814**	**0.814**
Biceps	Hudgins4	overall	0.486	0.486	0.481	0.486	0.558
	Hudgins4	personal	0.693	0.729	0.708	0.657	0.682
	Basic8	overall	0.579	0.686	0.618	0.471	0.637
	Basic8	**personal**	**0.843**	**0.843**	**0.843**	**0.843**	**0.843**

5 Discussion

The hypotheses stated that active movement entails voluntary neural commands and increases muscle activity and sEMG amplitude. Sensor outputs based on posture change were also expected to increase during active motion. The results align with these expectations and show sufficient contrast between active and passive states for classification. Under both RF and RBF-SVM, sEMG consistently surpasses OMG.

A key contextual factor is the difference in native sampling rates caused by device design. sEMG was acquired at 1,000 Hz with a 20450 Hz band-pass, which preserves sharp onsets before envelope formation. OMG is hardware-fixed at 27 Hz (~37 ms per frame) and observes slower mechanical deformation of muscle and skin.

Rate-driven comparability issues were mitigated by representing both modalities on a common temporal basis (len66: 6 pre + 54 core + 6 post; ~2.4 s). For sEMG, a 50 ms RMS envelope was formed to reduce the effective bandwidth before bin averaging. For OMG, ZC/SSC were computed from the baseline-corrected unsmoothed signal, whereas MAV, WL, and Basic8 were computed from the baseline-corrected smoothed signal. Thus, feature extraction in both modalities predominantly integrates information below a few hertz over the ~2 s window.

Within this aligned representation, the accuracy gap plausibly reflects sensor physics and signal-to-noise ratio (SNR) at onset rather than a mere sampling-rate mismatch. High-rate sEMG protects against aliasing of electrophysiological content and retains crisp activation transients. By contrast, 27 Hz OMG adequately tracks the movement envelope but cannot represent very fast transients, which tends to smooth activepassive contrast.

Model comparisons reveal slightly higher scores for RF with sEMG and slightly better RBF-SVM performance with OMG. These differences are small and do not change conclusions. Feature-set comparisons show generally higher values for Basic8, especially in the triceps. An exception occurs for sEMG biceps under RF overall, where Hudgins4 is marginally higher. Basic8 aggregates amplitude, dispersion, and range, capturing broad facets of activepassive differences. Across metrics (F1, specificity, precision, recall), trends move with accuracy, indicating robustness to the choice of index.

Across evaluation settings, personal exceeds overall in all conditions. Within-subject training absorbs constant factors such as electrode placement, skin impedance, donning shifts, and range-of-motion differences. Under the personal setting, both sensors reach practical levels, suggesting that short individual adaptation in clinical or interaction contexts can markedly raise performance.

Global "optimal" sampling rates are not claimed in this study. For surface EMG with a 450 Hz upper cutoff, 1 kHz remains a standard, conservative choice that enables precise onset timing before envelope formation. For the OMG hardware used here, 27 Hz is fixed and adequate for the 2 s envelope analyzed. A systematic sweep of acquisition and resampling rates remains valuable future work. Examples include testing whether envelope-domain features saturate above 50100 Hz for sEMG and whether higher-frame-rate optical arrays improve OMG transients. Several limitations remain: modest participant and trial counts constrain inter-subject generalization, and rater variability may enter labeling and preprocessing. Future studies should employ multiple independent raters and evaluate feature reproducibility, label agreement, and model stability (e.g., ICC for continuous features and Cohen's κ for binary labels). Cross-validation stratified by rater or mixed-effects models can help identify sources of performance variance. Extensions include recurrent sequence models such as Long Short-Term Memory (LSTM) networks [30], and fusion of sEMG with OMG. Regularization and semi-supervised learning may further improve cross-subject performance while limiting the burden of personal adaptation.

6 Conclusion

This study compared sEMG and OMG for binary classification of active and passive elbow movements and evaluated performance using RF and RBF-SVM. As shown in Tables 2, 3, 4 and 5, sEMG consistently outperforms OMG across classifiers. Basic8 generally yields higher scores, with clearer advantages in the triceps. An exception occurs for sEMG biceps under RF overall, where Hudgins4 is slightly higher; this does not alter overall trends.

Beyond accuracy, F1, specificity, precision, and recall show aligned differences, supporting conclusions that are robust to metric selection. For evaluation settings, personal exceeds overall in every condition. Clearer decision boundaries emerge within individuals, suggesting that brief personal adaptation is effective for deployment. Within this study's scope, sEMG should be prioritized as the sensor for active–passive discrimination, and Basic8 should serve as the baseline feature set.

Future work will expand participants, standardize acquisition procedures, and verify inter-rater reliability. Further extensions will consider time-structure models, such as LSTM, and fusion of sEMG with OMG. These steps aim to raise cross-subject reproducibility and enhance practical utility in clinical and interaction scenarios.

References

1. Proske, U., Gandevia, S.C.: The proprioceptive senses: Their roles in signaling body shape, body position and movement, and muscle force. Physiol. Rev. **92**(4), 1651–1697 (2012). https://doi.org/10.1152/physrev.00048.2011
2. Marasco, P.D., de Nooij, J.C.: Proprioception: A new era set in motion by emerging genetic and bionic strategies? Annu. Rev. Physiol. **85**, 1–24 (2023). https://doi.org/10.1146/annurev-physiol-040122-081302
3. Han, J., Waddington, G., Adams, R., Anson, J., Liu, Y.: Assessing proprioception: A critical review of methods. J. Sport Health Sci. **5**(1), 80–90 (2016). https://doi.org/10.1016/j.jshs.2014.10.004

4. Tamaki, E., Miyaki, T., Rekimoto, J.: PossessedHand: Techniques for controlling human hands using electrical muscle stimuli. In: Proceedings of SIGCHI Conference on Human Factors in Computing System, pp. 543–552. ACM, New York (2011). https://doi.org/10.1145/1978942.1979018
5. Azmandian, M., Hancock, M., Benko, H., Ofek, E., Wilson, A.D.: Haptic retargeting: Dynamic repurposing of passive haptics for enhanced virtual reality experiences. In: Proceedings of CHI 2016 Conference on Human Factors in Computing System, pp. 1968–1979. ACM, San Jose, CA, USA (2016). https://doi.org/10.1145/2858036.2858226
6. Xie, T., Leng, Y., Xu, P., Li, L., Song, R.: Mapping of spastic muscle activity after stroke: Difference between passive stretch and active contraction. J. NeuroEng. Rehabil. **21**(1), 102 (2024). https://doi.org/10.1186/s12984-024-01376-z
7. Kalckert, A., Ehrsson, H.H.: Moving a rubber hand that feels like your own: A dissociation of ownership and agency. Front. Hum. Neurosci. **6**, 40 (2012). https://doi.org/10.3389/fnhum.2012.00040
8. Moore, J.W.: What is the sense of agency and why does it matter? Front. Psychol. **7**, 1272 (2016). https://doi.org/10.3389/fpsyg.2016.01272
9. Harb, A., Margetis, K., Kishner, S.: Modified Ashworth Scale. StatPearls. StatPearls Publishing, Treasure Island, FL, USA (2025)
10. Zheng, Z., Wu, Z., Zhao, R., Ni, Y., Jing, X., Gao, S.: A review of EMG-, FMG-, and EIT-based biosensors and relevant human–machine interactivities and biomedical applications. Biosensors **12**(7), 516 (2022). https://doi.org/10.3390/bios12070516
11. Naik, G.R., Selvan, S.E., Gobbo, M., Acharyya, A., Nguyen, H.T.: Principal component analysis applied to surface electromyography: A comprehensive review. IEEE Access **4**, 4025–4037 (2016). https://doi.org/10.1109/ACCESS.2016.2593013
12. Tamaki, E., Hosono, S., Iwasaki, K.: FirstVR: FirstVR: A Muscle Deformation Sensors Array Device to Detect Finger Gestures and Noise Reduction Case. In: Proceedings of the 2019 2nd International Conference on Electronics, Communications and Control Engineering, pp. 21–24. ACM, Phuket (2019). https://doi.org/10.1145/3324033.3324041
13. Shimabukuro, S., Miyake, T., Tamaki, E.: Time series analysis of muscle deformation during physiotherapy using optical wearable sensors. Sensors **25**(11), 3507 (2025). https://doi.org/10.3390/s25113507
14. Kato, H., Yamamoto, S.: Surface Electromyography for Clinical Use: A Motion Analysis Method for Therapists. Igaku-Shoin, Tokyo (2020)
15. De Luca, C.J.: The use of surface electromyography in biomechanics. J. Appl. Biomech. **13**(2), 135–163 (1997). https://doi.org/10.1123/jab.13.2.135
16. Howell, J.N., Chila, A.G., Ford, G., David, D., Gates, T.: An electromyographic study of elbow motion during postexercise muscle soreness. J. Appl. Physiol. **58**(5), 1713–1718 (1985). https://doi.org/10.1152/jappl.1985.58.5.1713
17. Hosono, S., Miyake, T., Miyake, S., Tamaki, E.: Feedback method of force controlled by electrical muscle stimulation based on infrared optical sensing. Front. Virtual Real. **3**, 880238 (2022). https://doi.org/10.3389/frvir.2022.880238
18. Miyake, S., Miyake, T.: CNN-based gripping-force estimation using optical myography. In: Extended Abstracts of the 2025 CHI Conference on Human Factors in Computing System, pp. 1–8. ACM, Yokohama, Japan (2025)
19. Alvarez, J.T., de Marcillac, A., Jin, Y., Gerez, L.F., Araromi, O.A., Walsh, C.J.: Surface-level muscle deformation as a correlate for joint torque. Adv. Mater. Technol. **9**(15), 2400444 (2024). https://doi.org/10.1002/admt.202400444

20. Cho, S.G., Toyoda, M., Ding, M., Takamatsu, J., Yokota, C., Ogasawara, T.: Analysis of skin deformation differences on the upper arm between active and passive movements during elbow flexion and extension. In: Proceedings of 43rd Annual International Conference of the IEEE Engineering in Medicine & Biology Society, pp. 6187–6191. IEEE, Mexico City, Mexico (2021)
21. Kadavath, M.R.K., Nasor, M., Imran, A.: Enhanced hand gesture recognition with surface electromyogram and machine learning. Sensors **24**(16), 5231 (2024). https://doi.org/10.3390/s24165231
22. TS-MYO homepage. https://ts-myo.com. Accessed 23 June 2025
23. Hermens, H.J., Freriks, B., Disselhorst-Klug, C., Rau, G.: Development of recommendations for SEMG sensors and sensor placement procedures. J. Electromyogr. Kinesiol. **10**(5), 361–374 (2000). https://doi.org/10.1016/S1050-6411(00)00027-4
24. Bongiorno, G., Biancuzzi, H., Dal Mas, F., Miceli, L.: Evaluation of muscle energy in isometric maintenance as an index of muscle fatigue in roller speed skating. Front. Sports Act. Living **5**, 1153946 (2023). https://doi.org/10.3389/fspor.2023.1153946
25. Li, X., Rymer, W.Z., Li, G., Zhou, P.: The effects of notch filtering on electrically evoked myoelectric signals and associated motor unit index estimates. J. NeuroEng. Rehabil. **8**(1), 64 (2011). https://doi.org/10.1186/1743-0003-8-64
26. Carvalho, C.R., Fernández, J.M., del-Ama, A.J., Barroso, F.O., Moreno, J.C.: Review of electromyography onset detection methods for real-time control of robotic exoskeletons. J. NeuroEng. Rehabil. **20**(1), 141 (2023). https://doi.org/10.1186/s12984-023-01268-8
27. Heald, J.B., Franklin, D.W., Wolpert, D.M.: Increasing muscle co-contraction speeds up internal model acquisition during dynamic motor learning. Sci. Rep. **8**(1), 16355 (2018). https://doi.org/10.1038/s41598-018-34737-5
28. Miyake, T., Minakuchi, T., Sato, S., Okubo, C., Yanagihara, D., Tamaki, E.: Optical myography-based sensing methodology of application of random loads to muscles during hand-gripping training. Sensors **24**(4), 1108 (2024). https://doi.org/10.3390/s24041108
29. Hudgins, B., Parker, P., Scott, R.N.: A new strategy for multifunction myoelectric control. IEEE Trans. Biomed. Eng. **40**(1), 82–94 (1993)
30. Hochreiter, S., Schmidhuber, J.: Long Short-Term Memory. Neural Comput. **9**(8), 1735–1780 (1997). https://doi.org/10.1162/neco.1997.9.8.1735

Physical-Layer Techniques for Medical and Body-Centric Systems

Biometric Authentication in Galvanic Coupling Communications: A Physical Layer Approach for Secure Wearable Medical Systems

Stefano Caputo[1], Anna Vizziello[2], Antonio Coviello[3], Maurizio Magarini[3], Giacomo Borghini[1], Pietro Savazzi[2], Sara Jayousi[4], and Lorenzo Mucchi[1(✉)]

[1] Department of Information Engineering, University of Florence, Florence, Italy
{stefano.caputo,giacomo.borghini,lorenzo.mucchi}@unifi.it
[2] Department of Electronics, Computer and Biomedical Eng, University of Pavia, Pavia, Italy
{anna.vizziello,pietro.savazzi}@unipv.it
[3] Department of Electronics, Information and Bioengineering, Politecnico di Milano, Milan, Italy
{antonio.coviello,maurizio.magarini}@polimi.it
[4] Prato Campus of the University of Florence, Prato, Italy
sara.jayousi@pin.unifi.it

Abstract. This paper presents a biometric authentication framework based on Galvanic Coupling (GC) signals for secure communication in Wireless Body Area Networks (WBANs). Unlike traditional biometric systems that rely on handcrafted features, our approach leverages a Long Short-Term Memory (LSTM) neural network to classify raw GC signals directly, exploiting the subject-specific characteristics of the propagation channel. The system is designed for on-body configurations and integrates a lightweight authentication protocol that operates at the physical layer. Experimental results demonstrate the effectiveness of the proposed method in mitigating both over-the-air and direct contact attacks, achieving high classification accuracy and robustness through confidence-based rejection mechanisms. The solution is optimized for low-resource environments, making it suitable for real-time medical applications.

Keywords: Physical Layer Authentication · Wireless Body Area Network · Galvanic Coupling (GC) · On-Body Communications · Long Short-Term Memory Neural Network (LSTM) · Deep Learning signal classification

1 Introduction

Wearable technologies are increasingly shaping the future of healthcare by enabling real-time tracking of physiological parameters, personalized therapeutic

H. Tanaka et al. (Eds.): BodyNets 2025, LNICST 714, pp. 119–133, 2026.
https://doi.org/10.1007/978-3-032-38657-1_9

interventions, and enhanced recovery. These compact and intelligent devices are particularly beneficial in managing chronic illnesses such as cardiovascular and neuromuscular disorders. Their integration into clinical workflows allows continuous data acquisition and remote patient supervision. Despite these advantages, the reliability and security of wireless communication among devices remain a major concern, especially in scenarios involving sensitive medical data [1,2]. According to recent market analyses, the global wearable medical devices market was valued at USD 42.74 billion in 2024 and is projected to reach USD 168.29 billion by 2030, growing at a compound annual growth rate (CAGR) of 25.53% from 2025 to 2030 [3].

In parallel, the widespread use of mobile electronics, such as smartphones, tablets, and smartwatches, has significantly changed how users interact with digital services. These devices now serve as multifunctional platforms, supporting activities from financial transactions to health monitoring. As a result, the need for secure and user-friendly authentication systems has become increasingly important [4]. Traditional approaches relying on passwords or physical tokens often suffer from usability and security limitations. Biometric authentication, which leverages unique physiological traits such as fingerprints or facial features, offers a more robust alternative [5]. To enhance the reliability of these systems, artificial intelligence (AI) techniques are commonly employed. Machine learning (ML) models can define biometric features, while deep learning (DL) approaches allow automatic feature extraction and classification. Furthermore, recent research has explored privacy-preserving methods for continuous authentication using sensor-based data, aiming to balance usability with data protection [6].

Galvanic Coupling (GC) has recently emerged as a promising technique for Body Area Networks (BANs), enabling on-body and intra-body communication through electrodes placed on or implanted within the skin [7]. Unlike traditional wireless methods, GC uses low-power electrical signals that propagate primarily through biological tissues, with most of the signal confined within the body and a small portion extending into the near-body region [8]. This results in a transmission path that is largely internal but not strictly limited to the body. The predominant confinement of the GC signal within the body reduces vulnerability to external interference and eavesdropping. Additionally, the use of low-power electrical signals and the short-range nature of GC transmission contribute to lower energy consumption compared to traditional wireless methods.

Inspired by Electroencephalogram (EEG)-based authentication systems, this work investigates the potential of GC signals for biometric verification in wearable medical applications. The unique and stable nature of the GC propagation channel, influenced by individual physiological traits, suggests its suitability for subject-specific identification. The proposed approach aims to integrate biometric authentication directly into the physical communication layer, enhancing the security of intra-body data exchange.

1.1 Related Work

GC has been extensively studied as a secure and energy-efficient communication method for BANs. Its ability to propagate signals primarily through biological tissues has led to various applications in medical and biometric systems. Prior research has addressed physical layer design for authentication [9], transmission optimization for implantable devices [8], and experimental channel characterization [7], highlighting the subject-specific and stable nature of GC channels.

Building on these foundations, further studies have investigated the use of GC for cryptographic key extraction. Methods have been proposed to generate secret keys by exploiting the reciprocity of GC channels, enabling secure communication between on-body devices without the need for key exchange [10]. Earlier approaches have also leveraged channel randomness and movement-induced variations to enhance key entropy and authentication robustness [11,12]. The integration of authentication into the key extraction process has been shown to be effective in preventing impersonation attacks [13].

In parallel, biometric authentication using physiological signals, particularly EEG, has been extensively studied. Multi-class classifiers such as neural networks [14], multilayer perceptrons [15], and convolutional architectures [16–18] have demonstrated high accuracy in user identification. Other machine learning models, including decision trees, support vector machines, and probabilistic classifiers, have also yielded promising results [19]. One-class classifiers have been employed to detect intrusions and authenticate users based on specific EEG patterns [20–22], while anomaly detection techniques like Isolation Forest and Local Outlier Factor have been applied to physiological data, although not always in the context of authentication [23–27].

1.2 Our Contribution

This work introduces a biometric authentication framework based on GC for BANs. The approach leverages subject-specific characteristics of the GC propagation channel to enable secure user identification. A Long Short-Term Memory (LSTM) network classifies raw GC signals directly, without relying on handcrafted feature extraction. The system operates in on-body configurations, such as communication between an implantable or wearable sensor and a GC-enabled smartwatch receiver, aiming to verify the identity of the transmitting device from the intrinsic properties of the propagation channel.

In addition, a lightweight authentication protocol is integrated into the communication process between wearable devices. This protocol incorporates biometric verification at the physical layer and is validated through experiments involving human subjects. The proposed solution is optimized for low-resource environments, making it suitable for real-time applications in medical contexts.

The remainder of this paper is structured as follows. Section 2 introduces the overall methodology, presenting the considered threat models and the design of the authentication framework. The experimental campaign, together with the setup adopted for GC signal acquisition, is then described in Sect. 3. Numerical results and performance analysis are discussed in Sect. 4, while Sect. 5 concludes the paper and outlines possible directions for future research.

2 Methodology

In wearable medical systems, secure communication between on-body devices is essential to protect sensitive biometric data. Traditional wireless methods are vulnerable to interception, particularly in scenarios where adversaries attempt to compromise the system through physical proximity or direct interaction with the body. Two primary threat models are considered:

- Over-the-Air (OTA) attacks: the adversary places external antennas in the vicinity of the subject and attempts to intercept, inject, or modify wireless signals.
- Direct contact attacks: the adversary physically connects a pair of electrodes to the subject's body and transmits falsified data to the receiver.

To counter these threats, the proposed system integrates biometric authentication directly into the physical communication layer. The approach leverages the subject-specific nature of the GC propagation channel, which is influenced by physiological factors such as tissue composition, body geometry, and electrode placement. This results in a transmission path that is unique and stable over time, making it difficult to replicate or spoof.

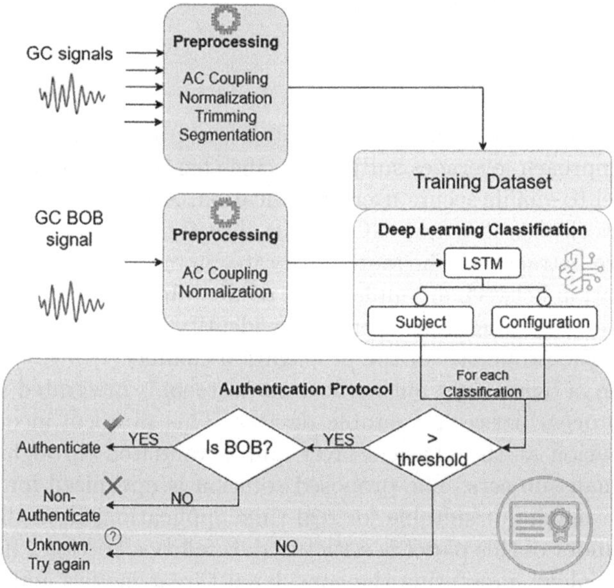

Fig. 1. Architecture of proposed authentication system

The authentication framework is designed to operate in on-body configurations, such as communication between a wearable or implantable sensor and a GC-enabled smartwatch receiver. It consists of two neural network classifiers:

- A subject classifier, which identifies the individual transmitting the signal, ensuring protection against OTA attacks by verifying the identity regardless of electrode placement.
- A configuration classifier, which determines the distance between electrodes, enabling detection of anomalies in electrode setup and mitigating direct contact attacks.

The following subsections describe the signal processing pipeline, the architecture of the deep learning models for classification, and the authentication protocol, which is designed to operate efficiently in low-resource medical environments, as shown in Fig. 1.

2.1 GC Signal Dataset for Neural Network

To enable biometric authentication based on GC signals, the raw data acquired during the experimental campaign is preprocessed and structured into a dataset suitable for training and evaluating a neural network classifier. The preprocessing pipeline is designed to preserve subject-specific signal characteristics while removing irrelevant or misleading components.

The first step involves removing the DC component from the acquired signal. This is achieved by applying AC coupling to the entire signal packet, effectively centering the signal around zero and eliminating any baseline offset introduced by the acquisition system. This ensures that only the dynamic variations of the signal are retained, which are more informative for classification.

Next, the signal is normalized with respect to its maximum absolute value. This operation scales the signal to the range $[-1, 1]$, removing amplitude variations caused by path loss and electrode placement. While path loss is a prominent and easily distinguishable feature, it is also the most vulnerable to estimation by an eavesdropper. By eliminating this dependency, the classifier is forced to rely on more subtle and robust features embedded in the signal structure.

The third step consists of trimming the signal to exclude portions where no transmission occurred. These segments contain only noise and do not contribute meaningful information for authentication. Removing them improves the signal-to-noise ratio and ensures the dataset contains only relevant samples.

The cleaned signal is then segmented into fixed-length portions of 100 samples, without overlap between segments. This segmentation allows the neural network to process consistent input sizes and facilitates batch training. Each segment is treated as an independent sample, capturing a snapshot of the GC signal under specific conditions.

Finally, each signal segment is annotated with two labels: one indicating the electrode configuration used during acquisition, and the other identifying the subject. This dual-labeling enables the network to learn both configuration-specific and subject-specific patterns, supporting evaluation of classification performance across different experimental setups.

2.2 Deep Learning Classifier

Recurrent Neural Networks (RNNs) are a class of artificial neural networks designed to process sequential data. Unlike feedforward networks, RNNs include internal memory states that allow them to retain information across time steps. This temporal structure enables RNNs to model dynamic behaviours and dependencies in time-series data, making them particularly suitable for tasks such as speech recognition, handwriting analysis, and physiological signal processing.

LSTM networks are a specialized type of RNN designed to overcome the limitations of standard RNNs, such as vanishing or exploding gradients. LSTMs introduce memory cells and gating mechanisms that regulate the flow of information, enabling the network to learn long-term dependencies more effectively. This makes LSTMs particularly well-suited for analysing biomedical signals like GC, where subtle temporal patterns may carry subject-specific information useful for authentication.

The LSTM network used in this work is designed to classify segments of GC signals into subject identities. The input to the network consists of signal segments of 100 samples, preprocessed as described in the previous section. The architecture includes a single LSTM layer with 120 hidden units, followed by fully connected layers and a final softmax output layer. The softmax layer outputs a probability distribution over the possible classes, corresponding to the subjects in the dataset.

The dataset used for training and evaluation consists of 78,240 signal segments. A random 90% of the dataset (70,416 segments) is used for training, while the remaining 10% (7,824 segments) is reserved for testing. This split ensures that the model is evaluated on unseen data, providing a reliable estimate of its generalization performance.

The network is trained using the Adam optimizer, which combines the advantages of adaptive learning rates and momentum. The learning rate is set to 0.002, and the model is trained for 200 epochs. The primary evaluation metric is classification accuracy, which measures the proportion of correctly identified signal segments. The training process is performed in batches, and early stopping is applied to prevent overfitting.

This architecture provides a balance between model complexity and computational efficiency, making it suitable for deployment on resource-constrained wearable devices. By learning directly from raw GC signals, the network avoids the need for handcrafted features and leverages the temporal dynamics of the signal for robust user authentication.

2.3 Authentication Protocol and Performance Evaluation

The authentication protocol is based on the output of two independent neural network classifiers. One classifier identifies the subject transmitting the signal, while the other determines the electrode configuration used during signal acquisition. Both networks operate on 100-sample GC signal segments and produce a probability distribution over their respective classes using a softmax activation function. The class associated with the highest probability is considered the most likely prediction.

However, in biometric authentication systems, a classification result alone may not be sufficient. A misclassification could be interpreted as a successful impersonation attempt. To mitigate this risk, the protocol introduces a confidence score threshold: if the highest predicted probability (i.e., the confidence score) does not exceed a predefined value θ, the system rejects the authentication attempt. This mechanism allows the system to respond with "uncertain" rather than forcing a potentially incorrect classification.

This threshold-based decision introduces a trade-off between responsiveness and security. Increasing θ improves the reliability of accepted predictions but leads to a higher rejection rate. Conversely, lowering θ increases the number of accepted segments but may reduce robustness against adversarial attacks. Given that each 100-sample segment corresponds to approximately 2 milliseconds of transmission time, the protocol can afford to discard uncertain segments and request retransmission without significantly impacting system performance.

To evaluate the effectiveness of the protocol, two key performance indicators are defined:

- Reliability: the proportion of signal segments that are accepted by the system, i.e., those for which the confidence score exceeds the threshold θ. It is defined as:

$$Reliability = \frac{N_{\text{accepted}}}{N_{\text{total}}},$$

  where N_{accepted} is the number of segments with confidence score above θ, and N_{total} is the total number of transmitted segments.
- Security: the proportion of correctly classified segments among those that are accepted. It reflects the system's robustness against impersonation and is defined as:

$$Security = \frac{N_{\text{correct}}}{N_{\text{accepted}}},$$

  where N_{correct} is the number of accepted segments that are correctly classified.

In the results section, the threshold θ is varied from 0 (inclusive) to 1 (exclusive) to analyse the trade-off between reliability and security, and to identify optimal operating points for different application scenarios.

3 Experimental Campaign

GC enables on-body communication by transmitting low-power alternating currents (below 1 mA) through biological tissues using surface electrodes. The signal is applied differentially between a pair of transmitting electrodes, while a pair of receiving electrodes detects the attenuated signal after propagation through the body. The human body acts as a conductive medium, allowing signal transmission in the frequency range of 1 kHz to 100 MHz.

In previous work [10], the GC channel was characterized through estimation of the Channel Impulse Response (CIR) for cryptographic key extraction. In contrast, the present study focuses on biometric authentication and directly uses the received signal segment as input to a classification model. This approach eliminates the need for channel estimation, reducing computational complexity and enabling faster processing suitable for real-time applications.

3.1 Measurement Setup and Experimental Protocol

The experimental platform (see Fig. 2) consists of two battery-powered laptops acting as transmitter (TX) and receiver (RX), connected via LINE OUT and LINE IN ports, respectively. Signal generation and acquisition are performed using MATLAB. The analog signal is transmitted through the TX sound card and injected into the body via two Ag/AgCl surface electrodes (PG10C, FIAB, CE-certified). The received signal is captured by two electrodes and digitized at 48 kHz with 16-bit resolution.

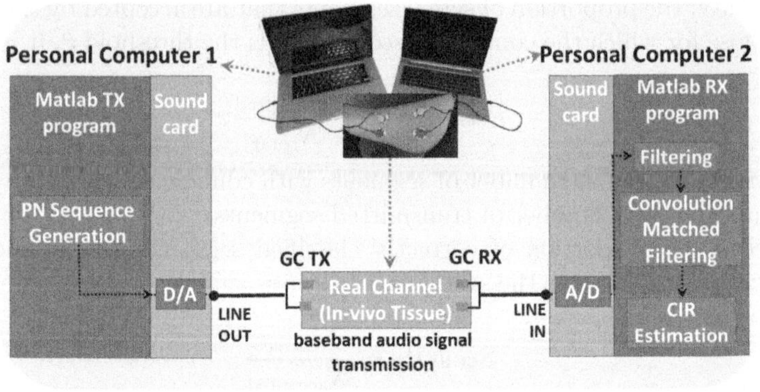

Fig. 2. Experimental setup for GC signal acquisition, showing the connection between transmitter and receiver, and the placement of electrodes on the forearm.

To ensure galvanic isolation and avoid shared ground paths, both laptops operate on battery power. A 50 Hz notch filter is applied to suppress power line interference. The transmitted signal is a pseudorandom noise (PN) sequence generated using a linear-feedback shift register, representative of arbitrary data exchanged between wearable devices.

Experiments were conducted on eight healthy volunteers (ages 24–30). All experiments involved voluntary participation of university research staff only. All participants were informed about the study purpose and signed a written informed consent prior to participation.

Electrodes were placed on the inner forearm, with multiple configurations tested to evaluate signal variability. As illustrated in Fig. 3, the longitudinal distance (d_l) between TX and RX pairs was set to 3, 5, 10, and 15 cm, while the transverse distance (d_t) within each pair was 3 or 5 cm. Each configuration was repeated five times to ensure statistical consistency.

Before each test, the system was configured to ensure optimal signal transmission and acquisition. The following steps were followed:

- Cable connection: TX connected to LINE OUT, RX to LINE IN.
- Audio settings: LINE IN and LINE OUT volumes set to 80% of maximum; all other channels disabled.
- Format configuration: Both laptops set to "16-bit, 48000 Hz"; audio enhancements disabled.
- Power isolation: Laptops disconnected from power supply to avoid ground loops.
- Electrode placement: Electrodes applied to the skin with distances as specified.
- Transmission: RX software started approximately 2 s before TX to ensure synchronization.

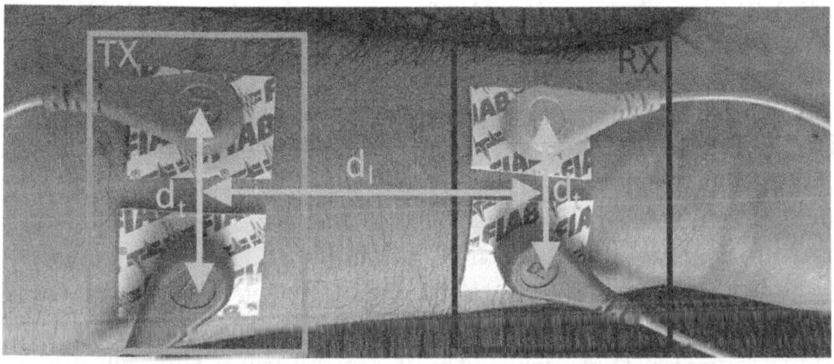

Fig. 3. Electrode placement scheme illustrating longitudinal distance (d_l) between TX and RX pairs, and transverse distance (d_t) within each pair.

Although electrode attachment and skin hydration can influence the galvanic coupling channel, their effects were not explicitly varied in this study. All measurements were conducted under stable indoor conditions, with consistent electrode placement and contact ensured before each acquisition. Furthermore, the proposed system shows adaptive behaviour, as the model compensates for small variations in propagation characteristics after a short calibration phase, indicating robustness to moderate physiological and environmental changes.

If the signal was not properly acquired, the test was repeated. This procedure ensures consistent and reliable acquisition of GC signals for biometric analysis under controlled conditions.

4 Numerical Results and Discussion

This section presents the performance evaluation of the proposed biometric authentication system based on GC signals. The analysis focuses on the system's ability to withstand two distinct threat models previously introduced: direct contact attacks, which are addressed through classification of the electrode configuration, and OTA attacks, mitigated by identifying the subject transmitting the signal.

For each scenario, the system's behaviour is studied by varying the confidence score threshold θ in the range $[0, 1)$, and observing how this affects the two key performance indicators: reliability and security. As defined earlier, reliability measures the proportion of signal segments accepted by the system, while security quantifies the accuracy of classification among those accepted segments.

To complement the analysis of these metrics, we also present confusion matrices for two representative operating conditions. The first corresponds to $\theta = 0$, where the confidence-based rejection mechanism is disabled and all segments are accepted. The second refers to the case where θ is set such that the system achieves a reliability of 0.8, meaning that 2 out of 10 segments are rejected.

4.1 Reliability and Security Performance for Contact Direct Attack

The evaluation of the system under the Direct Contact Attack scenario focuses on its ability to correctly classify the electrode configuration used during signal acquisition. This classification is crucial to detect unauthorized physical connections to the body, where an adversary attempts to transmit falsified data by mimicking the legitimate electrode setup.

Figure 4 illustrates the behaviour of reliability and security as the confidence score threshold θ is varied. When the threshold is set to zero, meaning that all segments are accepted regardless of confidence, the system achieves a security of 82%. This indicates that even without any filtering, the classifier is able to correctly identify the configuration in the majority of cases. By increasing θ to a value that yields a reliability of 0.8, the security improves to 88%, showing that discarding low-confidence segments enhances the robustness of the classification. However, achieving perfect security (100%) requires setting θ so high that only 0.02% of the segments are accepted. Given that each segment corresponds to approximately 2 milliseconds of transmission time, this implies that authenticating with absolute certainty would require around 10 s of continuous transmission, which is impractical for real-time applications.

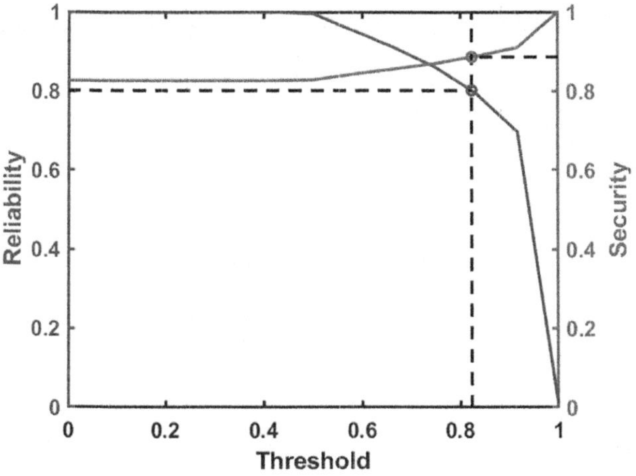

Fig. 4. Reliability and Security Performance

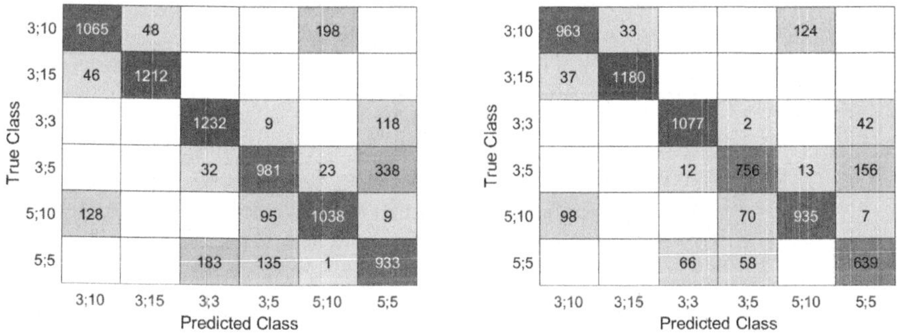

(a) Reliability = 100%

(b) Reliability = 80%

Fig. 5. Confusion Matrix

Figure 5 provides further insight into the classification performance by comparing the confusion matrices for two operating points: $\theta = 0$ and the threshold corresponding to 80% reliability. In both cases, the system demonstrates high overall accuracy, but struggles to distinguish between configurations with similar electrode placements. Misclassification events are more frequent when the longitudinal and transverse distances between electrodes are close, suggesting that the signal features become less discriminative in these conditions.

Despite these limitations, the authentication system remains effective in detecting adversarial configurations, provided that the attacker is not positioned too close to the legitimate transmitter. The results confirm that the GC signal retains sufficient spatial sensitivity to support configuration-based authentication, especially when low-confidence segments are filtered out.

4.2 Reliability and Security Performance for OTA Attack

In the context of OTA attacks, the authentication system is evaluated based on its ability to correctly identify the subject transmitting the GC signal. This classification is essential to prevent adversaries from impersonating legitimate users by injecting signals wirelessly through their own GC transmission channel.

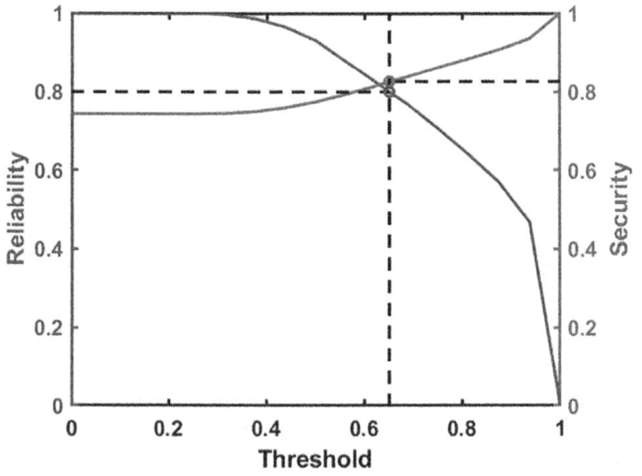

Fig. 6. Reliability and Security Performance

Figure 6 shows the variation of reliability and security as the confidence score threshold θ increases. When the threshold is set to zero, meaning that all segments are accepted, the system achieves a security of 74%. This baseline performance indicates that the classifier is able to distinguish users with reasonable accuracy even without filtering. By increasing θ to a value that yields a reliability of 0.8, the security improves to 82%, confirming that discarding low-confidence segments enhances the system's resistance to impersonation. As in the previous scenario, achieving perfect security (100%) requires a threshold so strict that only 0.02% of the segments are accepted, resulting in an impractical authentication time of approximately 10 s.

The confusion matrices in Fig. 7 provide additional insight into the classification behaviour. Unlike the Direct Contact Attack scenario, where errors are concentrated among similar configurations, the misclassifications in the OTA case are more evenly distributed across the matrix. As the threshold increases from 0 to the value corresponding to 80% reliability, the number of errors gradually decreases across all classes. This suggests that the classifier is able to refine its predictions uniformly, without being disproportionately affected by specific subject pairs.

Although some subjects exhibit signal characteristics that are more similar to others—leading to occasional misclassifications—the differences are less

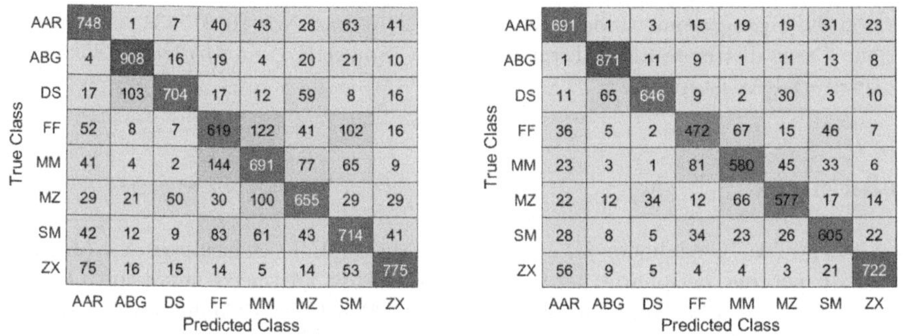

(a) Reliability = 100% (b) Reliability = 80%

Fig. 7. Confusion Matrix

pronounced than in the configuration classification task. Overall, the system demonstrates strong discriminative capability in identifying users, and the use of a confidence-based rejection mechanism significantly improves its robustness against OTA attacks.

5 Conclusion and Future Directions

This work presents a physical-layer biometric authentication framework for BANs based on GC signals. By leveraging a deep LSTM network trained on raw GC data, the system successfully exploits the subject-specific features of the propagation channel, providing robust protection against both direct contact and over-the-air attacks. Experimental results confirm that the confidence-based rejection mechanism significantly improves security while maintaining acceptable reliability, making the approach suitable for real-time applications in medical environments.

Future work will focus on expanding the experimental dataset to include a larger and more diverse subject population, improving generalization and reducing bias. Additional research will explore the integration of multimodal biometric features and adaptive thresholding techniques to dynamically balance security and usability. Moreover, reliability assessment through repeated measurements and cross-session analysis will be conducted to further validate system consistency over time.

Acknowledgments. This work was supported in part by the Italian Ministry of Foreign Affairs and International Cooperation, grant number US23GR04 (CUP: D43C23000350001). This work was also partially supported by the European Union under the Italian National Recovery and Resilience Plan (NRRP) of NextGenerationEU, partnership on "Telecommunications of the Future" (PE00000001 - program "RESTART"), by the European Telecommunication Standard Institute (ETSI), Smart Body Area Networks (SmartBAN) Technical Committee, by the European Union's

Horizon 2020 programme under grants No. 872752 and No. 101017331, and by Fondazione Cassa di Risparmio di Firenze (project: SmartHUB on Medical & Social ICT for Territorial Assistance).

References

1. Coviello, A., Cavigliano, C., Tasso, V., Tavassi, E.T., Giacalone, Y., Magarini, M.: Emerging peripheral nerve injuries recovery: advanced nerve-cuff electrode model interface for implantable devices. In: 2024 Global Conference on Wireless and Optical Technologies (GCWOT), pp. 1–7. IEEE (2024)
2. Mucchi, L., Jayousi, S., Martinelli, A., Caputo, S., Marcocci, P.: An overview of security threats, solutions and challenges in wbans for healthcare. In: 2019 13th International Symposium on Medical Information and Communication Technology (ISMICT), pp. 1–6. IEEE (2019)
3. Grand View Research. Wearable medical devices market size, share & trends analysis report by product (diagnostic, therapeutic devices), by site (handheld, headband, strap, shoe sensors), by application, by region, and segment forecasts, 2025–2030. https://www.grandviewresearch.com/industry-analysis/wearable-medical-devices-market. Accessed 10 Sep 2025
4. Hastie, T., Tibshirani, R., Friedman, J.: The Elements of Statistical Learning. Springer, Berlin/Heidelberg, Germany (2009)
5. Obaidat, M., Trore, I., Wougang, I.: Biometric-Based Physical and Cybersecurity Systems. Springer, Berlin/Heidelberg, Germany (2019)
6. Hernández-Álvarez, L., De Fuentes, J., González-Manzano, L., Hernández Encinas, L.: Privacy-preserving sensor-based continuous authentication and user profiling: A review. *Sensors* **21**, 92 (2021)
7. Vizziello, A., Savazzi, P., Guerra, R.R., Dell'Acqua, F.: Experimental channel characterization of human body communication based on measured impulse response. IEEE Trans. Commun. **72**(7), 3970–3984 (2024)
8. Swaminathan, M., Vizziello, A., Duong, D., Savazzi, P., Chowdhury, K.R.: Beamforming in the body: Energy-efficient and collision-free communication for implants. In: IEEE INFOCOM 2017 - IEEE Conference on Computer Communications, pp. 1–9. IEEE (2017)
9. Tomlinson, W.J.: Physical layer design and implementation of a biometric authentication system using galvanic coupling intra-body communication, Ph.d. thesis. Northeastern University (2018)
10. Caputo, S., et al.: Secret key extraction using galvanic coupling in wireless body area networks. In: 2025 19th International Symposium on Medical Information and Communication Technology (ISMICT) (2025)
11. Shi, L., Yuan, J., Yu, S., Li, M.: Ask-ban: authenticated secret key extraction utilizing channel characteristics for body area networks. In: Proceedings of the sixth ACM conference on Security and privacy in wireless and mobile networks, pp. 155–166. ACM (2013)
12. Shi, L., Yuan, J., Yu, S., Li, M.: Mask-ban: Movement-aided authenticated secret key extraction utilizing channel characteristics in body area networks. IEEE Internet Things J. **2**(1), 52–62 (2015)
13. Yuan, J., Shi, L., Yu, S., Li, M.: Authenticated secret key extraction using channel characteristics for body area networks. In: Proceedings of the 2012 ACM conference on Computer and Communications Security, pp. 1030–1032. ACM (2012)

14. Gui, Q., Jin, Z., Xu, W.: Exploring eeg-based biometrics for user identification and authentication. In: 2014 IEEE Signal Processing in Medicine and Biology Symposium (SPMB), Philadelphia, PA, USA, pp. 1–6. IEEE (2014). https://doi.org/10.1109/SPMB.2014.7002950
15. Kaur, B., Singh, D., Roy, P.: A novel framework of EEG-based user identification by analyzing music-listening behavior. Multimedia Tools Appl. **76**, 25581–25602 (2017)
16. Wu, Q., Zeng, Y., Zhang, C., Tong, L., Yan, B.: An EEG-based person authentication system with open-set capability combining eye blinking signals. Sensors **18**(11), 335 (2018)
17. Schons, T., Moreira, G.J.P., Silva, P.H.L., Coelho, V.N., Luz, E.J.S.: Convolutional Network for EEG-Based Biometric. In: Mendoza, M., Velastín, S. (eds.) CIARP 2017. LNCS, vol. 10657, pp. 601–608. Springer, Cham (2018). https://doi.org/10.1007/978-3-319-75193-1_72
18. Bidgoly, A., Bidgoly, H., Arezoumand, Z.: Towards a universal and privacy preserving eeg-based authentication system. Sci. Rep. **21**, 1–12 (2022)
19. Valsaraj, A., Madala, I., Garg, N., Patil, M., Baths, V.: Motor imagery based multimodal biometric user authentication system using EEG. In: 2020 International Conference on Cyberworlds (CW), pp. 272–279. IEEE (2020)
20. Zuquete, A., Quintela, B., Cunha, J.: Biometric authentication using brain responses to visual stimuli. In: Third International Conference on Bio-inspired Systems and Signal Processing (BIOSIGNALS), pp. 103–112 (2010)
21. Gupta, E., Agarwal, M., Sivakumar, R.: Blink to get in: Biometric authentication for mobile devices using EEG signals. In: 2020 IEEE International Conference on Communications (ICC), pp. 1–6. IEEE (2020)
22. Moctezuma, L., Molinas, M.: Multi-objective optimization for EEG channel selection and accurate intruder detection in an EEG-based subject identification system. Sci. Rep. **10**, 5850 (2020)
23. Guo, Y.: Epileptic seizure detection by cascading isolation forest-based anomaly screening and easyensemble. IEEE Trans. Neural Syst. Rehab. Eng. **30**, 915–924 (2022)
24. Ketu, S., Mishra, P.: Hybrid classification model for eye state detection using electroencephalogram signals. Cogn. Neurodyn. **16**, 73–90 (2022)
25. Kumaravel, V., Farella, E., Parise, E., Buiatti, M.: Near: An artifact removal pipeline for human newborn eeg data. Dev. Cogn. Neurosci. **54**, 1–14 (2022)
26. Saba-Sadiya, S.: Unsupervised eeg artifact detection and correction. Front. Digital Health **2**, 608920 (2021)
27. Chakravarthy, S., Rajaguru, H.: Effective breast tumor classification using k–strongest strength with local outlier factor algorithm. Int. J. Aquatic Sci. **12**, 1596–1603 (2021)

A Fundamental Study of Inductive/Capacitive Hybrid WPT for Implantable Devices: Coupler Misalignment Tolerance

Miyu Kodama and Dairoku Muramatsu(✉)

The University of Electro-Communications, 1-5-1 Chofugaoka, Chofu, Japan
dmuramatsu@uec.ac.jp

Abstract. Implantable medical devices require stable and efficient power delivery systems. Conventional approaches employ either inductive or capacitive wireless power transfer (WPT), but each has limitations. To overcome these limitations, we propose and evaluate a hybrid WPT coupler that combines inductive and capacitive coupling. In this study, we conducted electromagnetic field simulations with a numerical human body model at 13.56 MHz to evaluate the misalignment tolerance of the proposed design. The coupler was modeled as a double-sided printed circuit board containing both coils and comb-shaped electrodes, and its performance was compared with coil-only and electrode-only couplers. Results showed that the hybrid coupler exhibited the smallest efficiency degradation under displacement and achieved higher efficiency values than the other designs. These findings demonstrate that hybrid WPT can provide efficient and stable power transfer even under practical clinical conditions, where device positioning varies. The proposed approach has strong potential to enhance patient quality of life.

Keywords: Implantable Medical Device · Wireless Power Transfer · Electromagnetic Field Simulation

1 Introduction

Implantable medical devices (IMDs) require a reliable power source. Most IMDs rely on primary batteries. However, they must be surgically replaced before the battery is fully depleted. The need for repeated surgical battery replacement imposes physical and psychological burdens on patients. By using wireless power transfer (WPT) and recharging secondary batteries externally, it is possible to reduce the need for replacement surgery. WPT systems are classified into inductive and capacitive coupling. Inductive coupling achieves high power transmission efficiency [1]. However, it is highly sensitive to coil misalignment, and many studies have investigated ways to improve its robustness to misalignment [2]. Capacitive coupling, in contrast, tolerates electrode misalignment but suffers from limited transmission distance [3].

H. Tanaka et al. (Eds.): BodyNets 2025, LNICST 714, pp. 134–142, 2026.
https://doi.org/10.1007/978-3-032-38657-1_10

Recently, hybrid WPT combining inductive and capacitive coupling has attracted attention [4–6]. By using both coils and electrodes as couplers, hybrid systems enable simultaneous magnetic and electric coupling, taking advantage of the strengths of each method to compensate for their weaknesses [7, 8]. Previous studies on hybrid WPT have mainly targeted large-scale applications such as electric vehicles. In implantable environments, the transmitter and receiver are separated by biological tissues with different electrical properties, making the transmission path more complicated than in air. In particular, conductive and dielectric losses as well as impedance variations are expected to occur due to the presence of biological tissues. Moreover, implantable devices have much stricter dimensional constraints than large-scale systems such as vehicles, and minimizing potential biological effects associated with power loss is also critical; therefore, compact and highly efficient coupler designs are required. Considering this background, we aim to apply this hybrid WPT method to implantable devices [9]. In our previous work, hybrid WPT appeared suitable for implantable use, as it leverages both inductive and capacitive coupling to improve tolerance to misalignment [10].

Based on these findings, this paper presents a detailed evaluation of the misalignment tolerance of the hybrid WPT system for implantable devices. Using electromagnetic simulations with a numerical human body model, we compare the transmission efficiency of hybrid, inductive, and capacitive systems under misalignment conditions. This study confirms the effectiveness of the proposed hybrid approach.

2 Proposed Hybrid WPT Method

2.1 Requirements for Hybrid WPT for Implantable Devices

In this study, we investigate a WPT system that transmits power through biological tissue from an external transmitter to an implanted receiver, as illustrated in Fig. 1. The casing of the implanted unit was set to $50 \times 50 \times 10\ \text{mm}^3$ [10]. The coupler for WPT was designed with dimensions of $24 \times 24 \times 1.6\ \text{mm}^3$. The implanted receiver was assumed to be located beneath the subcutaneous fat layer of the abdomen. The external transmitter was positioned on the skin surface over the implant.

For the power transmission frequency, we considered the Industrial, Scientific, and Medical (ISM) band [11]. The ISM band allows license- exempt operation worldwide and includes several frequencies such as 13.56 MHz, 40.68 MHz, and 434 MHz. Among these, 13.56 MHz is one of the few frequencies that are globally available regardless of region. In addition, higher frequencies tend to increase inverter and rectifier losses [12] and intensify electromagnetic absorption in biological tissue [13]. Considering these factors, we adopted 13.56 MHz as the transmission frequency in this study. In addition, this frequency was selected as a representative ISM band typically used for power transfer applications, allowing our analysis to focus on a practically relevant and widely adopted operating condition.

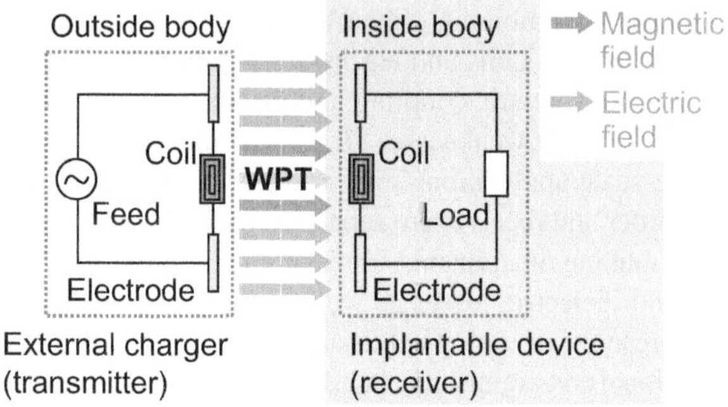

Fig. 1. Hybrid WPT for implantable medical devices.

2.2 Structure of Coupler

Figure 2 shows the structure of the hybrid WPT coupler used in the external transmitter and implanted receiver. The coupler was designed on a double-sided printed circuit board with dimensions of 24 × 24 × 1.6 mm^3. The transmitter and receiver had the same design, each consisting of two coils and two electrodes. On the surface facing the body, two electrodes were placed symmetrically with 8 mm spacing, and a single coil was positioned between them. On the opposite surface, another coil was placed. The transmitter feed and the receiver load were set between the centers of the two coils. In addition, one of the electrodes was connected to the coil on the opposite side via a wire.

The electrodes were designed in a comb-shaped configuration, formed by periodic slits in rectangular plates. This configuration avoids shielding of the magnetic flux by the electrodes. Although the comb structure reduces the electrode area to approximately half, the edge effect at the slit ends increases the coupling capacitance, so the impact of reduced area is considered negligible [14]. Each electrode had dimensions of 8 × 24 mm^2, with both the slit width and spacing set to 0.15 mm.

The coils were implemented in a helical configuration using both sides of the substrate to maximize inductance within the limited area [15]. Only the coil in contact with biological tissue was insulated. The coil located on the same side as the electrodes measured 8 × 24 mm^2 with 12 turns, while the coil on the opposite side measured 24 × 24 mm^2 with 39 turns. For both coils, the trace width and spacing were set to 0.15 mm.

For comparison and evaluation, we also fabricated coil and electrode couplers with the same dimensions as the proposed hybrid coupler. The coil coupler was a helical structure that supplied and received power at the center of the coils on both sides of the substrate. Its dimensions are the same as those of the 24 × 24 mm^2 coil of the hybrid coupler. The electrode coupler had the same dimensions as the hybrid electrodes but consisted of plain plates without slits. The feed and load were placed between the two electrodes.

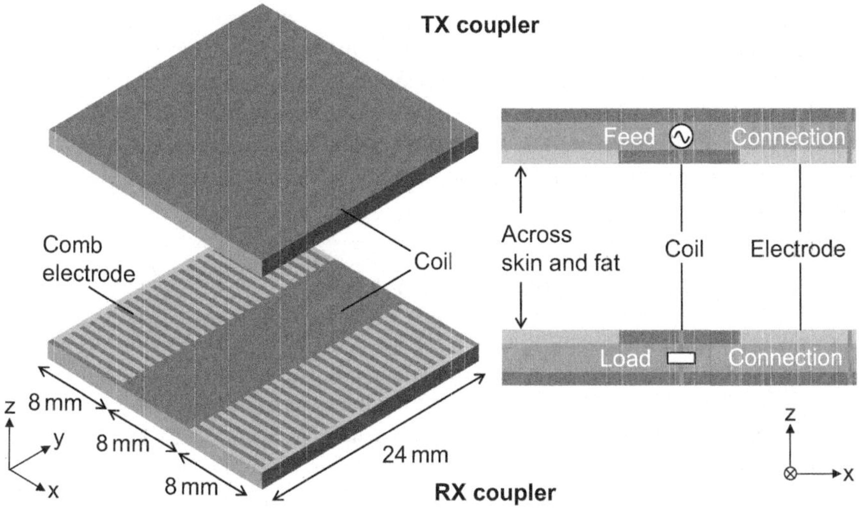

Fig. 2. Structure of proposed coupler for hybrid WPT.

3 Electromagnetic Field Simulation

3.1 Models for Electromagnetic Field Simulation

In this study, we evaluated the misalignment tolerance of the proposed hybrid coupler using electromagnetic field simulations. An overview of the simulation model is shown in Fig. 3. Referring to spinal cord stimulation devices in current clinical use, the implanted receiving coupler was positioned beneath the fat layer of the abdominal model, while the external transmitting coupler was placed on the skin surface.

As transmitting and receiving couplers, we used three structures described in Sect. 2.2: the hybrid coupler, the coil coupler, and the electrode coupler. A double-sided FR4 substrate with a relative permittivity of 4.6 was assumed, and coils and electrodes were modeled as perfect conductor patterns on each surface. Behind the implanted receiving coupler, a cavity of $50 \times 50 \times 10$ mm^3 was included to represent the implanted device casing [10]. A feed point was assigned to the transmitting coupler, and a load was assigned to the receiving coupler.

The abdominal model, shown in Fig. 3, was constructed as a three layer structure of skin, fat, and muscle, based on previous studies [16]. Dimensions were determined according to the average Japanese adult male [17, 18]: 2 mm for skin, 6 mm for fat, and 182 mm for muscle, with an overall size of $260 \times 210 \times 190$ mm^3. Voxels constituting each tissue layer were assigned frequency-dependent electrical properties [19].

Electromagnetic field simulations were performed using an FDTD-based solver (XFdtd, Remcom Inc.). The free-space distance from the model to the absorbing boundary was set to approximately 20 cells. A nonuniform mesh was employed, with a minimum cell size of 0.15–0.2 mm around the coils and electrodes and a maximum of 2 mm. Seven layers of PML were used as absorbing boundaries. The excitation source was a band-limited wideband pulse, and the time step was optimized for each coupler structure and configuration.

3.2 Method for Evaluating Misalignment Tolerance

We evaluated the misalignment tolerance of the proposed hybrid coupler in terms of power transmission efficiency. A misalignment of several millimeters is acceptable under the Qi standard for WPT [20]. To simulate this, the external transmitting coupler was shifted along the x- and y-directions, as shown in Fig. 3, by up to 12 mm. At this maximum displacement, the overlapping area between the transmitting and receiving couplers was reduced to one quarter of the total. In this situation, we compared the power transmission efficiency of the three coupler types and evaluated the misalignment tolerance of the hybrid design.

In this study, we calculated the maximum power transmission efficiency η for each coupler. The load impedance that maximizes η is uniquely determined by the two-port Z-parameters [21]. As the coupler position changes, the optimal load impedance also varies. However, it is impractical to adjust the impedance each time the coupler position shifts. Such an operation would require advanced control circuits and sensors. This would lead to increased complexity, higher power consumption, and response delays. Therefore, it is desirable to fix the load impedance in practical use. In this study, the load impedance was fixed at the optimal value at the reference position, and η was calculated using this fixed impedance. This approach enables the evaluation of misalignment tolerance under practical operating conditions.

The reference position was defined as $x = y = 0$ mm with an implantation depth of 8 mm. Misalignment tolerance was evaluated using two metrics:

(i) the transmission efficiency η at each position, and
(ii) the efficiency difference η_{diff} between each position and the reference position.

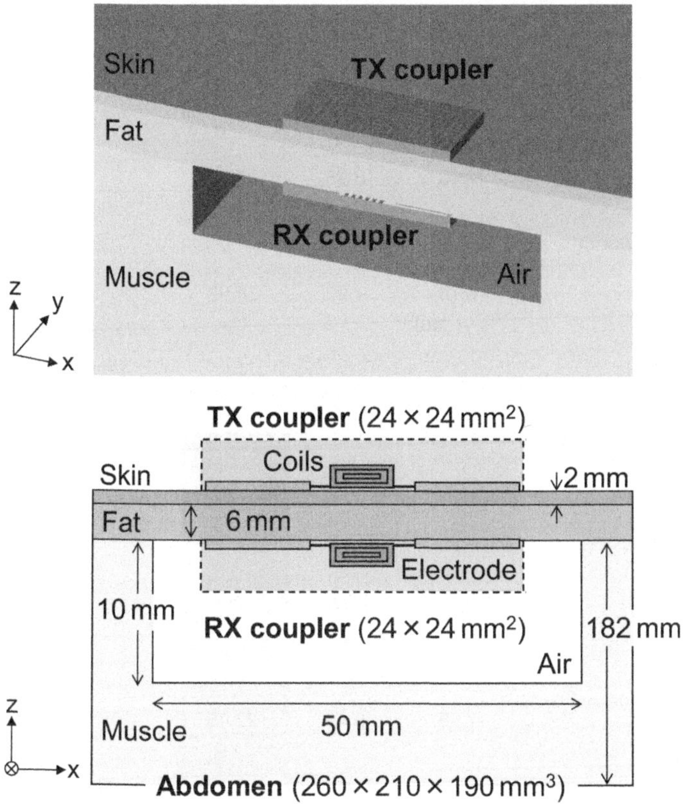

Fig. 3. Overview of electromagnetic field simulation model including human abdomen and couplers.

3.3 Results and Discussion

Figure 4 shows the power transmission efficiency of the three coupler types under misalignment. In each cell of the figure, the value represents the η at that position, while the color indicates η_{diff}.

For (i), the η of the hybrid coupler was higher than that of both the coil and electrode couplers at all evaluated positions. For (ii), the overall η_{diff} values were smallest for the hybrid coupler, indicating reduced efficiency degradation under misalignment. The maximum η_{diff} was 14.5 dB for the hybrid coupler, 29.2 dB for the coil coupler, and 20.6 dB for the electrode coupler. These results demonstrate that the hybrid coupler achieves higher transmission efficiency than coil- or electrode-only couplers by combining inductive and capacitive coupling. It also provides superior robustness to misalignment. The hybrid coupler exhibits highly practical advantages for WPT systems in implantable environments.

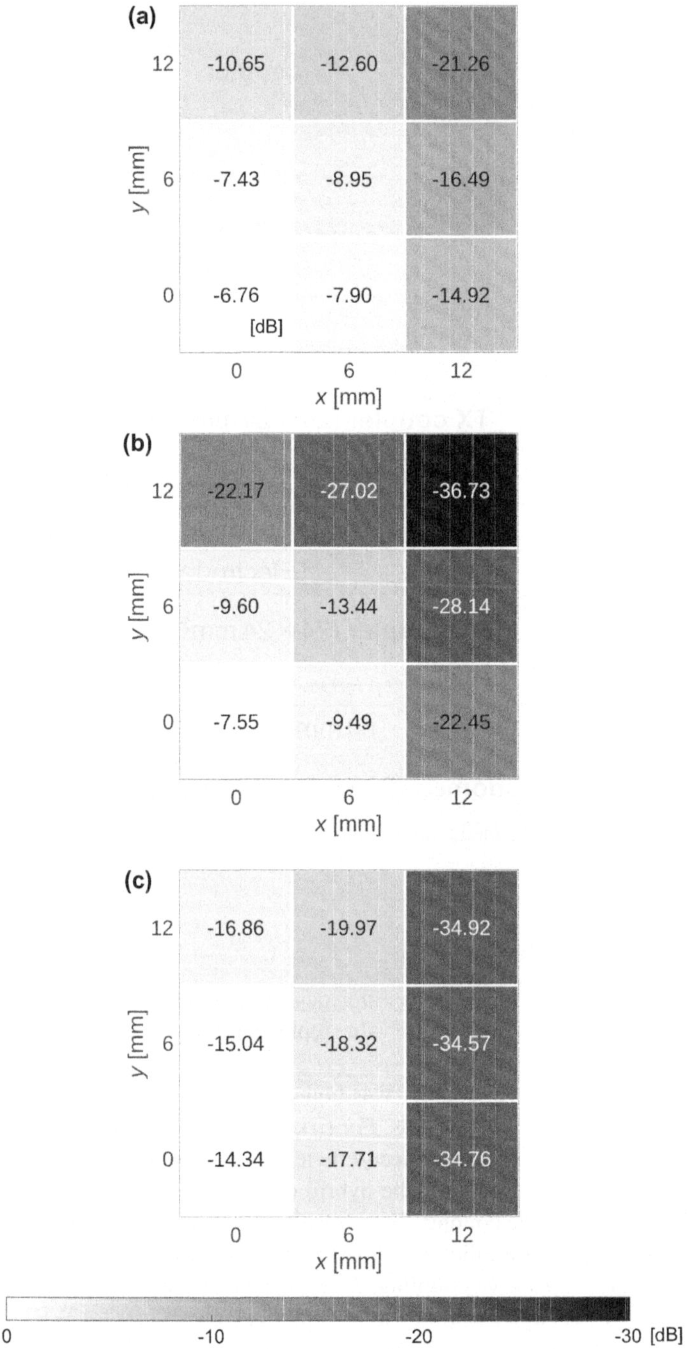

Fig. 4. Results of the power transfer efficiency under misalignment and its deviation from the reference position: (a) hybrid, (b) coil, (c) electrode coupler.

4 Conclusion

In this paper, we evaluated the misalignment tolerance of an inductive/capacitive hybrid WPT system for IMDs. Using electromagnetic field simulations with a numerical human body model, we demonstrated that the hybrid coupler achieved high transmission efficiency and excellent robustness against misalignment. These findings suggest that the hybrid approach can provide a robust and versatile power supply for implantable WPT systems, less affected by external transmitter placement. In future work, we will experimentally evaluate the performance of the hybrid coupler with prototypes and electromagnetic phantoms, comparing it against the numerical results.

Acknowledgments. A part of this research was funded by JSPS KAKENHI Grant No. JP23K25250, the Azbil Yamatake General Foundation, and the Japan Science Society.

References

1. Ye, Z., Yang, M., Chen, P.-Y.: Multi-band parity-time-symmetric wireless power transfer systems for ISM-band bio-implantable applications. IEEE J. Electromagn. RF Microwaves Med. Biol. **6**(2), 196–203 (2022)
2. Wang, Q., Che, W., Mongiardo, M., Monti, G.: Wireless power transfer system with high misalignment tolerance for bio-medical implants. IEEE Trans. Circuits Syst. II Express Briefs. **67**(12), 3023–3027 (2020)
3. Segawa, T., Aoyama, R., Tamura, M.: Electrode design theory using highly accurate equivalent circuits in biological capacitive WPT. IEEE Microw. Wirel. Technol. Lett. **33**(6), 943–946 (2023)
4. Luo, B., Long, T., Mai, R., Dai, R., He, Z., Li, W.: Analysis and design of hybrid inductive and capacitive wireless power transfer for high-power applications. IET Power Electron. **11**(14), 2263–2270 (2018)
5. Wang, F., Yang, Q., Zhang, X., Chen, T., Li, G.: Enhancing misalignment tolerance in hybrid wireless power transfer system with integrated coupler via frequency tuning. IEEE Trans. Power Electron. **39**(9), 11885–11899 (2024)
6. Wang, Y., Yang, J., Wang, K., Yang, Y.: Highly integrated hybrid inductive and capacitive power transfer system with asymmetrical printed-circuit-board-based self-resonator. IEEE Trans. Power Electron. **40**(7), 1–10 (2025)
7. Lu, F., Zhang, H., Hofmann, H., Mi, C.C.: An inductive and capacitive combined wireless power transfer system with LC-compensated topology. IEEE Trans. Power Electron. **31**(12), 8471–8482 (2016)
8. Lu, F., Zhang, H., Hofmann, H., Mi, C.C.: An inductive and capacitive integrated coupler and its LCL compensation circuit design for wireless power transfer. IEEE Trans. Ind. Appl. **53**(5), 4903–4913 (2017)
9. Kodama, M., Muramatsu, D.: Complementary capacitive/inductive wireless power transfer for implantable medical devices. In: The 46th international conference of the IEEE engineering in medicine and biology society, Copenhagen (2025)
10. St. Jude Medical: Proclaim implantable pulse generator clinician's manual (2017).
11. International Telecommunication Union, Radio Regulations, edition of 2020: Volume 1: Articles (2020)
12. Liu, Y., Pan, L., Yao, S., Zhang, J., Cui, S., Zhu, C.: A review on the recent development of high-frequency inverters for wireless power transfer. Energies. **17**(20), 5153 (2024)

13. Mauludiyanto, A., Hendrantoro, G., Nova, M.F.: The attenuation characteristics of the body tissue on frequency function in WBAN channel. JAREE. **5**(2), 107–113 (2021)
14. Li, S., Xia, K., Li, T., Lu, S., Xia, J., Liu, Z.: A novel comb-shaped coupler for hybrid inductive and capacitive wireless power transfer system. IEEE Trans. Power Electron. **40**(4), 4787–4792 (2025)
15. Konno, S., Yamamoto, T., Koshiji, K.: Study on wireless power transfer using printed spiral coil. IEICE Trans. Electron. **J97-C**(12), 528–534 (2014)
16. Kodama, M., Muramatsu, D.: Propagation analysis of implantable human body communication system for neurostimulators and structural evaluation of abdominal models. AIP Adv. **15**(6), 1–6 (2025)
17. Kouchi M., Mochimaru, M: AIST anthropometric database, National Institute of Advanced Industrial Science and Technology, H16PRO 287 (2005)
18. Southwood, W.F.: The thickness of the skin. Plast. Reconstr. Surg. **15**, 423–429 (1955)
19. Gabriel, S., Lau, R.W., Gabriel, C.: The dielectric properties of biological tissues: II. Measurements in the frequency range 10 Hz to 20 GHz. Phys. Med. Biol. **41**(11), 2251–2269 (1996)
20. Wireless Power Consortium, Inc.: Qi Specification Introduction, Version 1.3 (2021)
21. Ohira, T.: Power transfer theory on linear passive two-port systems. IEICE Trans. Electron. **E101.C**(10), 719–726 (2018)

Peripheral Nerve Injuries: Impact, Solutions and Innovation

Antonio Coviello[1(✉)], Giulio Franceschini[1(✉)], Davide Scazzoli[1], Manuela Crocco[1], Silvia Mura[1], Paolo Motto Ros[2], Danilo Demarchi[2], Federica Burinato[1], Anna Simeone[1], Virginia Tasso[1], Chiara Cavigliano[1], Andrea Cerutti[1], Yeshua Giacalone[1], Umberto Spagnolini[1], and Maurizio Magarini[1]

[1] Politecnico di Milano, Piazza Leonardo da Vinci 32, 20133 Milano, MI, Italy
antonio.coviello@polimi.it, giulio.franceschini@mail.polimi.it
[2] Politecnico di Torino, Corso Duca degli Abruzzi 24, 10129 Torino, TO, Italy

Abstract. Peripheral nerve injuries (PNIs) remain a significant clinical challenge, impacting both patients' quality of life and healthcare systems globally. This paper examines the individual and societal burdens of PNIs, reviewing current therapeutic strategies, including pharmacology, neuromodulation, surgery, and rehabilitation. Despite advancements, these approaches often fail to restore complex nerve functions, particularly in severe cases. We propose a novel implantable system that bypasses nerve lesions by recording neural activity proximally, processing the signals externally, and delivering precise stimulation distally. The system integrates multi-contact cuffs for both sensing and stimulation, ensuring minimal invasiveness and enhanced safety. We present a detailed analysis of the system's signal processing techniques, including noise reduction and feature extraction, and its potential for motor and sensory restoration. Furthermore, we explore the translational path for this technology, focusing on clinical trials, regulatory approval, and stakeholder alignment, including patients, clinicians, manufacturers, and payers. This solution aims to bridge existing gaps in PNI treatment by providing a functional bypass that restores nerve function while reducing long-term healthcare costs.

Keywords: Peripheral Nerve Injuries · Implantable Device · Stakeholder Engagement · Functional Bypass

1 Introduction

The peripheral nervous system is a crucial component of the human body, responsible for bidirectional communication between the brain and the rest of the organism. Through this network, peripheral nerves transmit electrical and

A. Coviello and G. Franceschini—Both authors contributed equally.

H. Tanaka et al. (Eds.): BodyNets 2025, LNICST 714, pp. 143–158, 2026.
https://doi.org/10.1007/978-3-032-38657-1_11

chemical signals that regulate not only movement but also sensory perception, allowing the body to interact with the surrounding environment. Since these structures are among the most delicate and vulnerable, they are particularly prone to trauma such as crushing, compression, and other forms of physical damage. These injuries disrupt communication between the brain and target organs, compromising vital motor and sensory functions. When a peripheral nerve injury (PNI) occurs, caused by various types of trauma, the disruption of signals between the brain and the body prevents proper motor and sensory function, severely impairing the patient's autonomy, Fig. 1. Given the significant impact of PNIs, both on patients' quality of life and healthcare costs, further research into these injuries is essential [1].

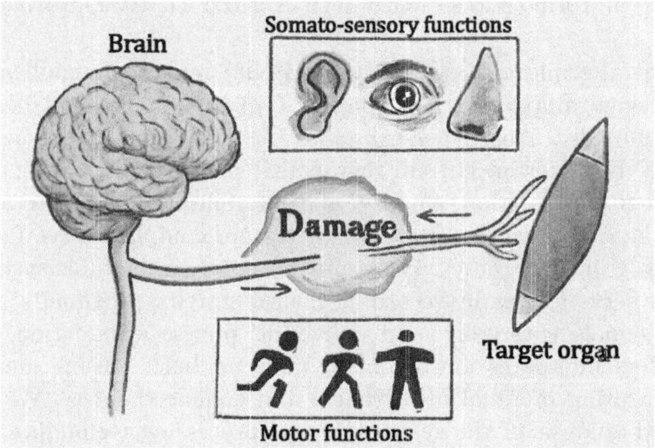

Fig. 1. Pictorial depiction of PNI showing how nerve damage disrupts the conduction of signals, impairing motor and somatosensory functions [3].

When nerves are damaged, Wallerian degeneration rapidly degrades the affected part, enabling surviving neurons to regenerate [2]. However, regeneration is often incomplete, with outcomes depending on factors such as age, injury severity, and neuronal survival. PNIs have a profound impact on both the physical and psychological health of patients, impairing motor skills, sensory perception, and independence, while often leading to anxiety, depression, and social isolation [4,5]. At a societal level, prolonged rehabilitation, long-term care, and reduced work capacity impose substantial economic costs on patients, families, and healthcare systems [6]. Given all those impacts, advancing treatment requires collaborative efforts among healthcare professionals, patients, caregivers, policymakers, and manufacturers to develop effective, sustainable solutions that restore function and quality of life.

This review synthesizes recent advances in diagnosis and treatment of PNIs, with emphasis on implantable technologies and future translational directions. Individually, it examines motor and sensory impairments, pain, and psychological consequences such as anxiety, depression, and reduced quality of life. Societally, it considers healthcare utilization, long-term care, productivity losses, and impacts on labor participation and tax contributions. The study reviews current diagnostic and therapeutic technologies, focusing on implantable solutions, analyzing their principles, mechanisms, advantages, and limitations. It also maps the stakeholder landscape—patients, caregivers, clinicians, payers, policymakers, regulators, manufacturers, and researchers—to identify challenges, innovation opportunities, and strategies for coordinated action to enhance outcomes and reduce costs.

The paper is organised as follows: Sect. 2 examines the physical and psychological effects of PNIs. Section 3 analyzes the socio-economic burden, including direct and indirect costs as well as impacts on labor participation and tax contributions. Section 4 reviews current diagnostic and therapeutic solutions. Section 5 focuses on implantable devices, outlining their operating principles, benefits, and limitations. Finally, Sect. 6 synthesizes the findings and discusses future developments, with particular attention to stakeholder perspectives and market considerations.

2 Individual Impact

PNIs can have a profound impact on patients, often leading to persistent and debilitating symptoms. These may include sensations such as tingling, paresthesia ("pins and needles"), and chronic pain. Depending on the severity of the injury, PNIs can also cause loss of somatosensation and dexterity, and in some cases, complete paralysis [7]. Such debilitating symptoms can severely affect patients' ability to perform daily activities and have a long-lasting impact on their overall well-being.

The most common effects of PNIs are outlined in Table 1 [4,8–11]. These outcomes underscore the devastating toll of PNIs on patients' physical, emotional, and psychological well-being, severely diminishing their quality of life and often leading to long-lasting personal and societal consequences.

Given the profound physical impact of peripheral nerve injuries, they also give rise to significant psychological challenges, affecting both traumatic and non-traumatic cases. Patients often experience high levels of anxiety, depression, and post-traumatic stress, as evidenced by various studies, as shown in Fig. 2 a.

In [12], a study that followed patients with median and ulnar nerve injuries in the forearm reported that early post-traumatic stress symptoms were present in 92% of patients at 1 month and 83% at 3 months. Among these patients, 24.6% and 13.3% met the thresholds for psychological treatment at 1 and 3 months, respectively.

Similarly, in [13], a database study of 1843 adults undergoing surgery for brachial plexus injury (BPI) found that preoperative depression and anxiety were present in 38% and 42% of patients, with new-onset depression and anxiety occurring within 12 months in 12% and 20%, respectively. Furthermore, the risk of developing depression and anxiety in patients with PNIs has been quantified using hazard ratios. Specifically, the hazard ratio for new-onset depression was

Table 1. Physical consequences and associated risks in patients affected by PNIs.

Possible PNI effects	Percentage of affected PNI patients (%)
Loss of sensation	95–100
Muscle weakness/paralysis	80–90
Neuropathic/acute pain	40–70
Autonomic dysfunctions*	5–15
Long-term disability**	25–50
Suicidal ideation	33.3
Suicide Risk	1.7x the general population

*Autonomic manifestations such as abnormal sweating,
gastrointestinal disturbances, and blood pressure alterations.
.**The risk of long-term disability varies greatly according to location,
severity, treatment efficacy, and patient characteristics.

found to be 1.3, indicating that patients with PNIs have a 30% higher risk of developing depression compared to matched controls. Similarly, the hazard ratio for new-onset anxiety was 2.1, meaning these patients are more than twice as likely (a 110% increased risk) to develop anxiety compared to the control group.

In [11], a clinical series of traumatic BPI cases was studied. 19% of patients met the criteria for Post-Traumatic Stress Disorder (PTSD), 19% for clinical depression, and 33% reported suicidal ideation. Focusing on suicidal ideation, it is evident that PNIs impose a severe psychological burden on patients. Alarmingly, 33.3% of PNI patients report suicidal ideation, which underscores the extreme emotional toll these injuries can take. In addition, patients with chronic pain are more likely to experience co-morbid depression and anxiety, with prevalence sharply increasing as the Chronic Pain Grade (CPG) worsens [5], as shown in Fig. 2 b. The psychological impact of PNIs—particularly the risk of suicide—is as critical as the physical consequences and demands urgent attention.

A study of 246 patients with cubital tunnel syndrome (CTS) [14] reported that depression and anxiety were found in 17.9% and 14.2% of the cases, respectively, as measured by the Hospital Anxiety and Depression Scale (HADS). The HADS is a widely used tool for assessing anxiety and depression in patients, consisting of 14 questions that evaluate emotional distress, with separate subscales for anxiety and depression.

Together, these findings quantify the high burden of PTSD, depression, anxiety, and stress responses in PNI patients, highlighting the urgent need for routine psychological screening and support alongside surgical and rehabilitative care.

3 Social Impact

The social impact of PNIs extends far beyond the physical and psychological consequences, influencing patients' ability to work, engage in daily activities, and maintain financial independence. Given the significant healthcare utilization and long-term care requirements, it is crucial to quantify the public cost of PNIs, highlighting the importance of investing in effective treatments to identify more cost-effective solutions.

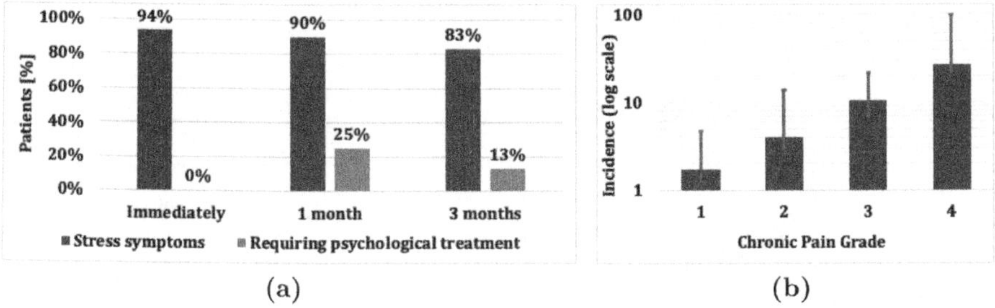

Fig. 2. Psychological burden of PNIs: (a) results of a prospective cohort of forearm median/ulnar PNIs [5]; (b) CPG correlation with co-morbid depression and anxiety, normalized to the general population incidence [5].

Across trauma populations worldwide, PNIs disproportionately affect working-age adults, with a strong male predominance. These injuries are most commonly caused by sharp trauma and motor vehicle accidents, particularly motorcycle crashes.

In [4], a study from the national Canadian trauma registry reports on 335 cases of PNIs and 64 cases of BPIs. The sex distribution of PNI cases was significantly male-skewed, with 81% of cases being male and 19% female. These data provide insight into the gender breakdown of nerve injuries in a contemporary trauma population, highlighting that PNIs and BPIs predominantly affect men in early-to-mid adulthood.

Contemporary registry and claims analyses [15] report cumulative PNI diagnoses following extremity trauma in $\sim$2.3% of cases overall (2.6% upper limb; 1.2% lower limb) in the United States and, in [4] a large Canadian trauma cohort (n=24,905), sharp injuries accounted for 39.4% of PNIs while motorcycle accidents were the leading cause of brachial plexus injury (32.8%). These epidemiologic profiles translate into substantial direct medical spending and even larger productivity losses borne by patients, employers, and public payers.

Direct acute and rehabilitation costs increase with the severity and complexity of the injury. In a nationwide workers' compensation cohort from Germany [6], which included 268 cases of upper-extremity PNIs (mean age 39.9 years; 85% male), mean in-patient reimbursement ranged from €3,418 to €5,360 per case, depending on the injury's location (distal to proximal). Additionally, 16% of patients required inpatient rehabilitation, averaging 41 ± 21 days, with €5,842 in extra costs. Sick leave averaged 147 days (range 11–1,109 days), with insurers covering €197 per day (€17,640 per case), and 26% of patients required a structured return-to-work program (mean duration: 21 days), highlighting the significant rehabilitation burden.

Procedure-specific studies show a similar cost gradient [16]: for surgically treated adult traumatic BPI in the USA, median 1-year direct payments amounted to $38,816 (IQR $18,209$72,411), representing only a fraction of the long-term costs.

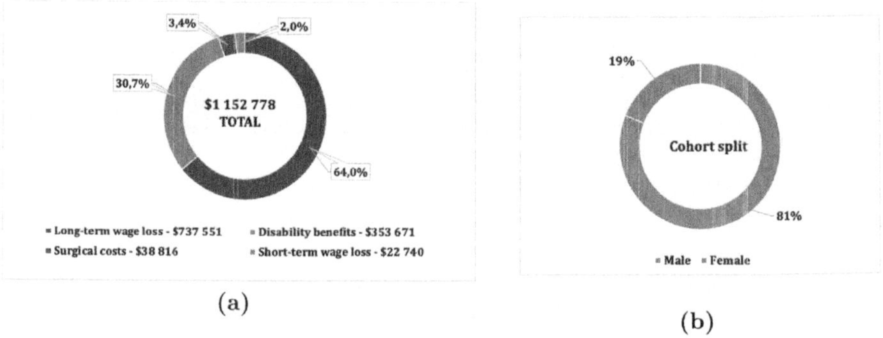

Fig. 3. Socio-economic aspects of PNIs: (a) breakdown of the lifetime cost for a traumatic brachial plexus injury in the USA [18]; (b) gender distribution of patients with PNIs [4].

In contrast, CTS incur much smaller direct costs. A Monte Carlo analysis in [17] estimated the mean total societal cost for operative CTS management at approximately $3,537, with surgery proving more cost-effective than nonoperative care. For patients with chronic nerve pain or injury, the financial burden is also significant: a cross-sectional USA study found considerable out-of-pocket expenses, missed workdays, and medical debt among individuals seeking surgery for chronic peripheral nerve injuries [18].

Indirect costs, including productivity loss and fiscal transfers, represent a significant portion of the overall economic burden of major PNIs. In particular, a USA lifetime BPI patient for a 26-year-old male manual laborer (base case) was estimated to incur substantial short-term and long-term financial losses [19]. These included short-term wage loss of $22,740, long-term wage loss of $737,551, and disability benefits amounting to $353,671, leading to a mean total indirect cost of $1,113,962 per patient (median $801,723), as shown in Fig. 3. This highlights the significant economic impact on individuals and society, underscoring the need for effective interventions to reduce long-term costs.

Crucially, this model demonstrated the sensitivity of indirect costs to return-to-work (RTW) outcomes. By doubling the probability of RTW into lower-paying employment, the model estimated a reduction in per-patient indirect costs to $867,987, resulting in savings of approximately $246,000 [19]. From a public payer perspective, disability transfers represent a significant fiscal expenditure. The same model attributed $353,671 to disability benefits alone [19]. Data from European insurers similarly reflect persistent public costs: in the German cohort, 30% of patients qualified for a work-disability pension, with an average annual payout of €3,187, leading to a projected lifetime liability of approximately €102,167 per recipient [6].

Broader social costs from upper-limb trauma—where PNIs are most commonly found—are substantial, even when averaged across a range of different injuries. In [20], a national study, hand and wrist injuries alone accounted for $740 million annually, with productivity losses making up 56% of the total costs. While these studies include various non-nerve injuries, they help contextualize the societal burden of upper-extremity morbidity. Taken together, contemporary evidence highlights the following key points:

- PNIs primarily affect men in their most productive years, with the injuries often resulting from motor vehicle accidents or sharp tools [4,15];
- While direct acute, surgical, and rehabilitation costs are significant, the long-term impact of productivity loss and disability payments outweighs these immediate expenses [6,16,19];
- Policies and treatments that yield even modest improvements in return-to-work (RTW) rates can result in large, quantifiable savings—both in terms of societal costs (hundreds of thousands of dollars per patient for major injuries) and government budgets through reduced disability transfers [6,19].

Consequently, timely referral, evidence-based surgical reconstruction, and access to rehabilitation and vocational reintegration should be viewed not only as clinical imperatives, but also as fiscal policy strategies with measurable returns on investment.

4 Current Therapeutic Solutions

Given the significant social and economic burden of PNIs, effective therapeutic strategies are essential not only for improving patient outcomes but also for reducing long-term healthcare costs and productivity losses. Currently, available solutions span pharmacology, noninvasive and implanted neuromodulation, manual neurodynamics, acupuncture, robotic exoskeletons, and surgery [1]. In this section, we provide an analysis of each modality, summarizing its mechanism, historical introduction, efficacy, adverse events (AEs), and innovation status. Figure 4 illustrates the trade-off between effectiveness and adverse effects for the existing solutions. In short, safety (low adverse effects) generally opposes efficacy across PNI solutions, with invasiveness and systemic exposure being the main drivers of adverse events.

Pharmacological Therapies. Drug strategies aim to enhance regeneration or control neuropathic pain. Following the discovery of nerve growth factor (NGF)

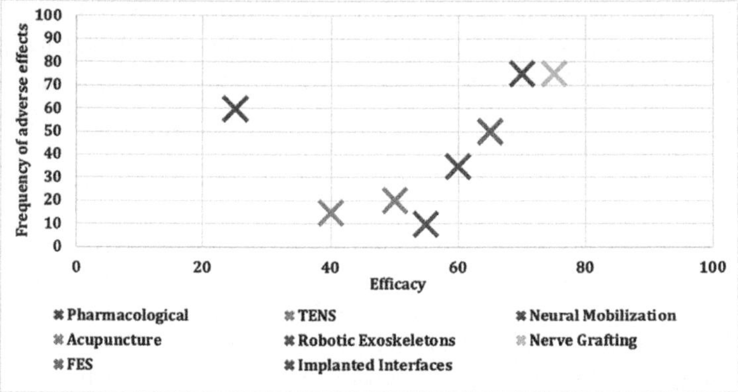

Fig. 4. Efficacy (higher is better) and adverse effects (higher is worse) trade-off, measured heuristically [1].

and other neurotrophins such as brain-derived neurotrophic factor (BDNF) (mid-20th century), agents including tacrolimus (FK506; identified for neurite outgrowth in the 1990s) have shown regeneration benefits (e.g., ∼12–15% axon-growth increases and faster reinnervation in preclinical/early studies) [21,22]. Clinical translation remains limited: no disease-modifying medication reliably restores nerve function; efforts now emphasize localized delivery (to mitigate systemic toxicities like infection risk, nephrotoxicity, seizures) and combination approaches [21,22]. Following the advances of the early 2000s, progress has been incremental [21,22].

Transcutaneous Electrical Nerve Stimulation (TENS). TENS (modern form late 1960s) delivers cutaneous pulses that activate large afferents and modulate pain pathways (gate-control and endogenous opioids) [23]. Evidence syntheses report modest-to-moderate pain reductions versus placebo with an excellent safety profile (mainly mild skin irritation); technology matured by the 1970s1980s with subsequent incremental refinements [23].

Neural Mobilization (neurodynamics). Formalized in the 1980s1990s, nerve "gliding" seeks to restore excursion, reduce edema/adhesions, and down-modulate mechanosensitivity. A 2024 systematic review and meta-analysis showed short-term physiological gains—motor conduction velocity (MCV) 3 m/s and sensory conduction velocity (SCV) 11 m/s—alongside symptom improvements in entrapment neuropathies [24]. AEs are rare; in one randomized clinical trial (RCT), mobilization had no reported side effects while 3/31 patients on ibuprofen discontinued for AEs [25]. Core methods have remained stable since the early 2000s [24].

Acupuncture for Painful Diabetic Peripheral Neuropathy (pDPN). Applied to neuropathic pain with proposed effects on microcirculation, neurotrophic signaling, and central neuromodulation, acupuncture has gained supportive evidence: recent reviews/meta-analyses report significant pain reduction and improvements in nerve conduction metrics (MCV, SCV) with favorable safety (no excess serious AEs) [26,28]. The technique is longstanding; contemporary work focuses on dosing/standardization rather than new procedural paradigms [26,28].

Exoskeletons for Motor Rehabilitation. After early concepts in the 1960s, clinically used lower-limb robotic exoskeletons emerged circa 20122015. In a 2023 randomized controlled trial (RCT) for incomplete spinal cord injury (SCI), exoskeleton training improved the Walking Index for Spinal Cord Injury II (WISCI-II) by ~ 3.5 points after 15 sessions versus < 1 in controls, with low serious-AE rates under supervision [29]. Devices restore task ability (gait practice, standing) and second-order benefits (conditioning, mood) but do not biologically repair nerves; innovation since the mid-2010s has been largely iterative (lighter frames, better control) [29].

Nerve Grafting and Surgical Repair. When tension-free neurorrhaphy is not possible, gaps are bridged with grafts. Decellularized allografts (introduced clinically in the late 2000s) preserve guidance architecture without chronic immunosuppression and now approach autograft sensory outcomes for moderate gaps: $\sim 87\%$ meaningful sensory recovery (Medical Research Council, MRC, sensory scale $S \geq 3$) for ≤ 50 mm, and $\sim 69\%$ for 5070 mm [27]. Donor-site morbidity limits autografts; typical surgical risks (infection, scarring) apply [27]. Major innovation plateaued after the adoption of processed allografts; current work explores adjuncts (bioactive cargos, tissue engineering) [27].

Electrical Stimulation and Neural Interfaces. Functional electrical stimulation (FES; in clinical use since the 1960s1990s) restores task-level functions (e.g., foot-drop correction, grasp) and confers physiological benefits despite fatigue-limited endurance; AEs are usually local (skin irritation, muscle soreness) with low serious-event rates for implanted systems [30]. Next-generation peripheral nerve interfaces enable bidirectional control and sensory feedback; human studies demonstrate stable, naturalistic tactile percepts over monthsyears with improved manipulation, indicating an active innovation frontier rather than a plateau [31].

In conclusion, noninvasive modalities (TENS, neural mobilization, acupuncture) offer symptom relief with excellent safety; exoskeletons restore function at the activity level; surgery (especially processed allografts) improves anatomic continuity with gap - and context - dependent outcomes; FES provides functional gains; and invasive neural interfaces are rapidly advancing toward finer, more durable bidirectional control. Most modalities, such as TENS, neural mobilization, and grafting, reached their main innovation plateau between the 1980s and 2010s, while neural interfaces remain under active development

5 A Prospective Implanted Device

As part of this review, we summarize a representative example of an implantable bypass concept, illustrating how current research trends may converge toward future therapeutic solutions. While current therapeutic strategies for PNIs offer a range of solutions, from pharmacological treatments to advanced surgical interventions, many of these approaches focus primarily on symptom management or partial restoration of function. These treatments often fall short of fully restoring the complex functions of the peripheral nervous system, particularly in cases of severe or chronic injury. As such, there is a growing need for alternative approaches that not only address the symptoms but also offer more comprehensive, long-term solutions for nerve regeneration and functional recovery.

In this context, a fully implantable device is proposed as a possible solution. The proposed system acts as a functional bypass, restoring information flow across the impaired peripheral pathway [32]. By capturing neural activity on one side of the lesion, interpreting it externally thanks data analysis, and reinjecting a physiologically meaningful command on the other side. This innovative approach seeks to bridge the gap between damaged neural circuits and restore vital functions.

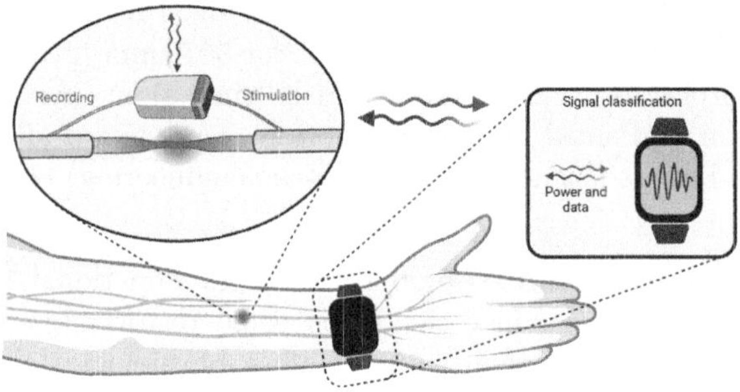

Fig. 5. Representative implantable bypass concept (illustrative example).

An example of a potential solution is illustrated in Fig. 5. The implant consists of non-penetrating, multi-contact nerve cuffs placed both proximally and distally to the lesion [3]. These cuffs gently encircle the nerve, ensuring long-term mechanical stability and a low-trauma interface for both sensing and stimulation [33].

Proximally, the cuff records neural activity associated with voluntary movements (efferent flow) or sensory signals traveling toward the brain (afferent flow). Distally, a similar cuff provides targeted electrical stimulation (neuromodulation)

to recruit the appropriate nerve fibers, while ensuring safety by controlling factors such as current density, pulse width, and duty cycle. The system uses a low-power, bidirectional telemetry link to connect the implant to an external processing unit, which handles computationally demanding tasks, minimizing heat dissipation and reducing the implant size [3].

The system works as follows [3]: The proximal cuff detects weak neural signals, typically in the range of 10–50 μV, which are often masked by noise from surrounding muscle activity and environmental interference. Given the small signal size, low-impedance electrodes are required for proper signal acquisition. These signals are processed through analog and digital filtering, reject interference, and suppress common-mode artifacts, such as motion and stimulation after-potentials.

The measured signals are characterized by a low signal-to-noise ratio of around 2 dB and a wide frequency band from 500 Hz and 7 kHz with a energy peak at about 2 kHz, ensuring minimal overlap with other biological signals. Due to the complexity and variability of the signal, the external processor performs signal analysis using advanced techniques as shown in [3, 34, 35].

Achieving near real-time classification is essential to ensure physiological responses remain natural, which makes feature extraction from ENG signals a critical step. Three main approaches dominate the literature: spike detection, which isolates action potentials but requires high signal quality [34]; window-based feature extraction, which characterizes activity in short temporal windows and is more robust to noisy signals [35]; and hybrid kernel methods, which combine local spike information with global activity patterns [3]. The latter, often implemented with convolutional or recurrent neural networks, has shown the best balance between accuracy and robustness.

After the residual neural signal has been classified—i.e., once the intended movement direction has been identified—the system generates a stimulation pattern that respects the natural timing and spatial selectivity of neural activity, ensuring that only the appropriate fibers are activated. The system enforces charge balance, monitors current compliance, and checks electrode impedance to detect unsafe conditions, using watchdog logic to silence output in case of uncertainty or anomalies [32, 36, 38].

For sensory restoration, the process is reversed: the distal cuff senses sensory events (e.g., touch or proprioception), the external processor interprets them, and the proximal cuff delivers the appropriate afferent stimulation to replace the lost sensory input. Since both acquisition and stimulation occur at each site, crosstalk between recording and stimulation can arise; to mitigate this, blanking circuits are commonly implemented to suppress stimulation artifacts during signal acquisition [32, 36].

To minimize latency between user intention (decoded motor command), its execution through stimulation, and the resulting sensory feedback (to give the sensation of the moviment), computation-heavy tasks are offloaded to a support external unit. This enables more sophisticated algorithms and remote updates without increasing the implant's complexity [37].

Comparable approaches have been demonstrated in recent literature. For instance, the SenseBack system provides a fully implantable 32-channel bidirectional interface for peripheral nerves, demonstrated in preclinical studies [36]. In humans, closed-loop sensory feedback via intraneural electrodes in human subjects has restored naturalistic sensations and improved function with lower-limb prostheses [38]. Together, these technologies outline the translational trajectory toward functional bypass systems capable of restoring bidirectional communication after nerve injury [32].

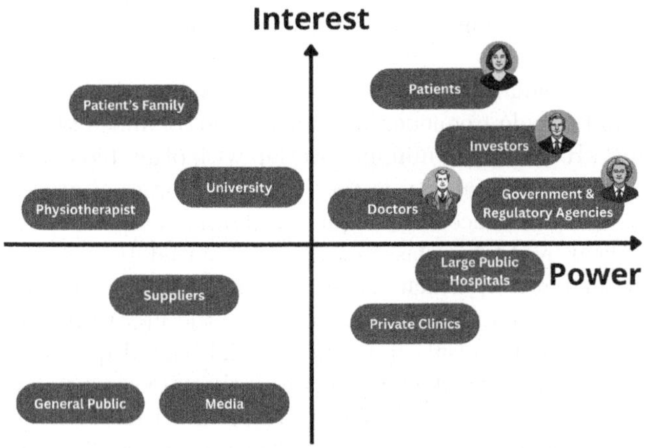

Fig. 6. Stakeholder ecosystem: Power Interest Matrix of Johnson & Scholes.

This proposed system represents a promising alternative to current therapies, offering a more comprehensive approach to treating peripheral nerve injuries. By bypassing the impaired pathways and restoring functional information flow, it not only addresses immediate symptoms but also facilitates long-term functional recovery. The integration of advanced computational processing, minimal invasiveness, and wireless communication underscores its potential to significantly enhance patient outcomes and reduce the overall burden on healthcare systems.

6 Conclusions

In summary, this review has outlined the multifaceted impact of PNIs and provided a structured overview of existing diagnostic and therapeutic solutions. By integrating evidence from clinical, engineering, and socioeconomic perspectives, it identifies current limitations and emerging opportunities for innovation. To move from promising therapeutic concepts to real-world impact, PNIs must be addressed not only at the technical and clinical level but also through coordinated engagement of the wider healthcare ecosystem. After outlining the dual burden of PNIs, the continuum of current care options, and the potential of a novel implantable bypass system, it becomes clear that long-term success will ultimately depend on the alignment of diverse stakeholders, each with each with varying degrees of interest and influence [39], as illustrated in Fig. 6.

Patients and caregivers are the primary beneficiaries and risk-bearers: they balance potential functional recovery and quality-of-life gains against surgical burden, device maintenance, and the psychological demands of a hybrid implantedexternal system. Clinicians oversee indication, implantation, programming, and follow-up, so they require clear workflows and seamless integration with existing practice. Hospital administrators and ethics committees evaluate operational fit, liability, and governance. Payers and health-technology assessment bodies prioritize cost-effectiveness, equity of access, and evidence quality. Regulators assess safety, performance, and benefitrisk across pre- and post-market phases. Manufacturers and suppliers must ensure product quality, resilient supply chains, and field serviceability. Standards organizations and cybersecurity experts promote interoperability and secure communication. Researchers depend on ethically governed data and updatable algorithms, while public agencies, advocacy groups, and investors shape diffusion through funding, education, and transparency. Effective adoption hinges on alignment around a shared value proposition: meaningful, measurable restoration of function delivered safely and sustainably.

The analysis of stakeholders highlights that technical innovation alone is insufficient: lasting impact requires coordinated action across patients, clinicians, institutions, payers, and regulators. PNIs remain a major unmet need, and investing in solutions that are safe, effective, and economically sustainable is essential. The proposed implantable bypass exemplifies this potential, but its translation will depend on rigorous validation and early integration into healthcare systems. Addressing peripheral nerve injuries requires more than incremental progress: only sustained investment in translational solutions that unite engineering, medicine, and policy will deliver therapies capable of restoring autonomy and reducing the long-term burden on society. Future research should build upon those investigations through interdisciplinary collaboration and validation of the most promising approaches in real-world clinical contexts.

Acknowledgment. This work was supported by the Institute of Information & communications Technology Planning & Evaluation (IITP) grant funded by the Korea government (MSIT)(No.RS-202400508465). We thank Alta Scuola Politecnica for the educational and financial support, and professors Maurizio Magarini and Paolo Motto Ros for their mentorship. Thanks also to all the students who helped us for their invaluable contribution and collaboration throughout our work.

References

1. Coviello, A.: Emerging peripheral nerve injuries recovery: advanced nerve-cuff electrode model interface for implantable devices. In: Global Conference on Wireless and Optical Technologies, pp. 1–7. GCWOT (2024)

2. Koeppen, A.H.: Wallerian degeneration: history and clinical significance. J. Neurol. Sci. **220**(1), 115–117 (2004)
3. Coviello, A., et al.: Artificial neural networks-based real-time classification of eng signals for implanted nerve interfaces. IEEE J. Sel. Areas Commun. **42**(8), 2080–2095 (2024)
4. Zaidman, M., et al.: Epidemiology of peripheral nerve and brachial plexus injuries in a trauma population. Can. J. Surg. E261–E268 (2024). https://doi.org/10.1503/cjs.002424. PMID: 38925857; PMCID: PMC11230667
5. de Heer, E.W., et al.: The association of depression and anxiety with pain: a study from NESDA. PLoS One, 9(10), e106907 (2014). https://doi.org/10.1371/journal.pone.0106907. Erratum in: PLoS One **9**(12), e115077 (2014)
6. Bergmeister, K.D., et al.: Acute and long-term costs of 268 peripheral nerve injuries in the upper extremity. PLoS ONE **15**(4), e0229530 (2020). https://doi.org/10.1371/journal.pone.0229530
7. Chandrasekaran, S., et al.: Case study: persistent recovery of hand movement and tactile sensation in peripheral nerve injury using targeted transcutaneous spinal cord stimulation. Front. Neurosci. **17**, 1210544 (2023). https://doi.org/10.3389/fnins.2023.1210544
8. Magnéli, M., Axenhus, M.: Epidemiology and regional variance of traumatic peripheral nerve injuries in Sweden: A 15-year observational study. PLoS One **19**(10), e0310988 (2024). https://doi.org/10.1371/journal.pone.0310988
9. Erlangsen, A., et al.: Association Between neurological disorders and death by suicide in Denmark. JAMA **323**(5), 444–454 (2020). https://doi.org/10.1001/jama.2019.21834
10. Adu, Y., et al.: Psychology of nerve injury, repair, and recovery: a systematic review. Front. Rehabil. Sci. **5**, 1421704 (2024). https://doi.org/10.3389/fresc.2024.1421704. PMID: 39568638
11. Landers, Z.A., et al.: The psychological impact of adult traumatic brachial plexus injury. J. Hand Surg. Am. **43**(10), 950.e1-950.e6 (2018). https://doi.org/10.1016/j.jhsa.2018.02.019
12. Ultee, J., et al.: Early posttraumatic psychological stress following peripheral nerve injury: a prospective study. J. Plast. Reconstr. Aesthet. Surg. **66**(10), 1316–1321 (2013). https://doi.org/10.1016/j.bjps.2013.05.017
13. Yannascoli, S.M., et al.: A population-based assessment of depression and anxiety in patients with brachial plexus injuries. J. Hand Surg. Am. **43**(12), 1136.e1-1136.e9 (2018). https://doi.org/10.1016/j.jhsa.2018.03.056
14. Jia, S., et al.: Determinants of anxiety and depression in patients with cubital tunnel syndrome. BMC Psychiatry **20**, 540 (2020). https://doi.org/10.1186/s12888-020-02934-0
15. Padovano, W.M., et al.: Incidence of nerve injury after extremity trauma in the United States. Hand (N Y) **17**(4), 615–623 (2022). https://doi.org/10.1177/1558944720963895
16. Dy, C.J., et al.: Direct cost of surgically treated adult traumatic brachial plexus injuries. J. Hand Surg. Global Online **2**(2), 77–79 (2020). https://doi.org/10.1016/j.jhsg.2019.12.001
17. Gabrielli, A.S., et al.: The direct and indirect costs to society of carpal tunnel release. Hand (N Y) **15**(2), NP1–NP5 (2020). https://doi.org/10.1177/1558944718810855
18. Felder, J.M., Ducic, I.: Cross-sectional evaluation of the economic burden on patients seeking surgical treatment for chronic nerve injuries. Ann. Plast. Surg. **88**(5), 485–490 (2022). https://doi.org/10.1097/SAP.0000000000002924

19. Hong, T.S., et al.: Indirect cost of traumatic brachial plexus injuries in the United States. J. Bone Joint Surg. (Am.) **101**(16), e80 (2019). https://doi.org/10.2106/JBJS.18.00658
20. de Putter, C.E., et al.: Economic impact of hand and wrist injuries: health-care costs and productivity costs in a population-based study. J. Bone Joint Surg. (Am.) **94**(9), e56 (2012). https://doi.org/10.2106/JBJS.K.00561
21. Bolandghamat, S., et al.: Recent findings on the effects of pharmacological agents on the nerve regeneration after peripheral nerve injury. Curr. Neuropharmacol. **18**(11), 1154–1163 (2020). https://doi.org/10.2174/1570159X18666200507084024
22. Millesi, F., et al.: Localized tacrolimus therapy: innovations in peripheral nerve regeneration through advanced drug delivery systems. Expert Rev. Neurother. **15**(10), 743–748 (2024). https://doi.org/10.1080/20415990.2024.2392481
23. Vance, C.G.T., et al.: Using TENS for pain control: update on the state of the evidence. Medicina **58**(10), 1332 (2022). https://doi.org/10.3390/medicina58101332
24. Bittencourt, J.V., et al.: Neural mobilisation effects in nerve function and nerve structure of patients with peripheral neuropathic pain: A systematic review with meta-analysis. PLoS One **19**(11), e0313025 (2024). https://doi.org/10.1371/journal.pone.0313025
25. Rodriguez-Sanz, D., et al.: Effectiveness of median nerve neural mobilization versus oral ibuprofen in subjects with cervicobrachial pain: a randomized clinical trial. Arch. Med. Sci. **14**(4), 871–879 (2018). https://doi.org/10.5114/aoms.2017.70328
26. Wang, L., Wang, L.-M.: Perspective on acupuncture treatment for diabetic peripheral neuropathy: A perspective. Medicine **104**(23), e42646 (2025). https://doi.org/10.1097/MD.0000000000042646
27. Buncke, G.: Peripheral nerve allograft: how innovation has changed surgical practice. Plast. Aesthet. Res. **9** 38 (2022). https://doi.org/10.20517/2347-9264.2022.08
28. Liu, J.: Efficacy and safety of acupuncture for painful diabetic neuropathy: a systematic review and meta-analysis. Front. Neurol. **15**, 1402458 (2024). https://doi.org/10.3389/fneur.2024.1402458
29. Gil-Agudo, Á., et al.: Exoskeleton-based training improves walking independence in incomplete spinal cord injury patients: results from a randomized controlled trial. J. NeuroEng. Rehabil. **20**, 36 (2023). https://doi.org/10.1186/s12984-023-01158-z
30. Harkema, M.S., et al.: Physiologic effects of electrical stimulation for rehabilitation and regeneration after spinal cord injury. J. Neurotrauma **25**(2), 201–210 (2008). https://doi.org/10.1089/neu.2007.0487
31. Graczyk, J.M.: A neural interface provides long-term stable natural touch perception. Sci. Transl. Med. **10**(439), eaao3252 (2018). https://doi.org/10.1126/scitranslmed.aao3252
32. Denison, T., Morrell, M.J.: Neuromodulation in 2035: the neurology future forecasting series. Neurology **98**(2), 65–72 (2022)
33. Rijnbeek, E.H., et al.: Update on peripheral nerve electrodes for closed-loop neuroprosthetics. Front. Neurosci. **12**, 350 (2018)
34. Koh, R.G., et al.: Selective peripheral nerve recordings from nerve cuff electrodes using convolutional neural networks. J. Neural Eng. **17**(1), 016042 (2020)
35. Brunton, E.: Identification of sensory information in mixed nerves using multichannel cuff electrodes for closed loop neural prostheses. In: International IEEE/EMBS Conference on Neural Engineering, pp. 391–394. NER (2017)
36. Williams, I., et al.: SenseBack-an implantable system for bidirectional neural interfacing. IEEE Trans. Biomed. Circ. Syst. **14**(5), 1079–1087 (2020)

37. Coviello, A., et al.: Comparison of data compression methods for implanted real-time peripheral nervous system. In: IEEE International Conference on Metrology for eXtended Reality, Artificial Intelligence and Neural Engineering (MetroXRAINE), pp. 110–115 (2023)
38. Petrini, F.M., et al.: Enhancing functional abilities and cognitive integration of the lower limb prosthesis. Sci. Transl. Med. **11**(512), eaav8939 (2019)
39. Hogg, H.D.J., et al.: Stakeholder perspectives of clinical artificial intelligence implementation: A qualitative systematic review. PLoS Digit. Health **25**, e39742 (2023)

Modeling of Propagation Characteristic for VHF-High Maritime Broadband System

Takahiro Ito[1(✉)], Masaaki Yamanaka[2], Daisuke Anzai[3], and Hirokazu Tanaka[1,3]

[1] Hiroshima City University, Hiroshima 731-3194, Japan
ito-t@hiroshima-cu.ac.jp
[2] Japan Coast Academy, Hiroshima 737-0832, Japan
[3] Osaka Metropolitan University, Osaka 599-8531, Japan

Abstract. The VHF-High band in Japan, covering the 170-222 MHz range, has undergone a major shift in its role. It was once dedicated to analog television broadcasts, but after those services ended, the band became available for new broadband communication applications. Because these frequencies are lower than those used by cellular networks or wireless LANs, they are particularly well-suited for creating links that can maintain stability over long distances. This property makes the VHF-High band a strong candidate for supporting maritime broadband systems, which must function in expansive oceanic areas where other technologies may struggle. However, wireless communication at sea faces an inherent limitation: the Earth's curvature restricts the reach of line-of-sight signals, creating natural boundaries on transmission range. To better understand how far signals in this band can actually travel across water, this research begins with a detailed investigation of radio propagation in marine environments. By modeling and analyzing these characteristics, the study seeks to quantify feasible communication distances and clarify the potential benefits of using the VHF-High spectrum at sea. The outcomes of this work could contribute to the development of more reliable and far-reaching maritime broadband infrastructure.

Keywords: Maritime broadcast · VHF-High band · Propagation model

1 Introduction

Providing appropriate medical services for seafarers is essential to prevent illness from worsening and to ensure quick response in emergencies. Since medical resources on ships are limited, initial care often depends on self-treatment or basic aid from officers with medical duties. However, these officers usually have only limited medical knowledge, which makes accurate diagnosis difficult. In

H. Tanaka et al. (Eds.): BodyNets 2025, LNICST 714, pp. 159–166, 2026.
https://doi.org/10.1007/978-3-032-38657-1_12

such cases, remote consultation with onshore doctors becomes crucial, and ICT enables telemedicine by connecting ships and land.

For Beyond 5G/6G, wide-area coverage including maritime regions is an important objective [1,2]. While terrestrial networks are well established, oceans remain outside the coverage of mobile communication services. Traditionally, ship communication in open seas has relied on satellites, which suffer from low throughput and high cost. Recently, low Earth orbit (LEO) satellites have made broadband communication at sea more feasible.

In Japan, the VHF-High band (170-222 MHz), formerly used for analog TV broadcasting, has been reassigned to public broadband mobile services. Applying this band to maritime communication offers the potential for low-cost and long-distance broadband. For example, telemedical assistance services (TMAS) using the VHF Data Exchange System (VDES) have been studied [3] and services in the EU already provide medical support via email or telephone [4]. Advanced systems such as the Marine Doctor (M Doc) [5] further improve support quality.

This paper focuses on constructing and analyzing a one-to-one maritime propagation model using the VHF-High band. This model serves not only to clarify basic propagation characteristics, but also as a foundation for future relay transmission systems, where multiple ships act as relay nodes to cover wider sea areas.

The paper is organized as follows. Section 2 describes the system configuration. Section 3 presents the propagation model and simulation results. Section 4 concludes the paper with a summary and discussion of future developments including relay systems. Figure 1 illustrates the conceptual diagram of the proposed maritime broadband system. It includes land-based endpoints, maritime endpoints, and either ships or UAVs in between them. A VHF-High band signal transmitted from land is received by an intermediary ship, as a relay node, which then retransmits the signal towards the next relay ship. This transmission scheme forms a relay network in maritime wireless communications.

2 System Model

When transceivers are placed only a few meters above the sea surface, line-of-sight (LOS) communication is possible up to approximately 30 km. This can be modeled as a two-ray system consisting of a direct wave and a sea-surface reflected wave. Beyond this distance, the direct wave is blocked by the horizon, resulting in non-line-of-sight (NLOS) conditions. In maritime environments, NLOS communication is mainly governed by spherical diffraction, which introduces much higher propagation loss than LOS transmission. Whether LOS can be achieved depends on the distance between the transmitter and receiver and their respective heights, as illustrated in Fig. 2. The horizon distance d_h is given by

$$d_h = \sqrt{h_t^2 + 2rh_t} \tag{1}$$

where r is the Earth's radius and h_t is the transmitter height. LOS communication is possible if the receiver height h_r is equal to or greater than h_t.

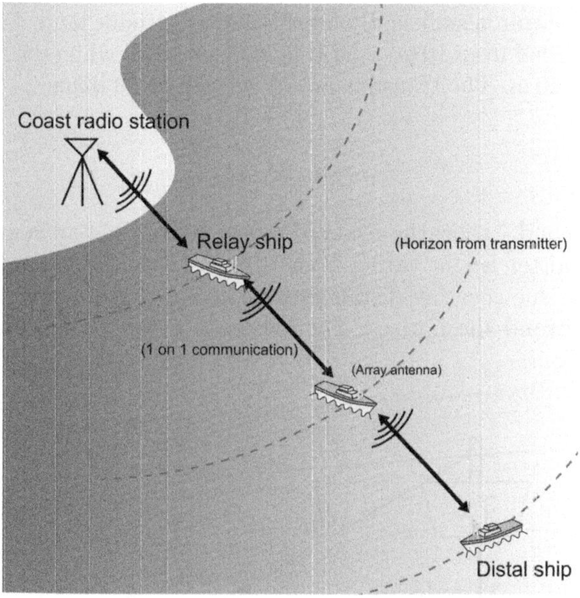

Fig. 1. Conceptual diagram of the maritime broadband system. A coast radio station and ships can communicate directly in a one-to-one link. By configuring a relay structure with intermediate ships, distant vessels can also establish broadband communication.

In this study, propagation characteristics were analyzed using a ray-tracing approach that considers both sea-surface reflection and spherical diffraction. Transmitter and receiver heights were specified, and isotropic antennas were assumed. The transmission distance was randomly varied up to 100 km, and propagation loss was calculated for each case. In addition, because the refractive index of the atmosphere decreases with altitude, electromagnetic waves are slightly bent downward rather than traveling in perfectly straight lines. This effect can be approximated by assuming an equivalent Earth radius of 4/3 the actual value, which is commonly used for linear modeling. Figure 2 shows a comparison between analytical and theoretical values of LOS distance under this model.

The received signal power P_r is expressed as

$$P_r = \frac{1}{L_p} G_t G_r P_t \tag{2}$$

where L_p is the propagation loss, G_t and G_r are the transmit and receive antenna gains, and P_t is the transmit power. When using an isotropic antenna, both G_t and G_r are equal to 1.

Propagation characteristics were further evaluated using the commercial software RapLAB with a ray-tracing method. Transmit and receive points were randomly selected within a sufficiently large sea area without land. The transmitter height h_t was varied from 10 m to 50 m in steps of 10 m, while the receiver height h_r was fixed at 10 m. The transmit power was set at 30 dBm.

3 Results

Figure 3, 4, 5, 6 and 7 show the received power when using an isotropic antenna, with the transmitter height varied from 10 m to 50 m. Two approximate fitting lines are drawn: one covering distances from 10 km to the horizon, and another for distances beyond the horizon. For distances below 10 km, an extrapolated curve is applied.

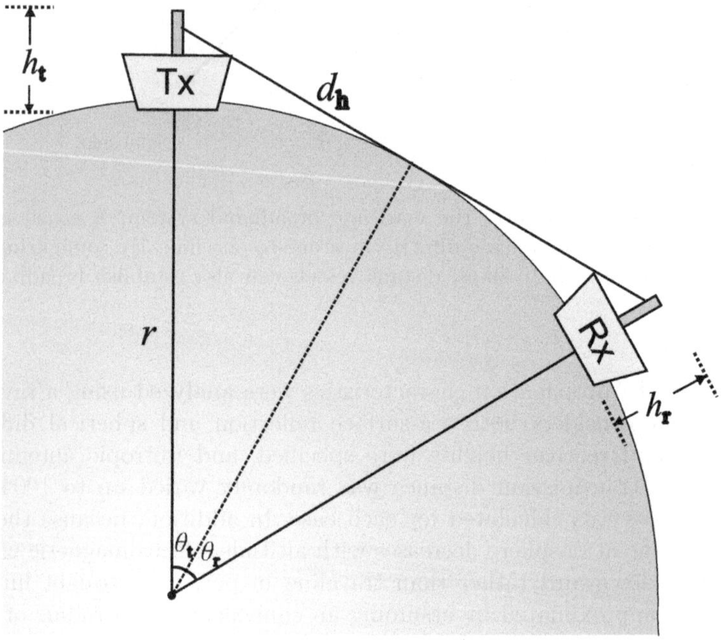

Fig. 2. NLOS condition caused by horizon shadowing. Increasing the transmitter height h_t extends the horizon distance, enabling LOS communication over longer ranges. Beyond the horizon, signals propagate in NLOS conditions through diffraction.

The higher the transmitter is placed, the farther the distance to the horizon becomes. Up to the horizon distance, the received power follows a two-wave propagation model consisting of a direct wave and a sea-surface reflected wave. This results in large fluctuations due to destructive interference. Beyond the horizon, the propagation shifts to a single-wave diffraction model, where the received power decreases linearly on a logarithmic scale. As the transmitter height increases, the horizon distance also extends.

For distances up to the horizon, the fitting curve is expressed by Eq. (3), and for distances beyond the horizon, by Eq. (4):

$$P_r = ad^b + c \tag{3}$$

$$P_r = PL_0 + 10n \log d/d_0 \tag{4}$$

Here, d is the distance and PL_0 is the path loss at the reference distance ($d_0 = 1$ km). The coefficients for each equation are listed in Table 1.

Table 1. Parameters of propagation model for VHF-High maritime communication

h_t [m]	a	b	c	n	PL_0
10	−0.299	1.601	−81.37	−1.983	−70.42
20	−0.0878	1.862	−81.68	−1.977	−70.57
30	−0.0513	1.937	−81.46	−1.972	−70.70
40	−0.0256	2.063	−82.40	−1.966	−70.84
50	−0.0102	2.249	−84.15	−1.961	−70.96

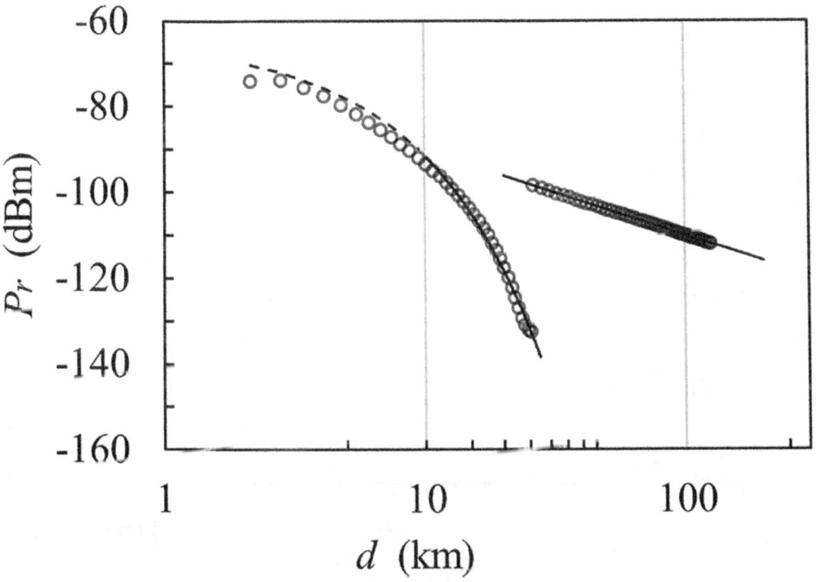

Fig. 3. Received power with $h_t = 10$.

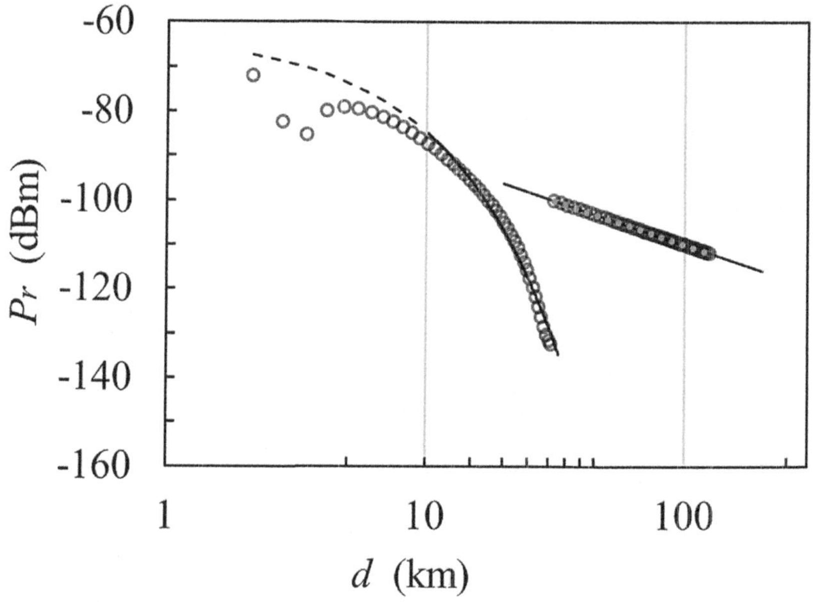

Fig. 4. Received power with $h_t = 20$.

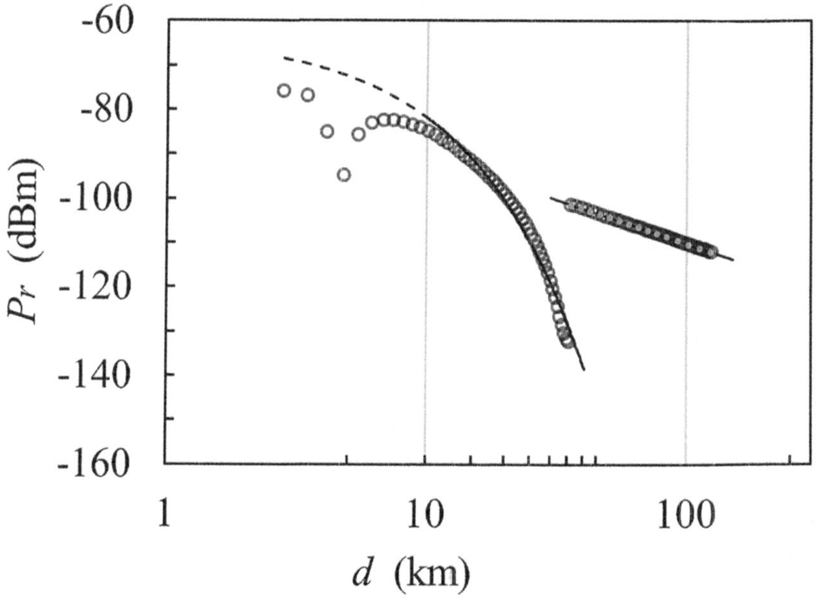

Fig. 5. Received power with $h_t = 30$.

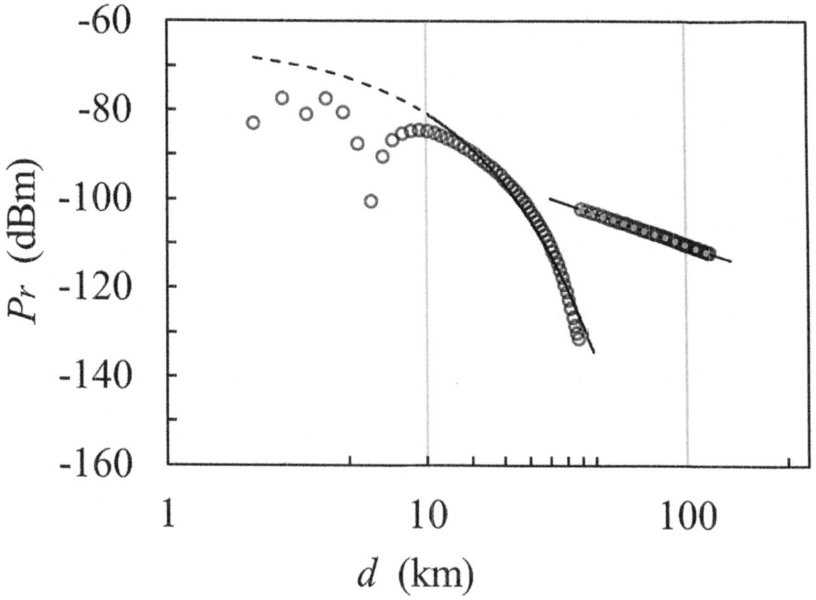

Fig. 6. Received power with $h_t = 40$.

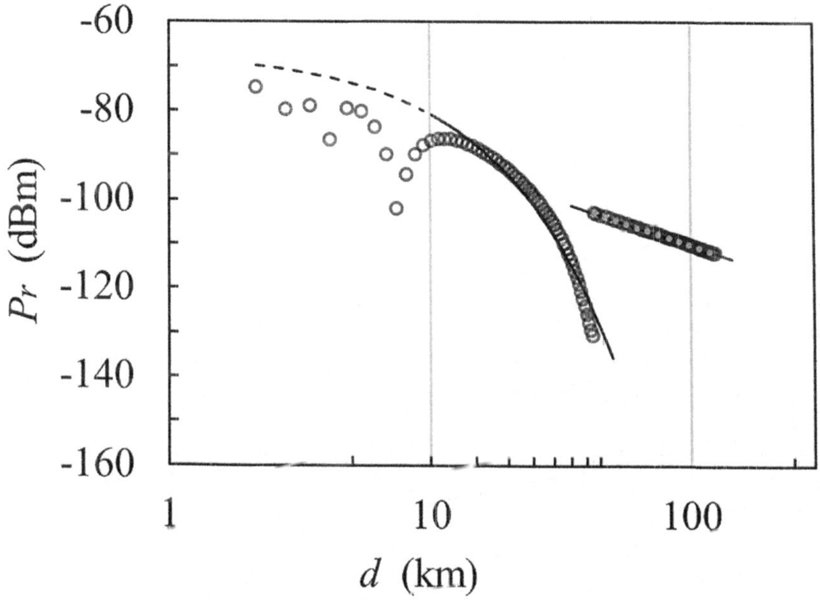

Fig. 7. Received power with $h_t = 50$.

4 Conclusion

This paper presented a study on maritime broadband communication using the VHF-High band. A one-to-one propagation model at sea was developed and analyzed, considering both sea-surface reflection and spherical diffraction. The analysis showed that line-of-sight communication can be achieved up to the horizon, following a two-wave model with significant power fluctuations caused by interference. Beyond the horizon, propagation is governed by diffraction, leading to higher path loss that can be represented by a logarithmic decay model.

Simulation results confirmed that the received power strongly depends on the transmitter height, which determines the distance to the horizon. Empirical fitting equations were derived for both LOS and NLOS conditions, providing a practical way to estimate propagation loss in maritime environments. These results serve as a fundamental step toward the design of broadband systems at sea using the VHF-High band.

Although this study focused on one-to-one communication, the propagation model established here forms the basis for more advanced schemes. In particular, the insights gained can be extended to multi-hop relay transmission systems, where multiple ships act as relay nodes to enable reliable broadband coverage over wide oceanic areas. Future work will include validating the model through field measurements and applying it to the design and optimization of relay-based maritime communication systems.

Acknowledgement. This research and development work was supported by the MIC/FORWARD #JPMI250830001.

References

1. Wang, C.X., et al.: On the road to 6G: visions, requirements, key technologies, and testbeds. IEEE Commun. Surv. Tutorials **25**(2), 905–974 (2023)
2. White Paper 5G Evolution and 6G. https://www.docomo.ne.jp/english/. Accessed 19 Sep 2025
3. IALA, G1117 VHF Data Exchange System (VDES) Overview. https://www.iala.int/. Accessed 19 Sep 2025
4. Getu Gamo Sagaro and Francesco Amenta: Past, present, and future perspectives of telemedical assistance at sea: a systematic review. Int. Marit. Health **71**(2), 97–104 (2020)
5. Battineni, G., Chintalapudi, N., Amenta, F.: Maritime telemedicine: design and development of an advanced healthcare system called marine doctor. J. Personalized Med. **12**(5), 832 (2022)

Advanced Sensing and Signal Processing for Health Monitoring

Trade-Offs in FMCW Radar-Based Respiration and Heart Rate Variability

Silvia Mura(✉), Davide Scazzoli, Lorenzo Fineschi, and Maurizio Magarini

Dipartimento di Elettronica, Informazione e Bioingegneria, Politecnico di Milano, Milan, Italy
{silvia.mura,davide.scazzoli,lorenzo.fineschi, maurizio.magarini}@polimi.it

Abstract. This study presents a comprehensive experimental assessment of a low-cost frequency-modulated continuous-wave (FMCW) multiple-input multiple-output (MIMO) radar for non-contact vital sign monitoring, focusing on respiratory rate (RR) and heart rate (HR) estimation. The influence of sensing distance and number of transmitted chirps on measurement accuracy is systematically quantified. Results exhibit a U-shaped error profile with optimal performance near 70 *cm*, achieving mean absolute errors of 0.8 *bpm* for RR and 3.2 *bpm* for HR. Accuracy deteriorates at short ($<$ 60 cm) and long ($>$ 100 cm) distances due to multipath, near-field, and signal-to-noise effects. Increasing chirp count enhances performance: RR errors converge asymptotically for $\geq$ 96 chirps, while HR requires at least 96 chirps for stable detection. Variability metrics, including heart and respiratory rate variability, remain less accurate ($>$ 15–30% error), indicating limited capability in capturing instantaneous fluctuations. These findings define a fundamental trade-off: the radar ensures robust estimation of average RR and HR but exhibits restricted precision in high-resolution beat-to-beat and breath-to-breath monitoring.

Keywords: FMCW Radar · Non Contact Vital Sign Monitoring · Signal Processing · Heart Rate · Respiration Rate

1 Introduction

Continuous monitoring of vital signs, particularly heart rate (HR) and respiratory rate (RR), is crucial for the early detection of physiological anomalies, as subtle fluctuations in these parameters often precede acute clinical events. Timely recognition of such changes substantially improves patient outcomes. Conventional monitoring relies on wearable devices, which provide continuous assessment during daily activities [1,2].

In specific clinical scenarios, wearable sensors are impractical or contraindicated. Patients with contagious diseases risk increased infection or disrupted

H. Tanaka et al. (Eds.): BodyNets 2025, LNICST 714, pp. 169–183, 2026.
https://doi.org/10.1007/978-3-032-38657-1_13

isolation protocols, while individuals with severe burns or skin injuries experience pain, hindered healing, or contamination from sensors. Patients with psychiatric or cognitive disorders often demonstrate poor compliance, and trauma or emergency care settings limit wearable use due to urgent interventions and equipment constraints. These limitations highlight the need for reliable, contactless vital sign monitoring solutions.

Radar-based systems offer a promising approach for non-contact vital sign (NCVS) monitoring by detecting thoracic micro-movements induced by cardiac and respiratory activity, enabling non-invasive estimation of HR and RR [3]. Early studies demonstrate the feasibility of extracting respiratory signals using short-range radar, and subsequent research confirms detection of both respiratory and cardiac-induced motion [4,5].

Radar systems for vital sign monitoring fall into continuous-wave (CW) and pulsed categories, including CW Doppler, frequency-modulated continuous-wave (FMCW), step-frequency CW (SFCW), and impulse-radio ultra-wideband (IR-UWB) [3]. CW Doppler radars are simple and cost-effective but limited in range estimation, whereas wideband techniques such as FMCW, SFCW, and IR-UWB provide more accurate distance measurements. Architectures employ single-input single-output (SISO) or multiple-input multiple-output (MIMO) configurations. SISO systems reduce complexity and cost, while MIMO designs enhance detection accuracy, extend range, and enable multi-target discrimination. Selecting an appropriate radar architecture requires balancing range, accuracy, target separation, complexity, and cost for the intended clinical application [3].

Millimeter-wave (mmWave) FMCW radar proves particularly effective for NCVS due to higher sensitivity to micro-movements, smaller antennas, and improved target separation [6]. Phased-array implementations steer the beam to detect multiple subjects in distinct angular sectors [7], but angular resolution is limited by array aperture, sequential scanning reduces temporal resolution, and overlapping echoes from closely spaced targets impair accuracy. MIMO radars use multiple transmitter (TX) and receiver (RX) antennas, often with time-division multiplexing, to enhance spatial diversity and isolate targets [8]. Low-cost radars with fewer antennas have reduced spatial resolution and multi-subject discrimination. Hybrid phased-MIMO architectures combine beamforming and MIMO principles to improve angular resolution, target separation, and temporal precision [9].

Despite recent advances in radar-based vital sign monitoring, most existing systems focus primarily on estimating average heart rate (HR) and respiratory rate (RR), offering limited insight into beat-to-beat and breath-to-breath variability. However, variability metrics, such as heart rate variability (HRV) and respiratory rate variability (BRV), are essential clinical indicators of autonomic nervous system activity and cardiopulmonary regulation, providing early markers of stress, fatigue, and pathological conditions [10]. Clinical translation of radar-based monitoring remains constrained by motion artifacts, multi-subject interference, phase noise, and environmental clutter. Although techniques such as microprocessor-controlled clutter cancellation [11], complex demodulation, motion compensation, adaptive beamforming, harmonic cancellation, wavelet decomposition, and machine learning [3,9,12,13] have attempted to mitigate these challenges, the accuracy and reliability of HRV and BRV estimation remain largely unexplored, highlighting a critical gap in understanding the trade-offs between average-rate accuracy and instantaneous physiological variability.

This study addresses this gap by performing a comprehensive experimental evaluation of a low-cost FMCW MIMO radar for non-contact monitoring of RR and HR, explicitly including variability metrics. Our results reveal a clear operational trade-off: RR can be reliably estimated across a broad range of distances (50 – 120 cm) and chirp counts (96–256), whereas accurate HR detection requires optimal positioning near 70 cm and at least 96 chirps. Variability metrics, however, remain less precise, with errors typically exceeding 15–30%, underscoring the current limitations of radar systems in resolving instantaneous physiological fluctuations. These findings suggest that while FMCW MIMO radar is well-suited for robust estimation of average vital signs, achieving clinical-grade resolution of HRV and BRV demands further refinement. Potential improvements may include multi-domain data fusion or temporal super-resolution techniques to improve beat-to-beat sensitivity. By systematically quantifying these dependencies and trade-offs, this work provides actionable guidelines for radar configuration, establishes quantitative performance benchmarks, and extends the literature by explicitly addressing variability metrics as a key factor in non-contact vital sign monitoring.

2 System Model

This section presents a rigorous mathematical formulation of the MIMO FMCW radar system for contactless vital sign monitoring. We develop a comprehensive model that integrates electromagnetic wave propagation, human physiological dynamics, and signal processing theory to enable precise extraction of cardiorespiratory parameters.

2.1 Radar Model

We consider a MIMO FMCW radar system characterized by N_{TX} transmitting antennas and N_{Rx} receiving antennas arranged in a virtual array configuration. The transmitted signal from the nth TX antenna during the cth chirp is modeled as a linear frequency-modulated (LFM) waveform

$$s_n(t) = A_{\text{TX}} \exp\left\{ j2\pi \left(f_c t + \frac{K}{2} t^2 \right) \right\}, \quad n \in 1, 2, \ldots, N_{\text{TX}}, \tag{1}$$

where f_c denotes the carrier frequency, K represents the chirp rate (frequency sweep rate), and A_{TX} is the complex transmitted coefficient.

The human subject is modeled as an extended scatterer located at range $R(t)$ and azimuth angle $\theta(t) \in [-\pi/3, \pi/3]$ relative to the radar array center. The time-varying nature of these parameters captures the micro-motion induced by cardiorespiratory activity. The received signal at the mth RX antenna from the nth TX antenna is described by

$$r_{mn}(t) = \alpha_{mn}(t) \cdot s_n(t - \tau_{mn}(t)) + w_{mn}(t) \tag{2}$$

where $\tau_{mn}(t) = \frac{2R_{mn}(t)}{c}$, c denotes the speed of light, and $w_{mn}(t) \sim \mathcal{N}(0, \sigma_w^2)$ represents circularly symmetric complex additive white Gaussian noise with zero mean and variance σ_w^2. In this model, we assume a propagation environment with no external interference or multipath reflections, such that only the direct target echo contributes to the received signal.

The complex attenuation coefficient $\alpha_{mn}(\mathrm{t}) \in \mathbb{C}$ encapsulates the comprehensive channel response

$$\alpha_{mn}(t) = \sqrt{\frac{\lambda^2 \sigma_{\mathrm{RCS}}}{(4\pi)^3 R_{mn}^4(t)}} \exp\left\{-j\frac{4\pi}{\lambda}\Delta d(t)\right\} \tag{3}$$

where $\lambda = c/f_c$ is the wavelength, σ_{RCS} is the radar cross-section of the thoracic region, and $\Delta d(t)$ represents the chest displacement from the baseline position.

Radar measurements are systematically collected and organized into a four-dimensional complex tensor $\mathbf{R} \in \mathbb{C}^{F \times N_{\mathrm{RX}} \times N_c \times N_a}$, where F is the number of temporal frames, N_c is the number of chirps per frame, and N_a is the number of fast-time samples per chirp. The temporal resolution is governed by the frame repetition interval T_f, which determines the slow-time sampling frequency $f_s = \frac{1}{T_f}$.

2.2 Cardiovascular and Respiratory Physiology

The human cardiovascular system comprises two interconnected circuits operating in synchronized cardiac cycles. Each cycle involves coordinated contractions (systole) and relaxations (diastole) producing mechanical vibrations detectable by radar systems. The respiratory system facilitates gas exchange through cyclical ventilation with typical parameter ranges: HR $\in$ [60, 100] beats per minute RR $\in$ [12, 25] breaths per minute, $\delta_h \in$ [1, 9] mm (cardiac displacement) [14] and $\delta_b \in$ [10, 50] mm (respiratory displacement) [15]. The instantaneous chest displacement is modeled as:

$$\Delta d(t) = d(t) - d_0 = \delta_b(t) + \delta_h(t) + \epsilon(t) \tag{4}$$

where d_0 is the baseline distance, $\delta_b(t)$ and $\delta_h(t)$ are respiratory and cardiac displacements respectively, and $\epsilon(t)$ represents measurement noise and artifacts.

3 Radar Signal Processing

This section delineates the systematic signal processing pipeline that transforms raw MIMO FMCW radar measurements into robust estimates of respiratory and heart rates. The following framework, adapted from [3], has been used

- **Two-Dimensional Spectral Analysis**: for each temporal frame k and chirp j, we construct a range–azimuth map through two-dimensional Fourier analysis:

$$\mathbf{A}_{i,j}(r,a) = \mathrm{FFT}_{\mathrm{azimuth}}\{\mathrm{FFT}_{\mathrm{range}}(\mathbf{R}_{k,:,j,:})\}\,. \tag{5}$$

This transformation yields a spatially resolved representation of backscattered energy, enabling precise localization of the thoracic region.

- **Optimal Bin Selection Algorithm**: The selection of the optimal range-azimuth bin (r^*, a^*) is crucial for maximizing sensitivity to physiological micro-motions while minimizing noise and clutter interference. This process involves three systematic steps:
  - Step 1: We first restrict the search to physically meaningful locations by defining a feasible region Ω:

$$\Omega = \left\{(r,a) : r_{\min} \le r \le r_{\max}, \quad |\mathbf{A}_{k,j}(r,a)|^2 \ge P_{\mathrm{threshold}}\right\} \tag{6}$$

    where $r_{\min}$ and $r_{\max}$ define the valid range window (excluding near-field coupling and far-field low-SNR region,$P_{\mathrm{threshold}}$ is a power threshold to exclude low-power static clutter regions.
  - Step 2: For each candidate bin $(r,a) \in \Omega$, we compute two complementary metrics:
    Phase Variability Metric (measures temporal fluctuations):

$$\sigma_\phi(r,a) = \sqrt{\frac{1}{N_c - 1}\sum_{j=1}^{N_c}\left[\phi_j(r,a) - \bar{\phi}(r,a)\right]^2} \tag{7}$$

    where $\phi_j(r,a) = \arg(\mathbf{A}_{k,j}(r,a))$ is the phase for chirp j, and $\bar{\phi}(r,a) = \frac{1}{N_c}\sum_{j=1}^{N_c}\phi_j(r,a)$ is the mean phase.
    Power Concentration Metric (measures signal strength):

$$P_{\log}(r,a) = \log\left(\frac{1}{N_c}\sum_{c=1}^{N_c}|\mathbf{A}_{k,j}(r,a)|^2\right) \tag{8}$$

  - Step 3: The optimal bin maximizes a weighted combination of both metrics:

$$(r^*, a^*) = \arg\max_{(r,a)\in\Omega}\left[w_1\sigma_\phi(r,a) + w_2 P_{\log}(r,a)\right] \tag{9}$$

    with weights $w_1, w_2 \ge 0$ and $w_1 + w_2 = 1$. Typically, $w_1 = 0.7$ and $w_2 = 0.3$ to prioritize phase variability (which indicates motion) over raw power.
    The rationale is that chest micro-motions cause significant phase variations across chirps, while static objects exhibit stable phases.
- **Phase Extraction and Preprocessing**: Once the optimal bin (r^*, a^*) is identified, we extract the slow-time phase sequence by averaging the complex

signal across all chirps within each frame:

$$\bar{z}_k = \frac{1}{N_c} \sum_{j=1}^{N_c} \mathbf{A}_{k,j}(r^*, a^*) \tag{10}$$

$$\phi_k = \text{unwrap}\big(\arg(\bar{z}_k)\big) \tag{11}$$

The averaging operation in (10) improves the signal-to-noise ratio by reducing uncorrelated noise across chirps. The unwrapping operation in (11) removes 2π discontinuities to obtain a continuous phase trajectory that represents the chest displacement over time.

- **Respiratory Rate Estimation**: Respiratory activity manifests as large-amplitude, low-frequency oscillations in the unwrapped phase signal. The estimation procedure follows:

$$\phi_{\text{resp},k} = \mathcal{H}_{\text{BP}}^{(0.1,0.5)} \{\phi_k\} \tag{12}$$

$$e_{\text{resp},k} = |\phi_{\text{resp},k} + j\mathcal{H}\{\phi_{\text{resp},k}[\}| \tag{13}$$

$$\widehat{\text{RR}} = 60 \left\langle \frac{1}{\Delta t_{\text{peaks}}} \right\rangle \text{ bpm} \tag{14}$$

where $\mathcal{H}_{\text{BP}}^{(0.1,0.5)}$ represents band-pass filtering in the respiratory frequency band (0.1–0.5 Hz, corresponding to 6–30 breaths per minute), $\mathcal{H}\{\cdot\}$ is the Hilbert transform for envelope extraction [16], and $\langle\cdot\rangle$ denotes temporal averaging over detected inter-peak intervals Δt_{peaks}.

- **Heart Rate Estimation**: Cardiac signals have much smaller amplitude than respiratory signals and may be contaminated by respiratory harmonics. Therefore, additional preprocessing is required:

$$\phi_{\text{notch},k} = \mathcal{H}_{\text{notch}}^{(f_{\text{BR}})} \{\phi_k\} \tag{15}$$

$$\phi_{\text{cardiac},k} = \mathcal{H}_{\text{BP}}^{(0.9,3.0)} \{\phi_{\text{notch},k}\} \tag{16}$$

where $\mathcal{H}_{\text{notch}}^{(f_{\text{BR}})}$ is a notch filter that attenuates the fundamental respiratory frequency f_{BR} and its harmonics to reduce respiratory interference.
The heart rate is then estimated in the frequency domain using the discrete Fourier transform as in [3]

$$X[n] = \left| \sum_{k=0}^{N_{\text{FFT}}-1} \phi_{\text{cardiac},k}\, e^{-j2\pi nk/N_{\text{FFT}}} \right| \tag{17}$$

$$f_n = \frac{n f_s}{N_{\text{FFT}}} \tag{18}$$

$$n^* = \arg \max_{n: f_n \in [0.9, 3.0]} X[n] \tag{19}$$

$$\widehat{\text{HR}} = 60 f_{n^*} \text{ bpm} \tag{20}$$

where the frequency search is restricted to the cardiac band [0.9, 3.0] Hz (54–180 bpm) to avoid spurious detections.

It is important to remark that respiration and heartbeat exhibit different characteristics, motivating distinct processing methods. Respiration is a low-frequency, quasi-periodic signal with large amplitude; applying the Hilbert transform yields the analytic signal, from which instantaneous phase and frequency can be extracted for accurate breathing rate tracking [16]. Heartbeat, being higher-frequency and lower-amplitude, is masked by respiration; after removing the fundamental respiration frequency and its harmonics via a notch filter, Fourier analysis efficiently identifies the heart rate from spectral peaks. Hence, Hilbert transform suits slow, quasi-periodic respiration, while filtered Fourier analysis is better for fast, periodic heartbeats.

4 Cardiovascular Metrics

This section presents the metrics analyzed for NCVS monitoring, focusing on both HR and RR. In particular, the HR-related metrics characterize the instantaneous fluctuations within the cardiac cycle, encompassing not only the average values but also statistical descriptors such as the standard deviation. These metrics play a pivotal role in detecting and defining clinical anomalies in cardiac dynamics, providing more comprehensive diagnostic information than the sole estimation of average HR over the measurement period [10]. Analogous variability metrics are also evaluated for the respiratory signal to capture fluctuations in the breathing cycle.

4.1 Heart Rate Variability (HRV) Metrics

Although the estimation of the heart rate provides very important information, it represents only a limited view of cardiovascular dynamics. A richer characterization is obtained by analyzing the fluctuations in the duration of successive cardiac cycles, a quantity known as Heart Rate Variability (HRV). HRV reflects the interplay between the sympathetic and parasympathetic branches of the autonomic nervous system, and its analysis has become a cornerstone in cardiology, stress research, and psychophysiology.

From the cardiac-filtered signal, Inter-Beat Intervals (IBIs) are extracted and processed to compute standard HRV metrics [17]:

$$\overline{\mathrm{IBI}} = \frac{1}{N}\sum_{i=1}^{N} \mathrm{IBI}_i, \tag{21}$$

$$\mathrm{SDNN} = \sqrt{\frac{1}{N-1}\sum_{i=1}^{N}(\mathrm{IBI}_i - \overline{\mathrm{IBI}})^2}, \tag{22}$$

$$\mathrm{RMSSD} = \sqrt{\frac{1}{N-1}\sum_{i=1}^{N-1}(\mathrm{IBI}_{i+1} - \mathrm{IBI}_i)^2}, \tag{23}$$

$$\text{pNN50} = \frac{100}{N-1} \sum_{i=1}^{N-1} \mathbf{1}_{\{|\text{IBI}_{i+1} - \text{IBI}_i| > 50 \text{ ms}\}}, \tag{24}$$

where $\mathbf{1}_{\{.\}}$ is the indicator function. These metrics are defined as:

- **Mean IBI ($\overline{\text{IBI}}$):** the average cardiac period, directly linked to mean heart rate.
- **SDNN (Standard Deviation of NN intervals):** a global measure of overall variability.
- **RMSSD (Root Mean Square of Successive Differences):** sensitive to parasympathetic activity.
- **pNN50:** the percentage of successive IBIs differing by more than 50 ms, often adopted in clinical practice as an indicator of vagal tone.

4.2 Breath Rate Variability (BRV) Metrics

A parallel analysis can be carried out for respiratory activity, giving rise to Breath Rate Variability (BRV). Although less standardized than HRV, BRV has recently attracted attention as it reflects not only the mechanical dynamics of breathing but also its modulation by cortical and autonomic mechanisms. From the respiratory envelope, we detect consecutive inspiratory peaks and compute the Breath-to-Breath Intervals (BBIs). After discarding implausible values (outside the 1.5–10 s range) and rejecting outliers, the following indices are extracted as in [18]

$$\text{MIBI} = \frac{1}{M} \sum_{j=1}^{M} \text{BBI}_j, \tag{25}$$

$$\text{SDBB} = \sqrt{\frac{1}{M-1} \sum_{j=1}^{M} (\text{BBI}_j - \text{MIBI})^2}, \tag{26}$$

$$\text{RMSSD}_{\text{BBI}} = \sqrt{\frac{1}{M-1} \sum_{j=1}^{M-1} (\text{BBI}_{j+1} - \text{BBI}_j)^2}, \tag{27}$$

where

- **MIBI (Mean Inter-Breath Interval):** the average breathing period.
- **SDBB (Standard Deviation of BBIs):** a general descriptor of the dispersion of respiratory cycles.
- **$\text{RMSSD}_{\text{BBI}}$:** the short-term variability of breathing cycles.

These metrics provide a concise description of respiratory variability, complementing the average breathing rate. High BRV is often associated with resilience and healthy autonomic regulation, while reduced BRV may indicate stress, fatigue, or compromised respiratory control. Although clinical guidelines for BRV are not as standardized as those for HRV, including these indices enriches the overall physiological assessment from radar measurements.

Together, these metrics enable not only the comparison between radar-derived signals and ground truth measurements, but also the evaluation of the radar's ability to capture subtle physiological variability relevant to stress assessment, sleep analysis, and cardiovascular risk stratification.

5 Experimental Campaign

This section presents the experimental campaign designed to assess the performance of the proposed MIMO FMCW radar system in estimating respiratory and cardiac metrics under controlled conditions.

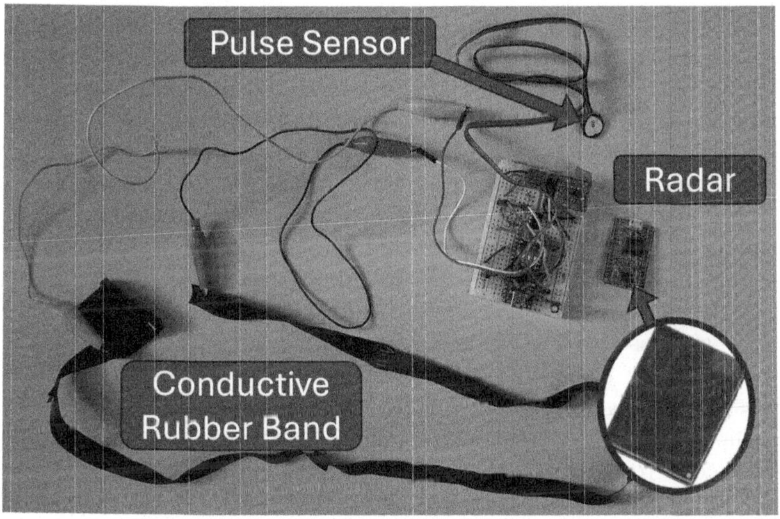

Fig. 1. Experimental setup showing the sensors used. An Arduino Nano is tasked with collecting the sensors outputs for ground truth. A python script synchronizes the captures from both radar and the Arduino.

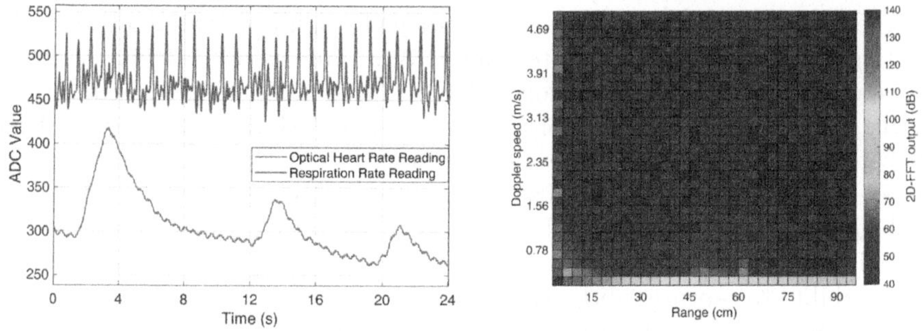

Fig. 2. Ground truth respiration and heart rate readings obtained from the Arduino (left), 2D FFT plot extracted from a single frame of the capture with the person placed at 50 cm from the radar (right).

5.1 Experimental Setup

Radar Setup: The experimental setup used for the results presented in this paper includes a wide-band mmWave radar sensor as well as two dedicated sensors for respiration rate and heart rate, used for the collection of the ground truth. The mmWave radar used is a BGT60TR13C from Infineon Technologies, which is a small size radar for which an evaluation platform is available [19]. The radar IC implements a FMCW Radar with a bandwidth of 5 GHz between the frequencies of 58 and 63 GHz. The radar has one TX antenna and three RX antennas arranged in an L configuration to enable 3D DoA estimation, as can be seen from Fig. 1. The radar was configured with a chirp repetition time of 124 μ s, number of chirp pulse repetitions of 128 and number of ADC samples per pulse of 128. The chirp waveform was configured to sweep over $5GHz$ bandwidth from a starting frequency of 58 GHz to a final frequency of 63 GHz. Intermediate frequency gain was set to 28 dB and ADC sample rate was set to 3 MSPS. This resulted in a range resolution of 3 cm and a Doppler resolution of 0.1565 m/s. The measurements were conducted on an adult male subject seated comfortably on an office chair and instructed to remain still throughout the acquisition. Data were collected at distances ranging from 30 cm to 150 cm, in increments of 10 cm, with each recording lasting 2 min. These settings were chosen as they were the maximum supported by the sensor while fixing the frame rate at 30 frames per second as well as enable readings up to 2 m. To evaluate the effect of a higher number of chirps, resulting in improved Doppler resolution, the measures performed ar 30, 50, 70 and 90 cm were repeated with the number of chirps repetitions increased to 256 while samples per chirp were reduced to 64, all other settings were kept the same. This improved the Doppler resolution to 7.8 cm/s.

Ground Truth Sensors: The RR sensor was constructed from a sheet of conductive silicone rubber with resistivity of 120 Ω/cm, which was cut into strips of 1 cm connected together so as to surround the person. The ends of this rubber are connected to a differential amplifier which reduces DC bias and amplifies the signal to the dynamic range of the Arduino's ADC. The HR ground truth was obtained via an optical pulse sensor based on the APDS-9008 optical sensor. It uses a green LED as a source of light and measures how much light is reflected back which correlates to blood concentration which are driven by the heart.

These analog sensors were digitized using an Arduino Nano with a sample frequency of 50 Hz, a python script was used to automate and synchronize the capture from both Arduino and Radar. The first 24 s of a ground truth reading alongside an example of a 2D-FFT frame derived from a single antenna of the Radar are given in Fig. 2.

5.2 Numerical Results

The radar performance was evaluated for RR, HR, and their variability metrics (BRV and HRV). Errors are reported as mean absolute error (MAE, mean ± standard deviation) relative to ground truth from strain sensors (RR) and optical pulse sensors (HR).

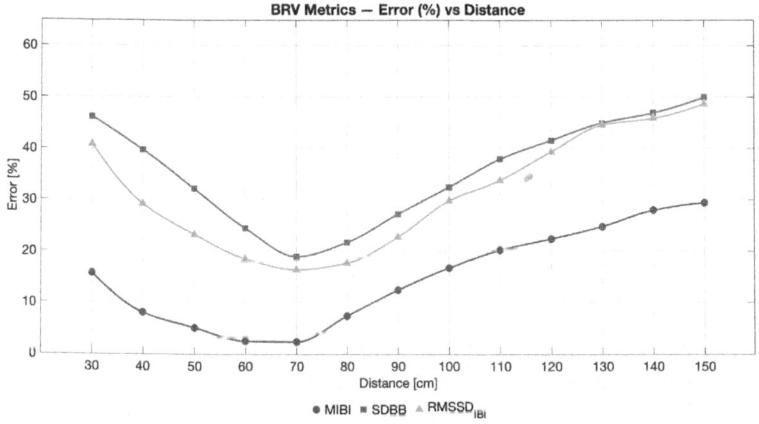

Fig. 3. RR estimation error versus distance of subject from the radar.

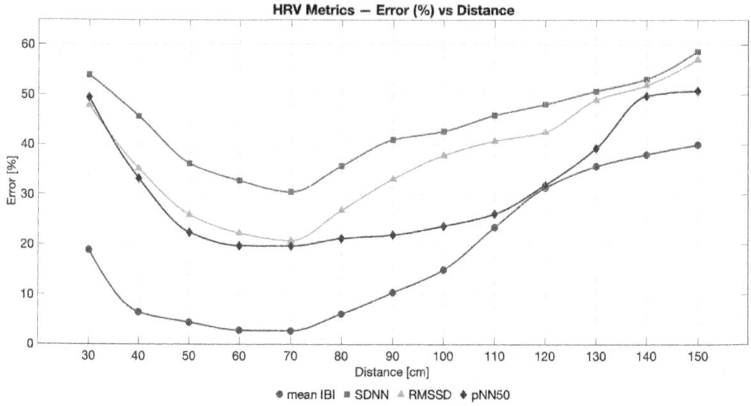

Fig. 4. HR estimation error versus distance of subject from the radar.

Figures 3 and 4 show the dependence of estimation accuracy on sensing distance. Both RR and HR exhibit a characteristic U-shaped error profile, with optimal performance at 70 cm. At this distance, RR estimation achieved a MAE of 0.8 $\pm$ 0.3 bpm ($\approx$ 4.5% relative error), while HR MAE was 3.2 $\pm$ 1.1 bpm ($\approx$ 4%). Respiratory variability metrics at 70 cm achieve a MAE of 2% error for MIBI, 17% for the standard deviation of breath-to-breath intervals (SDBB), and 20% for RMSSD. Heart rate variability metrics exhibited higher errors, with SDNN at 30%, RMSSD 20%, and pNN50 20%. Performance degrades at shorter distances. At 30 cm, RR MAE increased to 2.1 $\pm$ 0.7 bpm and HR MAE to 7.8 $\pm$ 2.3 bpm, with variability errors rising to 25–42%. Degradation at close range is attributed to multipath reflections, near-field coupling, and uneven beam illumination. Beyond 70 cm, errors increase gradually due to reduced SNR, reaching 1.9 $\pm$ 0.5 bpm for RR and 6.4 $\pm$ 1.9 bpm for HR at 150 cm. These results reflect the larger displacement of respiration (10–50 mm) relative to cardiac motion (1–9 mm), explaining the higher robustness of RR estimation.

The impact of the number of transmitted chirps was evaluated at 70 cm (Figs. 5 and 6). RR estimation improves monotonically with increasing chirp count, from 2.8 $\pm$ 0.9 bpm at 32 chirps to 0.9 $\pm$ 0.3 bpm at 256 chirps, with MIBI error decreasing from 3.2% to 2.0%. SDBB and RMSSD remain above 15–20% even at 256 chirps, indicating limited improvement in variability estimation.

HR estimation shows a pronounced threshold effect: below 96 chirps, measurements often fail, with MAE exceeding 15 bpm. Reliable HR estimation requires at least 96 chirps, reducing MAE below 5 bpm, and at 256 chirps, HR MAE stabilizes near 2.8 $\pm$ 0.9 bpm. HRV metrics also improve modestly with chirp count, with SDNN decreasing from 52% at 32 chirps to 28% at 256, RMSSD from 45% to 18%, and pNN50 from 48% to 19%.

These results highlight the operational trade-offs inherent to the radar system. Respiratory rate can be measured reliably with MAE below 1 bpm over a broad range of distances (50–120 cm) when using 96–256 chirps, demonstrat-

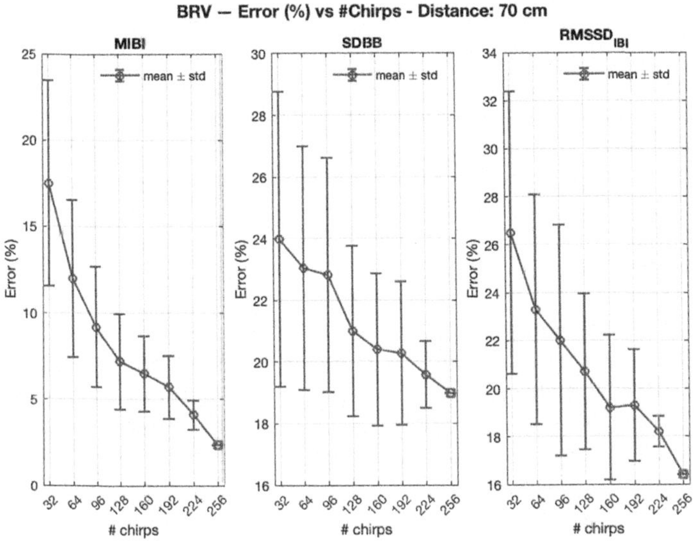

Fig. 5. RR estimation error versus number of chirps used for subject at a distance of 70cm.

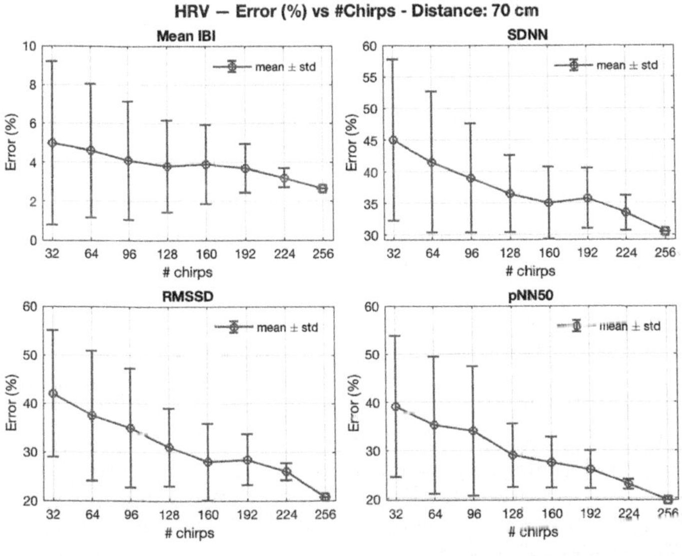

Fig. 6. HR estimation error versus number of chirps used for subject at a distance of 70cm.

ing robustness to both positioning and chirp count. In contrast, accurate heart rate estimation is more sensitive, requiring optimal positioning near 70 cm and at least 96 chirps to achieve MAE below 5 bpm. Variability metrics for both respiration and heart remain less precise, with errors typically above 15–30%, reflecting the challenge of capturing rapid, beat-to-beat or breath-to-breath fluctuations. These findings illustrate a trade-off: increasing chirp count and precise positioning enhance average rate estimation but provide limited gains for instantaneous variability metrics. The system excels at coarse, robust monitoring of RR and HR but is constrained in high-resolution autonomic analysis.

6 Conclusion

This study presents a systematic evaluation of a low-cost FMCW MIMO radar for non-contact vital sign monitoring, focusing on respiratory rate (RR) and heart rate (HR) estimation. Extensive experiments quantify how sensing distance and chirp count affect accuracy. RR can be reliably estimated across 50–120 cm and chirp counts ≥ 96, with mean absolute errors below 1 bpm. HR estimation shows stronger dependence on both parameters, requiring optimal positioning near 70 cm and at least 96 chirps for stable detection. Variability metrics, including HRV and RRV, remain less accurate (errors $\geq$15–30%), reflecting challenges in capturing instantaneous physiological fluctuations. Overall, the results reveal an inherent trade-off: the radar enables robust average vital sign estimation but limited beat-to-beat and breath-to-breath resolution. Future works will focus on expansion of the dataset with more subjects and different configurations, including subject movement, and relative algorithm adjustments to overcome these new scenarios.

References

1. Singh, A., Rehman, S.U., Yongchareon, S., Chong, P.H.J.: Multi-resident non-contact vital sign monitoring using radar: A review. IEEE Sens. J. **21**(4), 4061–4084 (2020)
2. Dias, D., Paulo Silva Cunha, J.: Wearable health devices—vital sign monitoring, systems and technologies. Sensors **18**(8), 2414 (2018)
3. Paterniani, G., et al.: Radar-based monitoring of vital signs: A tutorial overview. In: Proceedings of IEEE, Vol. 111, no. (3), pp. 277–317 (2023)
4. Gu, C., Li, C., Lin, J., Long, J., Huangfu, J., Ran, L.: Instrument-based noncontact doppler radar vital sign detection system using heterodyne digital quadrature demodulation architecture. IEEE Trans. Instrum. Meas. **59**(6), 1580–1588 (2009)
5. Islam, S.M., Fioranelli, F., Lubecke, V.M.: Can radar remote life sensing technology help combat covid-19? Front. Commun. Netw. **2**, 648181 (2021)
6. Alizadeh, M., Shaker, G., De Almeida, J.C.M., Morita, P.P., Safavi-Naeini, S.: Remote monitoring of human vital signs using mm-wave fmcw radar. IEEE Access **7**, 54 958–54 968 (2019)
7. Islam, S.M., Motoyama, N., Pacheco, S., Lubecke, V.M.: Non-contact vital signs monitoring for multiple subjects using a millimeter wave fmcw automotive radar. In: 2020 IEEE/MTT-S International Microwave Symposium (IMS), pp. 783–786 (2020)

8. Su, W.-C., Lai, Y.-C., Horng, T.-S., El Arif, R.: Time-division multiplexing mimo radar system with self-injection-locking for image hotspot-based monitoring of multiple human vital signs. IEEE Trans. Microw. Theory Tech. **72**(3), 1943–1952 (2023)
9. Xu, Z., et al.: Simultaneous monitoring of multiple people's vital sign leveraging a single phased-mimo radar. IEEE J. Electromagnet. RF Microwaves Med. Biol. **6**(3), 311–320 (2022)
10. Volterrani, M., et al.: Decreased heart rate variability in patients with chronic obstructive pulmonary disease. Chest **106**(5), 1432–1437 (1994)
11. Chen, K.-M., Huang, Y., Zhang, J., Norman, A.: Microwave life-detection systems for searching human subjects under earthquake rubble or behind barrier. IEEE Trans. Biomed. Eng. **47**(1), 105–114 (2000)
12. Zhu, F., Wang, K., Wu, K.: A fundamental-and-harmonic dual-frequency doppler radar system for vital signs detection enabling radar movement self-cancellation. IEEE Trans. Microw. Theory Tech. **66**(11), 5106–5118 (2018)
13. Guo, K., Zhai, T., Pashollari, E., Varlamos, C.J., Ahmed, A., Islam, M.N.: Contactless vital sign monitoring system for heart and respiratory rate measurements with motion compensation using a near-infrared time-of-flight camera. Appl. Sci. **11**(22), 10913 (2021)
14. Shafiq, G., Veluvolu, K.C.: Surface chest motion decomposition for cardiovascular monitoring. Sci. Rep. **4**(1), 5093 (2014)
15. Kaneko, H., Horie, J.: Breathing movements of the chest and abdominal wall in healthy subjects. Respir. Care **57**(9), 1442–1451 (2012)
16. Linschmann, O., Leonhardt, S., Vehkaoja, A., Hoog Antink, C.: Estimation of the respiratory rate from ballistocardiograms using the hilbert transform. BioMed. Eng. OnLine **21**(1), 54 (2022)
17. Shaffer, F., Ginsberg, J.P.: An overview of heart rate variability metrics and norms. Front. Public Health **5**, 258 (2017)
18. Soni, R., Muniyandi, M.: Breath rate variability: a novel measure to study the meditation effects. Int. J. Yoga **12**(1), 45–54 (2019)
19. AG, I.T.: Demo bgt60tr13c: Getting started with the xensiv™ 60ghz bgt60tr13c radar sensor demo board for advanced sensing (2024). https://www.infineon.com/cms/en/product/evaluation-boards/demo-bgt60tr13c/

A Systematic Comparison of Muscle Deformation Sensor Placement for Subject-Independent Cognitive State Classification

Tomo Akamine[1,2(✉)], Tamon Miyake[2,3], Satoshi Shimabukuro[1,2,4], Ryota Nishiguchi[2], Chihiro Okubo[2], Shinya Nakamura[2], and Emi Tamaki[1,2,5]

[1] Graduate School of Science and Engineering, University of the Ryukyus, Okinawa, Japan
[2] H2L Inc., Tokyo, Japan
k248586@ie.u-ryukyu.ac.jp
[3] Future Robotics Organization, Waseda University, Tokyo, Japan
[4] Okinawa Rehabilitation Welfare College, Okinawa, Japan
[5] Department of Systems Innovation, School of Engineering, The University of Tokyo, Tokyo, Japan

Abstract. The proliferation of remote work has highlighted a critical gap in digital communication: the absence of non-verbal and embodied cues, which can impede mutual understanding and productivity. This work addresses this challenge by systematically investigating an optimal anatomical site for cognitive-state estimation using non-invasive optical muscle-deformation sensors to classify states such as concentration and relaxation. To model and distinguish these muscle-deformation patterns, a Support Vector Machine (SVM) classifier was employed under a subject-independent evaluation protocol. A controlled four-site comparison across calf (gastrocnemius), trapezius, upper arm (biceps brachii), and neck (sternocleidomastoid; SCM) revealed that rather than a single best site, a trade-off was observed: calf yielded higher accuracy (66%), but trapezius demonstrated greater stability across participants (lower variance, standard deviation (SD) = 0.17), suggesting that optimal site selection depends on deployment context. Fine-grained confusion analysis further revealed complementary error tendencies between the two sites. For real-world deployments where robustness is paramount, trapezius is recommended; for controlled settings prioritizing peak accuracy, calf is preferable. These findings provide actionable guidance for sensor placement and motivate sensor-fusion designs that leverage complementary strengths.

This work was supported by Council for Science, Technology and Innovation, "Cross-ministerial Strategic Innovation Promotion Program (SIP), Development of foundational technologies and rules for expansion of the virtual economy" (JPJ012495). (Funding agency: NEDO).

H. Tanaka et al. (Eds.): BodyNets 2025, LNICST 714, pp. 184–199, 2026.
https://doi.org/10.1007/978-3-032-38657-1_14

Keywords: Wearable Sensors · Physiological Computing · Cognitive State Estimation · Muscle Deformation · Human-Computer Interaction · Remote Collaboration

1 Introduction

Recent progress in digital communication technologies and connectivity platforms has greatly expanded the feasibility of remote work and online learning [4]. This shift was significantly accelerated by global events such as the COVID-19 pandemic, which imposed severe restrictions on physical mobility and in-person interaction. Under such circumstances, the ability to continue professional and educational activities remotely has demonstrated not only practical convenience but also considerable social value, enabling inclusive participation regardless of geographic or health-related constraints.

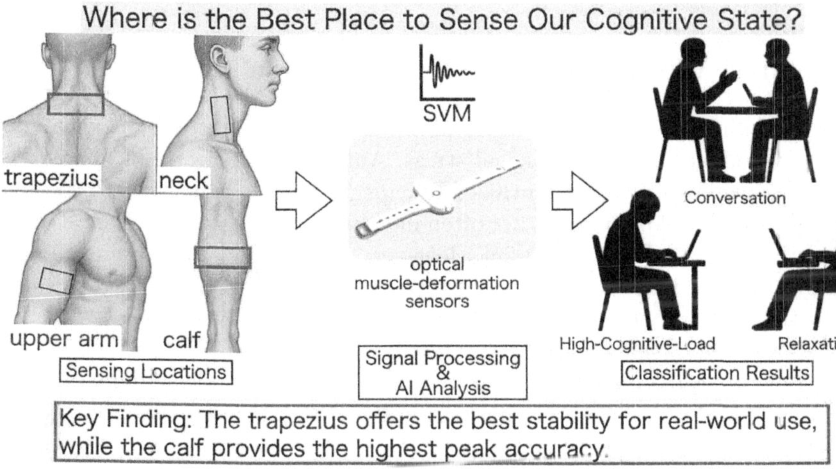

Fig. 1. Overview of the study. Four anatomical sites (trapezius, neck, upper arm, and calf) were monitored with non invasive optical muscle-deformation sensors. Red boxes indicate sensor placement sites. Signals were processed and classified with an SVM to estimate cognitive states (conversation, high-cognitive-load, relaxation). The key finding reveals a trade-off: the trapezius provides greater stability across participants, whereas the calf achieves the highest accuracy. (Color figure online)

Nevertheless, working remotely poses substantial limitations compared to face-to-face environments, particularly in the transmission of embodied and nonverbal information. Subtle cues—such as facial expressions, a concentration-relaxation state, or bodily tension—are often difficult to perceive through conventional video-based communication platforms. These cues, however, play a vital role in interpersonal understanding and efficient coordination. Their absence can impair the quality of interaction, lead to misunderstandings, and reduce overall productivity. In addition, in remote work environments, mental workload and fatigue tend to increase compared to face-to-face environments, raising concerns about productivity and overall well-being [18].

In this context, the present study systematically investigates the suitability of different anatomical sites for cognitive-state estimation using wearable optical muscle-deformation sensors. A four-site comparison across the calf (gastrocnemius), trapezius, upper arm (biceps brachii), and neck (sternocleidomastoid; SCM) is conducted under a subject-independent evaluation protocol to examine classification performance and error characteristics across Relaxation, Conversation, and High Cognitive Load (HCL) (Fig. 1).

The contributions of this study are twofold: (1) providing the first systematic evaluation of sensor placement for cognitive-state classification using optical muscle-deformation sensing, and (2) offering application-driven design implications for remote collaboration platforms. This vision also opens pathways for integration with immersive shared environments, such as metaverse office systems.

2 Related Work

A variety of physiological and behavioral markers have been studied to evaluate cognitive workload and psychological stress. Among them, electroencephalography (EEG) has been frequently utilized to capture brain activity, where spectral features in alpha and beta bands are often interpreted as proxies for mental effort and emotional strain [5,10,18,20,25]. However, the need for complex instrumentation and susceptibility to noise interference significantly hinders EEG's usability in real-world and non-laboratory settings.

Cardiovascular signals, particularly heart rate, have also been applied in estimating mental states during daily activities such as studying or light physical exertion [6,9,11,12,23]. Photoplethysmography (PPG), a widely adopted optical method, enables non-invasive tracking of heart rate variability (HRV), which is associated with stress levels [11,23]. Stress during driving is estimated not only using PPG, but also by incorporating respiratory signals [14]. Nonetheless, distinguishing HRV fluctuations caused by mental workload from those triggered by physical movement remains a significant unresolved issue [12]. A greater variety of bio-signals is important for more robust estimation of a worker's physiological state.

Another promising modality for assessing physiological state is muscle activity. Electromyography (EMG) has been employed to measure muscle tension with high temporal precision [1,13,19,26]. A wearable sensor was developed that integrates sweat cortisol and EMG to capture stress and physiological changes in real time [8]. However, EMG sensors require accurate electrode positioning and may cause discomfort over extended monitoring periods [24]. Optical myography sensors that detect changes in muscle geometry, such as contraction or expansion, have been introduced as a non-intrusive alternative with a capability of compensating for differences in attaching positions [15]. Prior implementations of optical myography have mainly targeted the forearm, an area prone to frequent voluntary movements like typing and gesturing, which compromises signal stability [7,15]. Although a previous study conducted estimation using calf muscle deformation [2], the investigation was limited. Identifying appropriate measurement parts of optical myography that allow for the unobtrusive acquisition of physiological data without disrupting task performance is essential.

In parallel, task design for inducing cognitive load has relied on well-established paradigms. Mental arithmetic under time pressure, exemplified by the Trier So- cial Stress Test (TSST) and the Paced Auditory Serial Addition Task (PASAT), is a standard procedure for eliciting sustained cognitive strain [22]. Beyond these classical paradigms, systematic evaluations have further highlighted mental arithmetic and N-back tasks as reliable indicators of high workload [3]. Recent frameworks additionally propose that high-load tasks should combine complex cognitive abilities with strict time constraints, thereby serving as robust paradigms for inducing mental fatigue [17]. Writing tasks similarly impose high demands on executive control and linguistic planning, while passive video watching has been reported to produce lower arousal and cognitive involvement, often making it difficult to distinguish from relaxed states [10,17]. These findings provide theoretical grounding for treating Arithmetic, Writing, and Watching as manifestations of a broader HCL condition when strong similarity among them is empirically observed.

3 Research Objectives and Contributions

In remote and metaverse work environments, the absence of embodied and non-verbal information—such as bodily tension, concentration, and relaxation—makes it difficult to share cognitive and emotional states, leading to reduced mutual understanding and collaboration efficiency. This study aims to establish a method for estimating human cognitive states through optical muscle-deformation sensing and to data-drivenly derive the optimal anatomical placement of sensors for such estimation. By integrating social and scientific perspectives, this research seeks to enable the transmission of embodied and affective information in remote collaboration environments, thereby building a foundation for empathic communication and adaptive humancomputer interaction systems that respond to inner states.

Building upon this objective, the study develops and validates a sensing and classification framework that captures muscle-deformation data from distinct anatomical regions using wearable optical sensors, and evaluates their effectiveness in distinguishing among cognitive states. Although prior work has demonstrated feasibility at single sites such as the calf [2], a systematic comparison across multiple candidate regions has not been conducted. Moreover, the potential integration of such physiological cues into networked environments to enhance socio-cognitive functions remains underexplored.

To address these gaps, an empirical study was conducted with 20 participants performing five structured tasks (Relaxation, Arithmetic, Writing, Watching,

Conversation) while wearing sensors on four body regions: calf, trapezius, upper arm, and sternocleidomastoid (SCM). Each task was designed to elicit distinct levels of cognitive engagement and physical stillness. A subject-independent evaluation protocol was applied to examine cross-user generalization performance and error characteristics.

Although the experimental design initially treated Arithmetic, Writing, and Watching as independent categories, subsequent similarity analysis and grid-search optimization revealed highly overlapping activation patterns among them. To ensure methodological rigor and reduce confusability, these tasks were consolidated into a unified HCL category for the main analysis. This refinement was not predetermined but was derived from systematic quantitative analysis, ensuring that the labeling scheme was data-driven rather than arbitrary. Importantly, the outcome is consistent with prior findings: arithmetic and writing are well established as prototypical high-load tasks [10]. While passive video watching has sometimes been described as closer to relaxation in previous literature, in the present dataset it clustered consistently with the high-load tasks [3,17]. Thus, the adopted HCL category is supported both by existing theoretical knowledge and by direct validation from the collected physiological data.

In addition, the study explored how physiological signals could be visualized and shared within a metaverse office platform. Using the BodySharing infrastructure, muscle-deformation states were mapped to avatar representations in a shared virtual space, demonstrating how subtle stress or engagement levels may be communicated implicitly to support coordination, empathy, and timely intervention in distributed collaboration.

In summary, the contributions of this study are threefold:

- Providing the first systematic within-study comparison of multiple muscle-sensor placements for subject-independent cognitive-state classification.
- Establishing empirical evidence for the feasibility of optical muscle-deformation sensing across distinct body regions, including the introduction of a data-driven task consolidation into a unified HCL category supported by prior literature.
- Proposing a pathway toward integrating muscle-based sensing into socially responsive metaverse platforms, thereby laying the groundwork for adaptive systems that respond not only to explicit user commands but also to latent cognitive and affective states.

4 Methodology

This study systematically compared the efficacy of muscle deformation data from four distinct anatomical sites for subject-independent cognitive state classification. This section details the participants, apparatus, experimental protocol, data processing pipeline, and the evaluation and statistical analysis methods.

4.1 Participants and Experimental Setting

This study collected data from 20 participants (10 males, 10 females), aged between 19 and 26 years (M = 22.7).

All participants were healthy, right-handed adults with no known neurological or musculoskeletal disorders. All participants provided written informed consent in accordance with the ethics approval of our institution. The experiment was conducted in a controlled laboratory setting. Participants were seated in an office chair while wearing muscle deformation sensors on four muscle sites. They performed five types of tasks, each designed to elicit one of three target cognitive-physiological states: HCL, Relaxation, or Conversation. The tasks were:

- Relaxation: Resting silently with eyes closed.
- Arithmetic: Performing simple calculations under time pressure.
- Writing: Composing a short text based on a given prompt.
- Watching: Viewing emotionally neutral video content.
- Conversation: Light verbal interaction with the experimenter.

Data for each task was recorded for 30 s. To eliminate potential artifacts from task onset and offset, the middle 24 s of each trial were extracted for analysis. The task order was pseudo-randomized across participants to mitigate fatigue and order effects. A short rest period was provided between tasks. The experimental procedure was explained in advance, and participants practiced each task once before data collection to ensure familiarity.

4.2 Sensor Configuration and Site Selection

We used the FirstVR sensor, a non-invasive optical device that observes muscle deformation via infrared reflection. Four sensors were simultaneously attached to the following muscle sites on the participant's body:

- Calf (gastrocnemius)
- Trapezius
- Upper Arm (biceps brachii)
- SCM (Sternocleidomastoid)

These sites were chosen for their accessibility and minimal interference during seated tasks. Data from all four sites were recorded simultaneously at a sampling rate of 27 Hz.

4.3 Data Preprocessing and Feature Engineering

- Windowing: Based on a preliminary analysis, the time-series data was segmented into 6-second non-overlapping windows.
- Feature Vector: The raw sensor values from all channels within each 6-second window were flattened into a single one-dimensional vector, which served as the feature vector for classification.

– Standardization: To prevent information leakage from the test set, data was standardized using scikit-learn's StandardScaler. The scaler was fit exclusively on the training data within each fold of the cross-validation, and the learned parameters were then used to transform both the training and test sets.

4.4 Classification Model and Task Definition

Classifier. The classification was conducted using SVM, a supervised learning algorithm that constructs hyperplanes to separate data in a high-dimensional space. An RBF (Radial Basis Function) kernel was employed with parameters C = 1 and gamma = 'scale'. To mitigate class imbalance, the class_weight = "balanced" option was applied, and reproducibility was ensured using a fixed random seed (random_state = 0).

Task Labels. The initial task design included five categories—Relaxation, Arithmetic, Writing, Watching, and Conversation (see Sect. 4.1 for detailed task descriptions). Quantitative inspection of inter-task confusion revealed substantial overlap among Arithmetic, Writing, and Watching, leading to frequent misclassifications; therefore, these tasks were consolidated into a unified HCL category. This data-driven refinement aligns with prior findings indicating that arithmetic and writing impose high cognitive demands, while passive video viewing, although sometimes resembling relaxation, can elicit overlapping physiological patterns with cognitively demanding activities [16,21]. The resulting structure—three consolidated task classes of Relaxation, Conversation, and HCL-serves as the basis for all subsequent analyses (see also Sect. 5.1 for validation of this consolidation).

4.5 Evaluation Protocol and Statistical Analysis

Evaluation Protocol. To rigorously evaluate the subject-independent generalization performance, we adopted a Leave-One-Subject-Out (LOSO) cross-validation scheme.

Statistical Analysis. Statistical tests were performed to compare LOSO accuracies across the four muscle sites. First, the normality of the data distributions was assessed using the Shapiro-Wilk test. As the data for several conditions significantly deviated from a normal distribution ($p < .05$), we opted to use non-parametric tests for all subsequent inferential statistics to ensure robustness. A Friedman test was conducted to test for overall differences among the four sites. For post-hoc analysis, Wilcoxon signed-rank tests were performed for all pairwise comparisons, with p-values corrected for multiple comparisons using the Bonferroni method. Hedges' g was reported as a measure of effect size. Furthermore, Levene's test was used to assess the homogeneity of variances to compare performance stability.

5 Results

This section first describes the process of optimizing the analysis parameters and their results. Subsequently, it reports in detail the results of the comparative analysis of generalization performance across the four muscle sites, which is the main objective of this study.

5.1 Optimization of Analysis Parameters

Determination of Window Length. To determine a suitable window length for the main analysis, a preliminary evaluation was conducted. The performance of 3 s, 6 s, and 12 s windows was assessed using a fundamental binary classification task: distinguishing the "Relaxation" state from all other active tasks ("Relaxation" vs. "All Tasks"). The results of this two-class LOSO accuracy are summarized in Table 1.

Table 1. Comparison of generalization performance (LOSO accuracy) by window length. The table shows the mean accuracy for each of the four muscle sites evaluated with 3 s, 6 s, and 12 s window lengths.

Muscle Site	3 s	6 s	12 s
Calf	92.7%	92.7%	88.4%
Trapezius	94.9%	94.0%	91.9%
Upper Arm	88.3%	87.2%	79.7%
SCM	87.4%	84.7%	75.0%

A one-way repeated measures ANOVA on these accuracies revealed a significant main effect of window length $F(1.3, 24.7) = 5.2$, $p = .025$, $\eta_p^2 = .22$ Post-hoc tests indicated that the performance of the 6 s and 3 s windows was significantly higher than that of the 12 s window ($p = .031$), while there was no statistical difference between the 3 s and 6 s windows ($p = 1.00$). Although their mean performances were statistically equivalent, we adopted the 6 s window for the main 3-class analysis, considering its potential for greater robustness against transient noise.

Following the task definitions introduced in Sect. 4.1 and the preliminary consolidation rationale described in Sect. 4.4, a binary LOSO classification was performed across all 10 task pairs to quantitatively validate inter-task similarity. The resulting similarity heatmap (Fig. 2) indicated substantial confusability among Arithmetic, Writing, and Watching (F1-scores of $0.45 - 0.55$), suggesting that their underlying muscle activation patterns were highly similar. A subsequent grid-search optimization confirmed that consolidating these three tasks yielded the highest classification performance. Accordingly, the final analysis

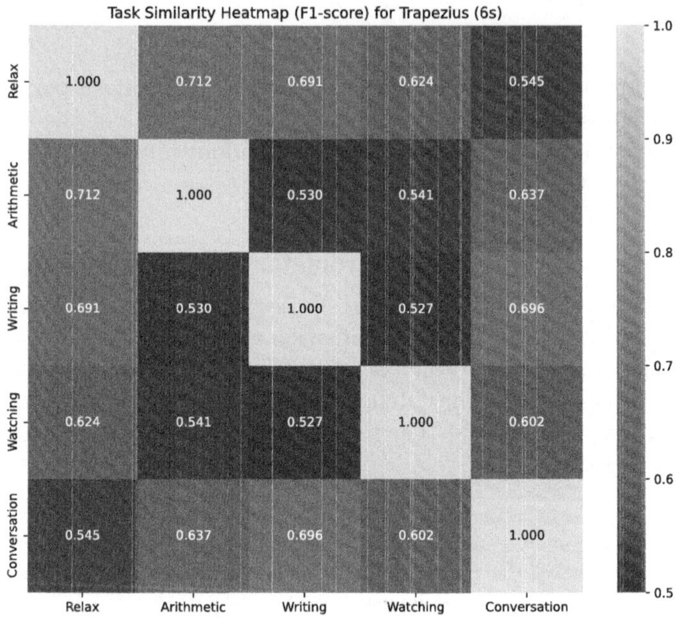

Fig. 2. Similarity heatmap of pairwise task classification for the trapezius muscle. Values represent the F1-score from a binary LOSO classification between each pair of tasks. Lower scores (darker colors) indicate higher similarity and confusability.

adopted a three-class framework: Relaxation, Conversation, and a unified HCL category. This consolidation was not predetermined but derived from systematic quantitative analysis, and its validity is reinforced by prior literature identifying arithmetic and writing as prototypical high-load tasks. Although passive video viewing has sometimes been associated with relaxation, its physiological patterns in the present dataset showed a stronger affinity with high-load tasks, supporting its inclusion in the HCL category.

5.2 Comparative Analysis of Generalization Performance Across Muscle Sites

The primary analysis focused on comparing the subject-independent generalization performance across the four muscle sites. Table 2 summarizes the descriptive statistics for the accuracy of each site, and the distributions are visualized in Fig. 3.

As presented in Table 2, the calf muscle yielded the highest mean accuracy. However, a descriptive analysis of the SD and the accuracy range (Max-Min) suggests that the trapezius model provided more consistent performance across participants, hinting at greater stability.

A Friedman test revealed a statistically significant difference in classification accuracy across the four muscle sites, $\chi^2(3) = 19.3$, $p < .001$, $W = 0.32$. Table 3

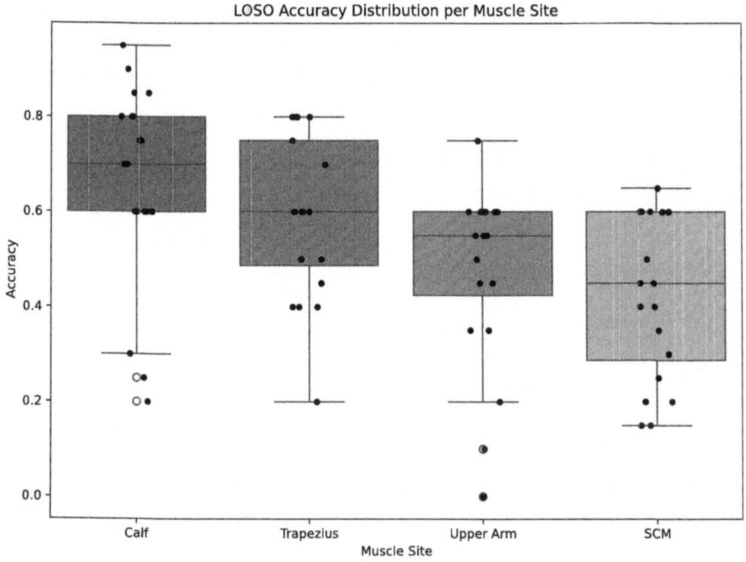

Fig. 3. Distribution of LOSO classification accuracies for each muscle site. Each boxplot shows the median, interquartile range, and overall range of accuracies across the 20 subjects. Individual data points are overlaid as dots.

Table 2. Generalization performance for the 3-class classification across the four muscle sites. Mean accuracy, SD, maximum accuracy (Max), and minimum accuracy (Min) from the LOSO cross-validation across 20 subjects are reported.

Muscle Site	Mean Accuracy	SD	Max	Min
Calf	66%	0.20	95%	20%
Trapezius	60%	0.17	80%	20%
Upper Arm	48%	0.19	75%	0%
SCM	43%	0.17	65%	15%

shows the results of the post-hoc pairwise comparisons, which were conducted with Bonferroni correction to break down this effect. The results indicated that only the difference between the calf and SCM was statistically significant after the strict correction ($p < .05$). However, a clear trend was observable from the descriptive statistics and effect sizes, presented in Table 2 and Table 3, respectively. These results show that the trapezius and calf substantially outperformed the arm and SCM.

Furthermore, a Levene's test indicated no significant difference in the variances of accuracy between the two top-performing sites ($F(1, 38) = 0.02$, $p = .88$).

Table 3. Results of non-parametric post-hoc pairwise comparisons for LOSO accuracy across muscle sites. Wilcoxon signed-rank tests were conducted, and p-values were corrected using the Bonferroni method (p-corr). The effect size is reported as Hedges' g.

Comparison A	Comparison B	p-corr*	Effect Size (Hedges' g)
Arm	Calf	0.068	–0.884
Arm	SCM	1.000	0.255
Arm	Trapezius	0.242	–0.584
Calf	SCM	0.015	1.162
Calf	Trapezius	1.000	0.375
SCM	Trapezius	0.083	–0.885

5.3 Detailed Analysis of Classification Performance for the Primary Candidate Sites

The analysis in Sect. 5.2 identified the trapezius and calf as the two primary candidate sites. To further understand their performance characteristics, we conducted a detailed comparative analysis of their per-class performance and confusion tendencies in the LOSO evaluation. Their respective confusion matrices are presented in Fig. 4.

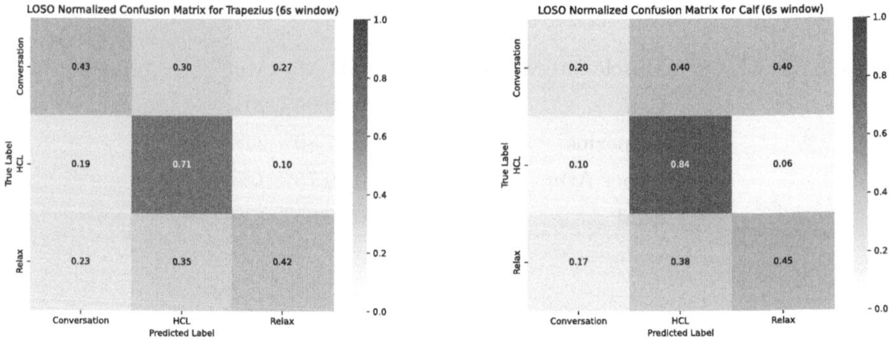

(a) Confusion matrices of Trapezius (b) Confusion matrices of Calf

Fig. 4. Confusion matrices for the two primary candidate sites, (a)Trapezius and (b) Calf, from the 3-class LOSO evaluation. Values are normalized by the true label count, with the main diagonal representing the recall for each class. The matrices show aggregated results across all 20 subjects.

While both models performed well in detecting the Relaxation state, qualitative differences were observed in their error patterns. As seen in Fig. 4a, the trapezius model was more likely to confuse Conversation with HCL. In contrast, in Fig. 4b, the calf model showed a stronger tendency to misclassify Conversation as Relaxation. This suggests a qualitative difference in the physiological information captured by the two sites, which will be elaborated upon in the Discussion.

6 Discussion

This study systematically compared the generalization performance of four muscle sites for subject-independent cognitive state estimation using a rigorous LOSO cross-validation protocol. In this section, we interpret the obtained results, discuss their physiological and practical implications, and acknowledge the limitations of our study.

6.1 Summary of Principal Findings

This study conducted a subject-independent evaluation of optical muscle deformation sensing across four anatomical sites - calf, trapezius, upper arm, and SCM - for three target states (Relaxation, Conversation, HCL). A systematic quantitative analysis (pairwise similarity heatmap and grid-search) indicated substantial overlap among Arithmetic, Writing, and Watching, motivating their consolidation into HCL for the main analysis (Fig. 2). Across sites, the calf and trapezius consistently ranked highest in average performance, whereas the upper arm and SCM lagged behind.

6.2 Physiological Interpretation of Site-Specific Patterns

The trapezius is associated with neckshoulder posture control and stress-related muscle tension, whereas the calf reflects global postural tone and subtle lower-limb adjustments even during seated tasks [1]. Consistent with these roles, the trapezius model exhibited fewer Relaxation-related false positives (i.e., lower propensity to map Conversation to Relaxation), while the calf model showed a stronger tendency to classify Conversation as Relaxation. By contrast, the trapezius more often confused Conversation with HCL, indicating heightened sensitivity to arousal-related neckshoulder activity. These complementary tendencies explain the divergence observed in confusion matrices.

6.3 Selection of the Optimal Site and Practical Implications

This section answers our primary goal by translating site-wise metrics into evidence-based placement guidelines for practical deployment. While mean accuracies of the calf and trapezius were comparable, the trapezius demonstrated lower across-participant variance and fewer Relaxation-related confusions - properties that are advantageous for real-world deployment, where stable readouts and conservative false-relaxation rates are critical. Accordingly, for applications prioritizing robustness and interpretability (e.g., ambient status sharing or remote collaboration dashboards), the trapezius constitutes a prudent default placement. Conversely, where mounting constraints permit and marginal gains in peak metrics are prioritized, the calf remains an attractive alternative. These recommendations align with the site-specific confusion tendencies reported in the Results (Fig. 4), indicating that design choices can explicitly leverage the complementary error profiles of the two sites.

These findings directly address the central objective of this study: identifying an optimal anatomical placement for robust cognitive-state estimation. The observed trade-off—between the trapezius offering stability and the calf achieving higher accuracy—demonstrates that optimality is context-dependent rather than absolute. Thus, the outcome fulfills the initial goal of providing evidence-based design guidelines that inform practical sensor deployment and future integration into adaptive systems.

Beyond remote collaboration and metaverse communication platforms, the proposed sensing approach has broader applicability across healthcare, education, and safety management. Continuous monitoring of muscle tension and relaxation can support fatigue detection, stress evaluation, or adaptive learning systems responsive to engagement levels. In safety-critical contexts such as driving or industrial operation, similar physiological cues may contribute to attention monitoring and early-warning mechanisms.

These potential applications illustrate the wider societal relevance of muscle-based cognitive sensing and motivate continued investigation into multimodal and longitudinal extensions.

6.4 Limitations of the Study

This study is subject to several limitations. First, only optical myography was considered, without integrating other physiological modalities such as PPG or respiration. While this ensured focus on mechanical correlates of cognitive state, multimodal fusion may further stabilize estimation under variable conditions. Second, the participant cohort was limited in size and diversity; long-term and cross-population validation remain necessary to evaluate generalizability. Third, the experimental tasks, although representative, were performed in controlled settings, and everyday scenarios such as extended remote work or mobile contexts were not examined.

These constraints highlight both the technical and practical boundaries of the present work. Nevertheless, the demonstrated differentiation between sites and the practical guidelines derived from it provide a foundation for future extensions. In particular, the broader societal relevance discussed above—spanning healthcare, education, and safety—underscores the importance of advancing this framework toward multimodal, longitudinal, and adaptive sensing pipelines. To address these limitations, longitudinal and multi-site validations are planned, as outlined in Sect. 7.2.

7 Conclusion and Future Work

7.1 Conclusion

This work established a subject-independent comparison of optical muscle-deformation sensing across four anatomical sites for cognitivephysiological state estimation. A data-driven consolidation of Arithmetic, Writing, and Watching into an HCL category—grounded in similarity heatmaps and grid-search—yielded a more reliable labeling framework consistent with prior literature that recognizes arithmetic and writing as prototypical high-load tasks. Considering mean accuracy, error profiles, and across-participant stability, the trapezius is recommended as a default placement for real-world deployment, whereas the calf remains a competitive option where mounting is feasible and marginal gains in peak metrics are targeted.

7.2 Future Work

First, multimodal fusion should explicitly leverage the complementary error tendencies of calf and trapezius observed in the confusion analyses, pairing global postural tone with neckshoulder tension signals. Second, longitudinal and ambulatory studies are required to evaluate robustness under naturalistic routines (e.g., extended remote work, mobility, and spontaneous speech). Third, adaptive personalization atop a subject-independent backbone may reconcile robustness with user-specific idiosyncrasies once multi-session data are available. Finally, integration into shared virtual environments (e.g., BodySharing-based metaverse offices) warrants systematic evaluation, including privacy-preserving visualizations, opt-in controls, and team-level utility assessed via communicative efficiency and task performance.

References

1. Ahmed, M., Grillo, M., Taebi, A., Kaya, M., Thibbotuwawa Gamage, P.: A comprehensive analysis of trapezius muscle emg activity in relation to stress and meditation. BioMedInformatics **4**(2), 1047–1058 (2024)
2. Akamine, T., Miyake, T., Shimabukuro, S., Tamaki, E.: Muscle-based monitoring system for classifying human concentration and relaxation states. In: HCI International 2025 – Late Breaking Papers, pp. 298–313 (2026). https://doi.org/10.1007/978-3-032-12660-3_22
3. Das Chakladar, D., Roy, P.P.: Cognitive workload estimation using physiological measures: a review. Cogn. Neurodyn. **18**(4), 1445–1465 (2024). https://doi.org/10.1007/s11571-023-10051-3
4. Ferreira, R., Pereira, R., Bianchi, I.S., da Silva, M.M.: Decision factors for remote work adoption: advantages, disadvantages, driving forces and challenges. J. Open Innov. Technol. Mark. Complexity **7**(1), 70 (2021)
5. Hayano, J., Barros, A.K., Kamiya, A., Ohte, N., Yasuma, F.: Assessment of pulse rate variability by the method of pulse frequency demodulation. Biomed. Eng. Online **4**, 1–12 (2005)

6. Heathers, J.A.: Smartphone-enabled pulse rate variability: an alternative methodology for the collection of heart rate variability in psychophysiological research. Int. J. Psychophysiol. **89**(3), 297–304 (2013)
7. Hosono, S., Miyake, T., Miyake, S., Tamaki, E.: Feedback method of force controlled by electrical muscle stimulation based on infrared optical sensing. Front. Virtual Reality **3**, 880238 (2022)
8. Hossain, N.I., Noushin, T., Tabassum, S.: Stressfit: A hybrid wearable physicochemical sensor suite for simultaneously measuring electromyogram and sweat cortisol. Sci. Rep. **14**(1), 29667 (2024)
9. Hwang, S., Seo, J., Jebelli, H., Lee, S.: Feasibility analysis of heart rate monitoring of construction workers using a photoplethysmography (ppg) sensor embedded in a wristband-type activity tracker. Autom. Constr. **71**, 372–381 (2016)
10. Katahira, K., Yamazaki, Y., Yamaoka, C., Ozaki, H., Nakagawa, S., Nagata, N.: EEG correlates of the flow state: A combination of increased frontal theta and moderate frontocentral alpha rhythm in the mental arithmetic task. Front. Psychol. **9**, 300 (2018)
11. Kawasaki, Y., Hossain, T., Yokokubo, A., Lopez, G.: Estimating the degree of mental state using heart rate while studying. In: Adjunct Proceedings of the 2021 ACM International Joint Conference on Pervasive and Ubiquitous Computing and Proceedings of the 2021 ACM International Symposium on Wearable Computers, pp. 126–130 (2021)
12. Lee, W., Lin, K.Y., Seto, E., Migliaccio, G.C.: Wearable sensors for monitoring on-duty and off-duty worker physiological status and activities in construction. Autom. Constr. **83**, 341–353 (2017)
13. Luijcks, R., Hermens, H.J., Bodar, L., Vossen, C.J., Os, J.v., Lousberg, R.: Experimentally induced stress validated by emg activity. PloS One **9**(4), e95215 (2014)
14. Mateos-García, N., Gil-González, A.B., Luis-Reboredo, A., Pérez-Lancho, B.: Driver stress detection from physiological signals by virtual reality simulator. Electronics **12**(10), 2179 (2023)
15. Miyake, S., Miyake, T.: CNN-based gripping-force estimation using optical muscle deformation sensors. In: Extended Abstracts of the 2025 CHI Conference on Human Factors in Computing Systems, Article 123, pp. 1–8 (2025). https://doi.org/10.1145/3706599.3719786
16. Puusepp, I., et al.: Changes in physiological arousal during an arithmetic task: profiles of elementary school students and their associations with mindset, task performance and math grade. Sci. Rep. **14**(1) (2024). https://doi.org/10.1038/s41598-024-51683-7
17. Ren, L., Wu, L., Feng, T., Liu, X.: A new method for inducing mental fatigue: A high mental workload task paradigm based on complex cognitive abilities and time pressure. Brain Sci. **15**, 541 (2025). https://doi.org/10.3390/brainsci15060541
18. Riedl, R., Kostoglou, K., Wriessnegger, S.C., Müller-Putz, G.R.: Videoconference fatigue from a neurophysiological perspective: Experimental evidence based on electroencephalography (eeg) and electrocardiography (ecg). Sci. Rep. **13**(1), 18371 (2023)
19. Schleifer, L.M., Spalding, T.W., Kerick, S.E., Cram, J.R., Ley, R., Hatfield, B.D.: Mental stress and trapezius muscle activation under psychomotor challenge: A focus on emg gaps during computer work. Psychophysiology **45**(3), 356–365 (2008)
20. Shriram, R., Sundhararajan, M., Daimiwal, N.: EEG based cognitive workload assessment for maximum efficiency. IOSR J. Electron. Commun. Eng. (IOSR-JECE), SICETE Special Issue, 34–38 (2013)

21. Stuldreher, I., Erp, J., Brouwer, A.M.: Robustness of physiological synchrony in wearable electrodermal activity and heart rate as a measure of attentional engagement to movie clips. Sensors **23**, 3006 (2023). https://doi.org/10.3390/s23063006
22. Tombaugh, T.: A comprehensive review of the paced auditory serial addition test (pasat). Archives of clinical neuropsychology : the official journal of the National Academy of Neuropsychologists **21**, 53–76 (02 2006). https://doi.org/10.1016/j.acn.2005.07.006
23. Tsunoda, K., Chiba, A., Chigira, H., Ura, T., Mizunq, O.: Estimating changes in a cognitive performance using heart rate variability. In: 2015 IEEE 15th International Conference on Bioinformatics and Bioengineering (BIBE), pp. 1–6. IEEE (2015)
24. Varghese, R.J., Pizzi, M., Kundu, A., Grison, A., Burdet, E., Farina, D.: Design, fabrication and evaluation of a stretchable high-density electromyography array. Sensors **24**(6), 1810 (2024)
25. Wen, T.Y., Mohd Aris, S.A.: Electroencephalogram (EEG) stress analysis on alpha/beta ratio and theta/beta ratio. Indones. J. Electr. Eng. Comput. Sci **17**(1), 175–182 (2020). https://doi.org/10.11591/ijeecs.v17.i1.pp175-182
26. Wijsman, J., Grundlehner, B., Penders, J., Hermens, H.: Trapezius muscle emg as predictor of mental stress. ACM Trans. Embedded Comput. Syst. (TECS) **12**(4), 1–20 (2013)

A Fundamental Study of Objective Color Blindness Evaluation Based on Brain Waves

Takumu Kobayashi(✉), Masaki Ohashi, and Akitoshi Itai

Graduate School of Engineering, Chubu University, Aichi, Japan
tp25004-3784@sti.chubu.ac.jp , itai@fsc.chubu.ac.jp

Abstract. The color vision deficiency slightly affects daily living. The evaluation of color blindness is typically conducted through a subjective assessment that utilizes color papers and color blocks. Therefore, the development of an effective and objective evaluation method for color blindness is desired. Now we focus on the estimation of personal characteristics using electroencephalogram (EEG) recorded from wireless electroencephalograph. EEG includes various components generated by vision, sound, attention, liking, and so on. Various researches are reported which estimates the human state from EEG that reflects visual information such as a visual evoked potential (VEP) and event-related potential (ERP). Steady-State Visually Evoked Potentials (SSVEP) is known as one of VEP evoked by gazing at a constant period of light flashes or flickering of checkerboard color pattern. The amount of SSVEP reflects a brightness, contrast, flashing frequency of flickering checkerboard. On the other hand, Kaneko showed the process of color information recognition in the human brain by changing the colors of checkerboard patterns. Results showed that the amount of SSVEP depends on the color combination of the checkerboard. Moreover, the amount of SSVEP was strongly related to color vision of the subject. These facts represent the SSVEP is a biological information which reflects color perception. If visual stimuli that induce different SSVEP depending on color recognition, a difference of color vision could be estimated. In this paper, we propose visual stimuli to evaluate color blindness using SSVEP.

Keywords: Color vision · SSVEP · EEG

1 Introduction

In the sustainable development goals, which have been the focus of attention recently, color blindness is an example of a target for eliminating disparities in all characteristics. Color blindness is a condition in which abnormalities or defects in cone cells make it difficult to distinguish colors. Currently, approximately 5% of men and 0.2% of women in Japan, and 7.4% of men and 0.5% of

H. Tanaka et al. (Eds.): BodyNets 2025, LNICST 714, pp. 200–212, 2026.
https://doi.org/10.1007/978-3-032-38657-1_15

women of European descent have color blindness, with some individuals unaware of their condition [1,2]. There are several commonly used methods for testing color blindness, such as the Ishihara color vision test, the standard color vision test, the Panel D-15 test, and the anomaloscope [3]. These methods are subjective tests that rely on the individual perception of the subject, and there is currently no practical method to assess color blindness. In addition, color blindness is classified into several types, and there are individual differences in color perception even among individuals with the same type. Therefore, color samples used in universal design that are visible to individuals with a specific type of color blindness typically serve only as representative examples. One reason for this issue is that color blindness is typically classified into only a few categories, such as severe, moderate, or mild. This classification system is insufficient for estimating individual differences. To address this problem, a practical method is required to quantitatively express color perception and the severity of color vision deficiency.

A brain-computer interface (BCI) is a system that uses brain waves reflecting a user's intention to control external devices. The electroencephalogram (EEG) used in BCI includes the steady-state visual evoked potential (SSVEP). The advantage of SSVEP over other brain waves for BCI is that it can be evoked without prior training. Therefore, SSVEP has been applied to computer input systems and wheelchair control as an assistive technology for individuals with physical disabilities [4,5].

In a previous study, Kaneko et al. investigated how color information is processed in the human brain by changing the colors of checkerboard patterns used as the visual stimulus to evoke SSVEP [6]. The results showed that the amount of SSVEP evoked depended on the color combinations of the visual stimuli and was strongly associated with the participants' subjective color perception.

Since subjective color perception is strongly related to the amount of SSVEP evoked, the color combinations in visual stimuli likely affect the evoked SSVEP depending on an individual's color vision characteristics. In this paper, we present fundamental research on an objective evaluation system for color blindness based on SSVEP. Specifically, we simulate visual stimuli perceived as different color combinations by individuals with normal trichromacy, type 1 dichromacy, and type 2 dichromacy. The SSVEP responses evoked by these stimuli are compared. We examine the feasibility of objectively evaluating color vision using SSVEP to detect color blindness.

2 Color Blindness

2.1 Cone Cells

When light enters the human eye, photochemical reactions occur between photons and photopigments in the photoreceptor cells of the retina. These reactions generate electrical signals. Among the photoreceptors, cone cells are categorized into three types based on the spectral sensitivity of their photopigments: L-cones (long-wavelength, ∼560 nm), M-cones (middle-wavelength, ∼530 nm), and S-cones (short-wavelength, ∼430 nm) [7]. Humans perceive color by integrating the neural signals transmitted from these three types of cone cells.

2.2 Congenital Color Blindness

Due to genetic factors, some individuals are born with deficient or altered function in specific cone cells, a condition known as congenital color blindness. Individuals with color blindness perceive colors differently from those with normal color vision. This makes it difficult to distinguish colors in designs created based on normal trichromatic vision. Color blindness is categorized by the number of functioning cone cell types: anomalous trichromacy, dichromacy, and monochromacy. When all three types of cone cells function normally, the condition is referred to as normal trichromacy. Furthermore, color vision is classified by the type of affected cone: type 1 if L-cones are abnormal or missing, type 2 if M-cones, and type 3 if S-cones. Type 3 color vision is extremely rare, while types 1 and 2 account for the most cased of congenital color blindness [8].

This paper focuses on types 1 and 2 dichromacy, which are characterized by the absence of one type of cone cell. These are the most common forms of color blindness among individuals with type 1 or type 2 dichromacy.

2.3 Color Blindness Test

The subjective test to detect color blindness is introduced here.

Ishihara Color Vision Test Chart. [9] It is a test chart in which letters or numbers are composed of color combinations that are difficult to distinguish for individuals with congenital color blindness. This chart enables classification of the type of color blindness.

Hue Array Check. [10] Color chips with varying hues are rearranged from a random order into a perceptual color sequence. This method is effective for identifying severe color blindness.

Anomaloscope. [11] This test method classifies color blindness and assesses its severity by having the subject adjusts the proportions of red and green light to match a reference yellow light.

2.4 SSVEP

The SSVEP is the periodic EEG response to a visual stimulus with a periodic blinking. The SSVEP is evoked by gaze or attention to a visual stimulus [12]. SSVEP is characterized by being evoked at the same fundamental frequency and its harmonics as the flickering frequency of the visual stimulus [13]. It is known that the visual stimulus of 15 Hz produces a greater SSVEP than other frequencies [14]. A typical visual stimulus that evokes SSVEP is the pattern reversal stimulus (Fig. 1) [15]. Pattern reversal stimulation is characterized by the strong induction of SSVEP at harmonic frequencies of the stimulation [16].

The amplitude spectrum of the EEG signal recorded by a 15 Hz pattern reversal stimulus is shown in Fig. 2. In this figure, the EEG signal includes peaks at 15 and 30 Hz In this paper, the 30 Hz amplitude spectrum was used as the measure of the SSVEP response, given that the stimulus frequency was 15 Hz.

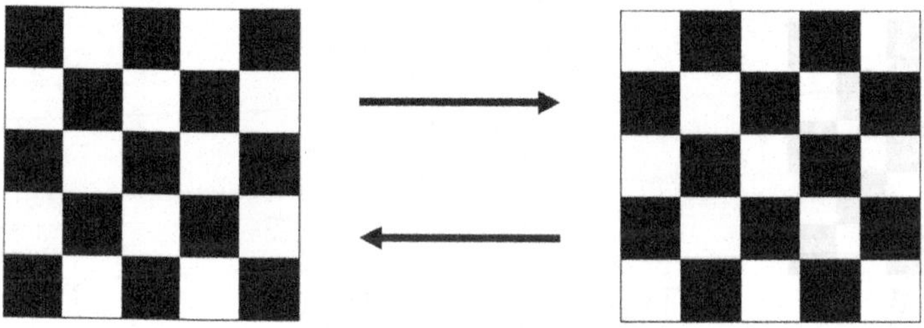

Fig. 1. Checkerboard for pattern reversal stimulus

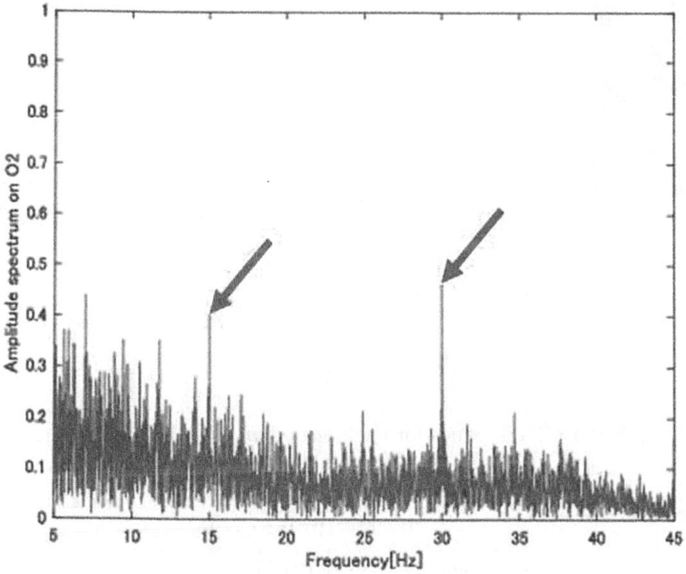

Fig. 2. Amplitude spectrum of EEG gazing 15 Hz pattern reversal stimulus

3 Experiment

3.1 Proposed Visual Stimulus

The visual stimuli used in this paper are shown in Fig. 3 and 4, and the RGB values of the visual stimuli, excluding the black-and-white pattern reversal stimulus, are shown in Table 1 and 2.

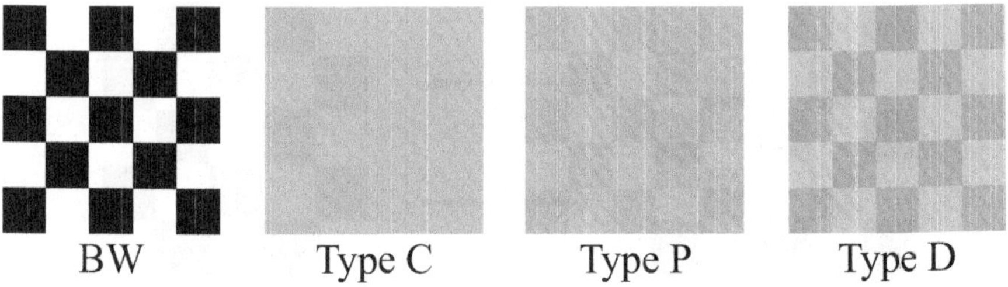

Fig. 3. Objective evaluation of type 1 dichromacy

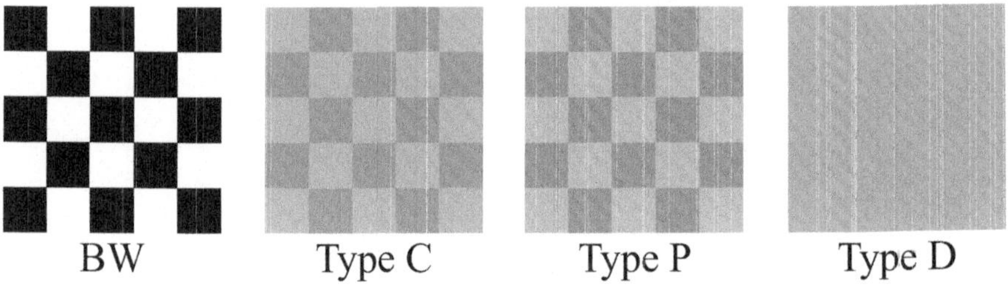

Fig. 4. Objective evaluation of type 2 dichromacy

Table 1. RGB values for each stimulus: type 1 dichromacy

	Light Blue			Pink		
	R	G	B	R	G	B
Type C	117	184	225	217	181	210
Type P	178	178	225	185	185	210
Type D	169	169	224	192	192	208

Table 2. RGB values for each stimulus: type 2 dichromacy

	Green			Pink		
	R	G	B	R	G	B
Type C	120	196	151	240	144	138
Type P	189	189	151	158	158	139
Type D	178	178	154	179	179	137

The black and white pattern reversal stimulus is referred to as BW (black-white). The color stimulus simulating color recognition for a normal color vision is defined as typeC (Common). The color recognition of typeC is different with a type of color blindness. Its for type 1 dichromacy is represented as typeP (Protanope), and that for type 2 dichromacy is typeD (Deuteranope). The type C color scheme shown in Fig. 3 is a consists of color combinations that are known to be difficult for individuals with color blindness to distinguish, based on the Color Universal Design Guidelines published by the Tokyo Metropolitan Government [17]. These colors appear distinctly different to individuals with type 1 and type 2 dichromacy. It is difficult to recognize the checkerboard of type C for Type 1 dichromacy people, since color contrast of type P is smaller than its type D and type C. Figure 4 consists of color combinations cited in the Color Universal Design Recommended Color Scheme Kit [18] as examples that should be avoided, particularly for individuals with type 2 dichromacy, due to the difficulty in distinguishing the colors. The type P and type D stimuli were generated by simulating how the type C colors would appear to individuals with type 1 and type 2 dichromacy, respectively, using the method proposed by Viénot et al. [19].

3.2 EEG Measurement

The recording conditions are listed in Table 3, the measurement environment is shown in Fig. 5, and an overview of the visual stimulus is shown in Fig. 6. The visual stimulus is a 5 cm square and is positioned 60 cm in front of the subject's nose. The subject sits in a chair with their head fixed in place using a chin rest. Subjects are instructed to fixate on a central point presented on the display and to pay attention to the entire visual stimulus. The experiment is conducted in a dark room, with no light sources other than the display.

The duration of visual stimulus presentation and EEG measurement are 65 s. The first 60 s EEG from the start of measurement is used for analysis. The visual stimuli consisted of four types 15 Hz flickering stimuli and one non-flickering stimulus (0 Hz, BW). Each stimulus is presented five times in a randomized order. The measurement electrodes are placed at O1 and O2 according to the 10–20 system [20], which are located in the occipital lobes and are often used to record better responses for visual stimulus [21]. The subjects are three adult males with normal trichromatic vision, as confirmed by a standard color vision test chart.

Table 3. Recording conditions

Electroencephalograph	Emotiv EPOC X
Output device	EX-LDGC251UTB
Sampling frequency	128 Hz
Frequency of stimulus	15 Hz
The electrode	O1, O2
Subjects	Three adult males (mean age: 22.7 years)
Number of measurements	5 times
Measurement duration	65 s

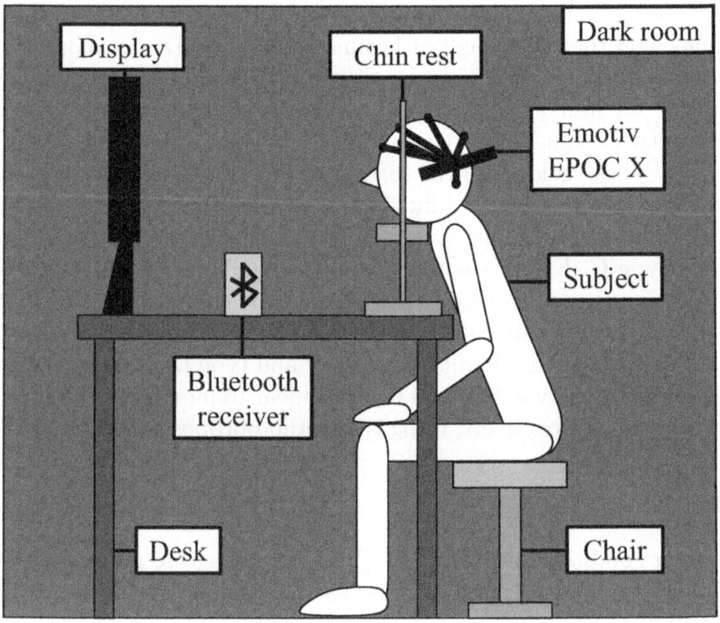

Fig. 5. Measurement environment

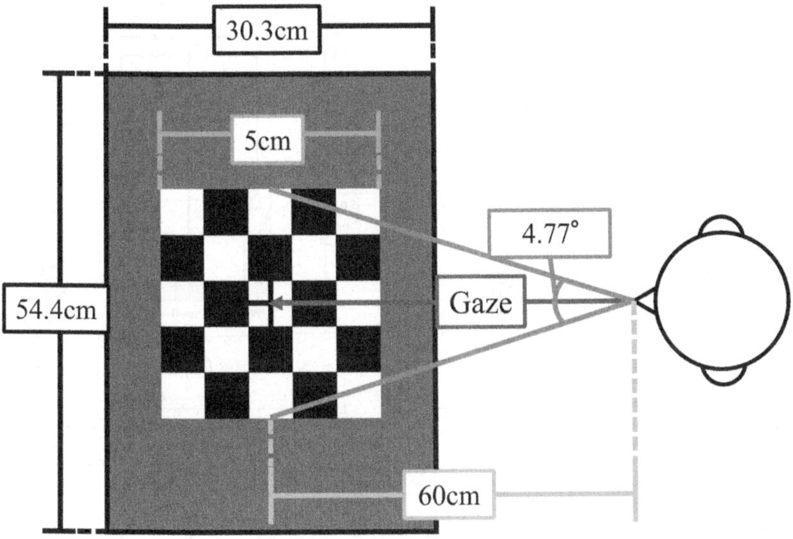

Fig. 6. Overview of Visual Stimulus Presentation

3.3 Analysis Method

The discrete Fourier transform (DFT) is applied to the recorded EEG signals. The SSVEP is defined as an amplitude at 30 Hz which is the second harmonic of flickering frequency of visual stimuli. SSVEP is detected using a threshold based on the 3σ method. The threshold X is calculated by Eq. (1).

$$X = \mu + 3\sigma \tag{1}$$

Here, μ is the mean of the amplitude spectrum of 30 Hz observed during the 0 Hz (non-flickering) stimulus condition. σ is the standard deviation. If the SSVEP amplitude in each experiment exceeds the threshold, it is considered that SSVEP is evoked.

A t-test is conducted to determine whether there are significant differences in the evoked SSVEP amplitudes among the visual stimuli.

3.4 Results

The SSVEP amplitudes and t-test results for each subject and each electrode, categorized by the type of color vision being evaluated, are shown in Fig. 7 and 8. The vertical axis indicates the SSVEP amplitude, The horizontal axis indicates the types of visual stimulus, Color bars are the averaged amount of SSVEP, error bars are the standard deviation of SSVEP. "*" indicates a significant difference ($p < 0.05$) between the connected pairs of stimuli.

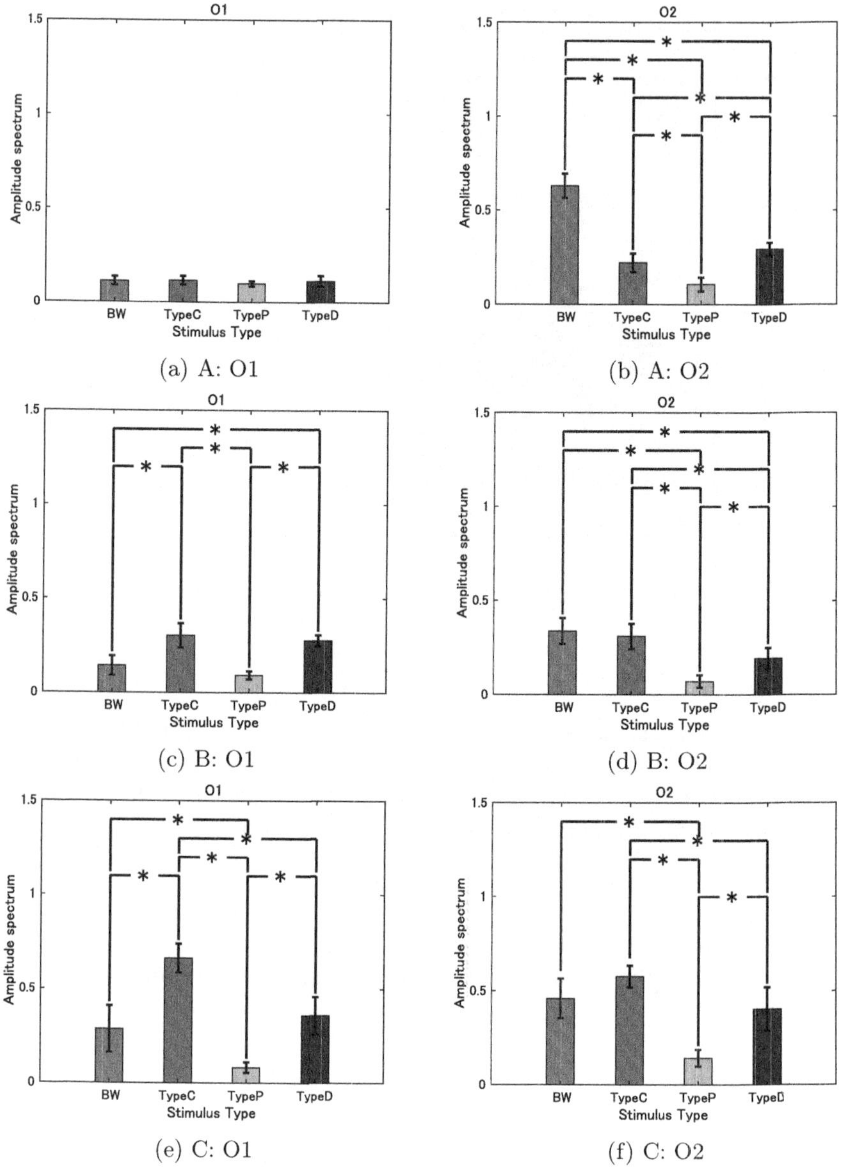

(a) A: O1 (b) A: O2 (c) B: O1 (d) B: O2 (e) C: O1 (f) C: O2

Fig. 7. Objective evaluation of type 1 dichromacy

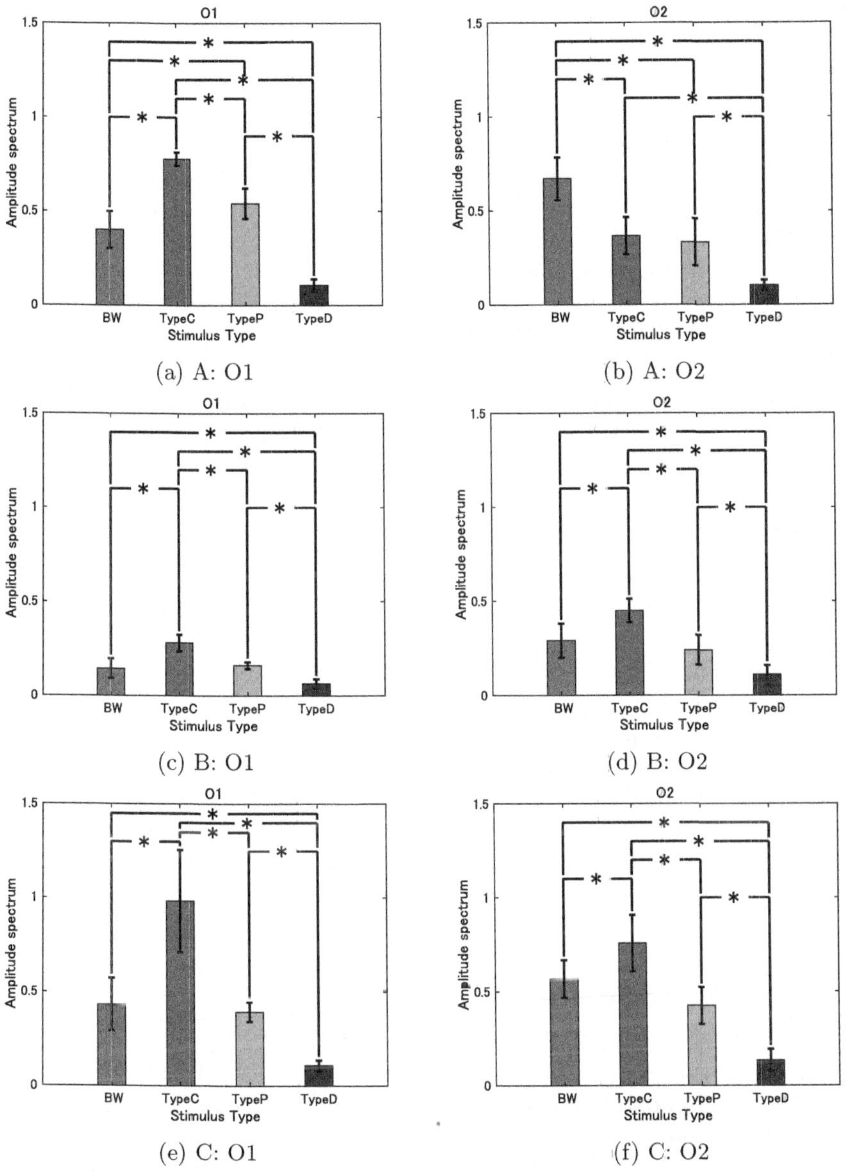

Fig. 8. Objective evaluation of type 2 dichromacy

4 Discussion

4.1 Objective Evaluation of Type 1 Dichromacy

Type P is a visual stimulus that simulates the visual appearance of a Type C stimulus for people with type 1 dichromacy. Therefore, it was assumed that the amount of SSVEP evoked by a Type C stimulus in subjects with type 1 dichromacy would be similar to the amount of SSVEP evoked by presenting Type P to subjects with normal trichromatic vision.

From Fig. 7, the mean amount of SSVEP evoked by Type P was the lowest across all subjects. Significant differences were observed between Type P and the other visual stimuli, except at electrode O1 in Subject B. Furthermore, Type P showed the lowest SSVEP elicitation rate across all subjects and electrodes. These results suggest that presenting the Type C stimulus (Fig. 3) to individuals with type 1 dichromacy may result in a lower amount of SSVEP evoked compared to other types of color vision.

4.2 Objective Evaluation of Type 2 Dichromacy

Type D is a visual stimulus that simulates the appearance of a Type C stimulus for individuals with type 2 dichromacy. It was assumed that the amount of SSVEP evoked by presenting Type C to subjects with type 2 dichromacy would be similar to the amount of SSVEP evoked by presenting Type D to subjects with normal trichromatic vision.

From Fig. 8, the mean amount of SSVEP evoked by Type D was the lowest across all subjects. Significant differences were observed between Type D and the other visual stimuli. Furthermore, Type D showed the lowest SSVEP elicitation rate across all subjects and electrodes. These results suggest that presenting the Type C stimulus (Fig. 4) to individuals with type 2 dichromacy may result in a lower amount of SSVEP evoked compared to other types of color vision.

4.3 Color Combinations of Visual Stimuli and Corresponding Amount of SSVEP Evoked

SSVEP is enhanced when the contrast between visual stimuli is high, which affects human visual perception [22]. Therefore, in general SSVEP elicitation experiments, visual stimuli composed of high-contrast color combinations such as black and white are commonly used.

However, Fig. 7c, 7e and 7f show that the average amount of SSVEP evoked by Type C, a visual stimulus composed of light blue and pink, is higher than that evoked by BW, a visual stimulus composed of black and white. In the objective evaluation for type 2 dichromacy, the average amount of SSVEP evoked by Type C (a green and pink stimulus), is higher than that evoked by BW (a black and white stimulus), except for the results shown in Fig. 8b. These results suggest that the influence of the color used in the visual stimuli is more significant than the magnitude of the luminance contrast. However, it is difficult to determine from the measurements in this experiment whether these factors originate from photoreceptors or from processing between the optic nerve and the visual cortex.

5 Conclusion

In this paper, we proposed an objective method for evaluating color blindness using SSVEP. To this end, we investigated whether objective evaluation is possible by modifying the color combinations used in visual stimuli to evoke SSVEP and by simulating how each type of color vision perceives these stimuli. We analyzed the tendencies of SSVEP evocation for each type of color vision by using visual stimuli composed of a color combination (light blue and pink) that is difficult to discriminate for individuals with type 1 dichromacy, simulated for both type 1 and type 2 dichromacy. These results suggest that type 1 dichromacy can be objectively distinguished based on SSVEP evocation tendencies by using visual stimuli composed of color combinations that are difficult to discriminate for individuals with type 1 dichromacy.

We also analyzed SSVEP responses using visual stimuli with a color combination of green and pink, which is difficult to discriminate for individuals with type 2 dichromacy. The results shows that type 2 dichromacy can be objectively distinguished based on SSVEP evocation tendencies by using visual stimuli composed of color combinations that are difficult to discriminate for individuals with type 2 dichromacy. These results suggest that the Type C visual stimulus developed in this study can be used to distinguish among normal trichromacy, type 1 dichromacy, and type 2 dichromacy.

Furthermore, the results of the two visual stimulus experiments suggest that the color composition of the stimuli plays a more significant role than the magnitude of contrast in increasing SSVEP evocation.

Future tasks include validation with participants who have actual color vision deficiencies without using simulated visual stimuli, as well as the development of a testing method to quantify and identify the degree of color blindness. In addition, it is necessary to investigate the factors that contribute to the increased amount of SSVEP evoked by the colors used in the visual stimuli.

Acknowledgment. This work was supported by JSPS KAKENHI Grant Number JP23K11292.

References

1. Zhang, Y., Shinoda, H.: Construction of a color-vision barrier-free environment that considers individual and displays differences. J. Color Sci. Assoc. Japan **44**(3), 11–14 (2020). (in Japanese)
2. Sharpe, L.T., Stockman, A., Jägle, H., J.: Nathans: Opsin genes, cone photopigments, color vision, and color blindness, pp. 3–52. Cambridge University Press (1999)
3. Saito, H.: Modeling of higher-level color perception in different color vision characteristics, Yokohama National University (2019). (Doctoral Thesis in Japanese)
4. Wolpaw, J.R., Birbaumer, N., McFarland, D.J., Pfurtscheller, G., Vaughan, T.M.: Brain comuputer interfaces for communication and control. Clin. Neurophysiol. **113**(6), 767–791 (2002)

5. Lebedev, M.A., Nicolelis, M.A.L.: Brain machine interfaces: past, present and future. Trends Neurosci. **29**(9), 536–546 (2006)
6. S. Kaneko, I. Kuriki, S. K. Andersen: Steady-state visual evoked potentials elicited from early visual cortex reflect both perceptual color space and cone-opponent mechanisms. Cerebral Cortex Communications, Vol. 1, Issue 1, tgaa059 (2020)
7. Bear, M.F., Connors, B.W., Paradiso, M.A.: Neuroscience exploring the brain. Nishimurasyoten (2021)
8. Ichikawa, K.: The hidden truth about color blindness. Gentosha (2019). (in Japanese)
9. Ishihara, S.: Ishihara's Tests for color deficiency 38 plates edition. Handaya (2019). (in Japanese)
10. Farnsworth, D.: The farnsworth dichotomous test for color blindness panel D-15. The psychological corp, New York (1947)
11. T. Yasuma: Fundamentals of anomaloscope. Japan. J. Visual Sci. **38**(2), 16–21 (2017). (in Japanese)
12. Morgan, S.T., Hansen, J.C., Hillyard, S.A.: Selective attention to stimulus location modulates the steady-state visual evoked potential. Proc. Natl. Acad. Sci. U.S.A. **93**(10), 4770–4774 (1996)
13. A. M. Norcia, L. G. Appelbaum, J. M. Ales, B. R. Cottereau, B. Rossion: The steady-state visual evoked potential in vision research: A review. J. Vision **15**(6) (2015)
14. Kus, R., et al.: On the quantification of SSVEP frequency responses in human EEG in realistic BCI conditions. PLoS One **8**(10) (2013)
15. Tobimatsu, S.: Key points in the interpretation of evoked potentials. Graduate School of Medical Sciences Kyushu University, Neurological Institute (2006). (in Japanese)
16. Ueda, S., Itai, A.: The analysis of SSVEP evoked by the modulated visual stimulus in medium and high frequencies. In: Proceedings of Soft Computing and Intelligent SystemsInternational Symposium on Advanced Intelligent Systems, pp. 1639–1642 (2014)
17. Bureau of Social Welfare Tokyo Metropolitan Government. https://jfly.uni-koeln.de/colorset/CUD_color_set_GuideBook_2018.pdf. Accessed 19 May 2025
18. Color Universal Desing Organization. https://cudo.jp/?page_id=1565, Accessed 19 May 2025
19. Viénot, F., Brettel, H., Mollon, J.D.: Digital video colourmaps for checking the legibility of displays by dichromats. Color. Res. Appl. **24**, 243–252 (1999)
20. Jasper, H.H.: The ten twenty electrode system of the international federation. Electroencephalogr. Clin. Neurophysiol. **10**, 371–375 (1958)
21. H. Shibasaki: Functional diagnosis of the brain by evoked potentials. Biomed. Eng. **1**(5) (1987). (in Japanese)
22. T. Yoshida, T. Naganawa, A. Itai: The difference of EEG between same contrast visual stimuli. IEICE Tech. Rep. **120**(176), SIS2020-24, 71–74 (2020). (in Japanese)

The Study on Health Status Assessment Technology Using a Foot-Pressure Mat

Momona Kikuzawa(✉), Miki Matsuura, Mayu Katsumoto, and Hideaki Kimura

Department of Computer Science, Graduate School of Engineering, Chubu University, 1200 Matsumotocho, Kasugai 487-0027, Aichi, Japan
{tp24005-7149,tp25012-0755,ep22050-0980}@sti.chubu.ac.jp, hideaki_kimura@isc.chubu.ac.jp

Abstract. In this study, we present a novel, non-invasive, and simplified health-assessment system based on a sensor-integrated foot-pressure mat. Our method eliminates the need for costly camera systems and elaborate imaging environments by allowing users simply to stand on the mat while wearing socks, capturing both plantar geometry and pressure distribution in a single measurement, with real-time data transmission and automated calibration features. Conventional approaches often require multiple cameras captures and introduce significant privacy concerns; in contrast, our system minimizes participant burden and preserves privacy. We employ a neuro-fuzzy inference model to estimate individual healthy-life expectancy, achieving a maximum estimation error of less than one year relative to theoretical benchmarks. The streamlined measurement protocol supports continuous monitoring for preventive care and daily health management, striking a balance between high usability and privacy protection. Ongoing work includes extensive validation across diverse age cohorts and investigation of the system's robustness for long-term, real-world deployment.

Keywords: Sole of the Foot · Neuro-Fuzzy · Healthy Life Expectancy.

1 Introduction

In recent years, Japan has entered a rapidly aging society, with the proportion of individuals aged 65 and older continuing to rise [1]. Meanwhile, there exists a gap of approximately ten years between "healthy life expectancy," during which one can lead an independent daily life, and "life expectancy," defined as the biologically sustained lifespan [2]. The financial burden on medical and long-term care services supporting this intervening period is increasing year by year [3]. To address this challenge, preventive approaches aimed at extending healthy life expectancy have become an urgent priority. In this study, we propose a novel method for estimating healthy life expectancy using a self-service "foot-pressure mat" sensor that requires no special wearable devices. By capturing plantar geometry and pressure distribution data and feeding them into a neuro-fuzzy inference model [4], our approach reduces estimation error from 1.3 years to within one year [5]. Furthermore, the system operates without cameras and allows measurement through socks, thereby achieving both privacy protection and user convenience.

H. Tanaka et al. (Eds.): BodyNets 2025, LNICST 714, pp. 213–227, 2026.
https://doi.org/10.1007/978-3-032-38657-1_16

2 Related Studies

This chapter describes the related studies [6, 7], the issues and the improvements of this study based on them.

2.1 Points of Issue

[6] employed an in-shoe system embedding five PVDF film sensors to capture plantar pressure during gait and perform biomechanical analysis. However, the limited sensor count provides insufficient coverage to comprehensively characterize pressure distribution and foot geometry across the entire plantar surface. Moreover, the in-shoe design is highly susceptible to sensor displacement and variability in fit pressure during walking, posing significant challenges for reproducibility and stability over extended, repeated use. Finally, although optimized for dynamic gait assessment, this approach cannot be readily adapted for static standing measurements or simple screening applications.

[7] reported a walking-energy-harvesting mat in which 35 piezoelectric elements are connected in series/parallel and encased beneath a wooden board. However, because the sensor layout and circuit design are optimized solely for power generation, this approach fails to meet the spatial-resolution and measurement-accuracy requirements necessary for detailed plantar pressure mapping and foot-shape estimation. Furthermore, although the system emphasizes rectification and storage of the generated electrical signals, the methods for raw data acquisition and analytical processing remain undeveloped, rendering it inadequate for gait-analysis applications. In addition, the wooden support structure induces variability in sensor response uniformity and durability, raising serious concerns regarding long-term reliability.

2.2 Points of Improvement

In contrast to [6], our system deploys a total of 36 piezoelectric sensors—24 27 mm-diameter "medium" elements arranged in a 4×6 grid and 12 30 mm-diameter "big" elements arranged in a 4×3 grid—on a mat-type platform, enabling high-resolution, simultaneous measurement of plantar pressure distribution and geometric information across the entire foot sole under both static stance and slow walking conditions. Foot length and width are estimated statically—without requiring any user movement—by applying Euclidean-distance rules between sensor contact points. Moreover, by incorporating each element's contact area into the calculation, the system reduces measurement burden while achieving high reproducibility and stability.

In contrast to [7], this study prioritizes measurement over power generation by optimally deploying 24 medium-sized (27 mm) and 12 large-sized (30 mm) piezoelectric elements according to application requirements, enabling high-density capture of plantar pressure distributions and geometric features on a single mat platform under both static and dynamic conditions. By integrating a neuro-fuzzy inference framework, our system markedly enhances the precision and robustness of foot-shape, body-weight/height, and healthy-life-expectancy estimations derived from the mat sensor.

3 Proposed Method

This chapter describes a piezoelectric device-based healthy life expectancy estimation and extension technique.

3.1 Health Status Monitoring System

Physical characteristics are estimated from plantar sensor data, and the resulting body mass index (BMI) is subsequently used to calculate healthy life expectancy (Fig. 1). The present algorithm was developed with reference to the methodologies described in prior studies [8–10], and the theoretical values for healthy life expectancy are determined in accordance with [5].

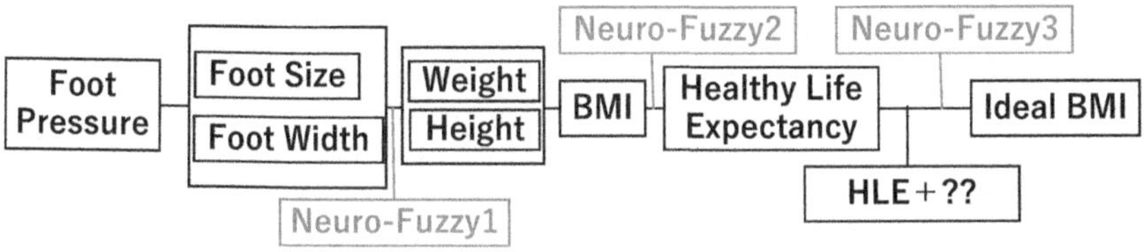

Fig. 1. Health Status Assessment Process.

In the third neuro-fuzzy model, we repurposed the inference engine from the second model and systematically configured the input parameters on a grid. Specifically, we generated all combinations of BMI values from 15 to 30 (in unit increments) and ages from 20 to 80 (in unit increments), input these points into the model, and organized the resulting outputs into a two-dimensional lookup table. We then performed an inverse search on this table to efficiently extract the BMI–age pairs corresponding to targeted healthy-life-expectancy or weight-estimation values. This approach enables quantitative derivation of the ideal physiological conditions indicated by the model.

3.2 Multipoint Arrangement of Piezoelectric Elements

In this study, to acquire high-precision plantar data, we designed a multipoint mat sensor incorporating 27 mm–diameter medium piezoelectric elements and 30 mm–diameter big piezoelectric elements. The medium elements are arranged in a 4 × 6 grid (24 sensors) and the big elements in a 4 × 3 grid (12 sensors) across the mat surface (Fig. 2), with no sensors placed within 10 cm posterior to the heel. This configuration exploits the fact that the minimum foot length of adult women exceeds 18 cm [11], allowing omission of unnecessary posterior measurements and concentration on regions of greatest geometric and load-bearing interest. Although the 27 mm medium elements provide a sufficiently fine inter-element pitch to resolve subtle variations in plantar geometry—thereby reducing error in static length estimation— the larger 30 mm sensors deliver enhanced sensitivity and a broader sensing area [12, 13], excelling at detecting load peaks and subsurface pressure distributions. By combining these heterogeneous elements, our system non-invasively captures both pressure distribution and geometric changes at high sampling rates, thereby bolstering the robustness and accuracy of our healthy-life–expectancy estimation model.

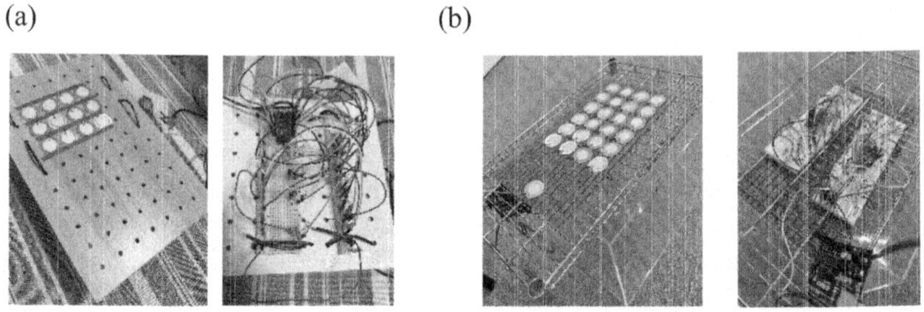

Fig. 2. Arrangement Diagram of Piezoelectric Elements. (a) Arrangement of medium-sized elements (left: front, right: back). (b) Arrangement of big-sized elements (left: front, right: back).

4 Experiment

In this chapter, we outline the experimental setup and methodology for estimating foot length and foot width using piezoelectric elements.

4.1 Devices for Reducing Measurement Error

In this study, the primary source of measurement error is attributed to the spatial-resolution constraints imposed by the effective detection diameters (27 mm and 15 mm) of the piezoelectric elements. Because each element's output voltage varies approximately in proportion to its contact area, we implemented a preprocessing normalization in which the maximum ground contact area of each element was defined as a baseline and all measured voltage responses were scaled relative to this reference. This normalization mitigates inter-element sensitivity differences and the influence of wiring resistance, thereby suppressing output variability under identical pressure (Fig. 3). Moreover, if an element's detected contact area falls below 70% of its baseline, the sensor is presumed to reside under the medial arch; such data points are excluded from foot-length and foot-width estimation, and local data gaps are filled via linear interpolation from adjacent sensor outputs. This approach eliminates aberrant values originating from the arch region and ensures robust forefoot shape estimation. Finally, by correcting boundary measurements based on the baseline values, we constrain the maximum absolute error during model training for foot-length and foot-width estimation to within the element diameters of 27 mm and 15 mm.

To clarify units and the readout chain, we use a 28-μm PVDF (polyvinylidene fluoride) film; the open-circuit voltage follows $V_{OC} \approx g_{33}\sigma t$ (typical $g_{33} \approx 0.2 - 0.3$ V · m/N, stance stress $\sigma \approx 0.3-$ 0.7 MPa). We digitized the signals with a 12-bit ADC (0–4095) at 100 Hz, configured with 11 dB attenuation. Data were stored as raw ADC counts and converted to voltage only when needed via V_{ADS}=(count/4095) V_{FS} and V_{sensor}=V_{ADS}/G. Figure 3 reports V_{ADS}; all other values are given in ADC counts.

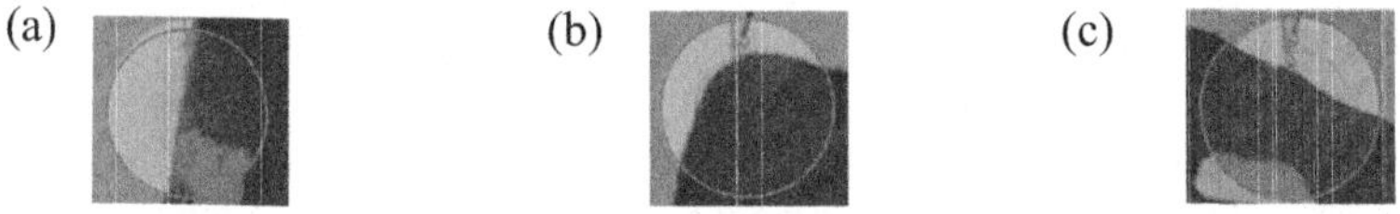

Fig. 3. Treaded area of piezoelectric element. (a) Percentage of sock area: 0.49, Output value of piezoelectric element: 0.521 V. (b) 0.69, 0.825 V. (c) 0.61, 0.795 V.

4.2 Length Estimation for Each Foot Section

In this study, foot length and width are estimated without rotation correction by computing the Euclidean distance between piezoelectric elements embedded in the mat. For the right foot using medium-diameter elements, the "toe point" is defined as the topmost, leftmost sensor whose output exceeds its reference threshold, and the "heel point" as the sensor located in the heel region; the Euclidean distance between these points constitutes the foot length. Foot width is determined by selecting, in the left most column, the highest-output sensor in the top row as the left-width point, and, in the rightmost column, the sensor three rows below the top row as the right-width point; the distance between these two points defines the foot width. For the big diameter elements, the foot-length procedure is identical, but the right-width point is taken as the sensor one row below the top row in the rightmost column, with its distance to the left-width point yielding the foot width. An analogous, mirror-symmetric rule set is applied to the left foot, ensuring algorithmic consistency and enabling realtime processing.

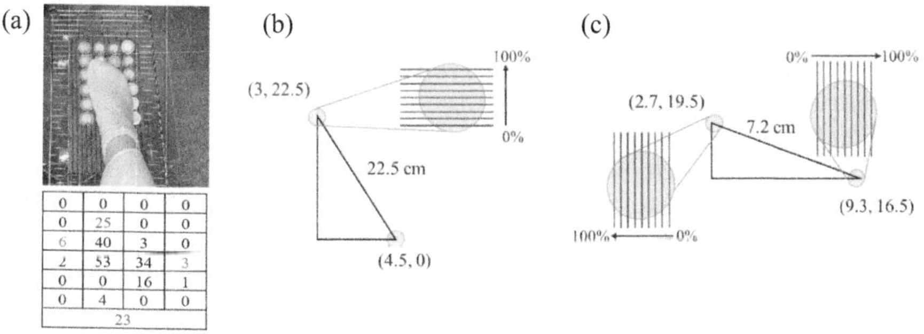

Fig. 4. Method of Estimating the Length of Each Foot from the Output Value of the Piezoelectric Element. (a) Output Value and Image of Piezoelectric Element. (b) Estimation of foot length ((a) in red). (c) Estimation of Foot Width ((a) in blue). "(color figure online)"

Figure 4(b) illustrates the Euclidean-distance approach for foot-length estimation, and Fig. 4(c) shows the corresponding method for foot-width estimation. Both procedures are founded on the relationship between plantar contact area and each piezoelectric element's output (Sect. 4.1) and employ segmentation of the sole into increments equal to the sensor diameters. For foot-length estimation, sensor rows aligned in the medial–lateral direction are processed by cumulatively summing the proportion of contact area in steps of one element diameter, beginning at the heel side. The sensors at which a predefined threshold is reached are identified as the heel point and toe point, respectively.

The Euclidean distance between these two points yields an accurate total foot-length estimate from partial ground-contact data on the mat.

Similarly, for foot-width estimation, vertically oriented sensor columns are cumulatively processed from both the left and right boundaries in element-diameter increments. The first sensor reached from the inner side of the left column is designated the left-width point, and the analogous sensor in the right column is designated the right-width point. Computing the Euclidean distance between these two points quantifies the optimal lateral spread of the foot.

This strategy obviates any need for rotational correction. By combining contact-area evaluation—derived from the piezoelectric outputs—with straightforward distance calculations, the method achieves high-precision estimation with minimal computational overhead.

5 Numeric Calculation

In this study, we employed the Adaptive Neuro-Fuzzy Inference System (ANFIS) implemented in MATLAB's Fuzzy Logic Toolbox to estimate physical characteristics. For body-weight and height estimation, the number of training epochs was set at three levels—1,500, 2,000, and 2,500—to compare the convergence behavior of the training error and the generalization performance at each stage, thus identifying the optimal epoch count that achieves adequate convergence while mitigating overfitting. For healthy-life-expectancy estimation, we adopted training epochs of 50, 100, and 150. In this study, the fuzzification design was optimized separately for each model as follows. For the weight–height estimation model, three linguistic labels were defined—SM (Small), MD (Medium), and BG (Big)—and two-term Gaussian membership functions (gauss2mf) were employed to capture broad data distributions while suppressing overfitting. For the healthy-life-expectancy estimation model, four labels were introduced—SM (Underweight/Young), MD1 (Moderate Obesity), MD2 (High Obesity), and BG (Severe Obesity)—with single Gaussian membership functions (gaussmf) applied to accurately discriminate subtle changes near class boundaries. These configurations achieve a balanced fuzzy-inference system that both generalizes well in weight–height prediction and sensitively resolves critical transitions in healthy-life-expectancy estimation.

5.1 Weight and Height Estimation

In this study, we used only foot-length and foot-width measurements obtained from the piezoelectric mat as input variables, and employed a neuro-fuzzy inference model to estimate participants' body weight. For model training, we utilized paired foot-length, foot-width, and weight data reported in the literature [Reference], whereas for testing, we fed the model with foot-length and foot-width values measured directly by our piezoelectric sensors to assess real-world applicability. To evaluate generalization performance, we conducted five-fold cross-validation, yielding a mean root-mean-square error (RMSE) of 5.6 kg and a mean coefficient of determination of 0.62. Figures 5 and 6 presents the training-loss trajectory, scatter plots comparing observed and predicted values, and the fuzzy-set structures used in inference.

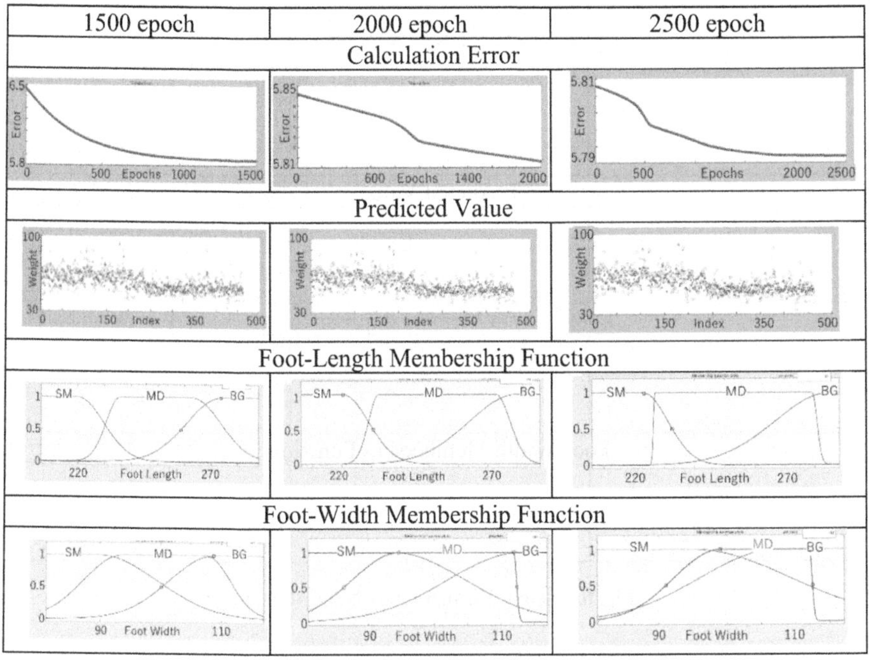

Fig. 5. Weight Estimation by Neuro-Fuzzy.

As shown in Fig. 5, increasing the number of training epochs yields only a marginal reduction in mean absolute error (MAE), which converges at approximately 5.85 kg, indicating that prolonged training fails to further improve estimation accuracy. Moreover, when plotting observed versus predicted values, the model consistently underperforms on outlier samples with exceptionally large or small foot lengths and widths.

A closer examination of the fuzzy-membership functions reveals that, in the foot-length "MD" (Medium) region, the left and right support widths both contract toward the center as epoch counts increase, resulting in an expanded, flat plateau around the mean. This behavior suggests that the model broadens its tolerance for midrange values while reducing sensitivity to extremes. Conversely, in the foot-width membership functions, the right support of the "SM" (Small) region gradually shifts outward, and the left support of the "MD" region similarly expands; this adjustment appears intended to encompass both central and peripheral width ranges but does not enhance performance on outliers.

These findings imply that merely increasing training epochs will not address outlier mispredictions and may in fact bias the model toward midrange tolerance. Future work should therefore involve redesigning the membership functions and reinforcing training on outlier samples, or otherwise revising the model architecture to improve robustness.

As shown in Fig. 6, the mean absolute error (MAE) converges to approximately 4.8 cm and 4.77 cm at 1,500 and 2,000 training epochs, respectively; however, at 2,500 epochs the MAE continues to decrease. Despite this apparent improvement, scatter-plot comparisons of observed versus predicted heights reveal two critical shortcomings:

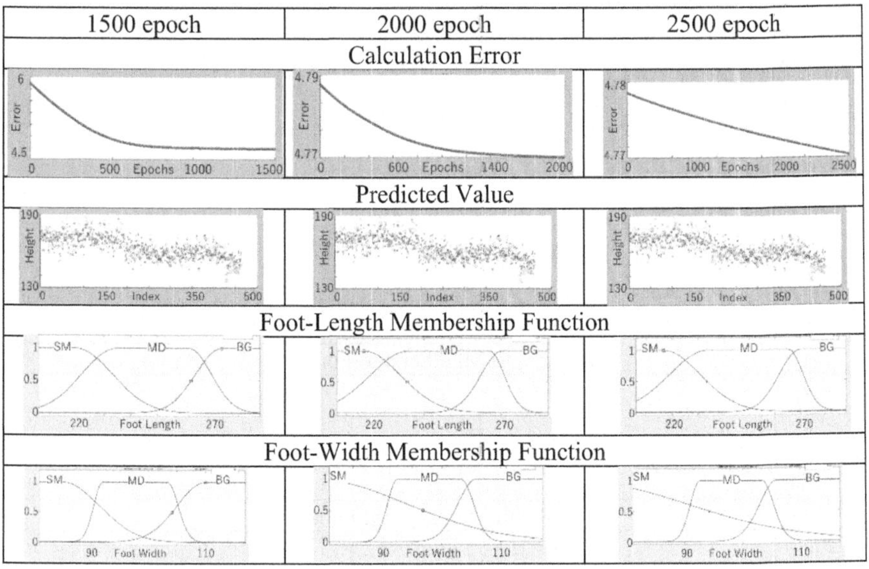

Fig. 6. Height Estimation by Neuro-Fuzzy.

- High-height region (Indices 50–200; height $\geq$ 180 cm):

  In this domain, the model's predictions deviate substantially from the true height distribution, exhibiting pronounced distortion.

- Low-height region (Index $\approx$ 450; height $\leq$ 150 cm):

  Similarly, for heights below 150 cm, predicted values tend to underestimate the actual measurements, indicating that the model fails to capture this range accurately.

These observations suggest that merely increasing the number of training epochs will not yield localized gains in predictive accuracy and may, in fact, exacerbate overfitting. Furthermore, the shapes of the fuzzy-membership functions employed for height estimation remain essentially unchanged beyond a certain epoch count, unlike those in the weight-estimation model. This indicates that the current model architecture offers minimal capacity for re-tuning fuzzy sets through additional training.

Accordingly, we identify two avenues for further investigation:

i. Redesign of membership functions:

Locally redefine triangular or single-Gaussian (gauss1) membership functions tailored to the extreme height ranges.

ii. Augmentation of training data:

Enrich the dataset with more extreme-value height samples and apply outlier-aware preprocessing to improve the balance of the training distribution.

By implementing these measures and re-evaluating model performance, we anticipate mitigating the observed prediction biases and achieving higher-precision height estimation.

We first verified the plotting conventions in Fig. 7: x = Foot Length [cm], y = Foot Width [cm], z = Weight [kg]. Predictions were inverse-transformed from any standardization before plotting, a common z-axis range was used across panels, and surfaces were clipped to the training domain; hence shape changes reflect training effects rather than axis/sign/scale artifacts. At 1500 epochs the surface is smooth and physically plausible. From 2000–2500 epochs spurious ripples and steep edge gradients appear—particularly near data-sparse boundaries—indicating overfitting and degraded generalization. In contrast, the height model's fuzzy membership functions stabilize beyond a certain epoch and change little, whereas the weight model continues to re-tune and oscillate. To address this we will (i) locally redesign membership functions (triangular or single-Gaussian with narrower widths at extreme ranges), and (ii) augment boundary/extreme samples with outlier-aware preprocessing. With these measures (in conjunction with early-stopping on a validation split), we expect to reduce the observed biases and recover a monotone, smooth surface.

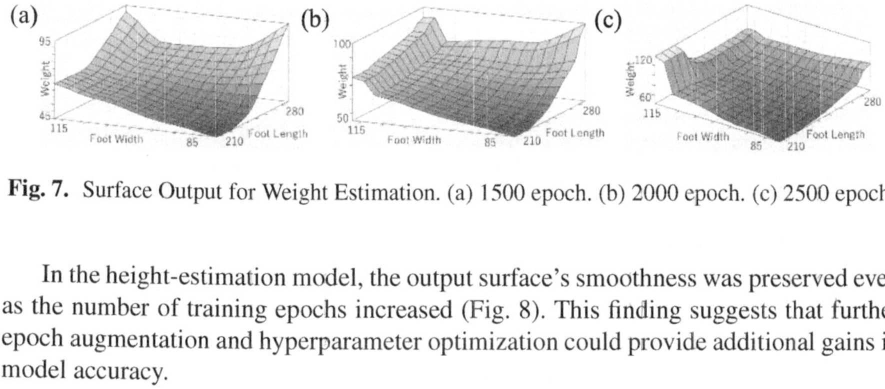

Fig. 7. Surface Output for Weight Estimation. (a) 1500 epoch. (b) 2000 epoch. (c) 2500 epoch.

In the height-estimation model, the output surface's smoothness was preserved even as the number of training epochs increased (Fig. 8). This finding suggests that further epoch augmentation and hyperparameter optimization could provide additional gains in model accuracy.

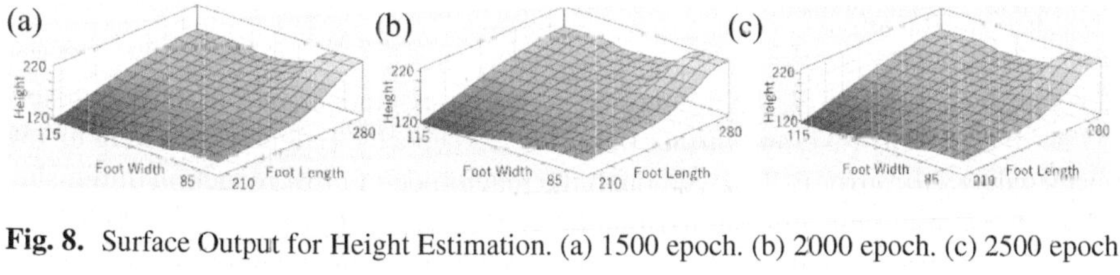

Fig. 8. Surface Output for Height Estimation. (a) 1500 epoch. (b) 2000 epoch. (c) 2500 epoch.

5.2 Healthy Life Expectancy Estimates

In this study, we constructed a neuro-fuzzy inference model as in the previous section, but additionally introduced age—an important determinant of healthy-life expectancy—into the antecedent alongside BMI. Since BMI alone cannot fully account for individual variability in body composition and metabolic state, we aimed to improve estimation accuracy by incorporating age-related physiological changes. Concretely, BMI was partitioned into three fuzzy sets ("Low," "Medium," and "High") and age into three fuzzy sets ("Young," "Middle-aged," and "Elderly"), yielding a total of nine fuzzy-inference rules. For training, we used the foot-length, foot-width, and weight correspondence data reported in [Reference], while for testing we input BMI values derived from our piezoelectric sensors along with participants' age information. We evaluated model performance using five-fold cross-validation, which produced a mean RMSE of 1.42 kg and a mean coefficient of determination (R^2) of 0.79. Figure 9 details the loss progression for each fold, scatter plots comparing observed and predicted values, and the parameter configurations of the fuzzy sets employed. These results confirm that integrating both BMI and age in the antecedent substantially enhances the explanatory power of healthy-life-expectancy estimation.

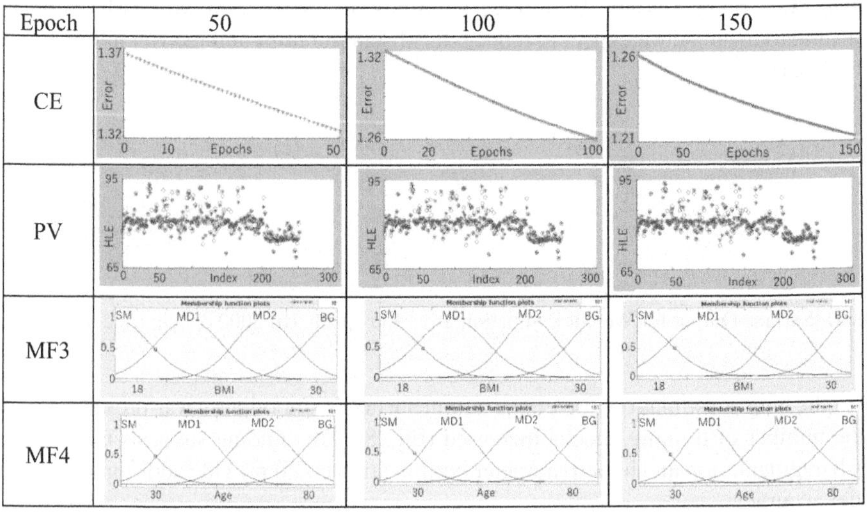

Fig. 9. Healthy Life Expectancy Estimation by Neuro-Fuzzy. MF3: BMI Membership Function, MF4: Age Membership Function

As presented in Fig. 9, the training error decreases gradually from approximately 1.37 at 50 epochs to 1.32, and further to 1.26 at 100 epochs. Extending training to 150 epochs reduces the error to 1.21, although the magnitude of error reduction diminishes with each interval, indicating an asymptotic convergence. However, scatter-plot comparisons of observed versus predicted values reveal that, while the model closely tracks measurements in the central output range (approximately 75–85), it exhibits substantial deviations for extreme samples—those above 90 and below 70. Notably, increasing the epoch count from 50 to 150 fails to improve the model's fit to these outlier regions.

Examining the age-input membership functions (MF4) further underscores this limitation. At 50 epochs, the SM function covers the young age range (~20–40 years), BG covers the elderly range (~60–80 years), and MD1/MD2 partition the middle-aged cohort in a canonical arrangement. By 100 epochs, the right support boundary of SM extends toward older ages, and the left support of MD1 broadens outward. These adjustments serve to widen the model's tolerance around the central age domain but do not enhance discriminative performance for age-extreme samples.

Collectively, these observations indicate that, despite continued reduction in training error and re-tuning of membership functions toward broader central-domain coverage, the model's ability to predict outliers remains unchanged. Therefore, merely increasing the number of epochs is insufficient for improving outlier accuracy; instead, targeted redesign of local membership functions and augmentation of outlier training samples are essential to bolster model robustness.

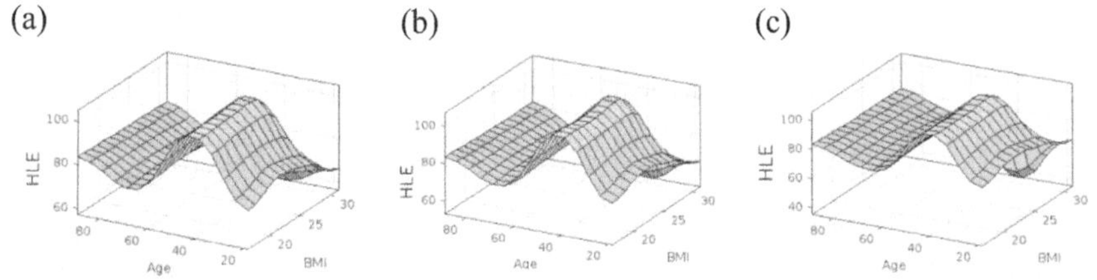

Fig. 10. Surface Output for Healthy Life Expectancy Estimation. (a) 50 epoch. (b) 100 epoch. (c) 150 epoch.

As illustrated in Fig. 10, although the overall surface shape appears to converge with increasing training epochs (50, 100, and 150), pronounced instability persists in the region around Age = 40–50 years. At 50 epochs, the surface exhibits coarse undulations and discontinuities, reflecting insufficient early-stage adjustment of the membership functions and the strong influence of sparse training samples. Increasing to 100 epochs sharpens the peak in the BMI $\approx$ 25–30 and Age $\approx$ 20–30 domain and yields a smoother appearance overall, yet the Age = 40–50 zone still contains irregular valleys and crests. After 150 epochs, the gradient around the primary peak becomes even steeper, but localized disturbances—such as abrupt drops and reverse-flow patterns—remain in the 40–50 age band. These artifacts arise because the model relies on fuzzy-membership weighting to interpolate and extrapolate in data-scarce regions, leading to reduced output reliability where no observations exist.

To eliminate this surface instability, it is essential first to collect sufficient samples for the 40–50 age cohort to fill the distribution gap. Additionally, introducing local shape constraints or penalty terms on the membership functions could suppress excessive curvature changes in missing-data regions. Implementing these measures should facilitate construction of a smoother, more trustworthy healthy-life-expectancy prediction surface.

6 Numerical Calculation Results

Tables 1, 2 and 3 present numerical results for a single healthy subject across multiple foot angles.

6.1 Estimated Value

For each device (MD, BD) and tilt condition (0°, +30°, −30°), we report the discrepancies between measured and theoretical values for height, weight, BMI, and the resulting estimated healthy life expectancy (HLE). Parentheses following each HLE denote the deviation from the theoretical anchor (ΔHLE; negative = underestimation, positive = overestimation). For comparability, Tables 4, 5 and 6 also summarize error magnitudes using MAE/RMSE alongside per-condition values. In addition, we present the ideal BMI required to achieve 1–3 years of HLE extension as ΔBMI relative to the baseline BMI (positive = increase, negative = decrease), obtained by inverting the HLE–BMI mapping under the measured height and the same model configuration (Fig. 11).

Table 1. When the Sole is Placed Vertically.

Tilt 0°	MD	MV (MD)	BD	MV (BD)
Foot Size [cm]	23.1	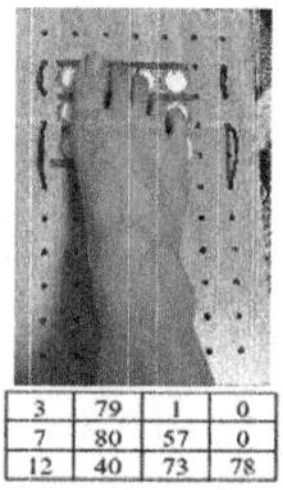	22.5	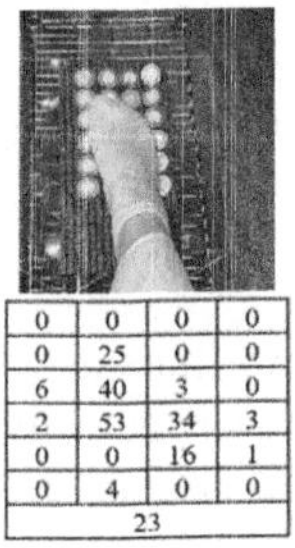
Foot Width [cm]	8.4		7.2	
Height [cm]	−2.0		−5.0	
Weight [kg]	−1.5		−4.7	
BMI	−0.7		−1.2	
HLE	81.3 (−0.9)		81.4 (−0.8)	
BMI1	+1.3		−0.3	
BMI2	+2.7		+1.6	
BMI3	+3.7		+2.9	

MD: Medium-Size Device, MV: Measured Value, BD: Big-Size Device, BMI1–3: Ideal BMI changes for 1–3 year healthy-life extension targets

6.2 Consideration

Based on Tables 4, 5 and 6 (parentheses after HLE denote deviation from the theoretical anchor), at 0° the MD shows small errors (height − 2.0 cm; weight − 1.5 kg; BMI −0.7), whereas the BD underestimates more markedly (−5.0 cm; −4.7 kg; −1.2). Under ±30° tilt, MD remains stable (height ≈ −2 cm; weight + 0.3–0.8 kg), while BD deteriorates (height − 12 to −13 cm; weight − 5.2 to −6.0 kg). This device gap is consistent with sensor geometry: MD's smaller elements better accommodate tilt-induced changes in contact area, whereas BD's larger elements are more susceptible to localized pressure bias and area quantization along the long axis of the foot.

HLE estimates stay close between devices—0°: 81.2 (−0.9) vs. 81.4 (−0.8); | 30°: 82.5 (+0.3) vs. 82.7 (+0.5); −30°: 82.2 (0.0) vs. 82.5 (+0.3)—with BD's slight overestimation plausibly arising from BMI underestimation propagating through the HLE mapping. For ideal BMI, the devices even diverge in sign at 0° (MD +1.3 vs. BD −0.3), but converge under tilt (both recommending increases of ≈ + 2.7 − +5.1 for 1–3-year

Table 2. When the Sole of the Foot is Placed on the Left Side of the Mat.

Tilt 30°	MD	MV(MD)	BD	MV(BD)
Foot Size	23.3	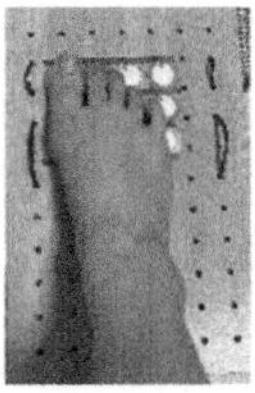	20.6	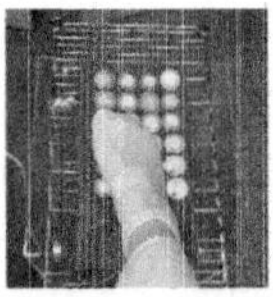
Foot Width	8.7		7.0	
Height	−2.0		−12	
Weight	+0.8		−5.2	
BMI	+0.2		+0.4	0 0 0 0 0 0 0 0 66 1 0 0 0 11 6 0 308 126 29 0 0 115 80 0 56
HLE	82.5 (+0.3)		82.7 (+0.5)	
BMI1	+3.0	91 4 0 0 88 2 13 0 90 81 84 2	+3.2	
BMI2	+4.0		+4.2	
BMI3	+4.9		+5.1	

Table 3. When the Sole of the Foot is Placed on the Right Side of the Mat.

Tilt −30°	MD	MV(MD)	BD	MV(BD)
Foot Size	23.1	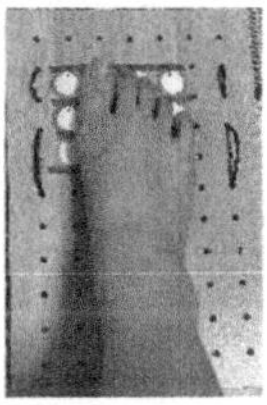	18.5	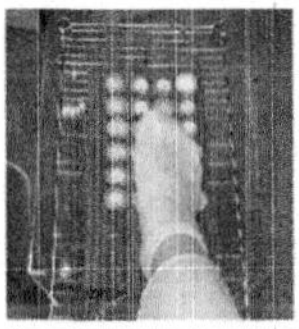
Foot Width	8.7		7.0	
Height	−2.0		−13	
Weight	+0.3		−6.0	
BMI	0.0		+0.2	
HLE	82.2 (0.0)		82.5 (+0.3)	0 0 0 0 0 0 0 0 0 10 0 0 0 11 6 2 0 0 134 270 0 1 88 21 56
BMI1	+2.7	0 90 72 0 1 95 55 40 0 86 91 94	+3.0	
BMI2	+3.7		+4.0	
BMI3	+4.6		+4.9	

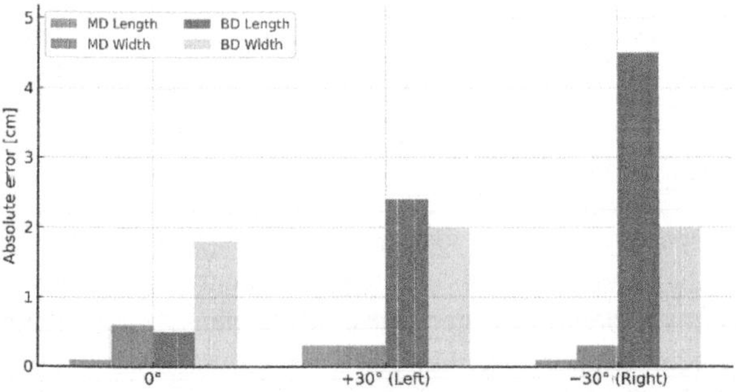

Fig. 11. Absolute Error (cm) to Ground Truth (23.0 cm, 9.0 cm) across Tilt Conditions

targets). Collectively, these results reveal a clear device×posture interaction and motivate inclination detection/compensation, reconsideration of element diameter/layout, and retraining with tilted data to harden membership functions.

These tendencies are visualized in the accompanying bar chart and lead to the following image-based interpretation.

Three patterns are evident in the bar chart: (i) MD errors stay sub-centimeter across all tilts (length ≤ 0.3 cm; width ≤ 0.6 cm); (ii) BD length error grows almost monotonically with tilt magnitude (0.5 cm $\rightarrow$ 2.4 cm $\rightarrow$ 4.5 cm for 0°, +30°, −30°), whereas BD width error remains roughly constant ($\approx$2.0 cm); (iii) the worst case occurs at −30° (right tilt). Mechanistically, the BD's larger element diameter yields coarser sampling: when the foot rotates, heel/toe boundaries intersect the sensor lattice obliquely and partial overlaps are quantized, producing systematic underestimation along the longitudinal axis. By contrast, lateral edges remain closer to the lattice orientation, so width bias is nearly constant. The −30° asymmetry is consistent with a small mounting/alignment offset and with the medial-arch masking rule (70%), which can remove medial cells and shorten the effective footprint. These image-level findings corroborate Tables 4, 5 and 6: MD is robust to tilt, while BD exhibits a strong device×posture dependence. Practically, this motivates (a) tilt detection/compensation in preprocessing, (b) smaller-diameter/denser elements or sub-cell area estimation to reduce quantization at heel/toe, and (c) rotation-augmented training so the estimator remains stable under off-axis contact.

7 Conclusion

7.1 Summary

In this work, we have developed a non-invasive, sock-friendly foot-pressure mat system that integrates 24 medium-diameter (27 mm) and 12 large-diameter (30 mm) piezoelectric sensors to capture high-resolution plantar geometry and pressure distribution under both static and slow-walking conditions. By combining fine-pitch medium elements for geometric accuracy with large-area big elements for load-peak detection, and by normalizing each sensor's contact area, our system achieves a maximum healthy-life-expectancy estimation error of less than one year relative to theoretical benchmarks. The streamlined measurement protocol obviates cameras and complex imaging setups, thereby ensuring user privacy and ease of use while maintaining robust performance.

7.2 Future Work

We will validate sensor designs across diverse users and foot morphologies (varying piezoelectric diameters/materials), extend the neuro-fuzzy model with dynamic gait features (temporal pressure trajectories, stride phase), and quantify/compensate environmental effects (temperature, humidity, sock thickness), enabling an adaptable foot-pressure platform for long-term preventive monitoring.

References

1. Inoue, M., Watanabe, T.: The future process of Japan's population aging: a cluster analysis using small area population projection data. Popul. Res. Policy Rev. **43**(5), 701–727 (2024)
2. Tokudome, S., Hashimoto, S., Igata, A.: Life expectancy and healthy life expectancy of Japan: the fastest graying society in the world. BMC. Res. Notes. **9**(1), 482 (2016). https://doi.org/10.1186/s13104-016-2281-2
3. Ministry of Health, Labour and Welfare: The current and future role of the public long-term care insurance system. Ministry of Health, Labour and Welfare, Tokyo (2018)
4. Jang, J.-S.R.: ANFIS: adaptive-network-based fuzzy inference system. IEEE Trans. Syst. Man Cybern. **23**(3), 665–685 (1993). https://doi.org/10.1109/21.256541
5. Kikuzawa, M., Kimura, H.: Research on technology for understanding health conditions using foot visualization shoes. IEICE Technical Report, vol. 125, no. 22, MICT2025-16, pp. 74–79, May 2025
6. Yang, B., Jia, B., Xin, Y., Zhu, K.: Plantar pressure distribution measurement system based on PVDF piezoelectric sensors. Integr. Ferroelectr. **230**(1), 40–47 (2022). https://doi.org/10.1080/10584587.2022.2102797
7. Suleiman, A.D., Abdulhamid, I.G.: Piezoelectric energy harvesting floor mat for low power applications. Int. Res. J. Mod. Eng. Technol. Sci. **3**(12), 118–124 (2021)
8. Kikuzawa, M., Kimura, H.: Study of the health condition estimation system using sole information. IEICE Technical Report, vol. 124, no. 98, EST2024-27, pp. 92–97, Jul. 2024
9. Kikuzawa, M., Kimura, H.: Study on step count optimization in foot color using HSV color system. IEICE Technical Report, vol. 124, no. 357, EST2024-100, pp. 34– 39, Jan. 2025
10. Kikuzawa, M., Kimura, H.: Research on gender estimation using foot information. IEICE Trans. Fundamentals, vol. J108-A, no.9, Sep. 2025 (to be accepted)
11. Gordon, C.C., Bradtmiller, B. (eds.) Anthropometric survey of U.S. Army Personnel: Summary Statistics (ANSUR II). Technical Report ARL-TR-5048. U.S. Army Research Laboratory, Natick, MA, (2012)
12. Guan, S., Zhang, D., Liu, Z., et al.: Screen-printed PVDF piezoelectric pressure transducer for acoustic spectroscopy. Micromachines. **15**(12), 1423 (2024)
13. Liu, X., Wang, Y.: Performance evaluation of medium-diameter PVDF piezoelectric sensors for dynamic load sensing. Sens. Actuators A Phys. **303**, 111846 (2024)

Motion Artifact Removal in R-R Interval Estimation of ECG Signal for Wearable Biomedical Sensors Using Empirical Mode Decomposition and High-Pass Filter

Aito Hirota and Tadao Nakagawa(✉)

Tottori University, 4-101 Koyama-cho Minami, Tottori-shi, Japan
nakagawa@tottori-u.ac.jp

Abstract. Clothing-type wearable electrocardiogram (ECG) sensors are effective for continuous long-term monitoring because they impose minimal burden on the body. However, these sensors are susceptible to noise (motion artifacts) caused by body movements. As a result, estimation accuracy may become unstable when the electrodes are not firmly attached to the skin. An adaptive filter using an accelerometer has been proposed as one method to remove motion artifacts. Nevertheless, biomedical sensors and accelerometers are not always integrated, and the use of a separately installed accelerometer complicates synchronization and increases overall system cost. A visual inspection of the frequency spectra of motion artifacts and ECG signals revealed that the ECG contains a fundamental frequency of 1.3 Hz along with its odd-numbered harmonics, whereas the frequency components of motion artifacts are concentrated primarily below 4 Hz. Based on this observation, we developed a new high-pass filter (HPF) design method. Although empirical mode decomposition (EMD) is effective for noise removal, EMD alone is insufficient to eliminate significant motion artifacts in wearable devices. Therefore, we propose a new configuration that combines the designed HPF with EMD.

Keywords: Wearable Biomedical Sensors · ECG · HPF · EMD.

1 Introduction

Approximately 50% of current causes of death are lifestyle-related diseases [1]. Regular checkups are essential for preventing, detecting early, and treating conditions such as cancer, heart disease, and cerebrovascular disease. However, regular visits to medical institutions can be burdensome, and lifestyle-related diseases often lack noticeable symptoms in their early stages, increasing the risk of unnoticed progression. Heart disease, one of the most significant lifestyle-related diseases, is the second leading cause of death [1]. Therefore, there is a growing demand for devices that allow individuals to conveniently and continuously measure their biomedical information and manage their

H. Tanaka et al. (Eds.): BodyNets 2025, LNICST 714, pp. 228–236, 2026.
https://doi.org/10.1007/978-3-032-38657-1_17

health without visiting medical institutions. Although commercially available smartwatches can measure heart rate, they cannot measure the R-R interval, which provides more detailed biomedical information, including indicators of autonomic nervous system activity. Consequently, there is a strong need for wearable biomedical sensors capable of continuously measuring the R-R interval.

2 Wearable ECG Sensor

Wearable biomedical sensors are valuable healthcare tools that continuously monitor biomedical information, such as electrocardiograms (ECG), and alert users to abnormalities. Recently, clothing-type wearable sensors have been developed using conductive fibers [2–4]. Figure 1 shows a clothing-type ECG sensor. This sensor enables long-term monitoring without placing a burden on the user. However, a major problem with clothing-type sensors is ECG distortion caused by body movements (motion artifacts). Figure 2 shows an ECG acquired from a clothing-type sensor. As shown in this figure, the ECG is recorded accurately when the user is at rest, but becomes distorted during movement. To remove such motion artifacts, signal processing techniques such as adaptive filters using accelerometers have been proposed [5]. However, adaptive filters impose a heavy computational load due to iterative calculations. Furthermore, in wearable devices where the biomedical sensor and accelerometer are not integrated, synchronizing the two sensors is difficult. Empirical mode decomposition (EMD) has been proposed as an alternative method that does not rely on adaptive filters [6], but its estimation accuracy is lower compared with adaptive filters using accelerometers. Therefore, in this study, we propose a new signal processing configuration to address these limitations.

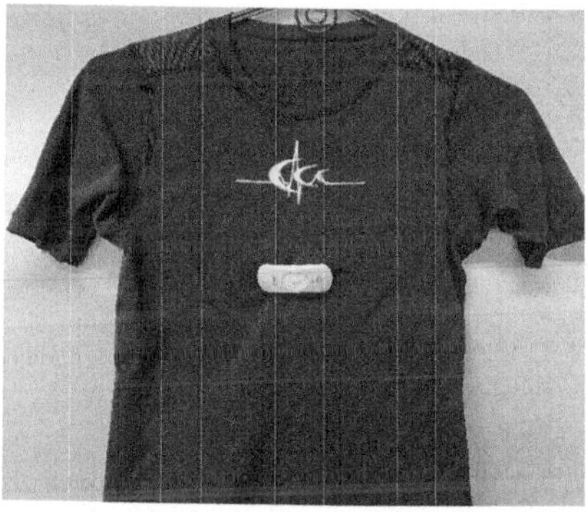

Fig. 1. Clothing-type wearable ECG sensor. (left)

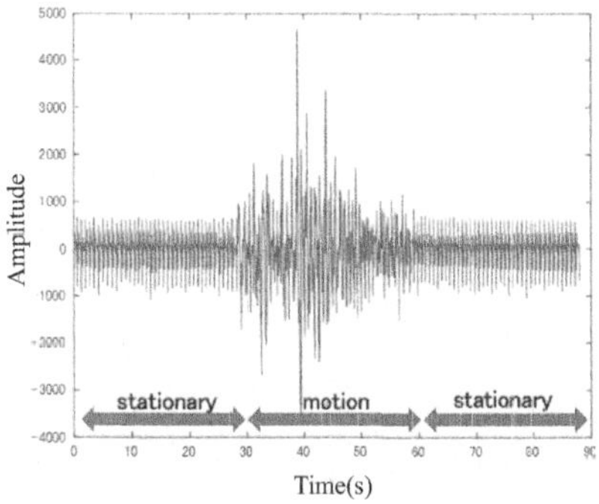

Fig. 2. ECG measured with a clothing-type wearable ECG sensor.

3 Adaptive Filter

An adaptive filter is a filter that sequentially updates its weighting coefficients. It is an effective method for noise removal in signals that continuously change, such as ECG waveforms [7]. Figure 3 shows the structure of the adaptive filter when the ECG waveform acquired from the wearable sensor at time k is denoted as $S_D[k]$, the number of taps is n, the acceleration acquired from the accelerometer is $\mathbf{x}[k]$, the filter output is $y[k]$, and the noise-removed ECG waveform is denoted as $S'_D[k]$. Furthermore, the weight coefficient w update formula is shown below when the least mean squares (LMS) adaptive algorithm is used. The acceleration $\mathbf{x}[k]$ is the square root of the sum of the squares of the accelerations along the X, Y, and Z axes obtained from a triaxial accelerometer. The update formula for the weight coefficient w is given by Eqs. (1), (2), (3), (4) and (5).

$$\mathbf{w}[k] = \mathbf{w}[k-1] + \mu\mathbf{x}[k]\left(S_D[k] - \mathbf{w}^{\mathrm{T}}\mathbf{x}[k]\right), \tag{1}$$

$$\mathbf{w} = [w_1, w_2, \cdots, w_n]^{\mathrm{T}}, \tag{2}$$

$$\mathbf{x}[k] = [x[k], x[k-1], \cdots, x[k-n+1]]^{\mathrm{T}}, \tag{3}$$

$$y[k] = \mathbf{w}^{\mathrm{T}}\mathbf{x}[k], \tag{4}$$

$$S'_D[k] = S_D[k] - y[k]. \tag{5}$$

Here, μ represents the step size.

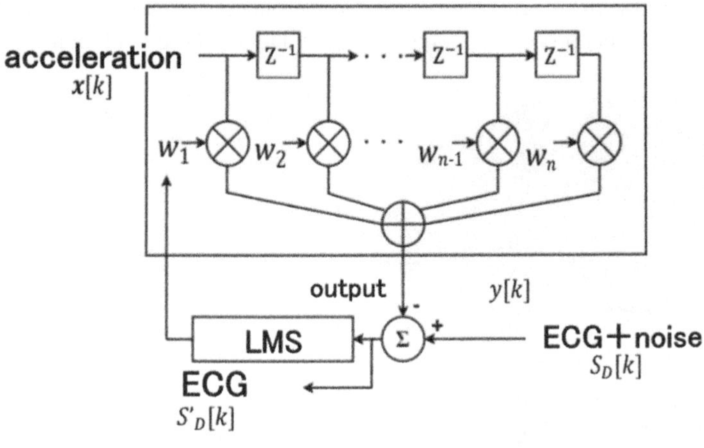

Fig. 3. Structure of the adaptive filter.

4 EMD

EMD is also effective for removing motion artifacts from ECG signals. EMD decomposes a signal into several highly orthogonal pseudo-monochromatic waves, known as intrinsic mode functions (IMF functions).

Motion artifacts are concentrated in the low-frequency portion of the signal. Therefore, it is possible to remove motion artifacts by extracting the high-frequency components of the signal using EMD. A noisy ECG can be decomposed into its respective IMF components using EMD according to the following procedure.

Step 1: Identify all local maxima in the signal $x_{(n)}$. Connect the maxima using a cubic spline and apply the same procedure to the local minima. This produces the upper envelope $e_{max}(n)$ and the lower envelope $e_{min}(n)$, from which the envelope mean $m_1(n)$ can be calculated (Eq. 6).

$$m_1(n) = \frac{e_{min}(n)+e_{max}(n)}{2}. \tag{6}$$

Step 2: Perform the shifting. The first component is obtained by subtracting $m_1(n)$ from the raw signal $x_{(n)}$, as given by Eq. (7).

$$h_1(n) = x(n) - m_1(n). \tag{7}$$

Verify whether $h_1(n)$ satisfies the two IMF criteria. If $h_1(n)$ is not an IMF, treat $h_1(n)$ as data and repeat all processing in Step 1 to obtain a new component $h_2(n)$.

$$h_2(n) = h_1(n) - m_2(n). \tag{8}$$

This screening process is repeated k times until the IMF criteria are met.

$$h_k(n) = h_{k-1}(n) - n_k(n). \tag{9}$$

This final component is defined as the initial IMF.

$$c_1(n) = h_k(n). \tag{10}$$

Step 3. Subtract the initial IMF from the original signal to obtain the residual data $r_1(n)$ (Eq. 11). This residual is treated as new data for further decomposition.

$$r_1(n) = x(n) - c_1(n). \tag{11}$$

Step 4. Repeat Steps 1–3 to find extract values for IMF $c_2(n)$, $c_3(n)$, $\cdots$, $c_i(n)$ until $r_n(n)$ becomes monotonically constant.

$$r_n(n) = x(n) - \sum_{n=1}^{K} c_1(n). \tag{12}$$

Subsequently, the filtering process is halted. The raw signal can be reconstructed by combining all IMF components with the final residual.

$$x(n) = \sum_{i=1}^{K} c_i(n) + r_n(n). \tag{13}$$

In this study, the signal was decomposed into 17 IMFs, and four high-frequency IMFs were extracted using EMD to obtain a noise-reduced signal. However, compared with an adaptive filter using an accelerometer, the estimation accuracy remained insufficient.

5 High-Pass Filter

To improve estimation accuracy, we implemented a high-pass filter (HPF). The frequency components of motion artifacts caused by body movements are primarily concentrated below 4 Hz [5]. Therefore, we applied an HPF with a cutoff frequency of 4 Hz.

As shown in Fig. 4, the frequency spectrum of the resting ECG waveform contains odd harmonics in addition to the fundamental frequency at 1.3 Hz. Consequently, when suppressing motion artifact components using the HPF, partial suppression of the fundamental R-wave is acceptable as long as the harmonics are preserved, thereby minimizing distortion of the time waveform. Figure 5 presents the frequency spectrum after applying the HPF to the resting ECG waveform. Figure 6 shows the time waveform during exercise before filtering, and Fig. 7 shows the time waveform during exercise after applying the HPF. These figures demonstrate that motion artifacts caused by exercise are effectively reduced, and the R-wave becomes more clearly visible.

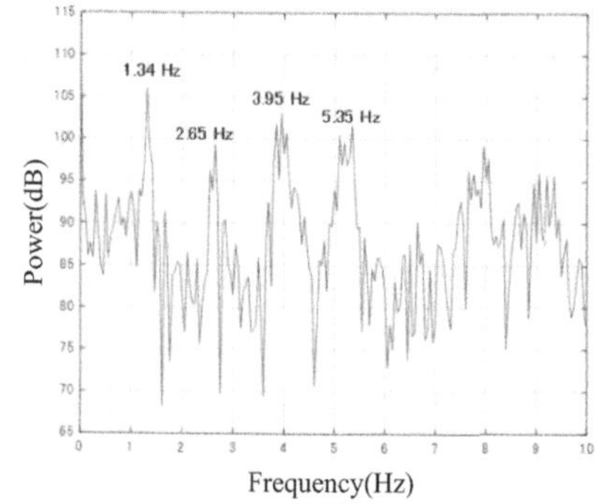

Fig. 4. Frequency spectrum of the electrocardiogram (at rest).

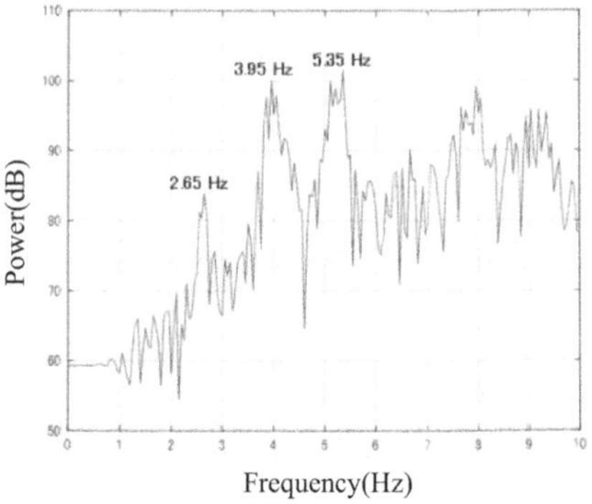

Fig. 5. Frequency spectrum of the ECG after HPF (at rest).

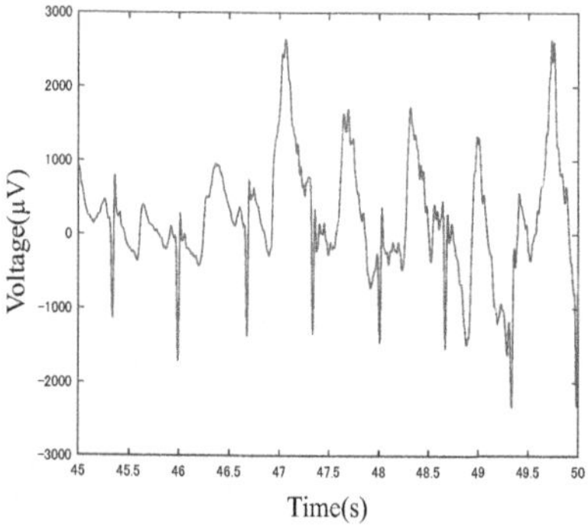

Fig. 6. Time waveform of the ECG before HPF (exercise).

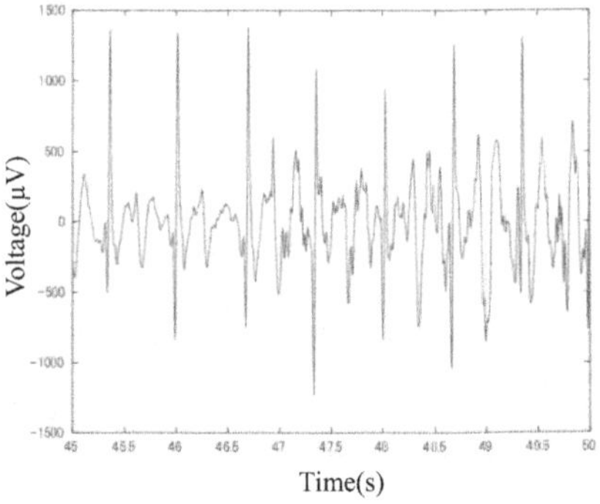

Fig. 7. Time waveform of the ECG after HPF (exercise).

6 Proposed Method

To overcome conventional limitations, we propose a method that enhances the estimation accuracy of R-waves by combining a high-pass filter with EMD, without requiring accelerometers. The flowchart of the proposed method is shown in Fig. 8.

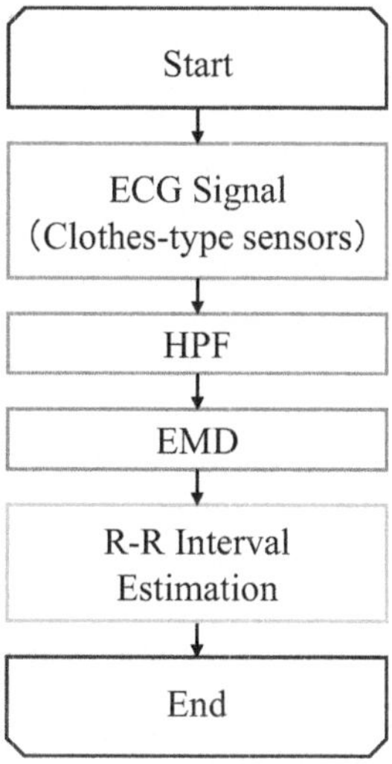

Fig. 8. Flowchart of the proposed method.

7 Experimental Method

For the experimental setup, both the clothing-type wearable ECG sensor and the belt-type ECG sensor [8] were worn simultaneously. In this state, participants performed Motion 1 (27 s stationary, 60 s stair climbing, 30 s stationary) and Motion 2 (27 s stationary, 30 s arm rotation, 30 s stationary). The accuracy of R-R interval estimation from the clothing-type sensor was evaluated using the belt-type R-R interval as the reference value (true value).

The mean absolute percentage error (MAPE) was adopted to assess estimation accuracy. When the belt-type R-R interval is denoted as $\mathrm{RRI}_{\mathrm{true}}$, the estimated R-R interval from the clothing-type sensor as $\mathrm{RRI}_{\mathrm{est}}$, the sample size as S, and the time as n, the MAPE is expressed as follows:

$$\mathrm{MAPE} = \frac{1}{S}\sum_{n=1}^{S}\frac{|RRI_{est}(n) - RRI_{true}(n)|}{RRI_{true}(n)}. \tag{14}$$

8 Experimental Results

Figure 9 shows the results when no processing was applied to the ECG acquired from the wearable sensor. Figure 10 shows the results when EMD was applied. Figure 11 shows the results when HPF and an adaptive filter using acceleration data from the accelerometer were combined. Finally, Fig. 12 shows the results of the proposed method, which combines EMD and HPF applied to the ECG. In these figures, the vertical axis represents the R-R interval (ms), and the horizontal axis represents time (s). The red signal represents the R-R interval estimated from the clothing-type sensor, whereas the blue signal represents the R-R interval estimated from the belt-type sensor. As shown in Fig. 9, estimation accuracy is maintained during rest but becomes disrupted by motion artifacts during exercise. Figure 10 demonstrates that applying EMD reduced noise during movement, but motion artifacts persisted. Figure 11 shows that combining HPF with an adaptive filter substantially reduced motion disturbance. Figure 12 presents the results of the proposed method with HPF and EMD added, demonstrating estimation accuracy comparable to that in Fig. 11, which uses the adaptive filter. Table 1 presents the MAPE values for Motion 1 and Motion 2. This indicates that the proposed method improves estimation accuracy compared to using EMD alone and achieves estimation accuracy comparable to that obtained by combining an accelerometer and an adaptive filter. Moreover, this method maintains stable estimation accuracy without requiring changes to filter parameters when the type of motion changes.

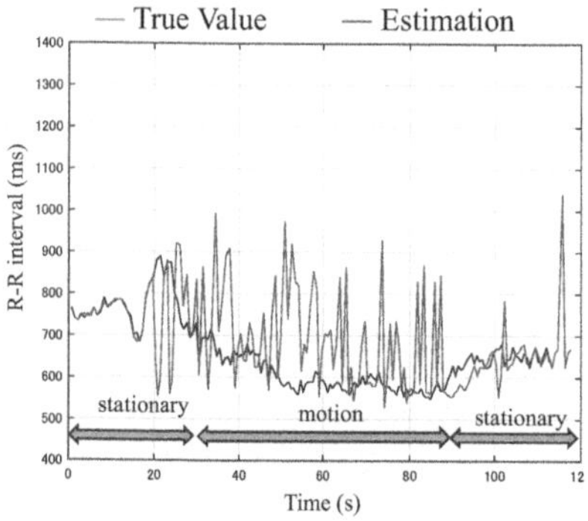

Fig. 9. Estimated R-R interval from unprocessed ECG (Motion 1).

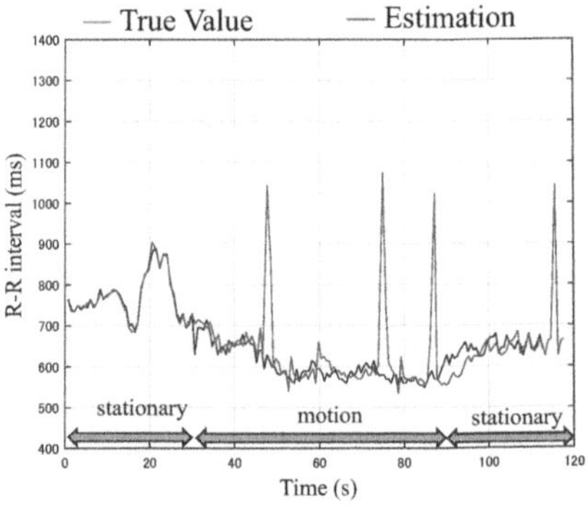

Fig. 10. Estimated R-R interval from ECG using EMD (Motion 1).

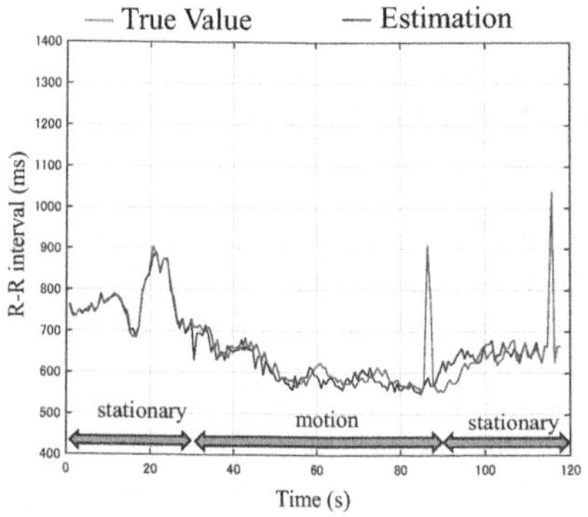

(Motion 1).

Fig. 11. Estimated R-R interval from ECG processed with HPF and an adaptive filter using acceleration data from the accelerometer (Motion 1).

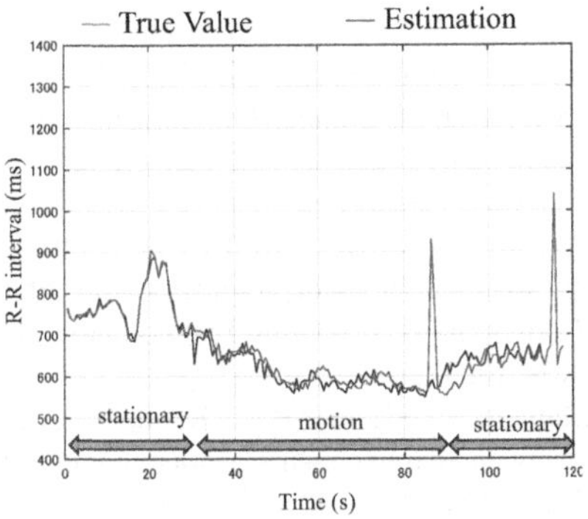

(Motion 1).

Fig. 12. Estimated R-R interval from ECG using the proposed method (Motion 1).

Table 1. Mean absolute percentage error (MAPE).

	Stair climbing (Motion 1)	Arm rotation (Motion 2)
Unprocessed	11.4%	8.87%
EMD	4.29%	0.99%
HPF, adaptive filter With an accelerometer	3.08%	0.96%
Proposed method	3.11%	0.90%

9 Conclusion

This study proposes a method for removing motion artifacts in wearable biomedical sensors without requiring an accelerometer. By combining a HPF with EMD, the proposed method improves estimation accuracy compared with EMD alone and achieves accuracy comparable to that obtained with an accelerometer and an adaptive filter.

Acknowledgements. This study was supported by JSPS KAKENHI (Grant number: JP25K07736).

References

1. Ministry of Health, Labour and Welfare: Annual summary of population dynamics statistics monthly reports for 2022 (preliminary figures), population dynamics survey, pp. 1–16 (2022)

2. Tsukada, Y.T., et al.: Validation of wearable textile electrodes for ECG monitoring. Heart Vessels. **34**, 1203–1211 (2019)
3. Fobelets, K., Hammour, G., Thielemans, K.: Knitted ECG electrodes in relaxed fitting garments. IEEE Sens. J. **23**(5), 5263–5269 (2023)
4. Hoxoskin, Hexoskin Connected Health Platform.
5. Arakawa, Y., Nakagawa, T.: Motion artifact removal in R-R interval estimation of ECG signal for wearable biomedical sensors using adaptive filter and high pass filter. In: 2023 International Conference on Emerging Technologies for Communications (ICETC 2023) Proc., Paper P2-29, Nov. 2023 (2023)
6. Ranjan, R., Sahana, B.C., Bhandari, A.K.: Motion artifacts suppression from EEG signals using an adaptive signal denoising method. IEEE Trans. Instrum. Meas. **71**, 1–10 (2022)
7. Yu, S., Song, Q., Liu, S.: Motion artifact cancellation from a single channel SCG using adaptive forgetting factor recursive least square filter. IEEE Access. **8**, 1–9 (2020)
8. Union-Tool company, mybeat heart rate sensor. https://www.uniontoolmybeat.com/SHOP/8600110.html

Clinical, Implantable, and Wearable Systems for Healthcare Applications

Improving Patient Care in the Emergency Wards of Bangladesh Through an RFID-Based Web Simulation

Hasan Md Mehedi[1(✉)], Hossain Shakil[1], and Eisuke Hanada[2]

[1] Saga University Graduate School of Science and Engineering, Saga 840-8502, Japan
mehedihasan.baiu22@gmail.com
[2] Saga University Faculty of Science and Engineering, Saga 840-8502, Japan
hanada@cc.saga-u.ac.jp

Abstract. Emergency wards in Bangladesh are often overcrowded, understaffed, and lack automated patient monitoring tools. As a result, critical events such as patient falls or sudden deterioration may go unnoticed until too late and essential medical equipment is often misplaced or unavailable when urgently needed. To address these challenges, this paper proposes a web-based system that integrates passive UHF RFID for patient location and chipless RFID for low-cost equipment tracking. The system features real-time patient location updates, automated fall detection alarms, and logging of equipment usage history. An edge–cloud architecture processes RFID data locally for fast alerts and stores records in a cloud database for long-term analysis. A simulation study was done using this system of 50 virtual patients and five tagged devices to evaluate location accuracy, alert latency, and operational reliability. Results showed an average location accuracy of 92%, fall detection sensitivity of 88%, alert latency below two seconds, and system uptime of 99%. Compared to traditional manual monitoring, this approach offers a scalable, cost-effective solution suitable for resource-constrained hospitals. The study highlights both the opportunities and challenges of deploying RFID in the emergency care system of Bangladesh and lays the groundwork for future real-world pilot trials.

Keywords: RFID · Patient Tracking · Fall Detection · Chipless RFID · Edge–Cloud · Bangladesh · BAN.

1 Introduction

The emergency departments of the healthcare system in Bangladesh suffer from very high patient-to-staff ratios, a lack of medical equipment, and manual tracking processes. Delays in patient care during emergencies can significantly reduce the chances of survival for the affected patients. The current patient management system in emergency wards heavily relies on verbal communication, handwritten notes, and manual updates to whiteboard systems, which are all prone to human error and delays. RFID (Radio

H. Tanaka et al. (Eds.): BodyNets 2025, LNICST 714, pp. 239–246, 2026.
https://doi.org/10.1007/978-3-032-38657-1_18

Frequency Identification) technology, which has been implemented in the hospitals of developed countries for logistics, patient identification, and real-time asset tracking, is a very low-cost and efficient solution for Bangladesh [1, 2]. But implementing RFID directly in hospitals without prior trials can be expensive and risky. The proposed online system will be a cost-effective method to assess performance, calculate ROI, and uncover possible integration issues [3, 4].

Our research Objectives are as follows:

1. To design a web simulation framework for RFID-based emergency ward operations in Bangladesh.
2. To assess patient flow efficiency and equipment tracking improvements using simulated data.
3. To propose a cost-effective implementation strategy tailored to developing country constraints.

2 Background and Related Works

RFID systems consist of tags, readers, antennas, and software for processing and visualization. Two common types—**passive** and **active** tags—offer tradeoffs between cost and range. RFID technology has been used in hospitals for [1–3] patient and asset tracking. Chipless RFID is a technology that can reduce the cost of tracking equipment, but is restricted by not being able to capture data over long distances and its low sensitivity [4]. Edge–cloud and hybrid architectures have been suggested for BANs to reduce latency and increase reliability [5].

- **Patient tracking**: Ensuring patients get to the correct treatment area [1].
- **Equipment tracking**: Reducing time spent locating essential tools like ECG machines and wheelchairs [5].
- **Staff coordination**: Improving task assignment and response times [3, 4].

In Table 1, we show a summary of related works on existing systems.

Table 1. Related works

Study	Country	Focus Area	Outcome	Limitations
Chen et al. (2019) [6]	Taiwan	RFID for ICU patient tracking	30% faster patient transfer	High deployment cost
Al Amin et al. (2021) [7]	Bangladesh	Hospital logistics tracking	Reduced lost equipment incidents	No simulation phase
Suzuki et al. (2022) [8]	Japan	RFID nurse coordination	Improved task completion speed	Limited to high-income settings

This paper builds on these concepts with a practical hybrid simulation tailored for a resource-constrained hospital environment.

3 Methodology

3.1 System Architecture

We constructed an RFID-based web simulation system to evaluate how hospital operations can be improved. Our system architecture includes [3, 5]:

- **RFID Tags**: Assigned to each patient and medical device.
- **RFID Readers**: Placed at critical checkpoints (entrance, treatment rooms, exit).
- **Database Server**: Stores location and status data.
- **Web Interface**: Displays patient queue, equipment status, and alerts.

The system Architecture is shown in Fig. 1 as an ASCII Diagram.

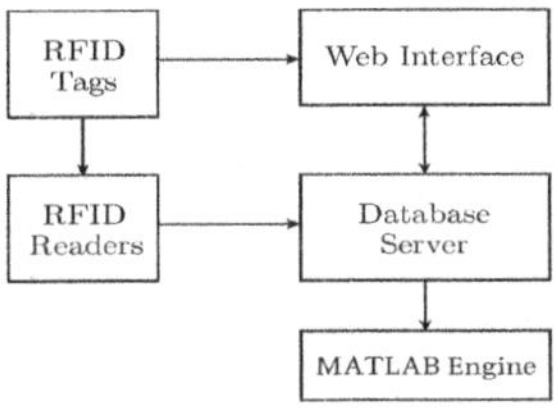

Fig. 1. System architecture of the proposed RFID-based hybrid MATLAB–Web simulation system.

This diagram illustrates the core architecture of the proposed RFID-based simulation system. Each patient and piece of medical equipment is tagged with a passive RFID tag. Readers placed at critical locations (entrance, treatment areas, and exit) capture real-time location data, which is sent to a centralized database server. The web interface allows staff to monitor patient flow, locate equipment, and receive alerts on bottlenecks or delays.

3.2 Workflow Diagram

The workflow shown in Fig. 2 is a diagram of the step-by-step process of patient management in an RFID-enabled emergency ward. Upon arrival, patients are assigned RFID tags that are scanned at the entry point. The system logs their arrival, directs them to the appropriate treatment area, and tracks the location of any required equipment. After treatment, patients are discharged, their RFID tags are removed, and all data is archived for analysis. This workflow enables real-time monitoring and reduces delays caused by manual tracking.

Using this system, we simulated how the RFID system improved hospital operations. Parameters for simulation are shown in Table 2.

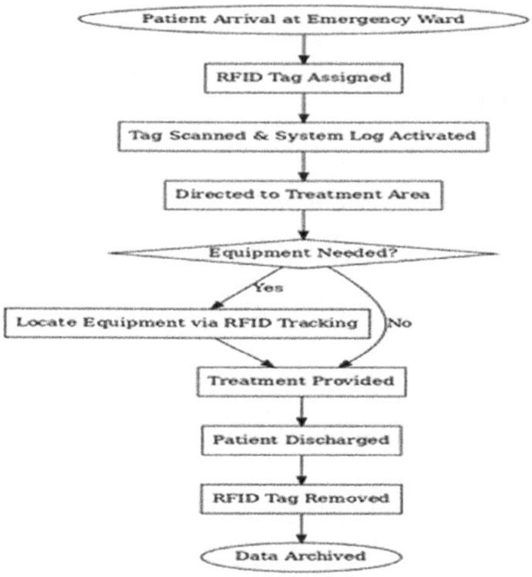

Fig. 2. Workflow of RFID-Based Patient Tracking in an Emergency Ward

Table 2. Simulation Parameters

Parameter	Value	Notes
Number of patients/hours	20	Peak emergency load
RFID reader coverage radius	5 m	Passive tag range
Avg. time to locate equipment (manual)	8 min	Observed baseline
Avg. time to locate equipment (RFID)	2 min	Simulated
Cost per passive RFID tag	USD 0.50	Reusable

4 Simulation and Calculation Procedure

4.1 Simulation Setup

The entire simulation was run on a personal computer with MATLAB in conjunction with a web-based visualization interface. A virtual ward layout was modeled in software to depict an emergency area of 20 m by 15 m, divided into four zones (A-D). Each zone represents a part of the hospital, such as patient beds, nursing stations, and emergency entrances. The simulation, rather than using actual RFID hardware, creates artificial RFID signals, simulating passive UHF tag readings and chipless equipment tags.

- Patients: The number of virtual patients is 50, and they are represented as moving objects (x,y coordinates) within the 2D map.
- Readers: The three simulated readers are positioned at the entrance and two key zone intersections.
- Movement Model: Random-walk trajectories with differing speeds regulate movement that illustrates usual patient or personnel mobility.

- Fall Events: The occurrence of fall accidents is based on the Poisson distribution ($\lambda = 0.05$ events/minute) with random time intervals for the fall events.
- Equipment Events: The usage of equipment and the reading of tags are done at intervals that coincide with the simulated clinical workflows.

The MATLAB simulation generates logs with timestamps for all tag reads and events. The web module displays these logs in real time through the use of simulated signal data instead of actual radio signals.

4.2 Hybrid Implementation

The hybrid structure links the MATLAB engine (computation and statistical analysis) to a local web interface (data visualization) through a network of interconnecting parts.

Data flow:

1. MATLAB either produces or takes in simulated RFID readings.
2. The edge-processing code eliminates duplicate readings and determines which zone each patient is in.
3. The web dashboard shows the outcomes, and they are also saved for future analysis.

With this system, researchers can fully experiment and evaluate their situation on a regular PC without the need for actual RFID hardware while keeping the functional equivalence to a hospital system on-site (Fig. 3).

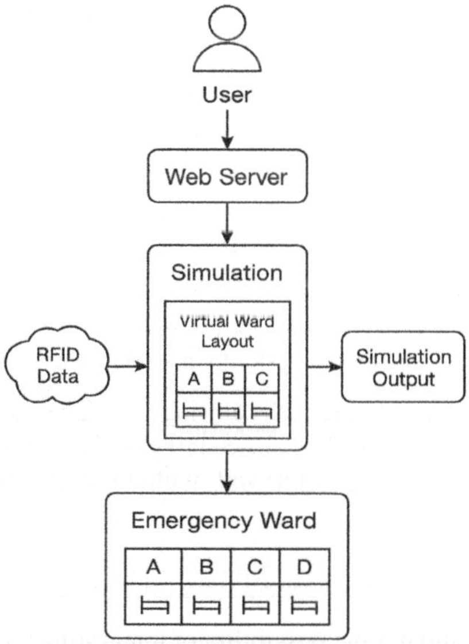

Fig. 3 Hybrid data flow between MATLAB computation and web-based visualization.

4.3 Calculation Formulas

The following formulas were implemented directly in MATLAB to calculate each performance metric across 20 simulation runs:

- **Localization Accuracy (LA)** $LA = \frac{N_{correct}}{N_{total}} \times 100$
- **Alert Latency (AL)** $AL = T_{alert} - T_{event}$
- **Fall Detection Accuracy (FDA)** $FDA = \frac{N_{detected}}{N_{falls}} \times 100$
- **System Uptime (SU)** $SU = \frac{T_{active}}{T_{total}} \times 100$

Each metric was computed automatically within MATLAB. The resulting values were exported to a CSV file, summarized in Table 3, and visualized through the web interface.

5 Results

Synthetic RFID read logs and patient movements were produced by the simulation based on MATLAB for 20 independent trials, each simulating a 30 min hospital emergency scenario. The average outcomes of all the simulation runs are represented in Table 3.

Table 3. Key Findings

Metric	Average Value	Observation
Localization Accuracy (%)	92	Stable detection of patients across four zones
Alert Latency (s)	2.06	Near-real-time alarm response within two seconds
Fall Detection Accuracy (%)	88	Minor false positives under random motion
System Uptime (%)	99	Consistent operation across all runs

All metrics computed from MATLAB output logs; mean values over 20 simulation runs.

The RFID-based localization and event detection system, combined with robust data filtering and hybrid edge computation, proved to be effective even in completely software-simulated conditions, as the system showed consistent performance.

- RFID significantly reduced bottlenecks at triage and treatment allocation.
- Equipment availability improved because staff could more quickly locate devices.
- Overall operational efficiency improved without requiring major infrastructure changes.

6 Discussion

This virtual simulation validates the possibility of integrating passive and chipless RFID concepts into an intelligent hospital workflow without the use of real hardware during early-stage research. The MATLAB + Web model allows the adjustment of parameters (reader coverage, read frequency, and movement speed) and instant observation of system response.

Even though the results indicate a slightly higher latency than laboratory hardware studies [3], the performance is well within the limits acceptable for hospital alert systems.

The simulated Localization Accuracy (92%) and Fall Detection Accuracy (88%) suggest that RFID data—when processed by an edge algorithm—can attain reliable patient tracking that is appropriate for emergency-ward conditions.

Advantages:

- Low-cost passive tags are affordable, even for public hospitals.
- Web-based systems avoid dependency on expensive proprietary hospital management software.

Challenges:

- RFID signal interference in metal-rich environments.
- Initial investment in readers may require donor funding.
- Scaling to larger virtual maps with multiple floors
- Integration with existing paper-based systems will need a carefully planned transition.

Comparison with Related Works While Taiwan and Japan have achieved efficiency gains with highly technical systems [3, 5], the resource constraints of Bangladesh require a low-budget adaptation, which can be addressed by prioritizing passive tags and open-source web interfaces.

7 Conclusion and Future Work

A simulation based on a web and MATLAB hybrid was developed for use on a PC to model an RFID-enabled emergency department for hospitals in Bangladesh.

The experiment illustrated that a completely virtual environment can realistically mimic hospital workflows and the necessary metrics, such as localization accuracy, alert latency, and system reliability.

Plans:

- Creating a MATLAB simulation that works with an Arduino-based RFID reader prototype for partial hardware validation.
- Adding a machine-learning module that will foresee high-risk fall events.
- Carrying out a pilot study in partnership with a Bangladeshi hospital under controlled conditions.

These extensions will connect the existing software prototype with a system for improving patient care that is ready for deployment.

Acknowledgments. The author sincerely expresses his gratitude to Professor Eisuke Hanada of Saga University, Japan, for his constant guidance and supervision throughout the research period.

Furthermore, the author extends his gratitude to Saga University, which played a crucial role in creating a conducive research environment and providing the necessary computational resources for the successful completion of this study.

References

1. Ajami, S., Rajabzadeh, A.: Radio frequency identification (RFID) technology and patient safety. J. Res. Med. Sci. **18**(9), 809–813 (2013)
2. Want, R.: An introduction to RFID technology. IEEE Pervasive Comput. **5**(1), 25–33 (2006)
3. Ngai, E.W., Moon, K.K., Riggins, F.J., Yi, C.Y.: RFID research: an academic literature review (1995–2005) and future research directions. Int. J. Prod. Econ. **112**(2), 510–520 (2008)
4. Al Ameen, M., Liu, J., Kwak, K.: Security and privacy issues in wireless sensor networks for healthcare applications. J. Med. Syst. **36**(1), 93–101 (2012)
5. Hu, F., Xie, D., Shen, S.: On the application of the internet of things in the field of medical and health care. In: Proceedings of IEEE International Conference on Green Computing and Communications, pp. 2053–2058. IEEE (2013)
6. Chen, T.-C., Lin, P.-H., Huang, J.-Y.: RFID-based ICU patient tracking for transfer efficiency. J. Healthc. Eng. **12**(4), 123–130 (2019)
7. Al Amin, M., Rahman, S., Ahmed, T.: RFID-enabled hospital logistics tracking in Bangladesh. Int. J. Healthc. Inf. Syst. Inform. **15**(2), 98–110 (2021)
8. Suzuki, K., Watanabe, Y., Tanaka, H.: RFID-based nurse coordination system for improved task efficiency. Sensors. **22**(15), 6789 (2022)

Development of Passive-Type Implantable VNS Device with Multiple Receive Coils

Kota Oku[1](✉), Jaakko Hyry[2], Takumi Kobayashi[2], Keita Saku[3], and Daisuke Anzai[2]

[1] Nagoya Institute of Technology, Graduate School of Engineering, Gokiso-cho, Showa-ku, Nagoya, Aichi 466-8555, Japan
cmj13042@ict.nitech.ac.jp

[2] Osaka Metropolitan University, Graduate School of Informatics 1-1, Gakuen-cho, Naka-ku, Sakai, Osaka 599-8531, Japan
{jaakko,kobayashi.takumi,d.anzai}@omu.ac.jp

[3] National Cerebral and Cardiovascular Center 6-1, Kishibesin-machi, Suita-shi 564-8565, Japan
saku.keita@ncvc.go.jp

Abstract. Neuromodulation is a treatment method, which aims to improve symptoms by stimulating abnormal nerve functions by using electricity or magnetism. Recently, implantable medical devices have ganered a great deal of attention as a method for neuromodulation, where devices are implanted both inside or outside the body for diagnosis, monitoring, and treating disease purposes. However, issues related to battery life and possible malfunctions from the battery usage, as well as issues from the angular and positional misalignment arise from the direct placement of a device inside a living body. In this study, we focused instead on implantable medical devices that use wireless power transmission and investigated a method by using multiple implantable communication terminals without batteries. As we assumed the developed device was used within the human body, we designed receiver coils considering the effects on the human body and conducted experimental evaluation of a neurostimulation device. In addition, a method to improve the receiving range when using multiple receiver coils was proposed and experimentally evaluated.

Keywords: Nerve stimulation · Magnetic field · Resonance coupling

1 Introduction

Implantable medical devices have been the focus of much attention due to the increase in chronic and neurological diseases associated with the rapid aging of the population, early detection and treatment of diseases in their early stages,

This work was supported in part by JSPS KAKENHI Grant Number JP21H01325 and Japan Agency for Medical Research and Development, Practical Research Project for Rare/Intractable Diseases, JP25ek0109791.

H. Tanaka et al. (Eds.): BodyNets 2025, LNICST 714, pp. 247–254, 2026.
https://doi.org/10.1007/978-3-032-38657-1_19

and prognosis and rehabilitation. Implantable medical devices are used for the diagnosis, monitoring, and treatment of diseases by implanting devices inside or outside the body. Examples of implantable medical devices include neuromodulation devices, cardiovascular implants, and defibrillators. Neuromodulation is a treatment method to improve symptoms by stimulating abnormal nerves with electricity or magnetism. Currently, cochlear implants [1] have been developed to assist the needs of patients with sensory hearing loss. It has recently shown promise in the treatment of conditions such as epilepsy, Parkinson's disease, obesity [2]. Vague nerve stimulation (VNS) is a type of neuromodulation that stimulates the vagus nerve, a cranial nerve that connects the brain to internal organs [3]. VNS is expected to be applied to depression, cardiovascular diseases, diabetes, myocardial infarction, heart failure. Currently, there are issues with batteries and angular and positional deviations caused by placing the receiver directly inside the living body. Therefore, we investigated using multiple implantable communication terminals that do not require batteries. Because receiver coils implanted in the body are affected by its surrounding tissue, we designed coils to account for this effects. We also conducted experimental evaluation using an assumed neurostimulation device as the target. Furthermore, we investigated a method to improve angular characteristics of misalignment, by using multiple receiver coils and performed an experimental evaluation.

2 Development of Passive-Type Implantable Neuromodulation System

2.1 Design of Wireless Power Transmission Systems Considering Resonant Frequencies

In general, a coil has inductance L [H], winding resistance R [Ω], and winding capacitance C [F]. Therefore, the characteristics of the coil may change depending on the electrical constants of the biological tissue. Figure 1 shows the frequency characteristics of impedance when the coil is placed in air, in a bioequivalent liquid phantom (relative permittivity: 49.3 S/m @13.56 MHz), and inside a living body.

The coil length is 10.4 mm, the coil radius is 7.80 mm, and the number of turns is 10. The Q values in the bioequivalent liquid phantom and inside the body are lower than those in air. This is due to a parallel resistive component added to the equivalent circuit of the coil by the conductivity of the bioequivalent tissue. It can also be confirmed that the resonance frequency is lower, and this is because a capacitor component is added in parallel due to the relative permittivity of the biological tissue. Therefore, the equivalent circuit of the coil inside the living body can be expressed as shown in Fig. 2. In this study, the magnetic field resonance method, a type of wireless power transmission, was employed [4]. The design of the resonant frequency of the receiver coil, taking into account the effect of the living body, using the magnetic field resonance method is expressed

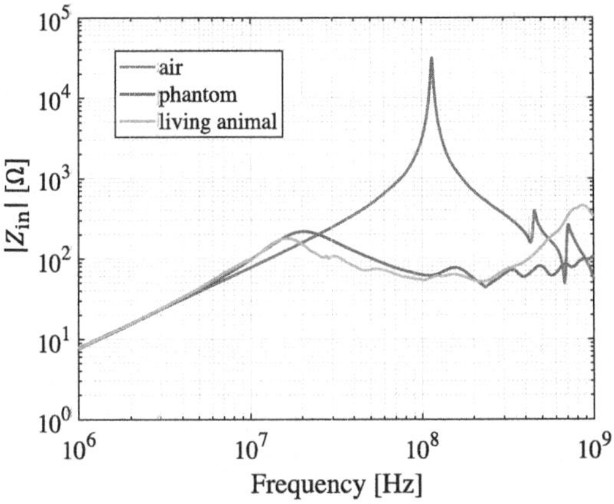

Fig. 1. Frequency response of coils

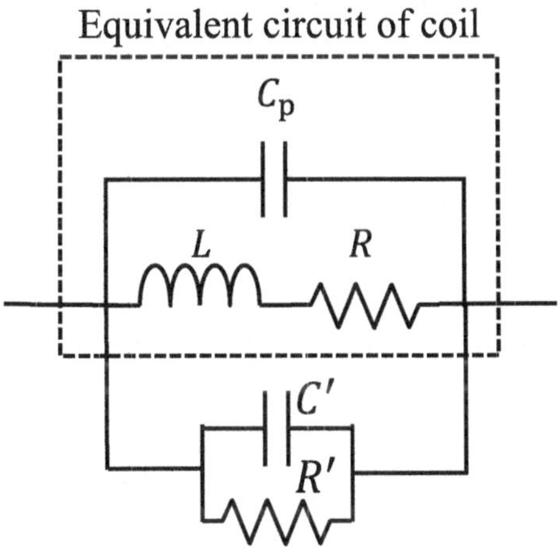

Fig. 2. Equivalent circuit model

by the following equation.

$$C = \frac{1}{4\pi^2 f_0^2 L} - C_p \tag{1}$$

where C is the capacitance of the capacitor to be installed to achieve the desired resonant frequency, L is the inductance value of the coil, f_0 is the resonant frequency, and C_p is the parasitic capacitance of the coil generated inside the body. Using (1), a receiver coil operating at 13.56 MHz in vivo was fabricated, and the effect of the design equation was confirmed experimentally.

2.2 Design of Passive-Type Neromodulation Devices

Figure 3 shows the circuit diagram of a transmitter/receiver coil for a neural stimulation device as an example of a passive receiver mechanism that combines information transmission and power transmission. The transmitter coil has a matching circuit. The receiving coil consists of a secondary coil and a load coil, and a total of three coils are used in the 3-coil system. Five parameters must be set appropriately for biostimulation: current value, frequency, pulse width, on-time, and off-time [5]. The signal generator emitted a 13.56 MHz signal for 0.3 ms followed by a 50 ms interval. The resonant frequency of the transmitter/receiver coil was set to 13.56 MHz. A rectifier unit was installed in the receiver coils to ensure the signal to be below 100 kHz. This is the boundary between thermal and stimulatory effects, where below 100 kHz the stimulatory action is dominant.

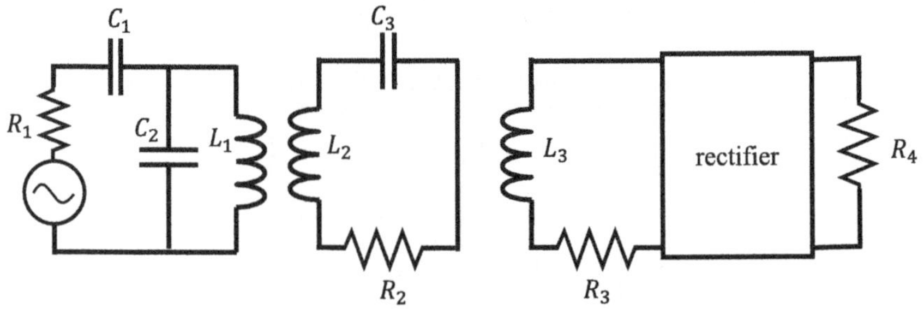

Fig. 3. Transmitter/receiver coil circuit diagram

3 Fundamental Experimental Evaluation

Figure 4 shows the experimental environment and Fig. 6 shows the receiver coil used. The circuit configuration of the receiver coils is shown in Fig. 5. The angle

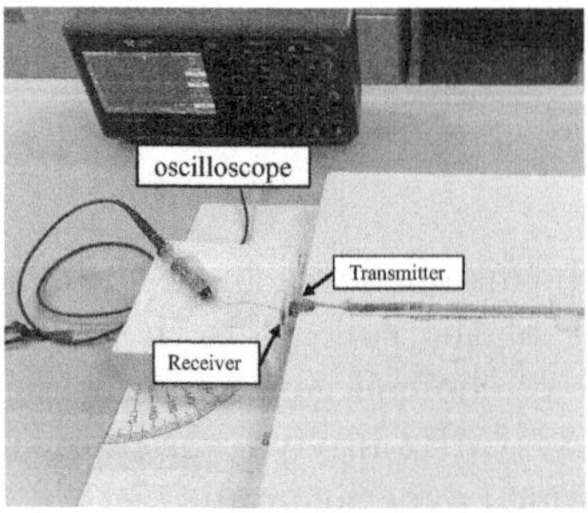

Fig. 4. Angular Characteristics Measurement Environment

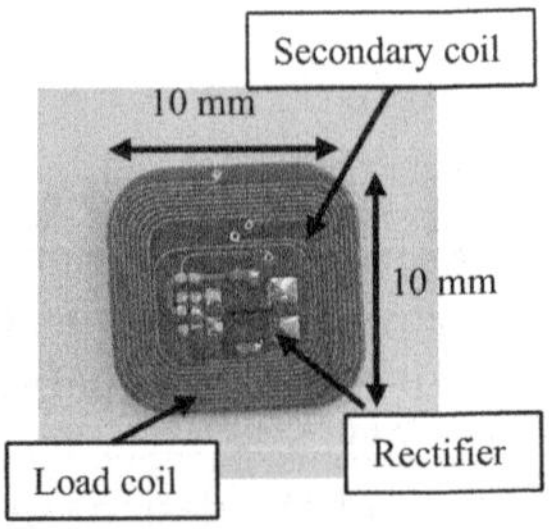

Fig. 5. Receiving coil

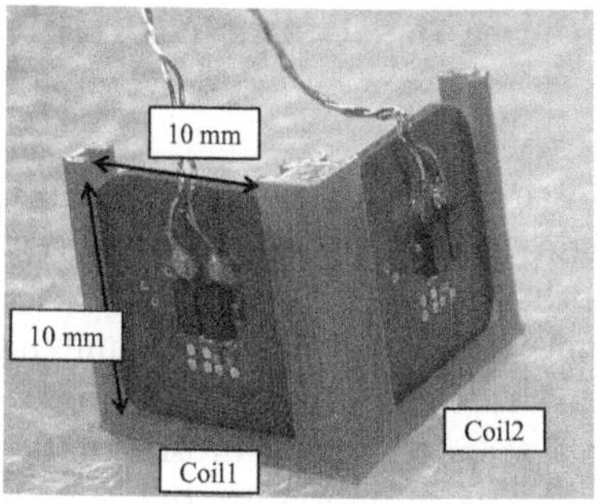

Fig. 6. Receiving system with 2 coils

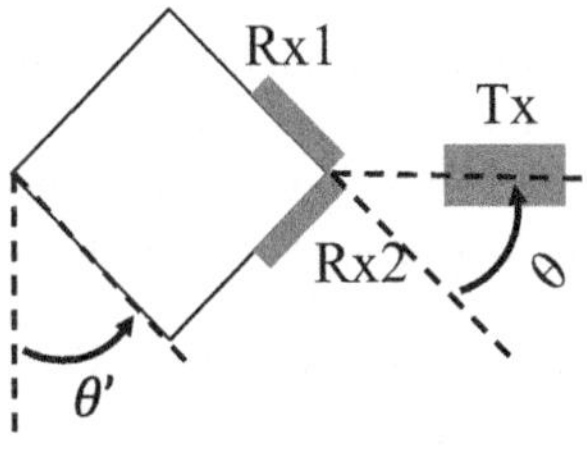

Fig. 7. Measurement method

between the two receiver coils was fixed at 90 degrees by fitting them into a mold made by a 3D printer. Furthermore, the angle-fixed receiver coils were attached to a styrene foam, and the angle θ was calculated by measuring the angle θ' shown in Fig. 7. The reason for using θ' in the derivation is to ensure the reproducibility of the experiment.

Figure 8 and 9 show the measurement results in air and in a bioequivalent liquid phantom, respectively. The maximum current value when using a single receiving coil (Rx1 only) is 1.5 mA, and the current flowing through the nerve-simulating resistor decreases as the angle θ becomes smaller. However, by combining two receiving coils, while the maximum current value remains almost unchanged, the minimum value becomes 0.7 mA, confirming that current flows even when the angle θ is small. This indicates that using multiple receiving coils improved the angular characteristics.

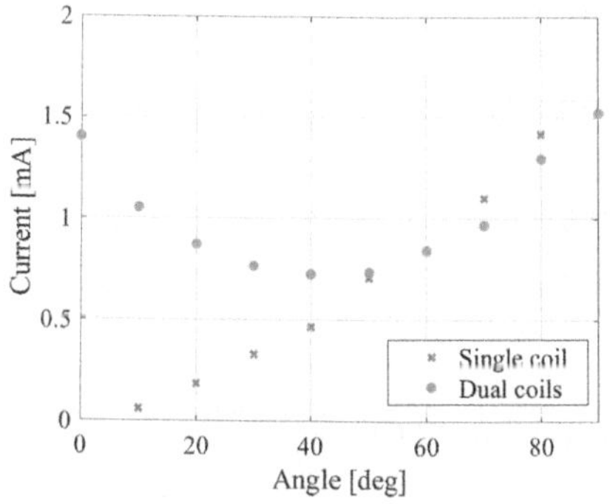

Fig. 8. Results measured in air

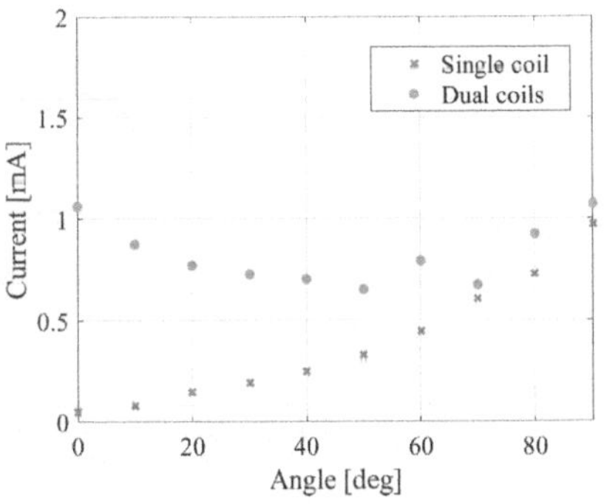

Fig. 9. Results measured in bioequivalent liquid phantom

4 In-Vivo Neurostimulation Experiments Using Multiple Receiver Coils

Figure 10 shows the results of an in-vivo neurostimulation experiment. An electrode connected to a receiver coil was place inside the neck area, near the exposed vaguse nerve, of a canine subject under anesthesia. After the placement, the subject's skin was surtured and the experiment was conducted by transmitting power from outside the body surface. The heart rate changes were used as the measurement evaluation. After anethesias was stopped, the neurostimulation response was done in the canine's awake state. As shown in Fig. 11, the angle at which the transmitter coil was applied was changed. Figure 12 shows the range of the neurostimulation response during anesthesia. Although it was not possible to determine the exact angle because the receiving coils were placed inside the body, the neurostimulation response was confirmed in the range from 15 deg to 165 deg when the center of the two receiving coils was set at 90 deg. Figure 13 shows some of the measurement results. When the signal generator was turned on, the heart rate decreased from 138 bpm to about 108 bpm. When the signal generator was turned off, the heart rate increased and converged to the original value. Figure 14 shows the results during awake state. Canine movements during arousal affected the heart rate waverforms. Making precise heart rate measurement difficult. Therefore, the waveform remained unstable after stimulation, but when the signal generator was turned on, the heart rate decreased from 135 bpm to about 44 bpm. When the signal generator was turned off, the heart rate increased and converged to the original value. Based on these measurement results, we confirmed that using multiple receiver coils improved angular characteristics and that neural stimulation responses in the awake state, which could not be achieved with a single receiver coil alone, were also detected.

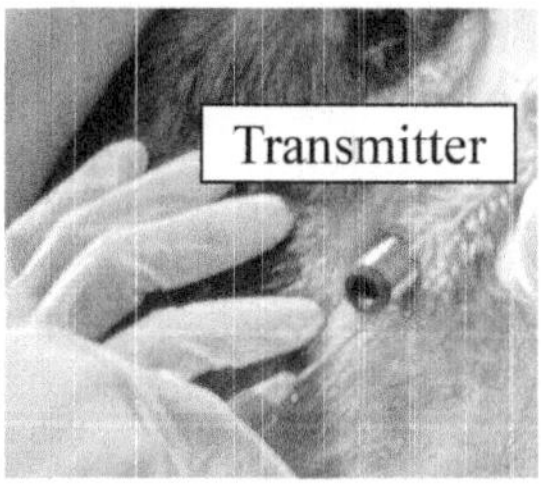

Fig. 10. In-vivo measurement environment

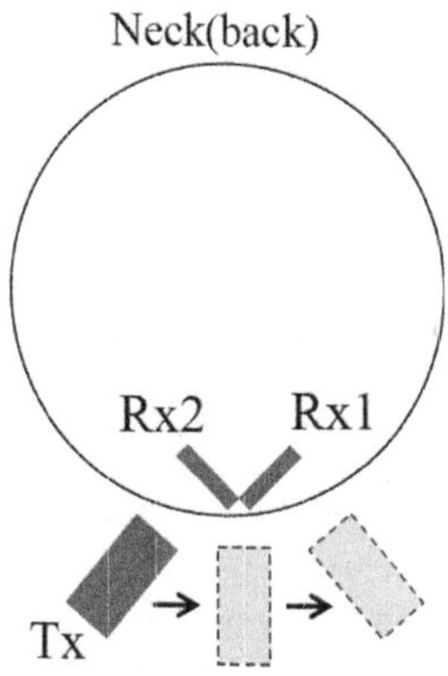

Fig. 11. Angular Characteristic Measurement

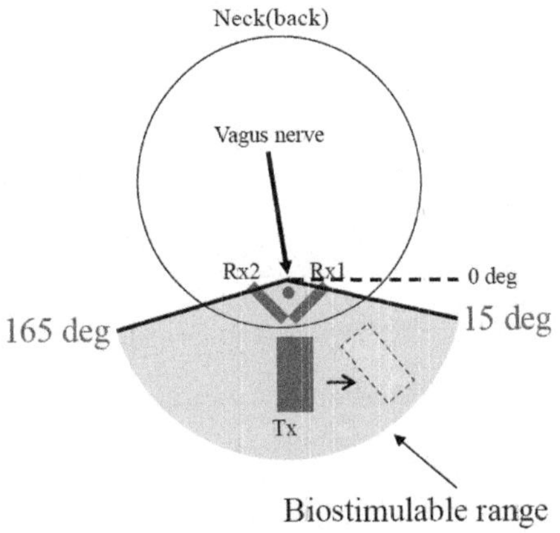

Fig. 12. Measurable range

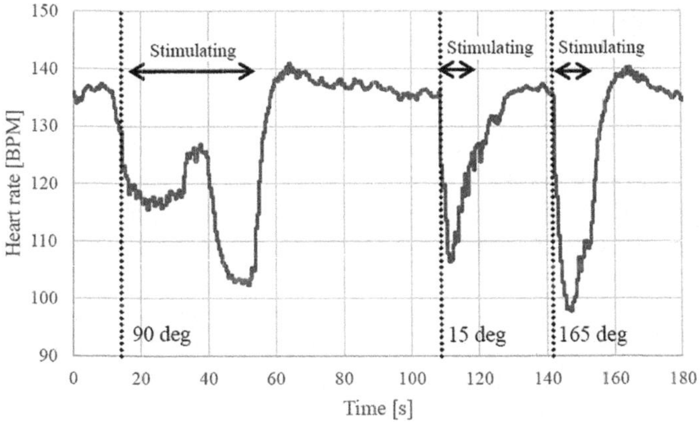

Fig. 13. Results of biostimulation experiments using multiple angles

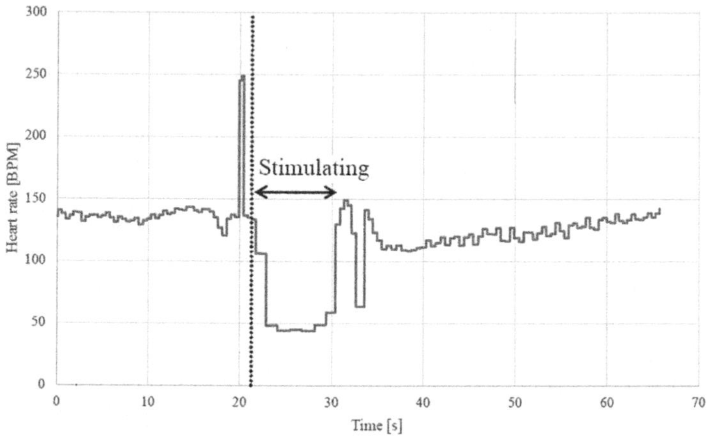

Fig. 14. Results of biostimulation experiments during arousal

5 Conclusion

To overcome the issues related to battery use in implants, and in wireless charging due to angular and positional misalignments. In this study, we designed a receiver coil considering the influence of the living body and conducted an experimental evaluation assuming a neurostimulation device. In addition, we investigated a method to improve the angular characteristics by using multiple receiver coils, and conducted experimental evaluations. By using multiple receiver coils, we confirmed the improvement of angular characteristics and the response to the bio-stimulation when the canine subject was in the awake state. Regarding future clinical applications, a reduction in power transfer efficiency is anticipated as the receiving coil is miniaturized, necessitating further optimization of the transmission and reception mechanisms. Moreover, the long-term durability of the implanted receiving coil should be evaluated to ensure stable operation in vivo. Future work include miniaturization of the receiver coils and design of a receiver coil that can receive power in all directions.

References

1. Testerman, R.L., Rise, M.T., Stypulkowski, P.H.: Electrical stimulation as therapy for neurological disorder. IEEE Eng. Med. Biol. Mag. **25**, 74–78 (2006)
2. Saku, K., Kamata, K.: Potential of vagal nerve stimulation as a treatment for heart failure. Nihon Rinsho **77**(Suppl.), 550–554 (2019)
3. Tubbs, R.S., Rizk, E., Shoja, M., Loukas, M., Barbaro, N., Spinner, R.: Nerves and nerve injuries. Elsevier, pp. 385 – 397 (2015)
4. Wei, X., Wang, Z., Dai, H.: A critical review of wireless power transfer via strongly coupled magnetic resonances. Energies **7**(7), 4316–4341 (2014)
5. Bonaz, B., Picq, C., Sinniger, V., Mayol, J.F., Clarencon, D.: Vagus nerve stimulation: from epilepsy to the cholinergic anti-inflammatory pathway. Neurogastroenterol. Motil. **25**, 208–221 (2013)

Fundamental Study of a Monitoring System for Clinical Settings Using LoRaWAN

Kai Ishida(✉)

Shonan Institute of Technology, 1-1-25, Tsujidonishikaigan, Fujisawa, Japan
gishikai310@gmail.com

Abstract. We investigated the application of long-range wide area network (LoRaWAN) in medicine and its associated challenges. First, we developed a prototype system that can remotely monitor the environment (temperature, humidity, and illuminance) and pulse rate of patients. This system consists of a gateway and an end node. The gateway receives sensor data from the end node via LoRaWAN communication. The received data are sent from a network server on the cloud to an application server. Users can access the data on the application server via an external line. Through simulation, we investigated whether LoRaWAN communication could be received when the transmission data rate and payload frame value were changed. The reception was good on the same floor of a building, even with obstructions and radio wave diffraction and reflection. Moreover, we evaluated the effective data reception rate while changing the data rate (spreading rate and transmission output) and payload size in LoRaWAN communication between an end node and a gateway. LoRaWAN uses frequency-spreading technology for long-distance transmission; however, increasing the spreading rate makes it impossible to transmit large amounts of data. In contrast, sensor data require only one byte if it is a two-digit integer value; therefore, even if multiple sensor data are sent from a single device, the amount of data is not considerably large. We believe that for low-volume data such as sensor data, highly reliable communication can be achieved by maximizing the spreading factor and improving reception characteristics.

Keywords: Low Power Wide Area · LoRaWAN · Monitoring System

1 Introduction

Low power wide area (LPWA) has been attracting attention as a wireless communication technology that enables low power consumption and long-distance transmission. In healthcare environments, LPWA is used to detect abnormal behavior and monitor vital signs in elderly people as well as to monitor the operating status of medical equipment [1–4]. In the modern medical environment, in which infectious diseases such as COVID-19 spread continuously, there is a high demand for contactless monitoring. Long-range

H. Tanaka et al. (Eds.): BodyNets 2025, LNICST 714, pp. 255–264, 2026.
https://doi.org/10.1007/978-3-032-38657-1_20

wide area network (LoRaWAN), a representative example of LPWA, does not require a license, has a maximum output of 20 mW, and can be used in the 920 MHz band frequency in Japan. Although LoRaWAN has a slow communication speed of 250—50 kbps, it is inexpensive and highly compatible with various IoT devices. Additionally, its reception performance and noise resistance can be improved using frequency-spreading technology. However, we are not aware of any studies that have reported the application of LoRaWAN in medical environments. Therefore, in this study, we investigate the application of LoRaWAN in medical settings and its associated challenges.

2 Medical Environment Monitoring System Using LoRaWAN

2.1 System Overview

In this study, we developed a prototype system that can remotely monitor the environment (temperature, humidity, and illuminance) and pulse rate of patients. Figure 1 shows an overview of the system. The system comprises an end node (sensor unit) and a gateway. Figure 2 shows the end node used in this study. The end node uses an Arduino-based microcontroller equipped with a LoRaWAN wireless chip to wirelessly transmit temperature, humidity, illuminance, and pulse rate data to the gateway. The gateway links the received data with an external application server, The Things Network (TTN), and is designed to enable remote data visualization. The end node is battery-powered and connected to environmental measurement and pulse rate sensors. Data measured by the sensors are transferred to the TTN via a gateway at 10-s intervals.

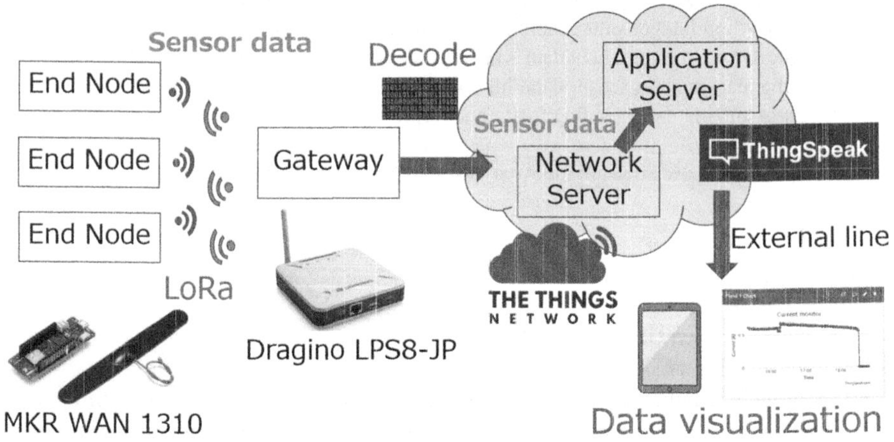

Fig. 1. Overview of the prototype system

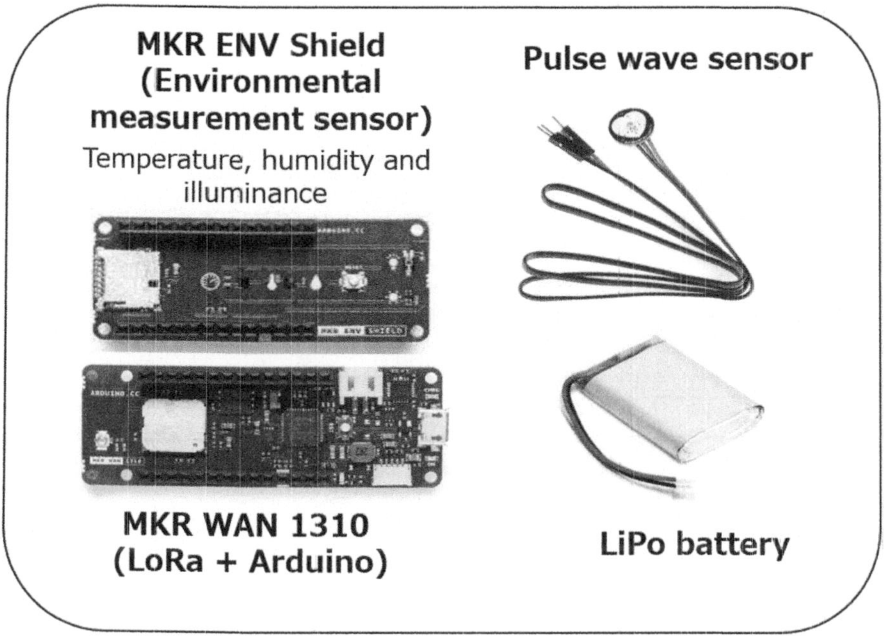

Fig. 2. Overview of the end node

Figure 3 shows the environmental measurement results, i.e., the temperature, humidity, and illuminance results, the vertical axis represents these results, and the horizontal axis represents time. The results are obtained via measurements and transmissions performed over approximately 14 h. Figure 4 shows the results obtained from measuring the pulse rate and transmitting it wirelessly. The vertical axis represents the pulse rate, and the horizontal axis represents time. Data were transmitted at 10-s intervals to enable the monitoring of pulse rate changes. In each measurement, sensor data were not lost because the end nodes and gateways were closely located; thus, the measurements, transmission, and visualization were accurate.

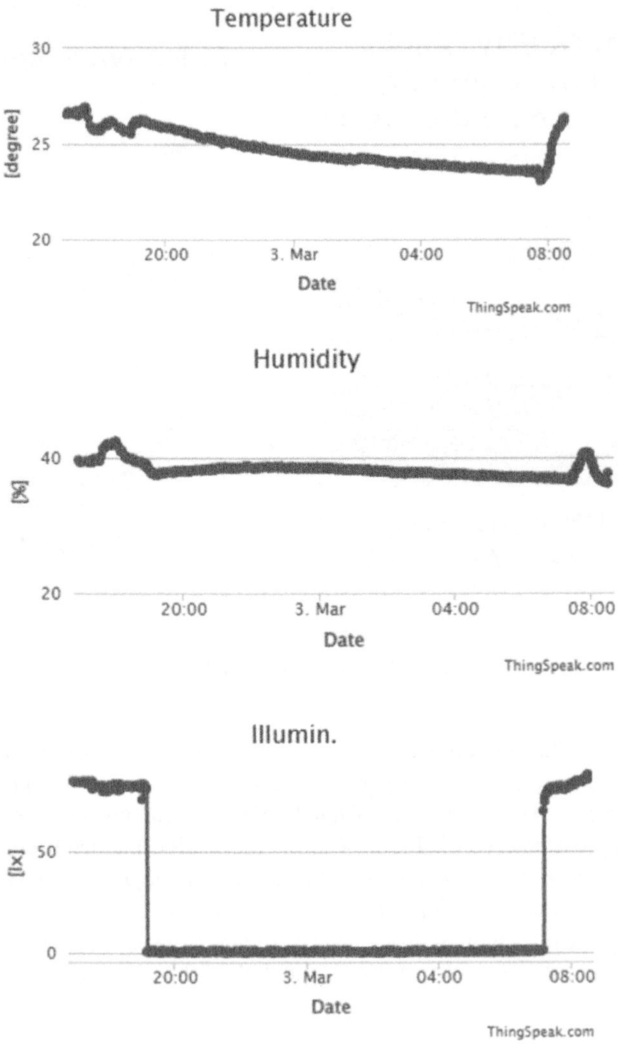

Fig. 3. Results of environmental measurements (temperature, humidity and illuminance) obtained via LoRaWAN transmission

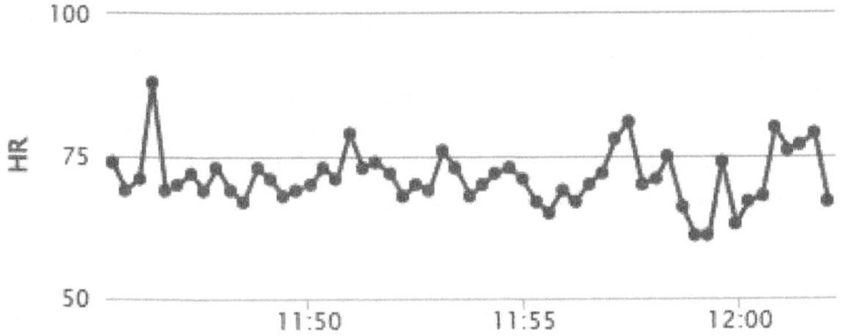

Fig. 4. Results of pulse rate measurements obtained via the LoRaWAN transmission

3 Communication Performance Evaluation of LoRaWAN

3.1 Reception Performance Evaluation in a Simulated Environment

To study the optimal communication parameters for LoRaWAN in healthcare, we investigated through simulation whether LoRaWAN communication could be received when the transmission data rate and payload frame value were changed. Figure 5 shows a floor plan of the simulation environment. The gateway was installed at point G, and the end nodes were installed at points A to C. The spreading factor (SF) of the end node was set to "7," and one byte of data was transmitted once per minute for approximately 19 h. At this time, the received signal strength indicator (RSSI) and signal-to-noise ratio (SNR) were measured from the signals received by the gateway from each end node.

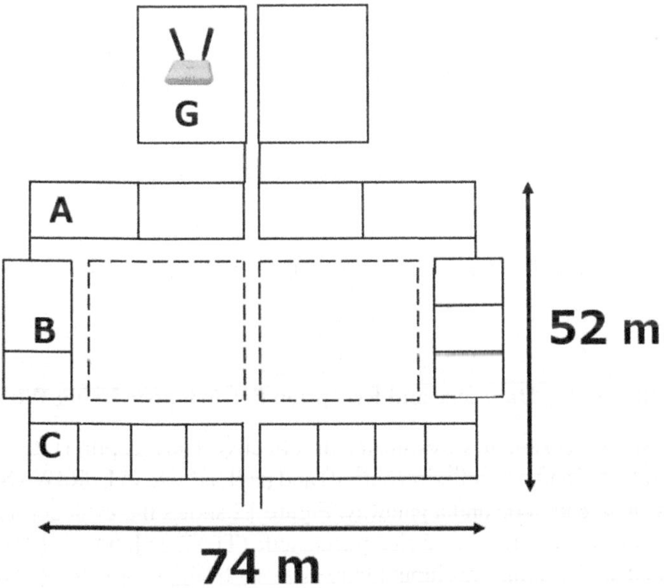

Fig. 5. Overview of the simulated environment

Figures 6, 7, 8, 9, 10 and 11 show the reception status from each end node. In all results, the valid data reception rate was over 98%. The average RSSI was −72.5 dBm at point A, −91.6 dBm at point B, and −111.2 dBm at point C. The average SNR was 8.4 dB at point A, 6.9 dB at point B, and −6.3 dB at point C. Point C was the furthest from the gateway and was in an environment with greater shielding than the other end nodes; however, normal reception was possible.

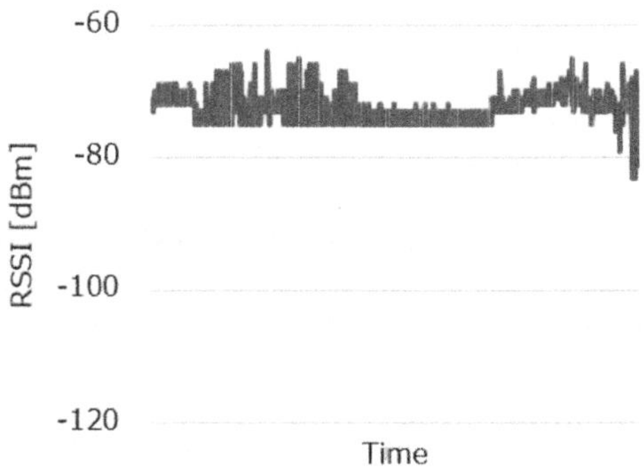

Fig. 6. Change in the RSSI of the end node at point A

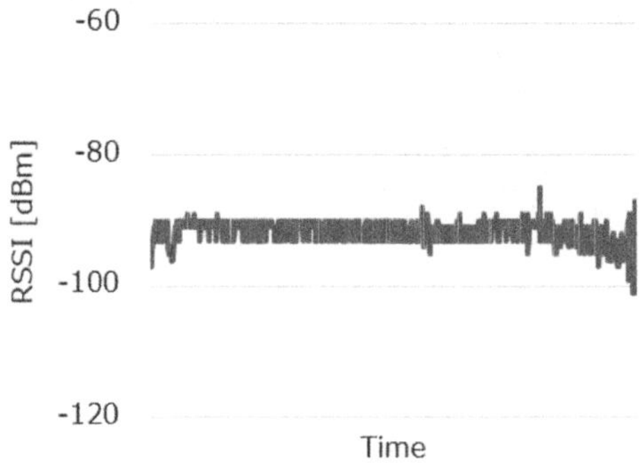

Fig. 7. Change in the RSSI of the end node at point B

3.2 Evaluation of the Data Size and Reception Performance Using Wired Systems

In a wired-system experiment, we evaluated the effective data reception rate when changing the data rate (SF and transmission output) and payload size in LoRaWAN communication between an end node and a gateway. Figure 12 shows the evaluation system. An end node was placed in a transverse electromagnetic (TEM) cell, one end of the terminal was terminated, and a signal was input to the gateway from the other end of the terminal via a variable attenuator (ATT). This made it possible to reproduce any signal strength and thereby simulate poor conditions with an extremely low SNR. We measured the

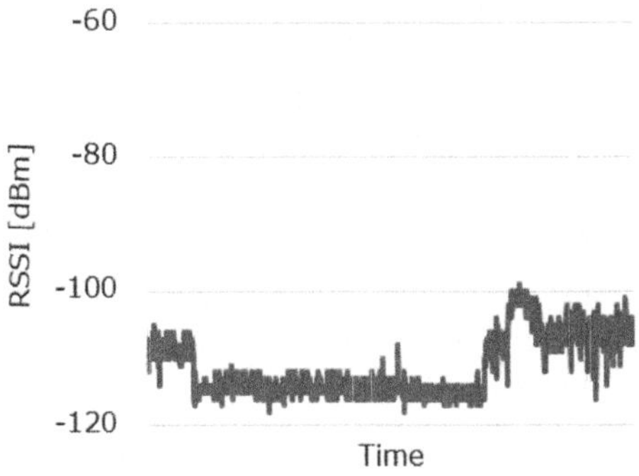

Fig. 8. Change in the RSSI of the end node at point C

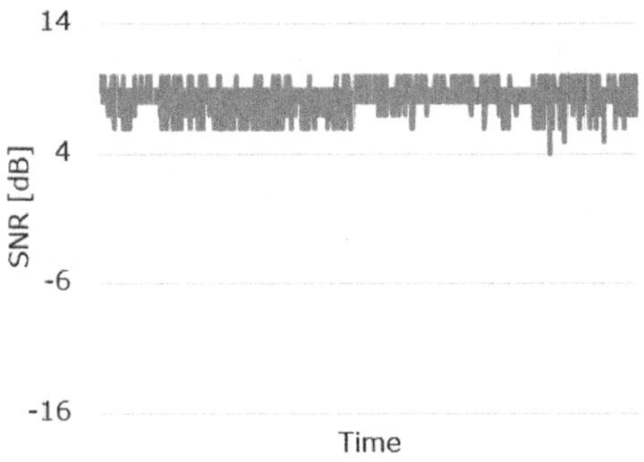

Fig. 9. Change in the SNR of the end node at point A

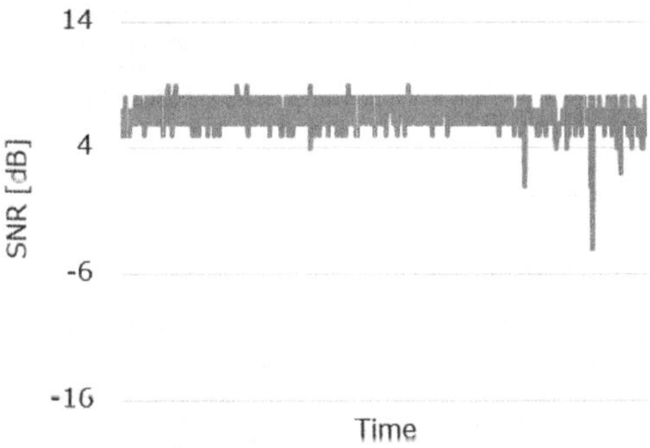

Fig. 10. Change in the SNR of the end node at point B

RSSI and SNR from the signals transmitted by the end node. Moreover, we evaluated the valid data reception rate. Herein, the valid data reception rate is expressed as the ratio of the number of signals transmitted from the end node to the number of signals received at the gateway.

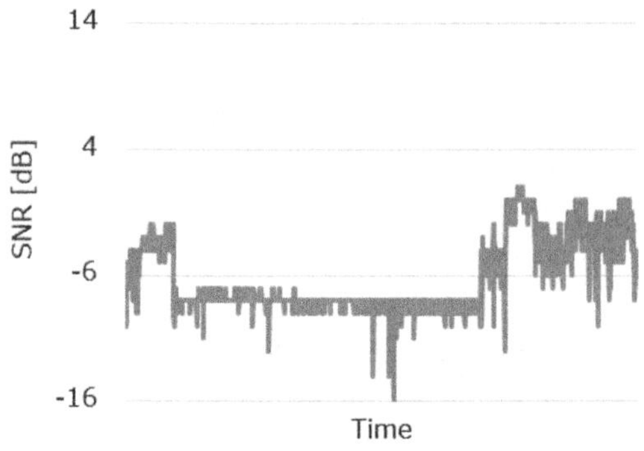

Fig. 11. Change in the SNR of the end node at point C

Table 1 shows the results obtained under each SF and data size The valid data reception rate tended to decrease as the data size increased. When the SF was 7 and the data size was 51 bytes or more, data were only successfully received approximately once in every four attempts (25% of the time). Furthermore, increasing the SF reduced the transmittable data size but made it possible to receive even signals with a low SNR. When the SF was 9, 100% reception was possible for all data sizes.

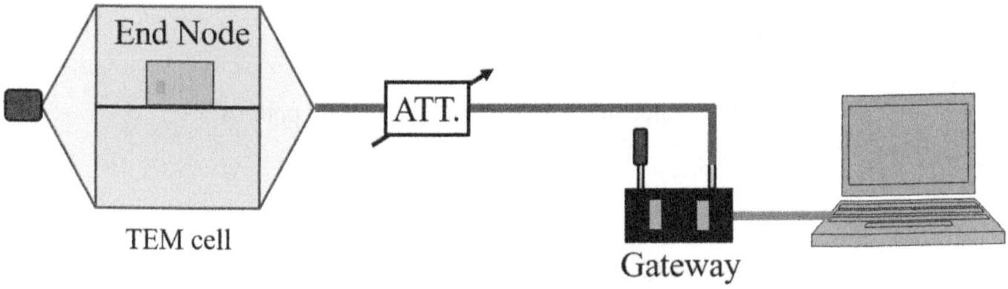

Fig. 12. Measurement setup for reception performance

Table 1. Evaluation results of the reception performance of each SF and data size

SF	Size (byte)	Mean RSSI (dBm)	Mean SNR (dB)	Valid data reception rate
7	1	−120.1	−7.6	82.1%
7	11	−120.8	−8.3	42.3%
7	51	−120.4	−7.9	27.1%
7	240	−120.7	−8.0	25.0%
8	1	−122.7	−10.3	78.3%
8	11	−123.8	−11.2	55.9%
8	51	−124.2	−10.9	39.4%

(continued)

Table 1. *(continued)*

SF	Size (byte)	Mean RSSI (dBm)	Mean SNR (dB)	Valid data reception rate
8	100	−123.6	−10.6	29.6%
8	240	−122.9	−10.3	28.6%
9	1	−122.4	−9.4	**100.0%**
9	11	−123.1	−10.2	**100.0%**
9	51	−122.9	−10.4	**100.0%**

4 Discussions

In this study, we used LoRaWAN to build an environment for aggregating sensor data. The environment can be built inexpensively and can handle a variety of sensor data because the end node is based on Arduino. Additionally, using an external server made it easy to aggregate and visualize data.

In tests performed in a simulated environment, the reception was good on the same floor of a building, even with obstructions and radio wave diffraction and reflection. In an actual medical environment, it would be possible to install a gateway at the staff station and end nodes in each patient room or corridor. Moreover, LoRaWAN employs frequency-spreading technology for long-distance transmission, but increasing the spreading rate makes it impossible to transmit large volumes of data. Conversely, sensor data require only one byte if it is a two-digit integer value; therefore, even if multiple sensor data are transmitted from one child device, the data volume is not considerably large. For low-volume data such as sensor data, we believe that highly reliable communication can be achieved by maximizing the SF and improving the reception characteristics.

Because the prototype system is not a medical device, it can be used for simple monitoring in nonmedical facilities such as at home or in hotels. During the COVID-19 outbreak, close contacts were forced to stay in hotels for long periods. In such nonmedical facilities, there is a shortage of vital sign monitoring equipment. Although it is difficult, sensor data can be transmitted remotely; therefore, we believe that the proposed system can be used in the event of an infectious disease outbreak. However, this research did not address the accuracy of the sensor, which can be verified in a future study.

5 Conclusion

We developed a prototype system that can remotely monitor the environment (temperature, humidity, and illuminance) and pulse rate of patients using LoRaWAN. Moreover, we evaluated the reception accuracy of LoRaWAN and experimentally demonstrated that if SF = 9, a high reception performance can be ensured even if the mean RSSI is approximately −122 dB.

References

1. Shima, K., Kawamura, T., Yamaguchi, M., Yoshida, T., Otsuka, T.: Implementation and layout optimization of motion sensor for anomaly detection in daily life of elderly persons. In: Proceedings of the 13th International Conference on Information & Communication Technology and System (ICTS) (2021)
2. Mdhaffar, A., Chaari, T., Larbi, K., Jmaiel, M., Freisleben, B.: IoT-based health monitoring via LoRaWAN. In: Proceedings of the IEEE EUROCON 2017 -17th International Conference on Smart Technologies (2017)
3. Abdulmalek, S., Nasir, A., Jabbar, W.A.: LoRaWAN-based hybrid internet of wearable things system implementation for smart healthcare. Internet Things. **25**, 101124 (2024)
4. Kakutani, K., Ito, N., Shima, K., Oyama, S., Otsuka, T.: Development of a location and operation monitoring device for medical device management. In: Proceedings of the 2023 International Conference on Consumer Electronics (2023)

Development of a Patient-Specific Cardiovascular Simulator for Tailored Cardiovascular Management

Takuya Nishikawa(✉)

National Cerebral and Cardiovascular Center, Suita, Japan
Nishikawa.takuya75@ncvc.go.jp

Abstract. Personalized cardiovascular medicine requires understanding individual patient cardiovascular characteristics. We developed a patient-specific cardiovascular simulator to reproduce hemodynamic characteristics of heart failure patients and quantify unmeasurable cardiac mechanical properties. We created 30 modified cases based on the SCG-RHC database from Physionet, including patients with heart failure with preserved ejection fraction (HFpEF) and reduced ejection fraction (HFrEF). The cardiovascular model utilized time-varying elastance for four cardiac chambers and vascular networks with compliance and resistance. Stepwise Bayesian optimization was employed to optimize nine parameters (ventricular contractility, stiffness, arterial resistance, compliance, and stressed blood volume) to match nine reference hemodynamic values. Parameter optimization achieved high accuracy with median error of 2.1% (1.7–2.8%). HFpEF patients increased significantly left ventricular contractility compared to HFrEF patients. Stressed blood volume remained unchanged between groups. Our approach successfully reproduced individual patient circulatory dynamics and enabled quantification of fundamental cardiac mechanical properties not measurable through conventional clinical methods. This represents an important advancement toward personalized cardiovascular medicine and optimized patient management.

Keywords: Cardiovascular simulator · parameter optimization · personalized medicine

1 Introduction

While evidence-based medicine has been based on population-level data of the same disease, personalized medicine that makes medical decisions for individual patients is now emerging [1]. To achieve personalized medicine in cardiovascular care, it is essential to understand the unique circulatory characteristics of each patient. The circulatory system that supplies blood throughout the body is characterized by the physical properties of organs such as the heart and blood vessels, including stiffness and resistance [2]. Circulatory disorders arise from mechanical loads on the system, such as oxygen

H. Tanaka et al. (Eds.): BodyNets 2025, LNICST 714, pp. 265–272, 2026.
https://doi.org/10.1007/978-3-032-38657-1_21

supply-demand imbalances due to thrombosis and mechanical stress from conditions like hypertension. Therefore, effective hemodynamic management requires understanding the mechanical properties of the heart and blood vessels and providing appropriate treatment accordingly. A detailed understanding of these properties is crucial for optimal clinical decision-making.

We have previously constructed a circulatory model as an integrated model of the circulatory system and demonstrated its applicability for pathophysiological understanding, prediction, and treatment [3–5]. In this study, we aimed to reproduce patients with heart failure with preserved ejection fraction (HFpEF) and heart failure with reduced ejection fraction (HFrEF) using cardiovascular models based on open data sources, and to evaluate the reproducibility, accuracy, and extract hemodynamic characteristics.

2 Methods

2.1 Patient Datasets

We created a set of 30 modified cases based on the SCG-RHC: Wearable Seismocardiogram Signal and Right Heart Catheter Database from Physionet (https://physionet.org/). This database contains comprehensive right heart catheterization parameters including cardiac output (CO), pulmonary artery wedge pressure (PAWP), pulmonary artery pressure (PAP), and right atrial pressure (RAP), as well as clinical information on underlying diseases such as HFpEF and HFrEF.

2.2 Preprocessing

Since EF information was unavailable, EF was set according to the underlying disease. EF for HFpEF was set to 50%, for HFrEF to 30%, and RVEF to 50%. Systemic arterial pressure (SBP) and diastolic blood pressure (DBP) were set to 120 and 80 mmHg. Volume at zero pressure (V_0) of cardiac chambers was set to 8 ml/m^2. We assumed PAWP equaled LAP.

2.3 Cardiovascular Model

The heart was represented by a time-varying elastance model with four chambers, and valves were represented by diodes. The vascular system was constructed as a network of compliance and resistance. The stressed blood volume (SBV) was set as the initial charge. As shown in Fig. 1, the circulatory system was constructed as a closed circuit.

Cardiac time-varying elastance was modeled by the following equations.

$$P(V, t) = P_{ed}(V) + e_N(t)[P_{es}(V) - P_{ed}(V)] \tag{1}$$

$$P_{ed}(V) = \alpha \times \{\exp[\beta(V - V_0)] - 1\} \tag{2}$$

$$P_{es}(V) = E_{es} \times (V - V_0) \tag{3}$$

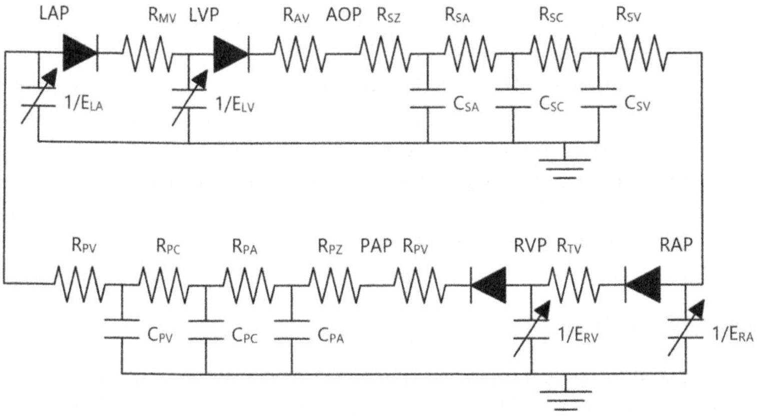

Fig. 1. Circuit diagram of the cardiovascular model.
Abbreviations: LAP, left atrial pressure; LVP, left ventricular pressure; AOP, aortic pressure; PAP, pulmonary artery pressure; RVP, right ventricular pressure; RAP, right atrial pressure; R_{MV}, resistance of mitral valve; R_{AV}, resistance of aortic valve; R_{TV}, resistance of tricuspid valve; R_{PV}, resistance of pulmonary artery valve; E_{LA}, elastance of left atrium; E_{LV}, elastance of left ventricle; E_{RA}, elastance of right atrium; E_{RV}, elastance of right ventricle; R_{SA}, resistance of systemic artery; R_{SC}, resistance of systemic capillary vessels; R_{SV}, resistance of systemic vein; R_{PA}, resistance of pulmonary artery; R_{PC}, resistance of pulmonary capillary vessels; R_{PV}, resistance of pulmonary vein; C_{SA}, compliance of systemic artery; C_{SC}, compliance of systemic capillary vessels; C_{SV}, compliance of systemic vein; C_{PA}, compliance of pulmonary artery; C_{PC}, compliance of pulmonary capillary vessels; C_{PV}, compliance of pulmonary vein.

and

$$e_N(t) = \frac{1}{2}\left\{\sin\left[\left(\frac{\pi}{T_{max}}\right)t - \frac{\pi}{2}\right] + 1\right\}, 0 < t \leq \frac{4}{3}T_{max} \tag{4}$$

$$e_N(t) = \frac{3}{4}\exp\left(-\frac{t-\frac{4}{3}T_{max}}{\tau}\right), t > \frac{4}{3}T_{max} \tag{5}$$

P, pressure; V, volume; es, end-systolic; ed., end-diastolic; $e_N(t)$, normalized time-varying elastance; T_{max}, time to maximum elastance; τ, the time constant of pressure decay; t, time.

2.4 Parameter Optimization

Heart rate was used as a measured value. Atrial function, capillary and venous resistance, and compliance were set as fixed values according to body surface area. Nine variables were used as reference values: systolic blood pressure (SBP), diastolic blood pressure (DBP), pulmonary artery systolic pressure (sPAP), pulmonary artery diastolic pressure (dPAP), left atrial pressure (LAP), right atrial pressure (RAP), cardiac output (CO), left ventricular ejection fraction (LVEF), and right ventricular ejection fraction (RV EF). Nine parameters were optimized: left and right ventricular contractility (LV E_{es}, RV E_{es}) and stiffness (LV end-diastolic pressure volume relationship: EDPVR β, RV EDPVR β), resistance (R_{SA}, R_{PA}) and compliance (C_{SA}, C_{PA}) of proximal arteries in systemic and pulmonary circulation, and SBV.

We performed stepwise Bayesian optimization. First, we established the initial parameter range based on cardiac mechanics and conducted Bayesian optimization. Based on the obtained Gaussian process, we estimated surrogate posterior probability distributions for each parameter. We then selected the search range based on the posterior probability distribution and iteratively repeated the subsequent Bayesian optimization process. We used MATLAB/Simulink 2024b.

2.5 Statistical Analysis

Data are expressed as median (interquartile range). Mann-Whitney U tests were used to assess statistical significance. We assumed $p < 0.05$ as significant. Statistical analyses were performed using R software.

3 Results

Table 1 shows the right heart catheterization data from Physionet. In HFrEF patients, dPAP was higher and cardiac index was lower than HFpEF patients. This suggests that cardiac pump function was more impaired in the HFrEF group.

Table 1. Basic characteristics of patients' data

	HFrEF (n = 21)	HFpEF (n = 9)	p value
Heart rate, beats/min	70 (67–78)	68 (58–77)	0.28
sPAP, mmHg	47 (35–53)	33 (31–49)	0.11
dPAP, mmHg	20 (15–26)	12 (11–23)	0.02
PAWP, mmHg	17 (12–28)	12 (10–21)	0.12
RAP, mmHg	6 (6–10)	6 (5–7)	0.27
Cardiac index, L/min/m^2	1.8 (1.7–2.4)	2.7 (1.9–3.2)	0.01

Figures 2, 3 and 4 show a representative case of a patient-specific simulation. Figure 2 shows the surrogate posterior probabilities of parameters at each step. While performing stepwise range convergence, when the probability distribution was skewed (yellow background), we extrapolated in that direction to determine the next range distribution. Figure 3 shows the deviation of the target variable across all trials of all steps. The variable represented by the blue circles is converging to the reference point represented by the orange line. Figure 4 shows the hemodynamics of a representative case. A patient-specific cardiovascular simulation reproduces pressure waveforms, flow waveforms, and PV loops, and can provide cardiovascular properties such as contractility and compliance, as well as energetics such as cardiac external workload.

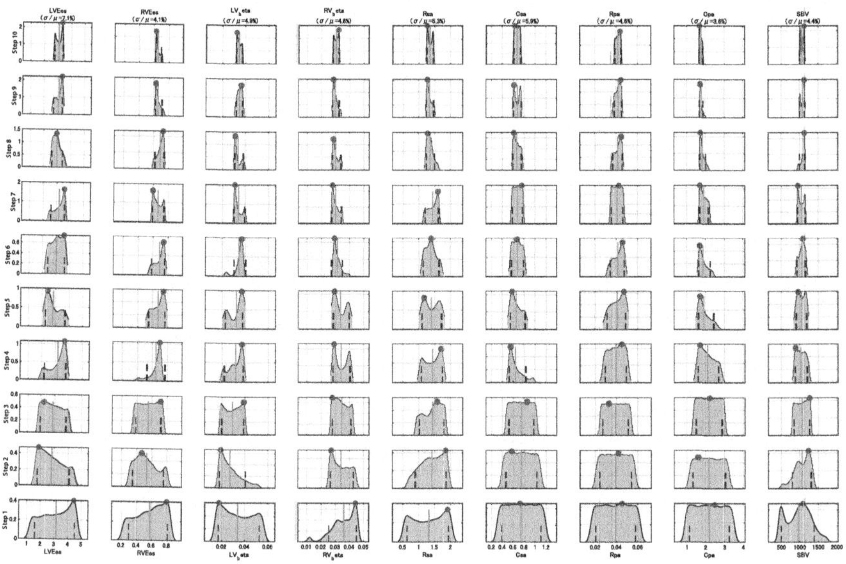

Fig. 2. Posterior probabilities of parameters at each step

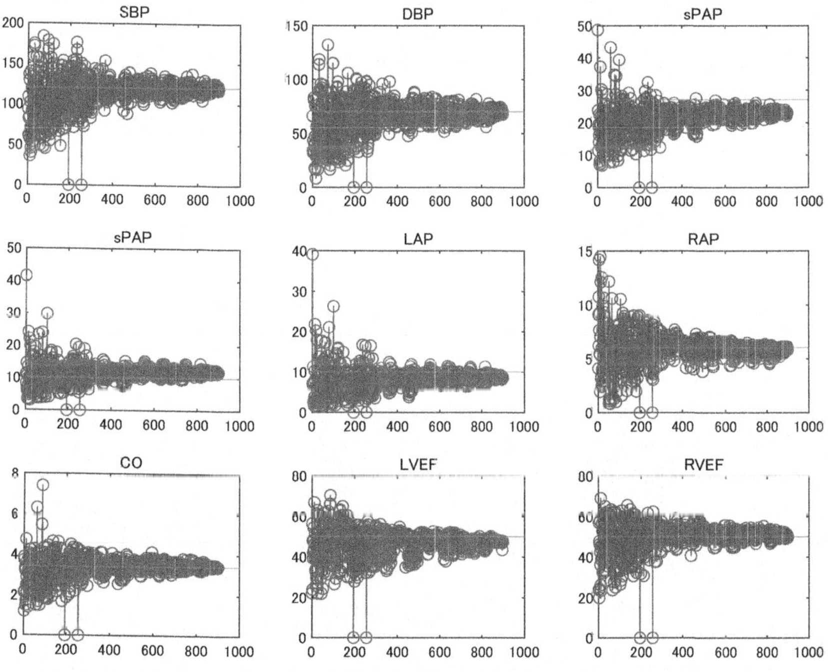

Fig. 3. The value of target variables across all trials of all steps

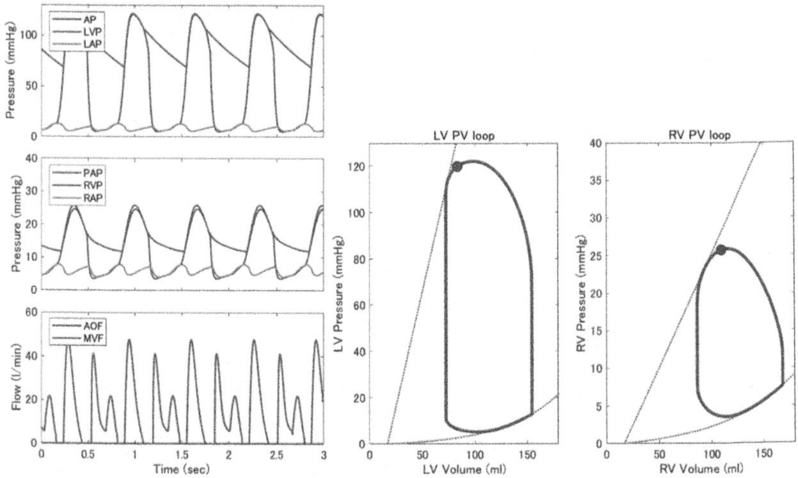

Fig. 4. Detailed hemodynamics of a representative patient-specific cardiovascular simulation. AOF, aortic valve flow; MVF, mitral valve flow; PV loop, pressure-volume loop

The entire error of parameter fitting was 2.1 (1.7–2.8) %. Figure 5 shows the contractility (E_{es}), chamber stiffness (EDPVR β) of LV and RV, and SBV. For LV, E_{es} was lower in the HFrEF group compared with HFpEF group, while EDPVR β remained unchanged. For RV, both E_{es} and EDPVR β were higher in the HFrEF group. There was no significant difference in SBV between the two groups. These findings represent important cardiac functions that cannot be measured in clinical practice.

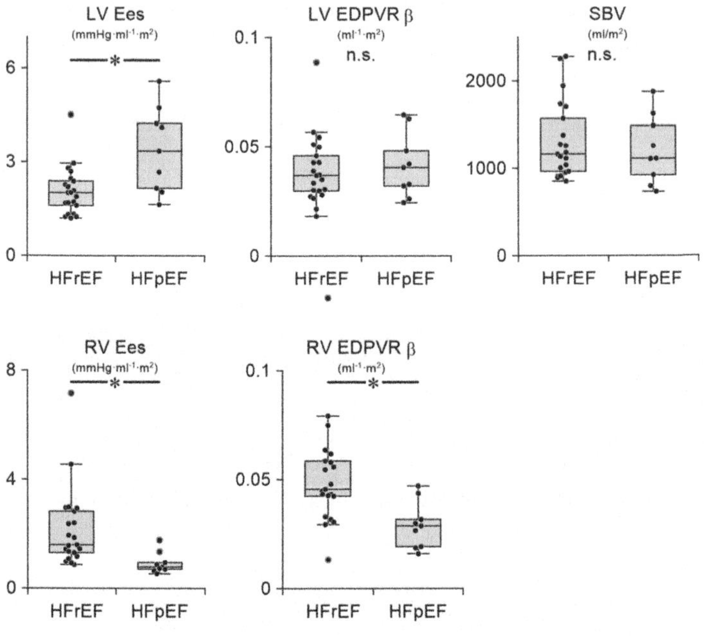

Fig. 5. Cardiovascular properties estimated from cardiovascular simulations

4 Discussions

In this study, we developed patient-specific cardiovascular simulators reproducing hemodynamic characteristics of HFpEF and HFrEF patients using stepwise Bayesian optimization. Our simulation approach enables quantification of fundamental cardiac mechanical properties that cannot be measured clinically, including ventricular contractility (E_{es}) and stiffness (EDPVR β), and SBV, representing an important advancement toward personalized cardiovascular medicine.

In most cases, parameter fitting errors were within 5%, demonstrating clinically acceptable accuracy. Patients with HFpEF exhibited significantly higher LV E_{es} compared to HFrEF patients, appropriately reflecting the preserved contractility characteristic of HFpEF [6]. In contrast, RV E_{es} and EDPVR were higher in the HFrEF group. Given the elevated dPAP and reduced cardiac output, pulmonary vascular resistance is likely increased. These findings suggest the development of pulmonary hypertension secondary to left HF, resulting in RV remodeling in response to pressure overload. However, given the differences in cardiac output and HF severity between groups, further research is needed to determine whether these findings represent inherent characteristics of HFrEF. Notably, despite the greater severity of HFrEF, SBV showed no significant difference between groups, which may be influenced by differences in diuretic management.

Our approach enabled direct quantification of cardiovascular properties such as increased LV Ees in HFpEF, which cannot be measured through conventional clinical methods. In clinical practice, physicians infer changes in cardiac function, vascular properties, and blood volume from measured hemodynamic parameters to guide therapeutic decisions. Patient-specific simulation enables direct visualization of these underlying pathophysiological conditions. The ability to quantify patient-specific cardiac mechanical properties through simulation has important implications for clinical decision-making, potentially guiding optimal therapy selection and risk stratification.

However, several limitations should be acknowledged, including the assignment of ejection fraction values based on disease classification, preprocessing modifications of several parameters, and the relatively small sample size, particularly for the HFpEF group ($n = 9$).

5 Conclusions

In this study, we developed patient-specific cardiovascular simulations by combining simulation models with parameter optimization methods. Our approach captured and quantified the contractility differences between patients with HFrEF and HFpEF. This patient-specific simulation framework can provide cardiovascular properties that cannot be clinically measured and has the potential to optimize therapeutic strategies in HF management.

References

1. Horwitz, R.I., Charlson, M.E., Singer, B.H.: Medicine based evidence and personalized care of patients. Eur. J. Clin. Investig. **48**(7), e12945 (2018)

2. Sunagawa, K., Sagawa, K., Maughan, W.L.: Ventricular interaction with the loading system. Ann. Biomed. Eng. **12**(2), 163–189 (1984)
3. Nishikawa, T., et al.: Development of a framework for the hemodynamic impact of positive end-expiratory pressure in normal and heart failure conditions. Am. J. Phys. Heart Circ. Phys. **328**(2), H361–H376 (2025)
4. Nishikawa, T., et al.: Automated control of Impella maintains optimal left ventricular unloading during periods of unstable hemodynamics and prevents myocardial damage in acute myocardial infarction. Int. J. Cardiol. **410**, 132244 (2024)
5. Nishikawa, T., et al.: Prediction of haemodynamics after interatrial shunt for heart failure using the generalized circulatory equilibrium. ESC Heart Fail. **7**(5), 3075–3085 (2020)
6. Zile, M.R., Brutsaert, D.L.: New concepts in diastolic dysfunction and diastolic heart failure: part I: diagnosis, prognosis, and measurements of diastolic function. Circulation. **105**(11), 1387–1393 (2002)

Applications of Wearable Devices in Motor Sport

Satoshi Maeda[1(✉)] and Ai Miura[2]

[1] Life Protection Sales Unit, Toyobo MC Corporation, Graduate School of Information Science, Hiroshima City University, Hiroshima, Japan
satoshim257@gmail.com, satoshi_maeda@toyobo.jp
[2] AIWIN, Gotemba, Japan
aimiura@aiwin.jp

Abstract. ANAIM® is a novel display method that plots autonomic nervous activity indices (logarithms of SNI: sympathetic nervous activity index and PNI: parasympathetic nervous activity index) derived from heart rate variability measured by a wearable device on an X-Y plane. This paper first provides an overview of ANAIM®, and then presents examples of how the method was used to observe the physical and mental state of professional racing drivers in various driving situations, including during motor racing.

ANAIM® is a registered trademark of Toyobo MC Co., Ltd.

Keywords: ANAIM · autonomic nerve · wearable device

1 Introduction

The method of calculating autonomic nerve activity from heart rate variability has been established since the 1980s [1]. Time-series data of RRI (interval between heartbeat peaks obtained from ECG: Electrocardiogram) is converted to frequency axis and separated into high frequency component (HF) and low frequency component (LF). LF/HF constitutes SNI: sympathetic nerve activity index while HF constitutes the PSI: parasympathetic activity index. Transformation to the frequency axis is used by FFT (Fast Fourier Transform).

Wearable devices can be used to measure heart rate variability, such as clothing-type devices that directly measure electrocardiograms using electrodes attached to the chest. Alternatively, wristwatch-type pulse monitors or pressure sensors can be used as a proxy for pulse. FFT requires a time window length appropriate for frequency resolution. From this perspective, electrocardiogram-based devices, which can measure RRI with a clear peak and high time resolution, are advantageous over pulse-based devices. Accelerometers built into chest-worn electrocardiograms provide data reflecting the trunk's movement state. Furthermore, a built-in thermometer can measure the temperature inside the clothing rather than the outside temperature. These are also advantages of clothing-type devices.

This paper first explains ANAIM®, a method for displaying autonomic nervous system activity indicators developed by the author while employed at Toyobo Co., Ltd.

H. Tanaka et al. (Eds.): BodyNets 2025, LNICST 714, pp. 273–286, 2026.
https://doi.org/10.1007/978-3-032-38657-1_22

[2], and then presents examples of using this method to observe the autonomic nervous system activity of professional racing drivers during various driving scenarios. ANAIM® allows even non-medical experts to interpret a subject's mental and physical state to some extent from autonomic nervous system activity.

2 Measurement of ECG by Clothing-Type Wearable Device

Figure 1 shows examples of clothing-type wearable devices made for athletes. They have electrodes and wiring formed inside the under bust part using the stretchable conductive film, and an ECG measuring device can be attached and detached via the snap fastener used as a connector [3].

In this study, the heart rate sensor "myBeat" WHS-1 manufactured by Union Tool was used as an electrocardiograph. For data analysis, Union Tool's software: RRI Analyzer (version 1.14) was used. Every minute or every 10 s, in each case, the FFT was calculated by a time window of the past 3 min, and the HF and LF were obtained with a boundary of 0.15 Hz. Graph plot intervals are 1 min unless otherwise noted. The heart rate sensor WHS-1 has a built-in thermometer and a 3-axis accelerometer, and the temperature inside the clothes obtained from them and the acceleration data obtained by vector summing the 3 axes were also used as a reference [4].

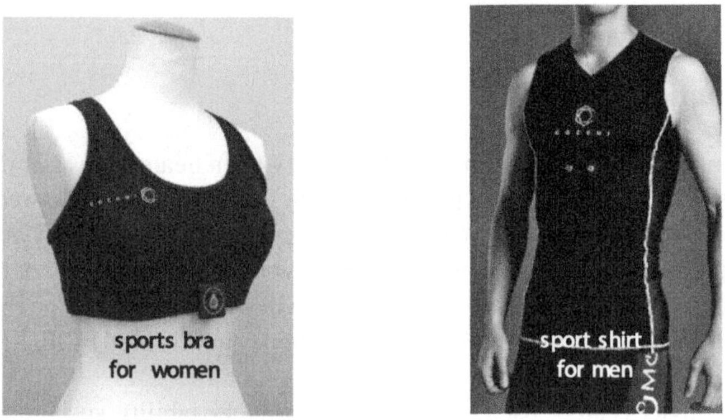

Fig. 1. Examples of a clothing-type wearable devices for athletes

3 Measurement of ECG by Clothing-Type Wearable Device

In general, the autonomic nerves are said to have a 24-h cycle rhythm in which SNI (sympathetic nerve activity) is dominant during the day and PNI (parasympathetic nerve activity) is dominant at night and at bedtime. However, observation by wearable devices in actual activities such as living, working, and playing sports reveals that autonomic nerve activity is more complicated.

Figure 2 shows time transitions of heart rate, autonomic nerve SNI (LF/HF), and PNI (HF) in the afternoon of a female subject. The FFT time window for obtaining LF and HF is set to the past 3 min, and the values calculated every minute are plotted.

It was her first presentation to executives that day. The area B in Fig. 2. is the period of sitting and waiting in the presentation room. The area P is the period during she is presenting on stage for about 20 min. The area A is the period during which she returned to her seats after the presentation and wait for other presentations to finish. Her heart rate reached nearly 150 in the area P. After her presentation, she left the office around 18:00 and returned to her home by her bicycle (around 18:30). At home, she appears exhausted after her first heavy presentation (her heart rate slows and her parasympathetic activity increases). Overall, it roughly shows SNI and PNI are moving in opposition to each other. However, both are observed to perform fairly small and they are complex and not simple movements.

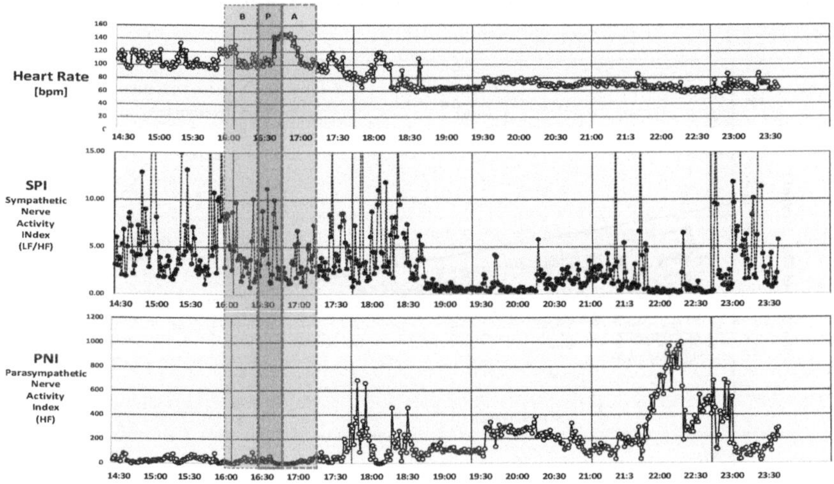

Fig. 2. Heart rate and autonomic nerve activity index over time (Conventional representation method of autonomic nerve activity index)

4 ANAIM®: A New Representation Method for Autonomic Nerve Activity

4.1 Cartesian Coordinate Representation

Figure 3 is a graph plotted the common logarithm of PSI on the vertical axis and the SNI on the horizontal axis using the same data as in Fig. 2. The upper left area of the graph is the area where the calmed SNI and the activated PNI, i.e. it is the relaxing area. Conversely, the lower right is the area where calmed PNI and activated SNI, ie it is exciting area.

If the SNI and PNI are just simply in conflicting relationships, the plot simply goes back and forth between the upper left and lower right in a 24-h cycle. However, the actual autonomic nerve activity has a wide distribution like this, moves in small steps, and very complex.

In Fig. 3, the thin dotted line corresponds to B, and the solid line to P (surrounded by a dashed line oval), and the thick dashed line to A in Fig. 1, light-gray plots are plots for other time periods.

The period during which the subject stayed at the presentation room was considered as a "special time period", and the other time period was considered as the subject's "ordinary living time period". The regression line is calculated for the "ordinary living time period" plot, and next, the standard deviation σ of the distance from the regression line for each plot is obtained. In Fig. 3, the thick straight line that descends to the right is the regression line, and the dashed lines are $\pm 3\sigma$ of the regression line. In other words, the interval of the parallelogram surrounded by this downward-sloping dashed line can be considered the 99.7% confidence interval of the subject's "ordinary living time period."

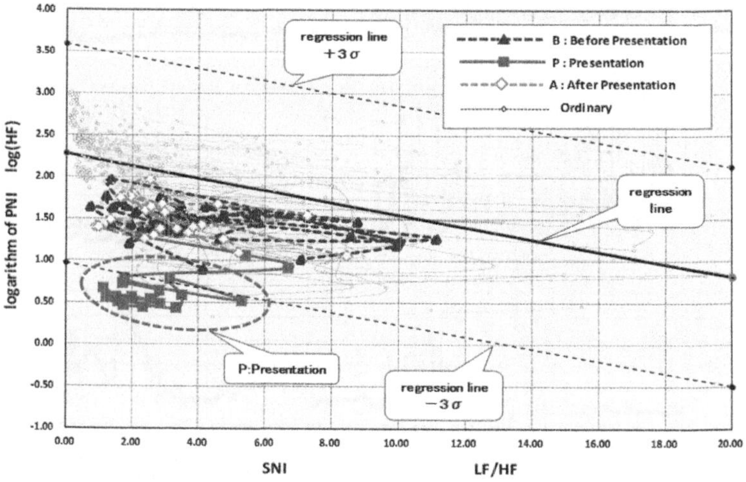

Fig. 3. A newly proposed representation method for the autonomic nerve activity index ANAIM®

Comparing subjects "ordinary living time period" and "special time period", plots during presentations within the special time period are continuously outside the 99.7% confidence interval of "ordinary living time period". In other words, it can be understood that the autonomic nerve activity during this period was clearly different from "ordinary".

Subject's heart rate reached 150 bpm during the presentation. Based on just heart rate, it seems the subject appeared to be very excited. However, Fig. 3 further shows that both the sympathetic and parasympathetic nerve activity of the subject decreased, deviating from the ordinary state. It expresses that the subject is in a very nervous state.

By expressing the autonomic nerve activity index in orthogonal coordinates in this way, it becomes possible to read mental factors that cannot be understood from just only heart rate. This expressing method is named ANAIM® (Autonomic Nervous Activity Index Mapping).

4.2 Example of ANAIM® During Music Performance

Figure 4 is the ANAIM® representation of the data obtained by the author (myself) as a subject. This is the result obtained from the ECG data acquired over about 40 h, and the sleep, desk work (ordinary work), and music playing time are selected and plotted. It is a plot of the autonomic nerve activity index obtained from the data for the past 3 min every 1 min during sleep and during desk work, however, during music performance, it is plotted every 10 s. The regression line and $\pm 3\sigma$ are calculated with the desk work as "ordinary".

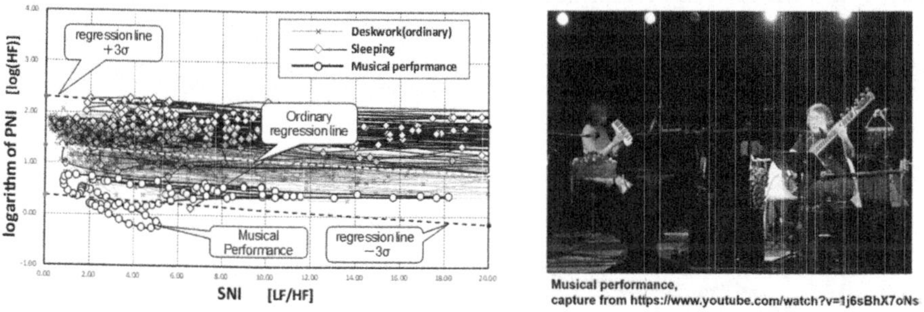

Fig. 4. Example of ANAIM® desk working, sleeping, and musical performance

Compared to the example in Fig. 3, the area of activity of the parasympathetic nerve is generally low, which is presumed to be an effect of age (64 years old at the time.). In my sleeping period, the plots have wide distribution, that may mean my sleeping quality is low.

Figure 5 is an enlargement during music performance in Fig. 4. And lower graph is the distance from the regression line to each ANAIM® plot (they are normalized by dividing by the standard deviation σ) on the vertical axis and time on the horizontal axis. Here, the author mainly plays strings instruments (Indian sitar and mandolin) and recorder, and my partner play several keyboard instruments. Each player switched between multiple instruments while playing 15 min of original music, including an improvisational performance section was played. A short movie of this musical performance has been on YouTube [5]. By synchronizing the time recorded in the movie with the time recorded in the heart rate sensor, it is possible to know what kind of autonomic nerve state was in which scene of the musical performance (there is an error of about ± 10 s).

An inflection point can be seen near the transition of the song or the transition of the instruments. This may reflect the mood at the time of playing music.

The improvisational performance section is a style in which the improvisational solo and accompaniment are exchanged for a predetermined number of bars while switching instruments. The order of chord progressions and instrument changes is pre-determined. At the point of "deviate from plan" in Fig. 5, the keyboard player was supposed to change the solo part to me. However, the keyboard player made a mistake and continued with her solo, so I was continuing to play with confused and uneasy. At that time, my parasympathetic nerve activity decreased quickly. after about one minutes, at "back to plan" point, when the keyboard player realized that her mistake, we made eye contact,

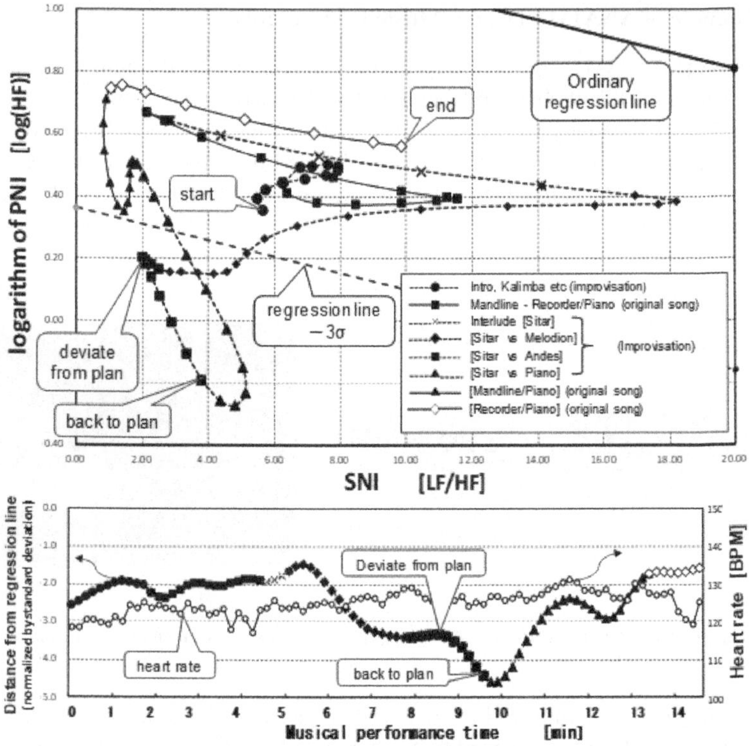

Fig. 5. Example of ANAIM®, enlargement during musical performance

and change solo part to me as planned. After that, my parasympathetic nerve activity was increasing, and returned to my ordinary state area. During this period, there was no significant change in heart rate.

This result shows the possibility that ANAIM® representation can visualize psychological movements of relatively short period.

4.3 Summary of ANAIM®

In this way, by applying ANAIM®, it has been shown that it is possible to express psychological and physiological states that cannot be read from changes in heart rate through autonomic nervous activity indices during various activities, based on electrocardiogram data obtained from a clothing-type wearable device.

Due to space constraints, it is not possible to show all experimental results, but the data that has been obtained in various situations so far can be summarized as shown in Fig. 6.

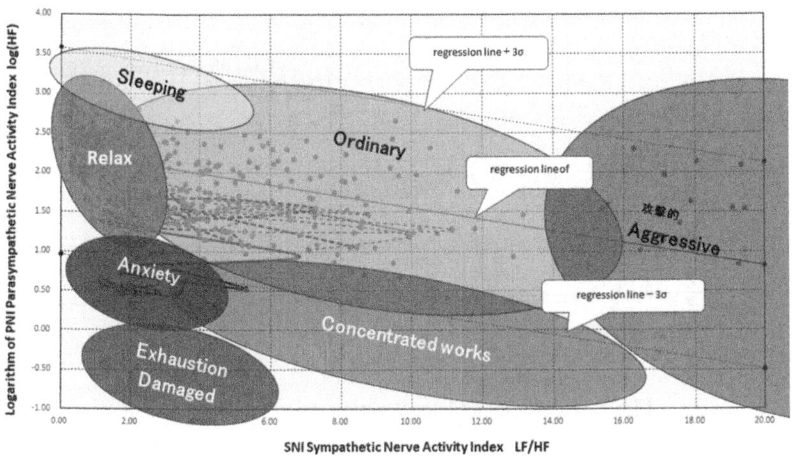

Fig. 6. Mental and physical states indicated by each area in the ANAIM® representation

5 Autonomic Nervous System Activity During Driving

5.1 Driver State Monitoring Technology

Research on driver state monitoring technology began in the 1980s. Since much of this work was carried out by automobile manufacturers, the technology was primarily developed for in-vehicle applications. In vehicles where only one driver is present at a time, such as private cars, high detection accuracy can be achieved through adaptive learning functions, and such systems are now becoming standard equipment in modern vehicles. However, from the driver's perspective, there are situations where one may need to operate multiple vehicles depending on time and circumstances. Therefore, it is desirable for drivers to have a monitoring system that can be used independently of the vehicle. In this context, personal driving state monitors using wearable devices have attracted growing attention [6].

5.2 Driver Physical Load During a Formula 3 Race

This section provides how ANAIM® can display a driver's physical and mental state during driving, highlighting its potential as a tool for monitoring driver condition. Data collection was made possible through the full cooperation of Ms. Ai Miura, representer and racing director of the AIWIN racing team, who both trains the next generation of drivers and competes as one of Japan's leading female racers.

Figure 7 presents the progression of Ms. Ai Miura's heart rate and acceleration during a Formula 3 race as an example of the physical load experienced by a driver in actual racing conditions. Figure 8 shows the racing car she drove during the event.

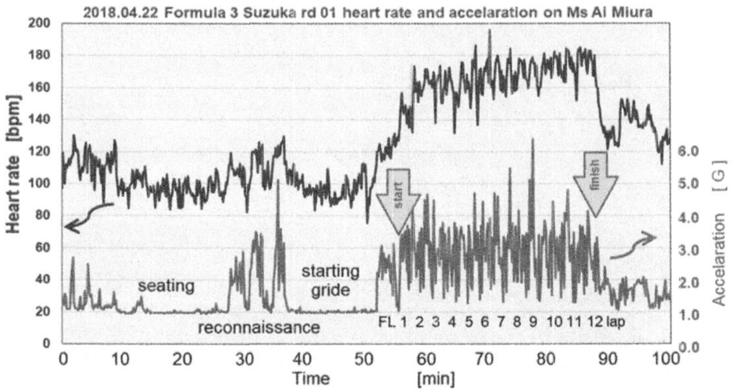

Fig. 7. Heart rate and acceleration during a Formula 3 race

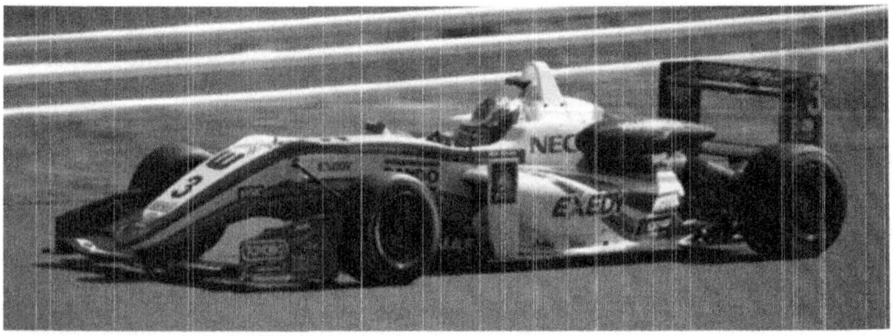

Fig. 8. Formula 3 Racing Car

5.3 ANAIM® from Specialized Tasks in the Lab, Ordinary, and F3 Races

Figure 9 shows an example of an ANAIM® display of data measured in the lab by Ai Miura during specific tasks, daily life, and the aforementioned F3 race. The downward-sloping straight line in the ANAIM® display is the regression line for autonomic nervous activity during daily activities, and the upper and lower dashed lines are the regression line $\pm 3\sigma$. Note that data from the time spent at home is considered "Ordinary."

Among the specific tasks, S: supine rest (10 min) and C: simple arithmetic problems (10 min) are plotted in the relaxation region in the upper left of the graph. In contrast, the task of sprinting on a treadmill for 10 min (R: all-out sprint) represents a level of exertion so intense that the subject "felt nauseous and nearly collapsed," with the heart rate rising to approximately 180 bpm. Autonomic nervous activity during this period is clearly plotted in the lower left region, far outside the ordinary activity range. This indicates that both sympathetic and parasympathetic activities were reduced, suggesting a state of autonomic nervous system imbalance.

"F3" data were collected during an actual Formula 3 race at Suzuka Circuit (Round 1 of the All-Japan F3 Championship, April 22, 2018 [7, 8]). During the race, the maximum speed exceeded 250 km/h, and the driver was subjected to accelerations of over 4G, resulting in a strenuous environment with a heart rate of approximately 180 bpm. In other words, based on heart rate, the physical load during the race was comparable to that of an all-out sprint. However, the autonomic nervous system activity showed a clearly different pattern. Although it was below the normal activity range, the distribution extended from the center to the right, indicating heightened sympathetic nervous activity.

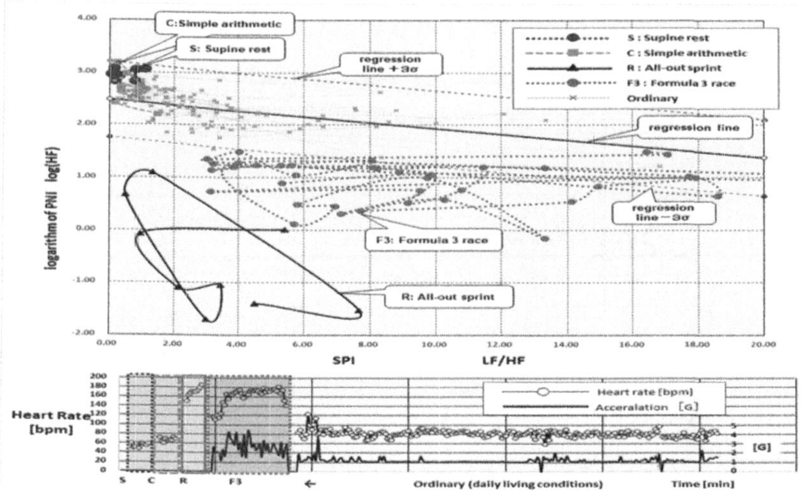

Fig. 9. ANAIM® Ms. Ai Miura (1) Lab, Formula 3, Ordinary

5.4 Racing Simulator

Figure 10 shows Ai Miura training in a racing simulator. The steering and pedal controls are identical to those of an actual racing car, and the weight of the steering wheel is faithfully reproduced. However, because the vehicle remains stationary, the driver does not experience the G-forces present in real races.

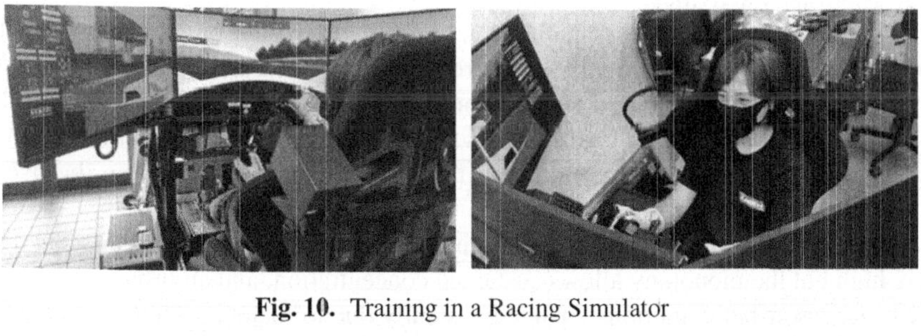

Fig. 10. Training in a Racing Simulator

Figure 11 presents data from simulator training, superimposed with data from specific laboratory tasks and a Formula 3 race. Her heart rate was approximately 120 bpm, which is significantly lower than during an actual race. This reflects the absence of major physical strain.

Nevertheless, her autonomic nervous system activity differed markedly from that of ordinary, shifting into a range similar to that observed during a Formula 3 race. This suggests that simulator training effectively reproduces the psychological and mental demands of actual racing.

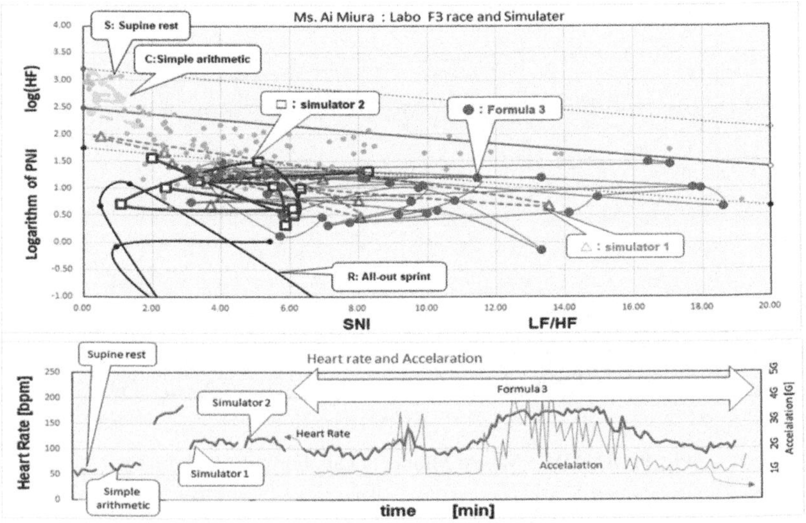

Fig. 11. ANAIM®: Ms Ai Miura (2) Racing Simulator

5.5 Express Way vs. Public Road

Figure 12 presents data from Ai Miura driving on an urban road, an express way, and a racing circuit. Both express way and urban road driving generally fall within the same range as ordinary activities.

On an express way, parasympathetic activity is lower than on an urban road, but sympathetic activity is also slightly lower, resulting in a concentrated distribution. This may represent a state of focused attention on driving.

On an urban road, parasympathetic activity is higher, indicating relaxation, but sympathetic activity is also more pronounced than on an express way, giving the overall impression of distraction.

This highlights the difference between an express way, where speeds are relatively high but the monotony allows sustained concentration, and an urban road, where speeds are lower but conditions change constantly due to factors such as traffic lights, pedestrians, and oncoming vehicles, requiring drivers to respond continuously.

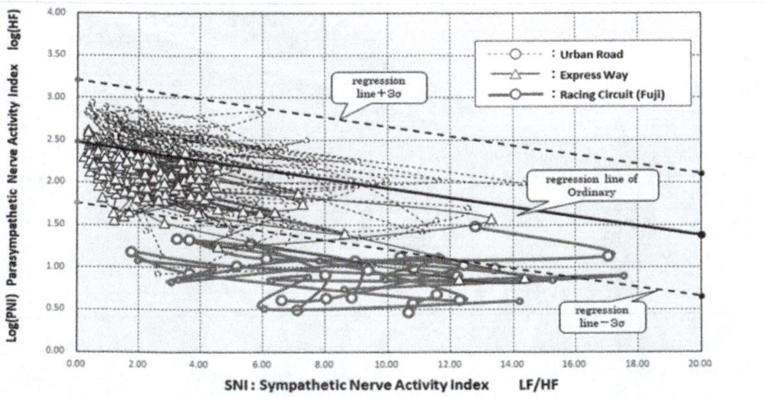

Fig. 12. ANAIM®: Ms. Ai Miura (3) on urban roads, express way, and racing circuits

5.6 Circuit Race by Racing car "VITA" (1)

Next, we present some notable data obtained from actual races performed by Ms. Ai Miura. All of these were sprint races held at Fuji Speedway in the fall of 2022. The vehicles used were open-top race vehicles, specifically designed for racing, called "VITA" [9], equipped with a 1500 cc production engine. All participants used the same specifications. Figure 13 shows a photograph of the VITA vehicle driven by Ms. Ai Miura.

Figure 14 shows data from Ai Miura's race in the final of the second round of the KYOJO CUP [10, 11] held on October 23, 2022. The autonomic nervous activity index calculated from the past three minutes of data is plotted every 10 s. Please note that the horizontal axis is three times larger than in previous examples. The graph below plots the y-axis distance from the regression line versus time trends in acceleration and heart rate.

Ms. Ai Miura placed second in the qualifying time trial held that morning and finished sixth in the final. In the final, cars lined up on the grid according to their qualifying positions. Before the start, a formation lap (FL) was conducted, during which the cars maintained the same order and completed one lap. After all cars returned to the starting grid, the countdown and race began.

In this race, the eventual winner quickly pulled away, while the second group—including Ms. Ai Miura—engaged in an intense battle for second place, with positions changing almost every lap. A peak in sympathetic nervous activity was observed between laps five and six, with data points exceeding the regression line +3σ. During this period, Her racing car made contact with another vehicle in a corner, leading to a fierce contest that caused a large crack in the FRP body cowling.

To date, this is the only instance in the author's testing where data exceeded the regression line +3σ threshold. This response is presumed to reflect an exceptionally aggressive psychological state. However, no notable changes in heart rate were observed.

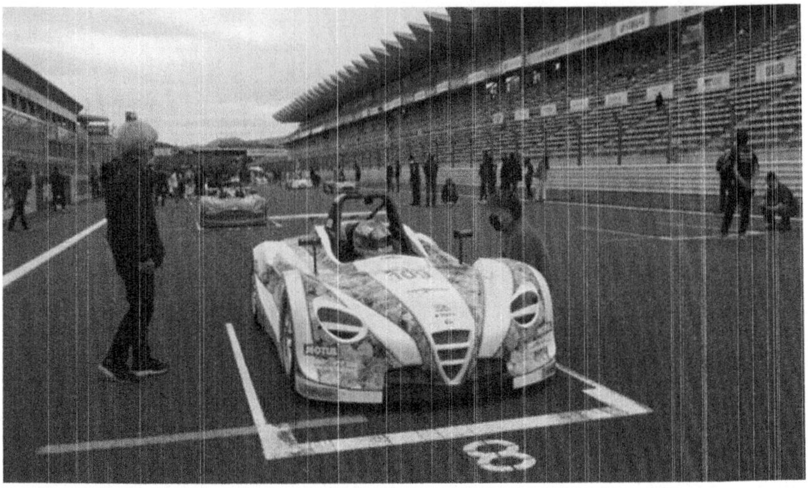

Fig. 13. Racing Car "VITA" at Fuji Speed Way

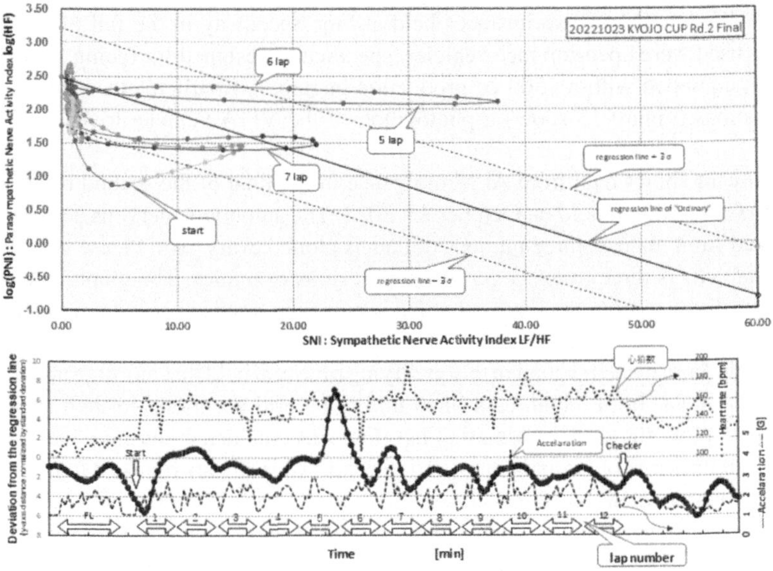

Fig. 14. ANAIM®: Ms Ai Miura (4) 2022 KYOJO CUP Rd.2 Final

5.7 Circuit Race by Racing Car "VITA" (2)

Figure 15 shows data for Ms. Ai Miura in the final of the third round of the Kyojo Cup, held on November 13, 2022 [12, 13]. Ai Miura qualified second out of 19 cars. In the final, she was overtaken by the third-place grid car at the first corner of the first lap and dropped to third place. However, she re-overtook the car on the third lap and regained second place. After that, the gap between the first and second-placed cars and the second and third-placed cars widened, and the order remained unchanged until the finish. The sympathetic nervous activity on the third lap is presumably a reflection of an extremely aggressive psychological state. Furthermore, no significant changes were observed in heart rate in this example.

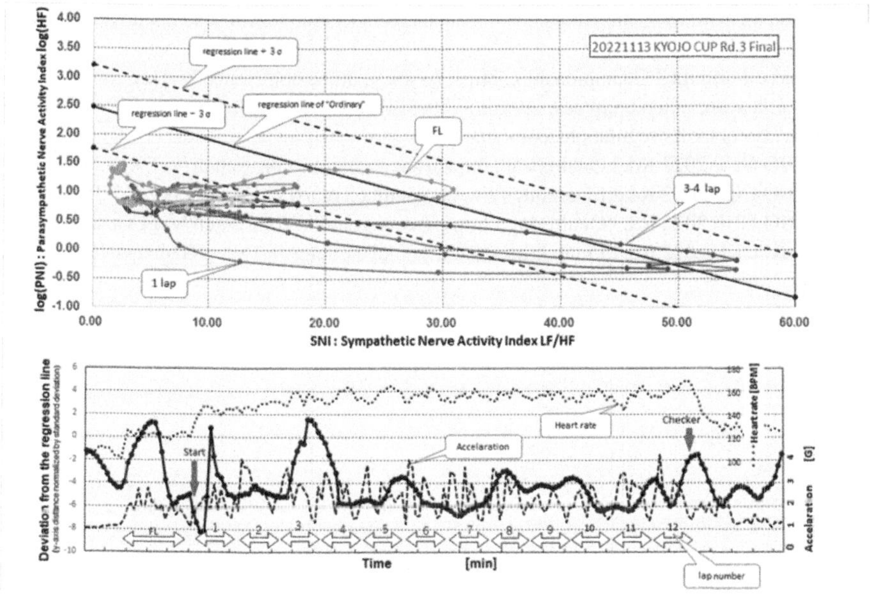

Fig. 15. ANAIM®: Ms. Ai Miura (5) 2022 KYOJO CUP Rd.3 Final

6 Summary

This method utilizes a known method for analyzing heart rate variability in the medical field, simply modifying the display method. However, with this simple modification, physiological and psychological states can be displayed in a way that is intuitively understandable to the general public, without using complex medical terminology. With the development of wearable devices, it will likely become possible to collect an even wider variety of vital data in the future, but in order to develop wearable devices as products for the consumer market (rather than just the medical field), it seems that this kind of accumulation of ingenuity will be essential.

Finally, we would like to thank racing team members of "AIWIN", who cooperated in the development of this method, as well as the many subjects.

References

1. Akselrod, S., et al.: Power spectrum analysis of heart rate fluction: a quantitative probe of beat-to-beat cardiovascular control. Science., New Series. **213**(4504), 220–222 (1981)

2. Maeda, S.: Autonomic nerve activity index representation method based on heartbeat information obtained from wearable devices. In: Proceedings of TBIS (2023)
3. Maeda, S.: Vital data measurement using clothing-type wearable devices and its applications. In: Digital Health in the 5G era and its Commercialization. Gijutsu Johō Kyōkai (2022)
4. https://www.uniontool.co.jp/assets/pdf/catalog/index_02_catalog_rri_analyzer_03.pdf
5. https://www.youtube.com/watch?v=1j6sBhX7oNs
6. Maeda, S.: Towards establishing health management techniques for solar car drivers. J. JSES. **51**(3) (2025)
7. Japanese Formula 3 Championship.: https://www.youtube.com/watch?v=DnGcu5Rrbjo
8. https://carview.yahoo.co.jp/news/detail/8736c5f5548ed4aef1eae3bcd87eb952f18305b6/
9. https://motorsports-regulations.com/vita
10. KYOJO CUP 2022 Rd.2 Qualifying.: https://www.youtube.com/watch?v=LXK-2q2Mi4I
11. KYOJO CUP 2022 Rd.2 Final: https://www.youtube.com/watch?v=LHSaVXl5vIU
12. KYOJO CUP 2022 Rd.3 Qualifying.: https://www.youtube.com/watch?v=gCQc4Zg2LPM
13. KYOJO CUP 2022 Rd.3 Final: https://www.youtube.com/watc1h?v=RT9hxqGrJq8

Molecular Communication and Bio-Inspired Networking Models

Extending a Parallel Boundary-Based CPM Algorithm Using a GPU-Accelerated Reaction-Diffusion Solver for Molecular Communication Simulations

Jiewen Wang(✉) and Tadashi Nakano

Graduate School of Informatics, Osaka Metropolitan University, Osaka, Japan
sh22295c@st.omu.ac.jp, tnakano@omu.ac.jp

Abstract. Molecular communication (MC) is an emerging paradigm in which bio-nanomachines exchange information via the diffusion of signaling molecules. To simulate MC systems, the Cellular Potts Model (CPM) provides a flexible framework that captures the morphological dynamics and spatial interactions of bio-nanomachines. In this paper, we extend the boundary-based (BL) algorithm of the CPM with a CPU–GPU hybrid framework to efficiently support MC simulations. Specifically, we incorporate a GPU–based reaction-diffusion partial differential equation (PDE) solver to model the propagation and degradation of signaling molecules emitted by transmitter bio-nanomachines. In the example simulations, receiver bio-nanomachines exhibit chemotactic migration toward the transmitter region, demonstrating that the proposed framework can simulate molecular communication in a drug delivery system (DDS) scenario. In addition, we show that the proposed framework reduces computational runtime compared with a CPU-based implementation.

Keywords: Molecular communication · Cellular Potts Model · GPU computing · molecular diffusion

1 Introduction

Molecular communication (MC) is an emerging paradigm in which bio-nanomachines, including both natural biological cells and artificially synthesized cells, exchange information through the emission, propagation, and reception of signaling molecules [1–3]. MC provides a basis for modeling information transfer within the body, enabling applications such as biomolecular sensing, targeted drug delivery, and synthetic cellular coordination. MC also plays a fundamental role in biological processes including immune signaling, tissue repair, and tumor development.

H. Tanaka et al. (Eds.): BodyNets 2025, LNICST 714, pp. 289–297, 2026.
https://doi.org/10.1007/978-3-032-38657-1_23

To examine the spatiotemporal dynamics of MC systems, computational modeling is essential [4,5]. The Cellular Potts Model (CPM) [6–8], widely used in cell biology, simulates the morphological dynamics and spatial interactions of biological cells. The flexibility of the CPM makes it a suitable framework for understanding the spatiotemporal dynamics of MC systems.

In CPM, each cell is represented as a connected domain of lattice sites, and the system evolves through stochastic copy attempts governed by an energy function that accounts for cell volume, cell surface area, and cellcell adhesion. The conventional CPM algorithm often performs redundant computations by evaluating the energy difference for every copy attempt, including those within cell interiors that do not alter the system configuration. To accelerate CPM, previous work proposed the boundary-based (BL) algorithm that reduces redundant computations by restricting copy attempts to cellcell interface sites and performing localized energy evaluations [9]. This algorithm was efficiently parallelized on CPUs, achieving up to a 40-fold speedup compared to the conventional algorithm, and was later extended to a CPUGPU hybrid framework [10], in which energy calculations are offloaded to the GPU, yielding an additional threefold acceleration over the CPU-based version.

Building on the previously developed CPUGPU hybrid BL algorithm, we extend the BL algorithm to simulate molecular communication among bio-nanomachines. Molecular diffusion and reaction are essential processes that underpin cell-based MC, enabling cellcell signaling and coordinated multicellular behavior.In CPM, diffusion is typically modeled by reactiondiffusion partial differential equations (PDEs), which simulate spatial concentration fields that influence cellular behavior and interactions. Existing platforms such as CompuCell3D integrate multiple GPU-accelerated PDE solvers directly within the CPM framework, efficiently supporting biochemical simulations [11]. In a similar manner, our extension incorporates a GPU-based reactiondiffusion PDE solver and chemotactic behaviors into the CPUGPU hybrid BL algorithm. This integration enables CPM to simulate both cellular morphology and molecular signaling in a unified manner while maintaining high computational efficiency through GPU acceleration.

The remainder of the paper is organized as follows. Section 2 describes the BL algorithm and its extension to a CPUGPU hybrid framework, including the integration of a GPU-accelerated reactiondiffusion PDE solver and the modeling of chemotactic behaviors. Section 3 presents simulation results for a drug delivery system (DDS) scenario, in which receiver bio-nanomachines migrate chemotactically toward the transmitter region. It also demonstrates that the proposed framework significantly reduces computational runtime compared with the CPU-based implementation. Finally, Sect. 4 concludes the paper with a summary of key findings and future research directions.

2 Boundary-Based CPM with GPU-Accelerated Reaction-Diffusion

In this section, we describe the main components of the proposed framework. We begin with the energy function in CPM. We then explain the BL algorithm, which restricts copy attempts to cellcell interfaces to improve computational efficiency. Next, we describe its extension to a CPUGPU hybrid framework for parallel energy evaluation. Finally, we introduce a GPUbased reactiondiffusion PDE solver and the implementation of chemotactic behaviors to simulate biological cell-based molecular communication.

2.1 Energy Function

In CPM, cell configurations evolve according to an energy function that encodes biophysical constraints. The energy E of the system is defined as:

$$E = E_{\text{area}} + E_{\text{peri}} + E_{\text{adh}}, \tag{1}$$

where E_{area} is the area energy, E_{peri} is the perimeter energy, and E_{adh} is the adhesion energy. Each energy term is defined as follows.

The area energy is defined as

$$E_{\text{area}} = \sum_{\sigma} \lambda_{\text{area}} \left(A_{\sigma} - A_{\sigma}^{\text{target}}\right)^2, \tag{2}$$

where A_{σ} is the area of cell σ, $A_{\sigma}^{\text{target}}$ is its target area, and λ_{area} is the area elasticity coefficient.

The perimeter energy is defined as

$$E_{\text{peri}} = \sum_{\sigma} \lambda_{\text{peri}} \left(P_{\sigma} - P_{\sigma}^{\text{target}}\right)^2, \tag{3}$$

where P_{σ} is the perimeter of cell σ, $P_{\sigma}^{\text{target}}$ is its target perimeter, and λ_{peri} is the perimeter elasticity coefficient.

The adhesion energy is defined as

$$E_{\text{adh}} = \sum_{\langle i,j \rangle} J(\sigma_i, \sigma_j)\left(1 - \delta_{\sigma_i,\sigma_j}\right), \tag{4}$$

where the sum runs over all neighboring site pairs $\langle i, j \rangle$, σ_i denotes the cell ID at site i, $J(\sigma_i, \sigma_j)$ represents the interfacial adhesion energy between cells, and δ is the Kronecker delta.

2.2 Boundary-Based Algorithm

In the conventional CPM, each cell is represented as a set of connected lattice sites sharing the same index. The system evolves through a series of Monte Carlo steps (MCS), each MCS consisting of N copy attempts where N corresponds to the total number of lattice sites. In each copy attempt, a source site i with index σ_i is randomly selected, and one of its neighboring sites j, with index σ_j, is designated as the target. Then the target site's index is proposed to be overwritten with σ_i of the source, and the proposed change is accepted or rejected based on the Metropolis criterion, which depends on the energy difference ΔE between the system states before and after the copy attempt.

As an optimization of the conventional CPM, the BL algorithm improves computational efficiency by limiting copy attempts to boundary sites [9]. A boundary site is defined as a lattice site whose neighboring index differs from its own. To support this approach, we maintain a dynamically updated boundary list during the simulation. This list records the positions of boundary sites along with relevant information such as the cell-cell adhesion and the surface area of the corresponding cell, enabling localized energy calculations restricted to regions affected by each copy attempt.

Each copy attempt then proceeds as follows:

1. Randomly select a boundary site i from the boundary list.
2. Randomly select a neighboring site j of site i. If site j has the same cell index as site i ($\sigma_i = \sigma_j$), skip the remaining steps, as the copy would result in no change.
3. Compute the energy difference ΔE resulting from the copy attempt $\sigma_j \leftarrow \sigma_i$, i.e., assigning the index σ_i of site i to site j.
4. Accept the copy attempt with probability

$$P(\Delta E) = \begin{cases} 1, & \Delta E \leq 0, \\ e^{-\Delta E/T}, & \Delta E > 0, \end{cases}$$

   where T is a dimensionless parameter called temperature controlling the stochasticity of cell membrane fluctuations.

As mentioned above, in conventional CPM, one MCS is defined as N copy attempts. However, since the BL algorithm restricts copy attempts to boundary sites only, we redefine one MCS as the number of copy attempts equal to the total number of boundary sites.

2.3 CPU-GPU Hybrid Framework of the BL Algorithm

To further accelerate CPM based on the BL algorithm, we extend our framework with parallel processing on both CPU and GPU. The execution flow of the BL algorithm is split between CPU-side preprocessing and GPU-side evaluation:

- **CPU (parallel and serial):**
  - **Parallel:** Randomly select boundary site-neighbor site pairs and check the validity of copy attempts in parallel. These checks ensure that the two sites belong to different cells ($\sigma_i \neq \sigma_j$) and that the copy attempt does not disconnect the target cell.
  - **Serial:** For each validated candidate pair, transfer the pair along with the relevant cell and lattice information required for local energy computation to the GPU. After receiving results from the GPU, update the

lattice, maintain the boundary list, and update associated cell properties accordingly.

- **GPU (parallel):**
  - Compute the energy difference (ΔE) and perform Metropolis acceptance or rejection for each validated candidate pair in parallel, executing all evaluations concurrently within a single kernel launch.

The CPU-GPU hybrid framework exploits the complementary strengths of different processors in modern computing platforms by parallelizing different steps of the BL algorithm according to their computational characteristics. The CPU handles candidate pair selection and connectivity checks, while the GPU performs massively parallel energy computations and stochastic acceptance decisions.

2.4 GPU-Based Reaction-Diffusion PDE Solver

We incorporate a GPU-based reaction-diffusion PDE solver into our CPU-GPU hybrid framework of the BL algorithm to simulate MC among bio-nanomachines. The concentration field of signaling molecules is modeled by the linear reaction–diffusion PDE:

$$\frac{\partial C}{\partial t} = D\nabla^2 C - \lambda C + S, \tag{5}$$

where C denotes the molecular concentration, D is the diffusion coefficient, λ is a degradation rate constant, and S is a spatially varying source term representing the localized emission of signaling molecules by transmitter bio-nanomachines. This PDE is discretized using the finite difference method and solved on the GPU to leverage parallel computation for high efficiency. As molecular diffusion operates on a faster timescale than bio-nanomachine movement, the PDE solver is executed multiple times per MCS to maintain numerical stability and accurately couple the diffusion field with bio-nanomachine dynamics.

In MC systems, some bio-nanomachines are designated as transmitters that emit signaling molecules, while others act as receivers that detect these molecules and migrate toward the transmitters by following the resulting concentration gradients. This biologically inspired movement, known as *chemotaxis*, is modeled by adding a chemotactic term to the energy function for each copy attempt involving a source site x_i and a target site x_j. The chemotactic energy contribution is defined as

$$E_{\text{chem}} = -\mu\left(C(x_j) - C(x_i)\right),$$

where μ is the chemotactic coefficient and $C(x)$ denotes the local concentration of signaling molecules at lattice site x. A positive ΔE_{chem} favors copy attempts that move cells toward regions of higher concentration, and this contribution is directly incorporated into the energy difference used in the Metropolis acceptance criterion.

Both the PDE solver and chemotactic energy computations run on the GPU as distinct kernels, while the CPU manages data transfer and kernel execution, minimizing CPU-GPU communication overhead and maximizing simulation efficiency. Integrating chemotactic energy terms with the GPU-based PDE solver enables accurate modeling of bio-nanomachine migration guided by molecular concentration gradients while ensuring computational efficiency.

3 Performance Evaluation

This section presents simulation results that evaluate both the functional behavior and computational performance of the boundary-based CPM algorithm with the integrated GPU-accelerated reaction-diffusion solver. We first examine whether the model simulate chemotactic aggregation behavior in response to spatial molecular gradients. Then, we compare the execution times of GPU-based and CPU-based implementations of the reaction-diffusion solver to evaluate computational efficiency.

3.1 Implementation

We implement the boundary-based CPM algorithm with the GPU-accelerated reaction–diffusion solver presented in Sect. 2 in Java SE 1.8.0_441 (Eclipse IDE), with GPU kernels dispatched via the Aparapi library [12]. All tests described in this section are run on a 16-inch MacBook Pro equipped with an Apple M4 Pro chip (14-core CPU, 20-core GPU) and 48 GB of unified memory. All simulations are conducted on a 500×500 lattice with 500 bio-nanomachines initialized as 2×2 lattice sites, placed uniformly at random.

In the simulations, we compute the concentration field of signaling molecules by numerically solving the linear reaction-diffusion PDE given in Sect. 2.4. We discretize the equation using the explicit Euler method with spatial and temporal resolutions $\Delta x = 1$ and $\Delta t = 1$. Let $C^n_{i,j}$ denote the concentration of signaling molecules at lattice site (i, j) and time step n. The update rule is then given by

$$C^{n+1}_{i,j} = C^n_{i,j} + \Delta t \left[D \left(\frac{C^n_{i+1,j} + C^n_{i-1,j} + C^n_{i,j+1} + C^n_{i,j-1} - 4C^n_{i,j}}{\Delta x^2} \right) - \lambda C^n_{i,j} + S_{i,j} \right], \quad (6)$$

where $S_{i,j}$ is the discrete source term representing the local production of signaling molecules at lattice site (i, j).

In our implementation, a bio-nanomachine is designated as a transmitter if its center of mass lies within a circular region of radius 20 lattice units centered on the lattice. Each transmitter emits signaling molecules at a constant rate of 5 units per time step. Accordingly, the source term is defined as:

$$S_{i,j} = \begin{cases} 5, & \text{if } (i, j) \text{ contains the center of mass of a transmitter bio-nanomachine,} \\ 0, & \text{otherwise.} \end{cases}$$

The emitted molecules undergo diffusion and degradation, with the diffusion coefficient and degradation rate constant set to $D = 20$ and $\lambda = 0.0002$, respectively. As molecular diffusion operates on a faster timescale than bio-nanomachine movement, the PDE solver is executed five times within each Monte

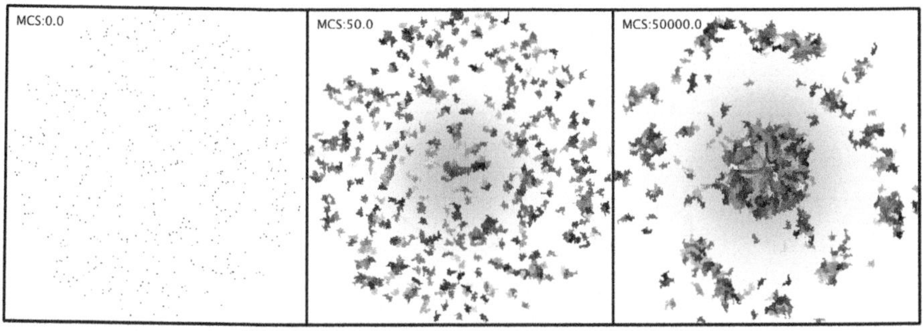

Fig. 1. Spatial distributions of bio-nanomachines and signaling molecules at 0, 50, and 50,000 MCS in the drug delivery system (DDS) scenario. Each bio-nanomachine is shown as a colored cluster of lattice sites, and the shading indicates the concentration of signaling molecules (darker green = higher concentration). Receiver bio-nanomachines migrate toward the tumor at the center via chemotaxis and form a localized cluster over time.

Carlo step (MCS) of the CPM. That is, one MCS corresponds to five diffusion time steps.

In the energy function, we use $\lambda_{\text{area}} = 1$ and $\lambda_{\text{peri}} = 0.5$ to weight area and perimeter constraints. The target area for each cell is set to $A^{\text{target}} = 100$, and the target perimeter is set to $P^{\text{target}} = 70$. Adhesion coefficients are assigned as $J(\sigma_i, \sigma_j) = 1$ for cell–cell interfaces and $J(\sigma_i, 0) = 0$ for cell–medium interfaces. The chemotactic sensitivity is set to $\mu = 5$, and the CPM temperature parameter is fixed at $T = 10$ throughout the simulation.

3.2 Emergence of Chemotactic Aggregation

In this simulation, we model a drug delivery system (DDS) scenario in which a tumor is located at the center of the lattice. Initially, 500 bio-nanomachines are uniformly distributed within a circular region centered on the lattice. Those whose centers of mass fall within a radius of 20 lattice units from the tumor detect its presence, become transmitters, and begin emitting signaling molecules at a constant rate. The remaining bio-nanomachines act as receivers that respond to the resulting concentration gradient and migrate toward the tumor via chemotaxis.

The simulation runs for 50,000 MCS to observe the emergence of chemotactic behavior and the formation of a localized cluster around the tumor. Signaling molecules diffuse from the transmitter bio-nanomachines and establish a radial gradient across the lattice.

Figure 1 shows the spatial distributions of bio-nanomachines and signaling molecules at selected time points. As the simulation progresses, receiver bio-nanomachines gradually migrate toward the tumor along the gradient. By the end of the simulation, a dense cluster of receiver bio-nanomachines has formed around the tumor. If drug molecules were to be released from this cluster, drug

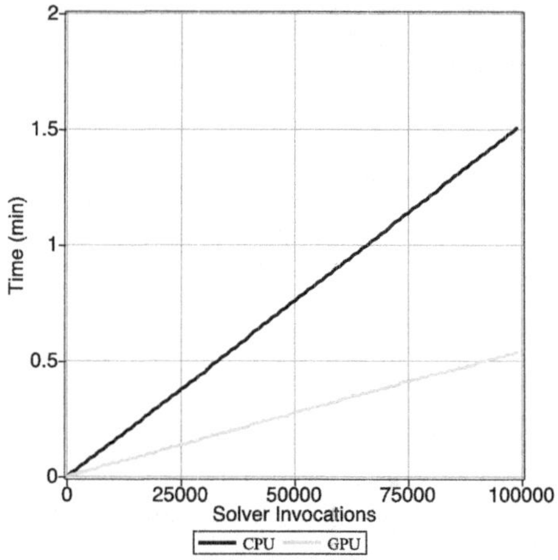

Fig. 2. Comparison of computation times between the CPU-based and GPU-based implementations of the reaction-diffusion PDE solver.

delivery would be spatially localized to the tumor site, demonstrating the potential of this collective behavior for targeted therapy applications.

3.3 Computational Efficiency

Next, we evaluate the computational efficiency of the proposed PDE solver by comparing the execution times of the GPU-based and CPU-based implementations under identical simulation conditions. To isolate the PDE solver's performance, we benchmark 100,000 consecutive PDE solver invocations during the simulation initialization phase, without any CPM updates or additional processing. Every experiment is repeated ten times to account for variability due to system load and hardware fluctuations.

Figure 2 shows experimental results. The CPU-based implementation took 1.51 min to complete 100,000 invocations, while the GPU-based implementation completed the same task in 0.54 min, which is approximately one-third of the CPU time. The computation time increases linearly with the number of invocations because each PDE solver invocation is performed independently, without inter-step dependencies.

4 Conclusion

In this paper, we extended the CPU–GPU hybrid framework of the BL algorithm to support molecular communication among bio-nanomachines by incorporating a GPU–based reaction-diffusion PDE solver and chemotactic behavior. The proposed GPU–based solver achieves approximately threefold speedup over a CPU–based implementation while maintaining consistent simulation results.

Future work will focus on further optimizing the solver, incorporating more complex biochemical reaction dynamics, and scaling the framework for larger and more heterogeneous bio-nanomachine systems.

Acknowledgment. This work was supported by JSPS KAKENHI Grant Numbers JP21H04876 and JP24KJ1910.

References

1. Bi, D., Almpanis, A., Noel, A., Deng, Y., Schober, R.: A survey of molecular communication in cell biology: Establishing a new hierarchy for interdisciplinary applications. IEEE Commun. Surv. Tutorials **23**(3), 1494–1545 (2021)
2. Farsad, N., Yilmaz, H.B., Eckford, A., Chae, C.-B., Guo, W.: A comprehensive survey of recent advancements in molecular communication. IEEE Commun. Surv. Tutorials **18**(3), 1887–1919 (2016)
3. Nakano, T., Eckford, A., Haraguchi, T.: Molecular Communication, second edn. Cambridge University Press (2024)
4. Noel, A., Cheung, K.C., Schober, R., Makrakis, D., Hafid, A.: Simulating with accord: Actor-based communication via reaction-diffusion. Nano Commun. Netw. **11**, 44–75 (2017)
5. Saiki, T., Imanaka, S., Kobayashi, S., Nakano, T.: A general-purpose simulation platform for multicellular molecular communication systems. IEEE Trans. Mol. Biol. Multi-Scale Commun. **11**(2), 152–165 (2025)
6. Glazier, J.A., Graner, F.: Simulation of the differential adhesion driven rearrangement of biological cells. Phys. Rev. E **47**, 2128–2154 (1993)
7. Graner, F., Glazier, J.: Simulation of biological cell sorting using a two-dimensional extended potts model. Phys. Rev. Lett. **69**, 2013–2016 (1992)
8. Hirashima, T., Rens, E.G., Merks, R.M.H.: Cellular potts modeling of complex multicellular behaviors in tissue morphogenesis. Dev. Growth Differentiation **59**(5), 329–339 (2017)
9. Wang, J., Nakano, T.: A parallel boundary-based algorithm for efficient cellular potts model simulation. In: Proceedings of the IEEE Global Communications Conference (GLOBECOM), IEEE (2025)
10. Wang, J., Nakano, T.: A CPU–GPU hybrid boundary based algorithm for accelerating cellular potts model simulations. In: Proceedings of the ACM International Conference on Nanoscale Computing and Communication (NanoCom), ACM (2025)
11. Swat, M.H. , Thomas, G.L., Belmonte, J.M., Shirinifard, A., Hmeljak, D., Glazier, J.A.: Chapter 13 - multi-scale modeling of tissues using compucell3d. In: Asthagiri, A.R., Arkin, A.P. (eds.) Computational Methods in Cell Biology, vol. 110 of Methods in Cell Biology, pp. 325–366, Academic Press (2012)
12. Aparapi Contributors: Aparapi: An api for expressing data parallel workloads in java (2024). https://github.com/Syncleus/aparapi. Accessed 27 June 2025

Model Based Error Rate Analysis of Electrical-to-Molecular Communication Interface via Redox Mechanisms

Karthik Reddy Gorla[1,2(✉)], Maurizio Magarini[1], and Massimiliano Pierobon[2]

[1] Department of Electronics, Information, and Bioengineering, Politecnico di Milano, Milan, Italy
{karthikreddy.gorla,maurizio.magarini}@polimi.it
[2] School of Computing, University of Nebraska-Lincoln, Lincoln, NE, USA
maxp@unl.edu

Abstract. Engineering bioelectrical interfaces to bridge electrical devices and biochemical elements (natural or synthetic) is a crucial step toward realizing the Internet of Bio-Nano Things (IoBNT) paradigm. In this paper, one such interface, which generalizes information transfer from the electrical domain to the molecular domain, is presented and analyzed. By leveraging molecular communication principles, the main electrochemical components of this interface are abstracted with reference to an experimental prototype that leverages redox mechanisms. In particular, every components capture the physical/chemical processes underlying the communication capabilities of this interface. Subsequently, a computational model based on the finite difference method is developed and implemented as a stochastic simulation in MATLAB. Through simulations, the communication performance of this interface are measured in terms of Bit Error Rate (BER) with respect to variations of design parameters such as initial concentration, input bit rate, and input length. The promising outcomes of this work will serve as a foundation for a thorough exploration of this novel kind of interfaces and their communication performance.

Keywords: Internet of Bio-Nano Things · Molecular Communication · Redox Electrochemistry · Non-return-to-zero · Bit Error Rate

1 Introduction

The Internet of Bio-Nano Things (IoBNT) is an emerging interdisciplinary field of nanotechnology, biotechnology, and communication engineering aimed at cre-

The current work is based upon work supported in part by the Italian Ministry of Foreign Affairs and International Cooperation, grant no. US23GR04 (CUP D43C23000350001).

H. Tanaka et al. (Eds.): BodyNets 2025, LNICST 714, pp. 298–310, 2026.
https://doi.org/10.1007/978-3-032-38657-1_24

ating nanoscale devices networks within biological environments [1]. These "bio-nano devices" are miniature sensors and actuators that can engage with biological systems on a molecular scale. Potential applications of IoBNT lie in healthcare through real-time monitoring and data acquisition, enabling sophisticated diagnostics, precise drug delivery, and personalized medical treatments. In addition, IoBNT has applications crucial for environmental monitoring, such as real-time identification of pollutants or pathogens with a high level of precision [2]. In order to understand the flow of information on the interaction with biological elements in such systems, Molecular Communication (MC) techniques are employed. MC is a branch of communication theory research that focuses on advancing tools to model, characterize, and control the communication performance of biological, chemical, and molecular-scale systems [3].

Recent advances in IoBNT have mainly been directed toward the development of advanced nanosensors [4,5] and the improvement of MC techniques [6,7]. This paper focuses on the latter through model analysis of a specific biochemical sensor. The biosensing component of the IoBNT paradigm can be achieved through various modalities such as optical, electrochemical, and piezoelectric, among others [8,9]. In our work, we utilize an electrochemical method called redox, which involves reduction and oxidation chemical reactions. The advantage of redox modality lies in its electrochemical nature of facilitating chemical reactions through the exchange of electrons, resulting in the generation of an electrical signal. Furthermore, the redox modality is a naturally occurring biochemical mechanism in the human body [10–12].

Previously, we developed a model of a redox-based interface that transmits information from the molecular domain to the electrical domain, conceptualized as a communication channel. Subsequently, we characterized the molecular-to-electrical (M2E) channel in terms of key performance metrics such as Signal-to-Noise Ratio (SNR), limit of detection, limit of quantification, mutual information, and the capacity [13,14]. In this paper, the objective is to renew our understanding of the redox-based interface, with information flowing in the reverse direction, forming an electrical-to-molecular (E2M) channel [15,16]. In [17], we presented an initial examination of the E2M channel, focusing on its SNR and eye diagram. The main contribution of this paper is to elaborate the E2M channel system model and to further analyze it in terms of Bit Error Rate (BER).

The rest of this paper is organized as follows. In Sect. 2, we describe the analytical system model of the redox-enabled E2M communication channel and detail each component. A computational model implementation of the E2M channel, which serves as the foundation for our simulation framework is presented in Sect. 3. In Sect. 4 we proceed to analyze the simulated results to estimate the BER of the channel across multiple scenarios, along with associated discussions. Finally, we conclude the paper in Sect. 5.

2 System Model of Redox-Based Molecular-Electrical Communication

This section outlines the key elements underlying the communication system evaluated for the E2M interface. The system facilitates the transfer of information from the electrical domain to the molecular domain through the diffusion of information-carrying redox-active species *i.e.*, substances that have the ability to lose (oxidize) or gain (reduce) electrons, and their redox reactions, *i.e.*, oxidation or reduction, with a transmitting electrode. In particular, as depicted in Fig. 1, we define a **Source** as an electrical element, *e.g.*, chip, processor, simple electrical circuit, which are mostly silico-based devices, producing an input information message; an **Electrical Transmitter**, where the voltage is applied at the electrode into the channel as modulated according to the input information message; **Redox Reactions**, where the redox-active molecules exchange electrons with the receiving electrode as function of the electrode voltage $V(t)$; a **Molecule Diffusion**, where molecules propagate by Brownian motion in the space between the transmitting electrode and the receiving surface; a **Molecular Receiver**, which receives the molecules of the redox-active species as they pass through the surface, forming the output information message that is then delivered to a **Destination** containing biological receptors and reaction networks. As mentioned earlier, this communication system is an abstraction of the main electrochemical components of the proof-of-concept experimental prototype presented in [18], and generalizes the idea of information transfer from the electrical domain to the molecular domain via redox mechanisms. In particular, this abstraction is intended to capture the underlying physical/chemical processes to understand the communication capabilities of a redox-enabled E2M communication channel, as experimented in [18]. The results of the research described in this section will be the basis for a simulation framework through which the communication performance of this channel will be characterized in

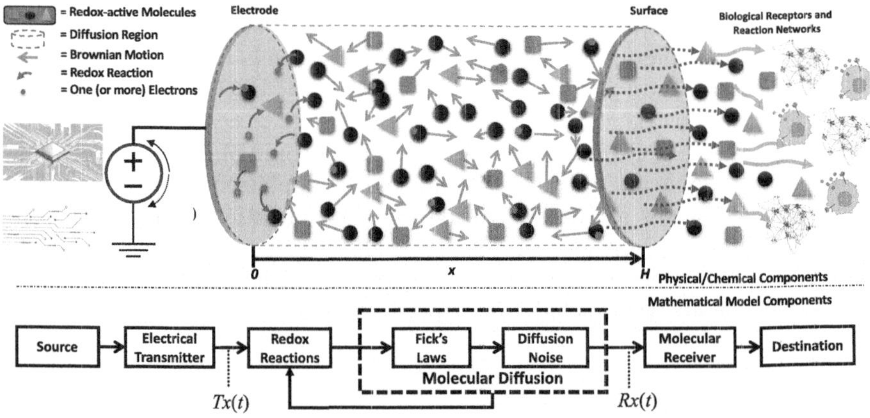

Fig. 1. Scheme of a redox-enabled E2M communication system.

terms of BER according to the mathematical models and simulation tools of the aforementioned abstraction.

2.1 System Model Components

Electrical Transmitter. It is the component of the system model that links to the electrical domain, which in our model is composed of a voltage generator connected to the electrode(s). The voltage generator functions based on the information (bitstream) received from the source in the electrical domain, as mathematically expressed in (1). This transmitted voltage is generally a pulse-shaped wave. Based on the voltage levels designated for each input symbol, the amplitude of the pulse modulates accordingly. As a result of the voltage applied, the redox-active species react at the electrode.

The input information from the source X_{in} as a n-symbol stream of length i can be expressed as:

$$X_{in}(t) = \sum_{i} s_i \delta(t - t_i), \tag{1}$$

where s_i represents the ith symbol, which when binary, simplifies to a value of '0' or '1' and t_i is the ith time sample.

The transmitted voltage signal, pulse amplitude modulated based on the input information from source is expressed as follows

$$Tx(t) = \sum_{i} v_i p(t - (i-1)\tau), \tag{2}$$

$$p(t) = \begin{cases} 1, & 0 \leq t \leq \tau \\ 0, & otherwise, \end{cases} \tag{3}$$

where $Tx(t)$ is a the rectangular pulse signal with amplitudes in the range $\{v_1, ..v_i, ..v_n\}$ based on the input symbol s from the input stream $X_{in}(t)$, $p(t)$ is a rectangular pulse shape signal which retains a value of 1 during the bit duration τ. The transmission signal's frequency depends on the input bitstream's frequency.

Redox Reactions. It refers to reduction-oxidation chemical reactions that involve the exchange of electrons, driven by the presence of a voltage in the environment. In our system model, these reactions are reversible and occur on the electrode surface. A typical reversible redox reaction can be expressed as follows [19]:

$$\mathrm{O} + \mathrm{ne} \underset{k_b}{\overset{k_f}{\rightleftharpoons}} \mathrm{R}, \tag{4}$$

where O is oxidized species, R is reduced species, e is an electron, n is number of electrons transferred, k_f is the forward reaction rate constant, and k_b is the reverse reaction rate constant. These reaction rate constants are related to voltage as follows [19]:

$$k_f(t) = k_0 e^{\frac{-\alpha nF}{RT}(V(t)-E_0)}, \tag{5}$$

$$k_b(t) = k_0 e^{\frac{(1-\alpha)nF}{RT}(V(t)-E_0)}, \tag{6}$$

where k_f is the forward reaction rate constant, k_b is the backward reaction rate constant, k_0 is the standard rate constant, α is the charge transfer coefficient, n is the number of electrons transferred per reaction, F is the Faraday constant, R is the Boltzmann constant, T is the absolute temperature, $V(t)$ is the voltage applied at time instant t at the electrode that corresponds to the input signal $Tx(t)$, and E_0 is the standard potential. The applied voltage signal $V(t)$ influences the forward and backward reaction rate constants (k_f and k_b), which in turn affect the redox reactions occurring at the electrode.

For a given specific redox-active species, the standard rate constant k_0, the charge transfer coefficient α ($0 < \alpha < 1$), the number of electrons transferred per reaction n, and the standard potential E_0 are constant. When $V(t) - E_0$ is positive, it leads to more oxidation reactions, whereas when $V(t)-E_0$ is negative, it leads to more reduction reactions.

In addition to the diffusion noise, there is also a reaction noise caused by the randomness of chemical reactions. Taking into account the current parameters, the scale of reaction noise is significantly lower by several orders of magnitude than that of diffusion noise, as similarly observed in the M2E communication channel [13,14]. Future investigations in various contexts will assess the impact and compare these two types of noise.

Molecule Diffusion. It is the region between the electrode and the surface that is occupied by a diffusive medium based on the design shown in Fig. 1, acting as a bridge between the electrical side at the electrode and the biological side at the surface. The size of this region is determined by the model design, and it can be filled with vacuum, air, liquid, hydrogel, or any other non-solid medium that supports diffusion. We use Fick's laws [20] to mathematically model diffusion.

At the electrode, the concentration gradient of the redox-active molecules is constantly changing as a result of the redox reactions that take place when a voltage is applied, which in turn influences diffusion. The molecular diffusion for the redox-enabled E2M communication channel in terms of an inhomogeneous Fick's equation [20] can be modeled as follows:

$$\begin{aligned}\frac{\partial C_{m,S}(\bar{x},t)}{\partial t} &= -\nabla\big(-D_{m,S}\nabla C_{m,S}(\bar{x},t)\\ &\pm J_O(\bar{x},t)\delta(\bar{x}-\bar{x}_e)\big),\ {}_{m=1,2,\ldots,M;S=O,R},\end{aligned} \tag{7}$$

where $C_{m,S}$ is the concentration of species m in a redox state S at time instant t in space $\bar{x}$, $D_{m,S}$ is the diffusion coefficient of species m in a redox state S, J_O is the flux of redox-active species in oxidised state at time instant t in space $\bar{x}$, and $\bar{x}_e$ are the Cartesian coordinates of a point on the electrode.

The diffusion in the model is affected at two boundaries, the surface and the electrode. In the scope of this paper, we assume the surface to be neither a sink nor a source, but to allow the free movement of redox-active molecules to interact with the biological elements in the biological domain in Fig. 1. The second boundary that is on the electrode, satisfies the Neumann boundary condition.

The stochastic motion of molecules caused by Brownian motion underlies the diffusion process [3,21], resulting in a random variation in molecular concentration. This introduces noise in a molecular communication channel, which can be accurately modeled by a Poisson process [22]. To analytically express the diffusion noise, we modeled it as a volume Poisson counting process, according to [22]. Consequently, the average number of molecules $N_{m,S}(t)$ is expressed as

$$N_{m,S}(t) = \nu N_A C_{m,S}(\bar{x}_e, t), \quad {}_{m=1,2,\ldots,M;S=O,R}, \tag{8}$$

where ν is an infinitesimal volume on the electrode, N_A is the Avogadro's number, $C_{m,S}(\bar{x}, t)$ is the concentration of molecules of species m in redox state S in space $\bar{x}$ at time instant t, and $\bar{x}_e$ are the Cartesian coordinates of a point on the electrode. We then express the effective redox-active molecule concentration $C'_{m,S}(\bar{x}_e, t)$ of species m in redox state S at location $\bar{x}_e$ on the electrode at time instant t as

$$C'_{m,S}(\bar{x}_e, t) \sim \frac{Poiss(N_{m,S}(t))}{\nu N_A}, \quad {}_{m=1,2,\ldots,M;S=O,R}, \tag{9}$$

where ν is an infinitesimal volume on the electrode at time instant t, and N_A is the Avogadro's number.

Molecular Receiver. It is abstracted here as a surface through which redox-active molecules are released from the redox-enabled E2M communication channel. As observed in Fig. 1, the right side of the surface is the biological domain, which contains natural or synthetic biological elements that interact with the redox-active molecules or participate in chemical reactions in the biological environment to produce signaling molecules such as green fluorescent protein (GFP) [15,23]. These signaling/redox-active molecules form the output signal as they pass through the surface *i.e.*, the molecular receiver.

The molecular receiver model is formulated as an ideal molecule receiver that measures the concentration of the chemical species passing through the surface, and it is expressed as follows:

$$\mathrm{Rx}(t) = \begin{bmatrix} \ldots\, C_{m,O}(\bar{x}_s, t)\, \ldots \\ \ldots\, C_{m,R}(\bar{x}_s, t)\, \ldots \end{bmatrix}, \quad {}_{m=1,2,\ldots,M}, \tag{10}$$

where $\mathrm{Rx}(t)$ is the molecular received signal in moles per volume, and $C_{m,S}(\bar{x}_s, t)$ is the concentration of redox-active molecules of species m in redox state S (oxidized O or reduced R) at time instant t and space $\bar{x}_s$, which are the Cartesian coordinates of a point on the **Surface**. M is the total number of redox-active molecular species considered in the system.

3 Model Implementation and Simulation Setup

3.1 Computational Model

A computational model for the redox-enabled communication channel has been implemented based on the analytical formulation of the model in Sect. 2.1, and in accordance with standard practice in electrochemistry simulation [19]. We built the computational model to provide a solution for the system model, as the concentration diffusion-reaction PDE (7) cannot be solved in closed-form. As a result, we opted to solve the model using computational methods, which in turn is formulated on the following assumptions:

1. Diffusion is one-dimensional and occurs along the axis perpendicular to the planar electrode surface. This reduces computational complexity while maintaining accuracy and is the approach typically used by electrochemists for modeling redox cells [19].
2. Without loss of generality, only one redox-active species is considered in the channel, *i.e.*, M = 1. This redox-based E2M model should allow different species to overlay their effects within the channel, provided that the selected redox species do not react with each other.
3. At the electrical transmitter, we assume the input information to be binary and modulate it using a binary pulse amplitude modulation, detailed in Sect. 3.2. This helps in a simpler design for a decoder at the molecular receiver. In the future, this can be extended to a multi-level pulse amplitude modulation.

The finite difference method is used to computationally solve partial differential equations that define the underlying electrochemical and diffusion processes and to obtain algebraic equations containing finite differences. Space and time are broken down into a finite number of steps to solve the algebraic equations and find the approximated solution at each discrete point. As diffusion is taken to be one-dimensional, the finite difference method assumes a 1D space, which compartmentalizes the model space into finite spaces of Δx (sampling space of the model). Assuming that J space blocks are between the surface and the electrode, and x_0 is the space block at the electrode location, the jth block is represented as $x_j = x_0 + j\Delta x$. Similarly, we sampled the time at an interval of Δt (sampling time of the model). With K time samples during a simulation starting at time t_0, the kth time sample can be calculated as $t_k = t_0 + k\Delta t$. Decreasing these sampling variables enhances the model's granularity; however, this comes with a rise in computational demand. To achieve a suitable compromise between accuracy and computational expense, it is essential to select optimal values for the sampling variables.

3.2 Simulation Setup

A simulation of the computational formulation of the redox-enabled channel model has been implemented in MATLAB. The simulation framework code used

Table 1. Chemical Parameters - Ferrocene

Parameter	Ferrocene
Oxidized Diffusion co-efficient (D_O)	3.79×10^{-6}cm^2/s
Reduced Diffusion co-efficient (D_R)	4.98×10^{-6}cm^2/s
Electrochemical rate constant (k_0)	1.75×10^{-2}cm/s
Charge transfer co-efficient (α)	0.55
Standard potential (E_0)	0.247V

*Initial state of Ferrocene is reduced.
*These parameters are specific for the gold-plated electrode surface.

to obtain the numerical results in this paper can be found in https://github.com/xneguvx7/RE-BIONICS-Code. For the simulation, the total time frame considered depends on the bit duration of each input bit and the length of the input bit stream. To ensure accuracy, we sample at every 0.1 sec (*i.e.* Δt). The spatial resolution of the computational model Δx was calculated using a constant model diffusion coefficient ($DM = 0.45$) [19], as

$$\Delta x = \sqrt{\frac{\text{Max}(D_O, D_R).\Delta t}{DM}}, \tag{11}$$

where Max(.) is a function that provides the maximum value among the input arguments, D_O is the diffusion coefficient of redox-active species in the oxidized state, D_R is the diffusion coefficient of redox-active species in the reduced state, Δt is the sampling time of the electrochemical setup, and DM is the model diffusion coefficient.

Table 2. Simulation Parameters

Parameter	Value
Sampling time (Δt)	0.1 s
Sampling space (Δx)	1.1 μm
Voltage high (v_1)	+0.5 V
Voltage low (v_0)	−0.3 V
Input length (L_{in})	$\{16, 32, 64, 128\}$ bits
Bit duration ($\tau = \frac{1}{rate}$) range	[1 – 1200] s
Electrode surface area (Ar)	0.0314 cm^2

*v_1 and v_0 taken from [18].

We ran simulations using the computational model developed in Sect. 3.1 with Ferrocene (1,1'-Ferrocenedimethanol) [24] a standard electrochemical species with distinctive redox properties. The value of three non-constant parameters, namely, the charge transfer coefficient α, the standard reaction rate constant k_0, and the redox-state-specific diffusion coefficients D_S were estimated from lab experiments performed for the M2E channel [14], while the others were obtained from the literature [19]. These values are reported in Table 1, and simulation-specific parameters are provided in Table 2.

The electrical input to the system is a pulse amplitude modulation of an incoming binary source as seen in Fig. 2. In particular, we use a bipolar PAM technique called non-return-to-zero (NRZ), where a bit '1' is represented by a high voltage and a bit '0' is represented by a non-zero lower voltage as tabulated in Table 2. Any given input signal has a length of L_{in} bits and each bit has a fixed duration of τ seconds.

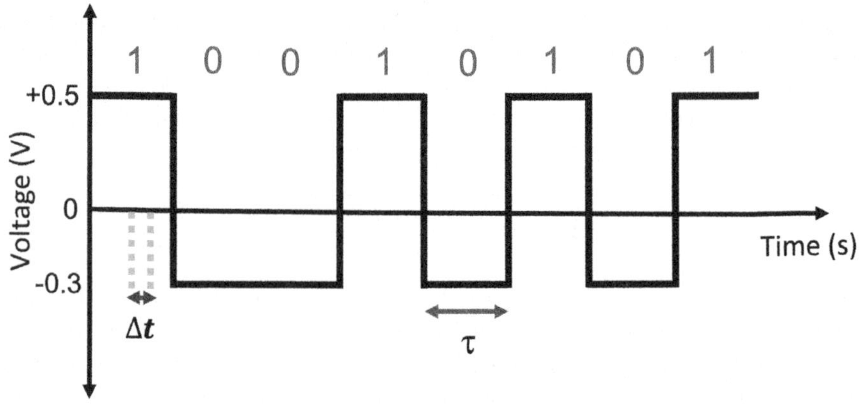

Fig. 2. An example of the input electrical signal

At the receiver end, the output concentration values are decoded through a straightforward binary classifier that utilizes a threshold. Any concentration exceeding the threshold is interpreted as bit '1', while a concentration below it signifies bit '0'.

4 Results

In this section, we characterize the redox-enabled E2M channel through its communication performance in terms of BER. Building upon [17], we furthered the analysis by simulating the model at concentrations that achieve an SNR of around 0dB to estimate the BER. Using the simulation model detailed in Sect. 3, we ran the simulations for initial concentrations in the range of [0.2 - 2]fM with increments of 0.2fM. In addition, the input bit rate and length were varied as tabulated in Table 2. These simulations use a randomized binary input and were executed 1000 times for each scenario.

As discussed in Sect. 3.2, accurately determining the threshold in the receiver's binary classifier is essential for preserving the integrity of the transmitted information signal. Initially, we set the threshold to the average of all measured concentrations for each input signal, but this approach did not produce satisfactory results. Considering that the system model has inherent memory, we transitioned to a sliding window averaging strategy. We explored various window sizes, initially fixed between 1 and 7 bits, and later as a fraction of the input length (L_{in}). Comparative analysis revealed that using a sliding window whose size is equal to half the input length resulted in improved classification accuracy. We label this approach the **half-window threshold** method, where the threshold for each point is set by averaging the prior concentrations received within the window. The corresponding algorithm with a detailed explanation is presented as:

Require: $C_{out} = [C_1, C_2, .., C_n]$ $\{n \leftarrow L_{in}\}$
  $window\_size \leftarrow n/2$
  $thresh \leftarrow mean(C_1 : C_{window\_size})$
  for $i = 1$ **to** n **do**
    if $i > window\_size$ **then**
      $thresh \leftarrow mean(C_{i-window\_size} : C_{window\_size-1})$
    end if
  end for

Figure 3 illustrates the BER values of the channel evaluated using the half-threshold method at various initial concentrations and a range of input bit rates with input lengths of 16, 32, 64, and 128 bits.

Analyzing all the figures, it is generally observed that the BER increases with higher input bit rates. In this diffusion-limited channel, at lower bit rates, the sufficient time available for the diffusion of redox-active molecules results in a significantly low BER. Conversely, at higher bit rates, the BER tends to stabilize around 0.5. This is attributed to the reduced time for bit transmission, leading to inadequate diffusion time, which introduces more noise; thus, the receiver is unable to accurately distinguish between 0 and 1. In the scope of a binary decoder, this causes the BER to average towards 0.5.

The behavior of BER can be further analyzed from Fig. 3, by considering either the input bit rate or the initial concentration to be constant:

- Input bit rate: For a given input bit rate, it can be observed that, as the initial concentration increases, BER decreases. The power of the received signal is determined by the initial concentration of redox-active molecules. Thus, a higher concentration enhances the quality of the received signal, consequently lowering the BER.
- Initial concentration: For a specific initial concentration of redox-active species, an increase in the input length corresponds to an increase in BER, particularly noticeable at lower concentrations. Given that this system operates as a diffusion-limited channel with memory, as the input length increases, the effect of noise becomes amplified due to the channel's memory, thereby increasing the BER.

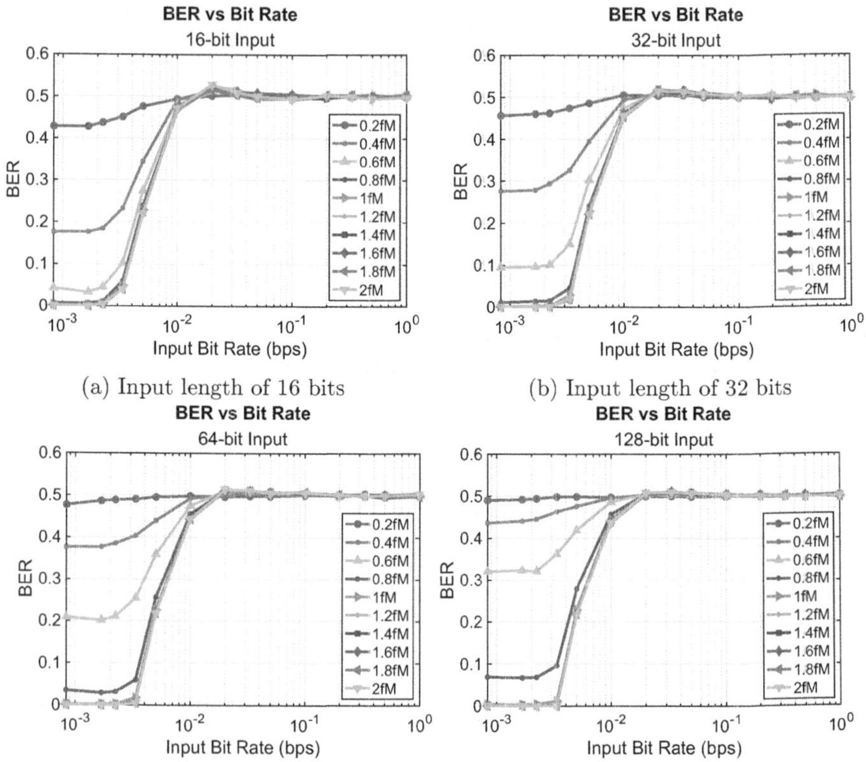

(a) Input length of 16 bits
(b) Input length of 32 bits
(c) Input length of 64 bits
(d) Input length of 128 bits

Fig. 3. BER plots with different initial redox-active concentrations across varying input bit rate for fixed input lengths of 16, 32, 64, and 128 bits.

This contrasting behavior offers valuable insight into the engineering of future redox-based E2M interfaces, with a trade-off between the minimum required initial concentration and the maximum input length.

The minor pertubations in the BER values for a given initial concentration are attributed to the restricted size of the channel, a hypothesis that will be investigated in future research. Overall, this E2M interface is suitable for applications operating at lower bit rates (≈ 0.001 bps).

5 Conclusion

In this paper, we provide an abstraction of an E2M communication interface based on redox processes. Continuing from our previous research on the M2E communication interface, we closed the loop by accounting for the information flow in the other direction. The computational model developed using finite difference methodology is stochastic in nature due to the noise in diffusion process.

Using the simulation framework built in MATLAB (based on the computational model), we analyzed the performance of the channel in terms of BER. Various threshold techniques were evaluated for the decoder at the receiver, and we decided on using the half-window threshold method. In this method, a sliding window of half the input length determines the threshold as the average of previously received concentrations within the window. We then compared the BER results across different scenarios with the numerical simulation data obtained by varying the input length, input bit rate, and initial redox-active concentration. The BER plots showed promising results with valuable insights into the influence of different system design parameters on interface performance.

References

1. Akyildiz, I., Pierobon, M., Balasubramaniam, S., Koucheryavy, Y.: The internet of Bio-Nano things. IEEE Commun. Mag. **53**(3), 32–40 (2015). https://doi.org/10.1109/MCOM.2015.7060516. http://ieeexplore.ieee.org/document/7060516/
2. Chang, L., Wu, J., Moustafa, N., Bashir, A.K., Yu, K.: AI-driven synthetic biology for non-small cell lung cancer drug effectiveness-cost analysis in intelligent assisted medical systems. IEEE J. Biomed. Health Inform. **26**(10), 5055–5066 (2022). https://doi.org/10.1109/JBHI.2021.3133455
3. Akyildiz, I.F., Pierobon, M., Balasubramaniam, S.: An information theoretic framework to analyze molecular communication systems based on statistical mechanics. Proc. IEEE **107**(7), 1230–1255 (2019). https://doi.org/10.1109/JPROC.2019.2927926
4. Zeng, Y., Zhu, Z., Du, D., Lin, Y.: Nanomaterial-based electrochemical biosensors for food safety. J. Electroanal. Chem. **781**(11), 147–154 (2016). https://doi.org/10.1016/j.jelechem.2016.10.030
5. Chen, D., Xu, T., Dou, Y., Li, T.: A calibration strategy for silicon nanowire field-effect transistor biosensors and its application in ultra-sensitive, label-free biosensing. ACS Nano **18**(33), 21873–21885 (2024). https://doi.org/10.1021/acsnano.4c01937. https://doi.org/10.1021/acsnano.4c01937, pMID: 39115266
6. Jamali, V., Ahmadzadeh, A., Wicke, W., Noel, A., Schober, R.: Channel modeling for diffusive molecular communication–a tutorial review. Proc. IEEE **107**(7), 1256–1301 (2019). https://doi.org/10.1109/JPROC.2019.2919455
7. Hofmann, P., Cabrera, J.A., Bassoli, R., Reisslein, M., Fitzek, F.H.P.: Coding in diffusion-based molecular nanonetworks: a comprehensive survey. IEEE Access **11**, 16411–16465 (2023). https://doi.org/10.1109/ACCESS.2023.3243797
8. Baranwal, J., Barse, B., Gatto, G., Broncova, G., Kumar, A.: Electrochemical Sensors and Their Applications: A Review (2022). https://doi.org/10.3390/chemosensors10090363
9. Wang, T.T., Huang, X.F., Huang, H., Luo, P., Qing, L.S.: Nanomaterial-based optical- and electrochemical-biosensors for urine glucose detection: a comprehensive review. Adv. Sens. Energy Mater. **1**(3), 100016 (2022). https://doi.org/10.1016/j.asems.2022.100016
10. Zhao, Z., et al.: Mediated electrochemical probing: a systems-level tool for redox biology. ACS Chem. Biol. **16**(7), 1099–1110 (2021). https://doi.org/10.1021/acschembio.1c00267

11. Liu, Y., et al.: Redox-enabled bio-electronics for information acquisition and transmission. IEEE Trans. Mol. Biol. Multi-Scale Commun. **9**(2), 146–166 (2023). https://doi.org/10.1109/TMBMC.2023.3274112
12. Lee, P.E., Demple, B., Barton, J.K.: DNA-mediated redox signaling for transcriptional activation of SoxR. Proc. Natl. Acad. Sci. **106**(32), 13164–13168 (2009). https://doi.org/10.1073/pnas.0906429106. https://www.pnas.org/doi/abs/10.1073/pnas.0906429106
13. Gorla, K.R., Barker, T., Pierobon, M.: Modeling diffusion and chemical reactions to analyze redox-based molecular-electrical communication. In: ICC 2020 - 2020 IEEE International Conference on Communications (ICC), pp. 1–7 (2020). https://doi.org/10.1109/ICC40277.2020.9148750
14. Gorla, K.R., Kim, E., Payne, G.F., Pierobon, M.: Modeling and characterization of a molecular-to-electrical communication channel enabled by redox reactions. IEEE J. Sel. Areas Commun. **42**(8), 2066–2079 (2024). https://doi.org/10.1109/JSAC.2024.3399254
15. VanArsdale, E., Pitzer, J., Payne, G.F., Bentley, W.E.: Redox electrochemistry to interrogate and control biomolecular communication. iScience **23**(9), 101545 (2020). https://doi.org/10.1016/j.isci.2020.101545. https://www.sciencedirect.com/science/article/pii/S2589004220307379
16. Wang, S., et al.: Redox-enabled Electronic Interrogation and Feedback Control of Hierarchical and Networked Biological Systems. bioRxiv (2023). https://doi.org/10.1101/2023.08.22.554301. https://www.biorxiv.org/content/early/2023/08/22/2023.08.22.554301
17. Gorla, K.R., Pierobon, M.: Preliminary characterization of a redox-based electrical-to-molecular communication channel. In: Proceedings of the 11th Annual ACM International Conference on Nanoscale Computing and Communication, NANOCOM 2024, pp. 124–125. Association for Computing Machinery, New York (2024). https://doi.org/10.1145/3686015.3689419
18. Tschirhart, T., et al.: Electronic control of gene expression and cell behaviour in Escherichia coli through redox signalling. Nat. Commun. **8**(1), 14030 (2017). https://doi.org/10.1038/ncomms14030
19. Bard, A.J., Faulkner, L.R.: Electrochemical Methods: Fundamentals and Applications. Wiley (2001). https://www.wiley.com/en-us/Electrochemical+Methods%3A+Fundamentals+and+Applications%2C+2nd+Edition-p-9780471043720
20. Fick, A.: On liquid diffusion. J. Membrane Sci. **100**(1), 33–38 (1995). https://doi.org/10.1016/0376-7388(94)00230-V. https://www.sciencedirect.com/science/article/pii/037673889400230V?via%3Dihub
21. Marcone, A., Pierobon, M., Magarini, M.: The Gaussian approximation in soft detection for molecular communication via biological circuits. In: 2017 IEEE 18th International Workshop on Signal Processing Advances in Wireless Communications (SPAWC), pp. 1–6 (2017). https://doi.org/10.1109/SPAWC.2017.8227764
22. Pierobon, M., Akyildiz, I.F.: Diffusion-based noise analysis for molecular communication in nanonetworks. IEEE Trans. Signal Process. **59**(6), 2532–2547 (2011). https://doi.org/10.1109/TSP.2011.2114656
23. Cooper, G.M.: The Cell: A Molecular Approach, 2nd edn. Sinauer Associates (2000)
24. Gagne, R.R., Koval, C.A., Lisensky, G.C.: Ferrocene as an internal standard for electrochemical measurements. Inorganic Chem. **19**(9), 2854–2855 (1980). https://doi.org/10.1021/IC50211A080/ASSET/IC50211A080.FP.PNG_V03. https://pubs.acs.org/doi/abs/10.1021/ic50211a080

Stochastic Modeling and Simulation of Collective Gradient Detection by Bio-nanomachine Clusters

Manaka Sugiyama[1] and Tadashi Nakano[2(✉)]

[1] Department of Engineering, Osaka Metropolitan University, Osaka, Japan
s122485h@st.omu.ac.jp
[2] Graduate School of Informatics, Osaka Metropolitan University, Osaka, Japan
tnakano@omu.ac.jp

Abstract. Gradient detection is a fundamental task for bio-nanomachines operating in molecular communication environments such as inside the human body. Due to their microscopic size, individual bio-nanomachines cannot reliably detect concentration gradients from pointwise measurements. To address this limitation, previous studies proposed a biologically inspired method in which a linear cluster of bio-nanomachines compares local and global molecular concentrations to infer gradient direction. This paper extends the previous deterministic model by incorporating stochastic fluctuations into the concentration dynamics of both local and global molecules. We develop a set of stochastic differential equations and numerically solve them using the EulerMaruyama method. Simulation results demonstrate how local and global concentrations evolve under molecular noise, how the coupling coefficient controlling molecule exchange affects detection accuracy, and how the cluster can move along a signal gradient in noisy environments. Our findings show that stronger coupling improves robustness and directional reliability through spatial averaging, enabling effective gradient detection even in the presence of noise.

Keywords: Molecular communication · Bio-nanomachine · Gradient detection · Collective behavior · Noise

1 Introduction

Molecular communication (MC) is a biologically inspired communication paradigm in which small-scale devices called bio-nanomachines exchange information using signaling molecules [1,3,6,8]. MC is particularly suited for operation in environments where conventional electromagnetic communication is not feasible, such as inside the human body. In such in-body environments, bio-nanomachines can be used for a wide range of applications, including targeted drug delivery, in-body diagnostics, and tissue-level coordination.

H. Tanaka et al. (Eds.): BodyNets 2025, LNICST 714, pp. 311–321, 2026.
https://doi.org/10.1007/978-3-032-38657-1_25

One of the key challenges in MC is gradient detection, that is, the ability of bio-nanomachines to sense spatial variations in the concentration of signaling molecules [9]. Gradient detection plays a central role in tasks such as chemotaxis [5], source localization [2], and targeted drug delivery [10]. For example, cancer cells may release specific signaling molecules into their surroundings, creating a concentration gradient. Bio-nanomachines deployed in the body can detect this gradient and move directionally toward the cancer site, enabling them to deliver therapeutic agents precisely where they are needed. However, because bio-nanomachines are extremely small, they can only sample molecule concentrations at a single point, making the differences in concentration difficult to detect reliably. As a result, accurate gradient detection becomes particularly challenging when performed by individual bio-nanomachines.

To address this challenge, a previous study applied a biologically inspired method for collective gradient detection [4]. In this method, a cluster of bio-nanomachines cooperatively infers the direction of a signal gradient. Each bio-nanomachine maintains two types of intracellular molecule concentrations: the concentration of local molecules, which reflects the signal level at its own position, and the concentration of global molecules, which represents a spatial average of signal levels obtained through diffusion with neighboring bio-nanomachines. By comparing these two concentrations, particularly at the two ends of the cluster, the bio-nanomachine cluster can determine whether the signal is increasing toward the left or the right.

In this paper, we extend the model in [4] by incorporating stochastic fluctuations into the concentration dynamics. Unlike the deterministic model in prior work, our stochastic model accounts for the inherent noise in molecular environments. Using this model, we first investigate how the concentrations of local and global molecules fluctuate over time due to noise. We then analyze how the coupling coefficient that governs the exchange of global molecules between neighboring bio-nanomachines affects the accuracy of gradient detection. Finally, we demonstrate that even in the presence of noise, a cluster of bio-nanomachines can detect the direction of the gradient and move accordingly.

The rest of this paper is organized as follows. Section 2 presents the stochastic model. Section 3 shows numerical results that illustrate the effects of molecular noise on concentration dynamics and gradient detection. Section 4 concludes the paper.

2 Stochastic Modeling of Collective Gradient Detection

A previous work investigates the performance of a biologically inspired collective gradient detection method [4]. Figure 1 illustrates the model where a linear cluster of N bio-nanomachines samples an external signal concentration profile $c(x)$ that increases linearly with spatial coordinate x. Each bio-nanomachine at position x_i maintains two intracellular molecule concentrations: the local molecule concentration l_i, and the global molecule concentration g_i. The local molecule concentration reflects the external concentration at the bio-nanomachine's own

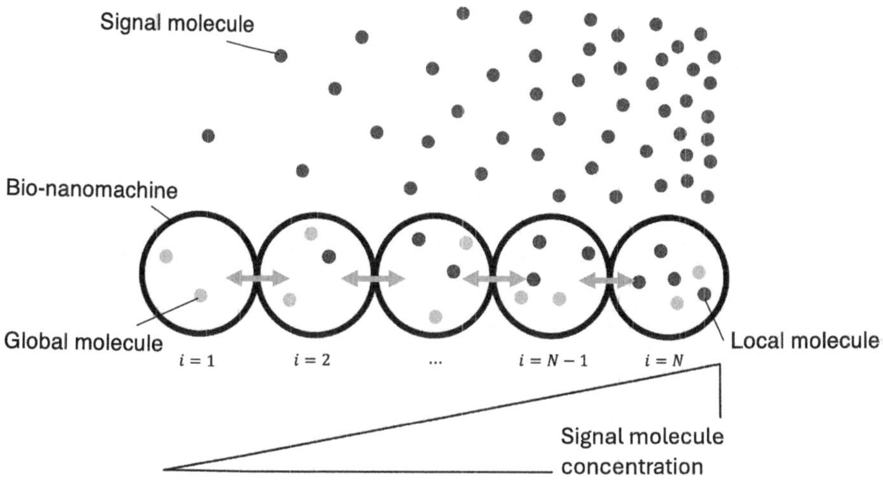

Fig. 1. A bio-nanomachine cluster that performs gradient detection [4]

position, while the global molecule concentration reflects a spatial average of external concentrations, aggregated from neighboring positions through diffusion. Together, these two concentrations allow each bio-nanomachine to compare local and spatially averaged molecule concentrations. Gradient detection is performed by the two end bio-nanomachines, specifically, $i = 1$ and $i = N$, which compare l_1 with g_1 at the left end and l_N with g_N at the right end, allowing the cluster to determine whether the signal concentration increases toward the right or the left.

Previous work employs deterministic coupled rate equations to describe the model. However, bio-nanomachines operate in noisy environments where fluctuations in molecular concentrations can impact detection accuracy. In this paper, we extend the model by explicitly incorporating stochastic effects into the rate equations governing both local and global molecule concentrations, following the general formulation used in [7].

Using a set of stochastic differential equations, we express the time evolution of l_i and g_i for $i \in \mathcal{N}$ as follow.

$$\frac{\mathrm{d}l_i}{\mathrm{d}t} = \beta c(x_i) - \gamma l_i + \eta_{l_i} \tag{1}$$

$$\frac{\mathrm{d}g_i}{\mathrm{d}t} = \beta c(x_i) - \gamma g_i + DM_i + \eta_{g_i} \tag{2}$$

$$M_i = \begin{cases} g_2 - g_1 & i = 1 \\ (g_{i-1} - g_i) + (g_{i+1} - g_i) & i \neq 1, N \\ g_{N-1} - g_N & i = N \end{cases} \tag{3}$$

The first terms on the right-hand side of (1) and (2) represent the production rates of local and global molecules, respectively. The production rates increase in proportion to the concentration of signal molecules, and β is the constant of proportionality.

The second terms on the right-hand side of (1) and (2) represent the decomposition rates of local and global molecules, respectively. The decomposition rates increase in proportion to the concentration of the two types of molecule and γ is the constant of proportionality. Note here that both production and decomposition rates (β and γ) are the same for local and global molecules.

The third term on the right-hand side of (2) represents the diffusion of global molecules between bio-nanomachines. D is the coupling coefficient that determines the rate of exchange and diffusion is driven by concentration differences, which are represented by M_i. Specifically, M_1 is the difference between bio-nanomachines 2 and 1; M_N is the difference between bio-nanomachines $N-1$ and N; and M_i for $i \neq 1, N$ is the sum of the difference between bio-nanomachines $i-1$ and i, and the difference between bio-nanomachines $i+1$ and i.

The third term on the right-hand side of (1) and the fourth term on the right-hand side of (2) represent the stochastic terms for the local and global molecules, respectively, which we newly introduce in this paper. These terms are further defined in (4) and (5) below.

$$\eta_{l_i} = \xi_{1,i}\sqrt{\beta c(x_i)} + \xi_{2,i}\sqrt{\gamma l_i} \tag{4}$$

$$\eta_{g_i} = \xi_{3,i}\sqrt{\beta c(x_i)} + \xi_{4,i}\sqrt{\gamma g_i} + \sqrt{D}F_i \tag{5}$$

$$F_i = \begin{cases} \chi_1(\sqrt{g_2} - \sqrt{g_1}) & i = 1 \\ \chi_{i-1}(\sqrt{g_{i-1}} - \sqrt{g_i}) + \chi_i(\sqrt{g_{i+1}} - \sqrt{g_i}) & i \neq 1, N \\ \chi_{N-1}(\sqrt{g_{N-1}} - \sqrt{g_N}) & i = N \end{cases} \tag{6}$$

The first terms on the right-hand side of (4) and (5) represent the stochastic fluctuations in the production of local and global molecules, respectively. Since the production process is modeled as a Poisson process, in which the variance equals the mean, the noise intensity increases in proportion to the square root of the production rate. The variables $\xi_{1,i}$ and $\xi_{3,i}$ represent independent Gaussian random variables with zero mean and unit variance.

The second terms on the right-hand side of (4) and (5) represent the stochastic fluctuations in the decomposition of local and global molecules, respectively. As with production, the decomposition process is also modeled as a Poisson process, implying that the noise intensity increases in proportion to the square root of the decomposition rate. The variables $\xi_{2,i}$ and $\xi_{4,i}$ represent independent Gaussian random variables with zero mean and unit variance.

The third term on the right-hand side of (5) represents the stochastic fluctuations in the diffusion of global molecules between bio-nanomachines. The noise intensity is scaled by the square root of the coupling coefficient D, and stochastic fluctuations are driven by differences in the square roots of global molecule concentrations, which are represented by F_i. Specifically, F_1 is the difference between the square roots of the concentrations at bio-nanomachines 2 and 1; F_N is the difference between those at bio-nanomachines $N-1$ and N; and F_i for $i \neq 1, N$ is the sum of the difference between bio-nanomachines $i-1$ and i, and the difference between bio-nanomachines $i+1$ and i, each taken in terms of square root concentrations. The variables χ_i $(i = 1, 2, \ldots, N-1)$ represent independent Gaussian random variables with zero mean and unit variance.

Table 1. Parameter values used in simulations

Parameter	Symbol	Value
Slope of external concentration	α	1.0
Number of bio-nanomachines	N	10
Bio-nanomachine length	L	1.0
Production rate constant	β	0.5
Decomposition rate constant	γ	0.02
Coupling coefficient	D	0.2
Time step	Δt	0.1

3 Simulations

In this section, we conduct simulations based on the stochastic model presented in Sect. 2 to examine how stochastic fluctuations affect the concentrations of local and global molecules over time, how the coupling coefficient influences gradient detection accuracy, and whether a cluster of bio-nanomachines can detect and move along a concentration gradient of external signals under noise.

3.1 Simulation Methods and Configurations

To conduct simulations, we numerically solve the stochastic model using the Euler–Maruyama method, which is a standard technique for approximating the solutions of stochastic differential equations (SDEs). In this method, time is discretized into small intervals of size Δt, and the values of molecular concentrations are updated iteratively based on both deterministic and stochastic terms in the model equations. The stochastic terms are approximated by drawing samples from Gaussian distributions scaled by the square roots of the corresponding reaction or diffusion rates.

In the simulations, the spatial position x_i of bio-nanomachine i is defined as $x_i = L \times i$, where L denotes the length of a single bio-nanomachine. The external signal concentration follows a linear profile given by $c(x) = \alpha x$, so that each bio-nanomachine samples the signal at its location as $c(x_i) = \alpha L i$. Table 1 lists the parameters used in the simulations. For each condition, we perform 1000 independent trials with different random seeds to evaluate statistical properties such as the mean and variance.

3.2 Simulation Results

3.2.1 Concentration Fluctuations Over Time

We first observe how the local and global molecule concentrations fluctuate over time due to stochastic noise at the rightmost bio-nanomachine ($i = N$). Figure 2 shows representative time courses of local and global concentrations in a single trial. Figures 3a and 3b summarize the mean and variance of these concentrations across 1000 trials.

The local molecule concentration exhibits Poisson-type fluctuations, where the mean and variance are approximately equal. This behavior reflects the stochasticity of molecular production and degradation processes at a single point. In contrast, the global molecule concentration shows a reduced variance, which results from spatial averaging due to molecule exchange with neighboring bio-nanomachines. This averaging effect leads to smoother fluctuations and enhances robustness to local noise.

These results highlight a key distinction between the two concentration types: while local signals reflect pointwise sampling with high variability, global signals benefit from collective smoothing through coupling, reducing the impact of stochastic perturbations.

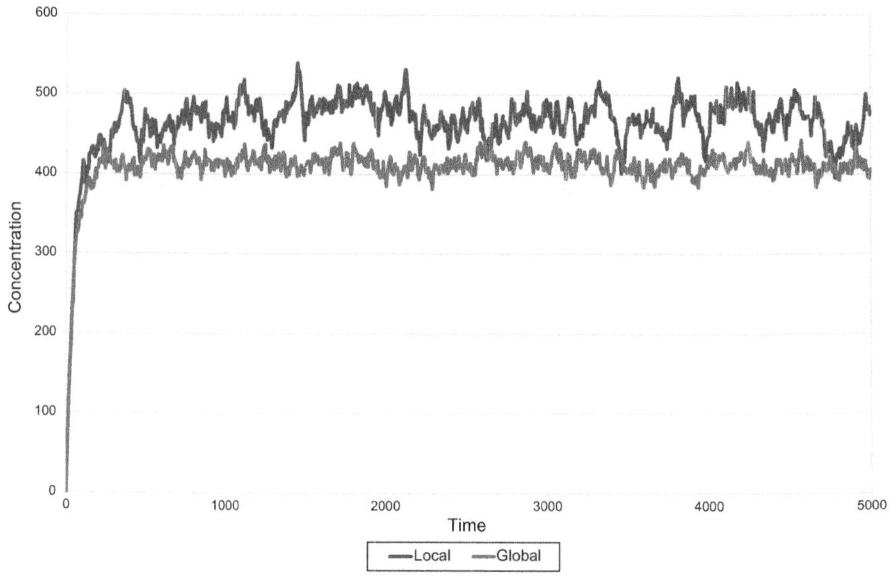

Fig. 2. Time evolution of local and global molecule concentrations at the rightmost bio-nanomachine ($i = N$) in a single simulation trial.

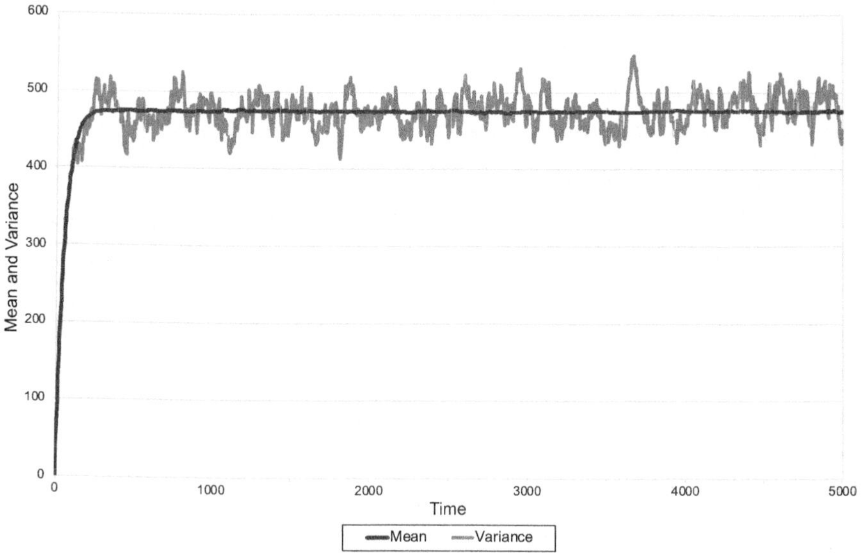

(a) Mean and variance of local molecule concentrations at $i = N$ across 1000 independent trials.

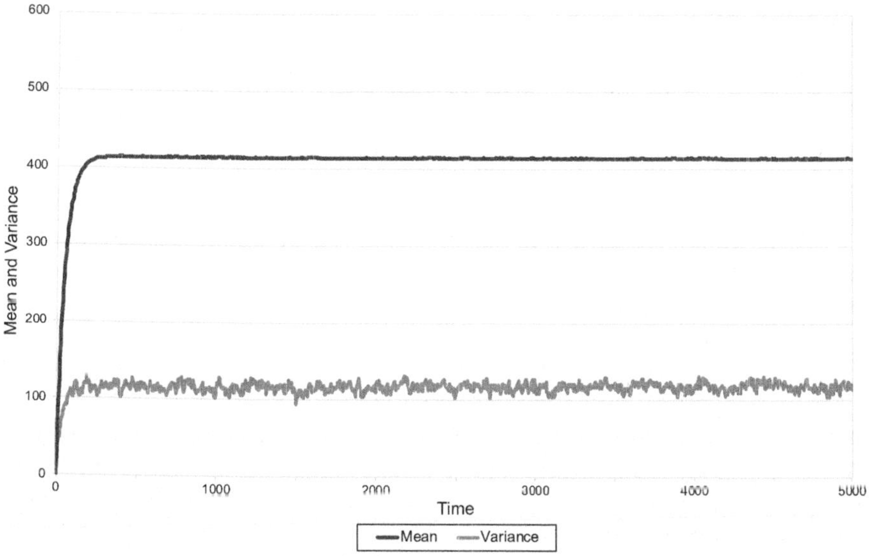

(b) Mean and variance of global molecule concentrations at $i = N$ across 1000 independent trials.

Fig. 3. Statistical properties of local and global molecule concentrations under stochastic fluctuations.

3.2.2 Impact of Coupling Coefficient on Detection Accuracy

As described in Sect. 2, the bio-nanomachine cluster detects the direction of the concentration gradient by comparing the local and global molecule concentrations at its ends. In particular, the difference $\Delta_N = l_N - g_N$ at the rightmost bio-nanomachine ($i = N$) serves as a decision signal: a positive or negative Δ_N indicates whether the external signal increases or decreases along the cluster.

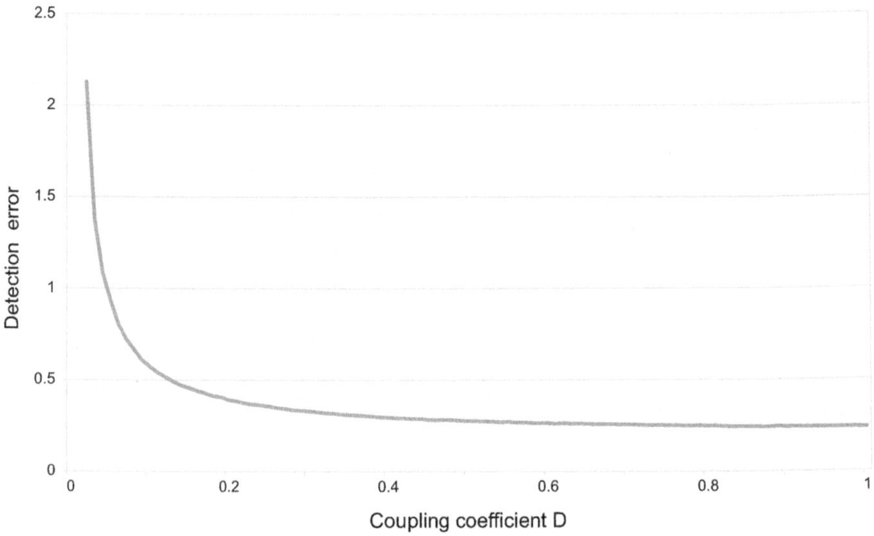

Fig. 4. Detection error $\sigma_{\Delta_N}/|\mu_{\Delta_N}|$ as a function of the coupling coefficient D.

To quantify how reliably a bio-nanomachine cluster can detect a concentration gradient, we define the detection error as the ratio between the standard deviation and the mean of Δ:

$$\text{Detection error} = \frac{\sigma_{\Delta_N}}{|\mu_{\Delta_N}|}, \quad \Delta_N = l_N - g_N, \tag{7}$$

where μ_{Δ_N} and σ_{Δ_N} denote the mean and standard deviation of Δ_N across independent trials. A smaller detection error indicates that the difference Δ_N is more consistently detectable despite stochastic fluctuations, and thus corresponds to more reliable gradient detection.

Figure 4 shows how the detection error varies with the coupling coefficient D, which governs the rate of global molecule exchange between neighboring bio-nanomachines. As observed in the figure, the detection error decreases monotonically with increasing D.

This trend can be understood from the role of D in shaping the global molecule concentration g_N. When D is small, diffusion between nanomachines is limited, and g_N largely reflects the local concentration at $i = N$. In this case, the difference $\Delta_N = l_N - g_N$ becomes small, making it difficult to distinguish the direction of the gradient. As D increases, global molecules incorporate information from neighboring bio-nanomachines, and g_N approaches a spatial average. This increases the magnitude of Δ_N, making gradient detection more reliable.

In addition, higher D values help suppress stochastic fluctuations in g_N through spatial averaging. This reduction in noise contributes further to the decrease in detection error.

3.2.3 Gradient Detection and Movement Under Noise

Finally, we evaluate whether a bio-nanomachine cluster can detect and respond to a concentration gradient in the presence of noise. To this end, we simulate the movement of the cluster in a spatially varying concentration field with a triangular profile:

$$c(x) = \begin{cases} \alpha x, & 0 \leq x < 30 \\ \alpha(60 - x), & 30 \leq x \leq 60 \end{cases} \tag{8}$$

Every 5000 units of time, the bio-nanomachine cluster computes two decision signals: $\Delta_1 = l_1 - g_1$ at the left end and $\Delta_N = l_N - g_N$ at the right end. The cluster then updates its position based on the signs of both $\Delta 1$ and Δ_N: if $\Delta_1 > 0$ and $\Delta_N < 0$, the cluster moves leftward; if $\Delta_1 < 0$ and $\Delta_N > 0$, it moves rightward; otherwise, it remains stationary.

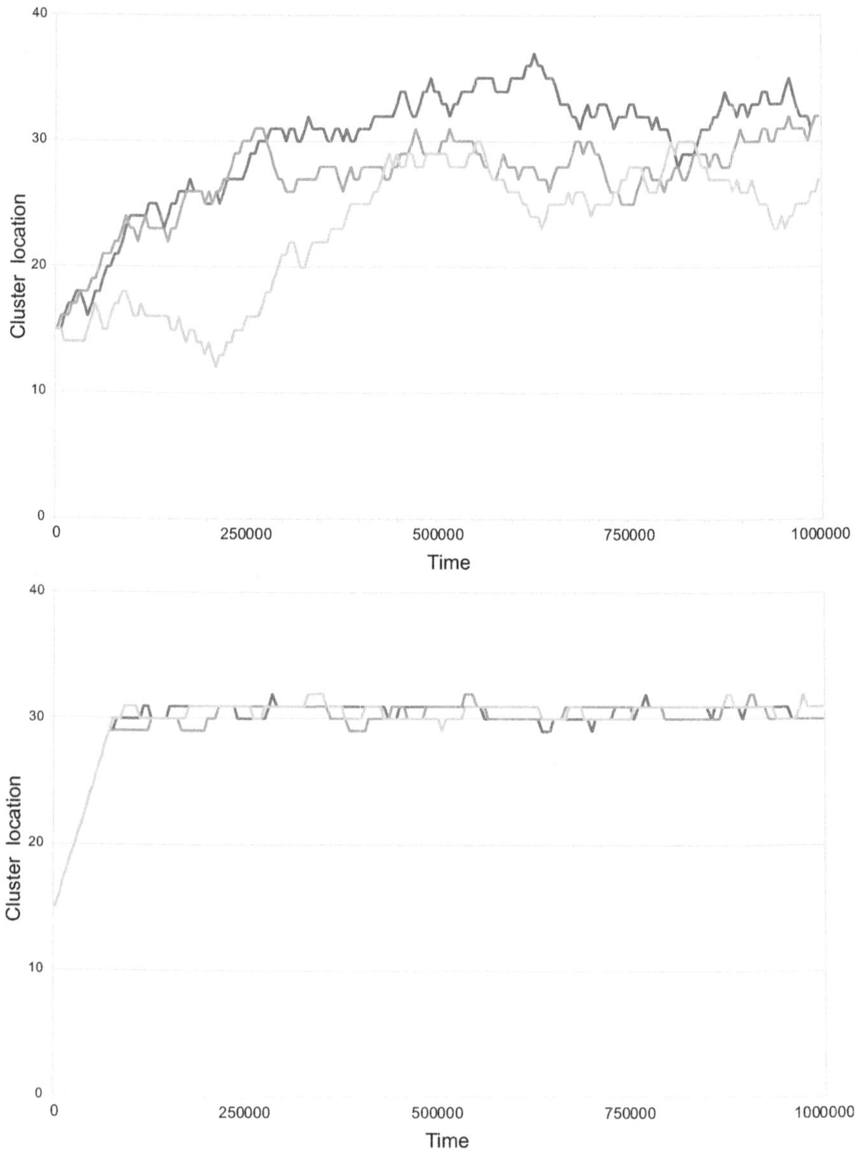

Fig. 5. Representative movement trajectories of the bio-nanomachine cluster in a triangular concentration profile. (Top) $D = 0.01$, (Bottom) $D = 0.5$.

Figure 5 shows representative trajectories of the cluster under different values of the coupling coefficient D and different noise realizations. When D is small ($D = 0.01$), fluctuations dominate the decision signal, and the cluster exhibits noisy motion: it repeatedly moves toward and away from the peak of the concentration profile before gradually settling near it with sustained fluctuations. In contrast, when D is large ($D = 0.5$), the cluster responds more deterministically, moving steadily toward the peak and remaining stably localized around it with reduced variability. These results indicate that stronger coupling improves directional consistency by suppressing noise.

4 Conclusion

This paper investigated a stochastic extension of a biologically inspired gradient detection model for bio-nanomachine clusters. Simulation results showed that molecular noise causes fluctuations in concentration signals, but spatial coupling through global molecules reduces variability and improves detection accuracy. As the coupling coefficient increases, spatial averaging becomes more effective, resulting in lower detection error and more consistent directional movement. These findings demonstrate that, even under noise, a bio-nanomachine cluster can detect and follow a concentration gradient.

Acknowledgment. This work was supported by JSPS KAKENHI Grant Number JP21H04876.

References

1. Akyildiz, I.F., Brunetti, F., Blázquez, C.: Nanonetworks: a new communication paradigm. Comput. Netw. **52**(12), 2260–2279
2. Balasubramaniam, S., Lio, P.: Multi-hop conjugation based bacteria nanonetworks. IEEE Trans. Nanobiosci. **12**(1), 47–59
3. Bi, D., Almpanis, A., Noel, A., Deng, Y., Schober, R.: A survey of molecular communication in cell biology: establishing a new hierarchy for interdisciplinary applications. IEEE Commun. Surv. Tutor. **23**(3), 1494–1545
4. Chiba, M., Nakano, T.: Performance analysis of a biologically inspired collective gradient detection method for a bio-nanomachine cluster. IEEE Commun. Lett. **28**(11), 2528–2532
5. Cobo, L.C., Akyildiz, I.F.: Bacteria-based communication in nanonetworks. Nano Commun. Netw. **1**(4), 244–256
6. Farsad, N., Yilmaz, H.B., Eckford, A., Chae, C.B., Guo, W.: A comprehensive survey of recent advancements in molecular communication. IEEE Commun. Surv. Tutor. **18**(3), 1887–1919
7. Mugler, A., Levchenko, A., Nemenman, I.: Limits to the precision of gradient sensing with spatial communication and temporal integration. Proc. Natl. Acad. Sci. U.S.A. **113**(6), E689–E695
8. Nakano, T., Eckford, A., Haraguchi, T.: Molecular Communication, 2nd edn. Cambridge University Press, Cambridge
9. Nakano, T., Suda, T., Okaie, Y., Moore, M.J., Vasilakos, A.V.: Molecular communication among biological nanomachines: a layered architecture and research issues. IEEE Trans. Nanobiosci. **13**(3), 169–197
10. Wei, G., Bogdan, P., Marculescu, R.: Bumpy rides: modeling the dynamics of chemotactic interacting bacteria. IEEE J. Sel. Areas Commun. **31**(12), 879–890

A Study on Coded Multiplexing Scheme for Optical Wireless Communications

Shochiro Yamasaki[1](✉), Hirokazu Tanaka[1], and Tomoko K. Matsushima[2]

[1] Hiroshima City University, 3-4-1 Otsukahigashi Asaminami-ku, Hiroshima-shi 731-3194, Japan
syamasa@mict.info.hiroshima-cu.ac.jp

[2] Yokohama College of Commerce, 4-11-1 Higashiterao, Tsurumi-ku, Yokohama-shi 230-8577, Japan

Abstract. Optical wireless communications using a light-emitting diode are unlikely to cause electromagnetic interference to electronic devices, then they are expected to be used in hospitals. Based on a communication scheme realizing data multiplexing and error correction coding simultaneously using discrete Fourier transform over finite fields, this study proposes a Reed-Solomon coded multiplexing scheme for optical wireless communications and shows evaluations of transmission characteristics. The scheme removes background light interference using a cancellation technique. And multiplexing user information data into a multiplexed symbol stream over the finite field contributes to symbol transmission with low peak-to-average power ratio characteristics.

Keywords: Optical wireless communications · Data multiplexing · Reed-Solomon coding

1 Introduction

Optical wireless communications using a light-emitting diode (LED) are unlikely to cause electromagnetic interference to electronic devices, then they are expected to be used in hospitals [1]. For example, LED light communication systems for enhanced control of mobile robots that perform transport operations in hospital has been presented [2]. Some of the advantages of optical communication systems over radio frequency communication systems is the high security provided by the optical systems, since lights do not penetrate through walls [3].

The authors have proposed variable-length orthogonal sequences based on discrete Fourier transform over finite fields, and the communication system using the proposed sequences realizes data multiplexing and error correction coding simultaneously [4]. This study proposes a Reed-Solomon coded multiplexing scheme for optical wireless communications, which has a function of reducing the degradation of communication quality caused by background light interference over channels, and shows evaluations of transmission characteristics.

Supported by JSPS KAKENHI Grant Numbers 22K04091, 22K04113, 23K11085, and 25K07755.

H. Tanaka et al. (Eds.): BodyNets 2025, LNICST 714, pp. 322–328, 2026.
https://doi.org/10.1007/978-3-032-38657-1_26

2 Discrete Fourier Transform

We define a vector $Y = \big(y(0)\ y(1)\ \dots\ y(n-1)\big)$ of length n. The discrete Fourier transform (DFT) transforms the vector Y to a vector $X = \big(x(0)\ x(1)\ \dots\ x(n-1)\big)$ of length n by

$$x(k) = \sum_{i=0}^{n-1} \omega^{ik} y(i), \quad k = 0, 1, \dots, n-1, \tag{1}$$

where ω is an element such that $\omega^n = 1$ and $\omega^i \neq 1$ for $i = 1, 2, \dots, n-1$. The inverse DFT (IDFT) transforms the vector X to the vector Y.

We review a finite field denoted as GF(q). When a prime field is selected, q is set to $q = p$ and p is a prime number of $p \geq 3$. When an extension field is selected, q is set to $q = p^r$, p is a prime number of $p \geq 2$, and r is an integer of $r \geq 2$. We set that $\omega^i \neq 1$ for $i = 1, 2, \dots, q-2$ and $\omega^{q-1} = 1$, then elements in GF(q) are in the set

$$F_q = \{0, 1, \omega^1, \omega^2, \dots, \omega^{q-2}\}. \tag{2}$$

An example, the extension field is selected, where the integers are set to $p = 2$ and $r = 8$. Then, q is set to $q = p^r = 2^8$. There exist 256 elements and they are in the set $F_{2^8} = \{0, 1, \omega, \omega^2, \dots, \omega^{254}\}$ over GF(2^8), where $\omega^{255} = 1$ and $\omega^i \neq 1$ for $i = 1, 2, \dots, 254$. And ω is defined as $\omega = \alpha$, where α is decided by a primitive root of the primitive polynomial $p(x) = x^8 + x^4 + x^3 + x^2 + 1$. In this case, $q - 1 = 2^8 - 1 = 255$ and the integer 255 is expressed as $255 = 3 \cdot 5 \cdot 17$, therefore the integer 255 is divided by the integers $3, 5, 15, 17, 51, 85$, and 255.

The DFT and the IDFT exist over finite fields. The number of the point for the DFT and the IDFT over GF(2^8) is selected from the set $\{3, 5, 15, 17, 51, 85, 255\}$ [5].

We set the vector $X = \big(x(0)\ x(1)\ \dots\ x(n-1)\big)$ of length n so that its k elements are assigned to information symbols and its $n-k$ elements are assigned to parity symbols which are equal to zeros as $x(k) = x(k+1) = \dots = x(n-1) = 0$, then the n-point IDFT transforms the vector X to the vector $Y = \big(y(0)\ y(1)\ \dots\ y(n-1)\big)$ of length n which is a codeword of non-systematic (n, k) RS code. Its minimum distance is $d_{\min} = n - k + 1$, then its decoder corrects any pattern of ν errors and ρ erasures where $d_{\min} \geq 2\nu + \rho + 1$ [5].

The authors have proposed variable-length orthogonal sequences based on the DFT and the IDFT over finite fields, and the communication system using the proposed sequences realizes data multiplexing and error correction coding simultaneously [4].

3 Scheme for Optical Wireless Communications

3.1 Transmitter and Receiver

An example of a configuration for the downlink system is illustrated in Fig. 1. A transmitter is equipped with the n-point IDFT over GF(q), where $q = 2^r$

and $n = 2^r - 1$. When an IDFT input vector over GF(2^r) is defined as $X_t = \big(x_t(0)\ x_t(1)\ \ldots\ x_t(n-1)\big)$, k information data symbols are input to $\big(x_t(0)\ x_t(1)\ \ldots\ x_t(k-1)\big)$, and $n-k$ parity symbols are input to $\big(x_t(k)\ x_t(k+1)\ \ldots\ x_t(n-1)\big)$ which are equal to zeros. Then, k and n are set to $k \leq n$.

An IDFT output vector is defined as $Y_t = \big(y_t(0)\ \ y_t(1)\ \ldots\ \ y_t(n-1)\big)$ over GF(2^r), then the IDFT output vector Y_t corresponds to a codeword of the non-systematic RS(n,k) codes. When a data symbol for a user is assigned to an input of IDFT, the n-point IDFT multiplexes data symbols for k users into the vector Y_t. Each IDFT output symbol in GF(2^r) is converted into r bits.

A mapper maps each bit to mapped signal V. When binary signaling is used, each bit is mapped to

$$V = \begin{cases} (1) & (\text{for Bit} = 1, \\ (0) & (\text{for Bit} = 0). \end{cases} \tag{3}$$

and when binary orthogonal signaling is used, each bit is mapped to

$$V = \begin{cases} (0\ 1) & (\text{for Bit} = 1), \\ (1\ 0) & (\text{for Bit} = 0). \end{cases} \tag{4}$$

This signaling is equal to Manchester signaling. In optical wireless communications, backgroud lights severely degrade communication quality. Manchester signaling has an advantage of cancelling influences of backgroud light in demapping process [6]. Then, we focus on the binary orthogonal signaling in this study.

The transmitter is equipped with an LED and turns the LED on and off according to the mapped signals. Optical signals yielded by the LED are fed to wireless channels.

The signals through the channels are fed to receivers. Each receiver is equipped with a photo detector (PD), and the PD converts the received optical signals to electrical mapped signals.

Demapping Scheme 1

A scheme which demapps the received Manchester signaling mapped signals to bits for optical communications is shown in [6]. As illustrated in Fig. 2, the mapped signals are demapped to bits by calculating the difference between the received mapped signals and the $\tau/2$ delayed received mapped signals and deciding the difference value greater or less than 0 in decision intervals, where τ is a bit time interval. The differential calculation cancels the interference caused by backgroud lights.

Demapping Scheme 2

The demapper has reference vectors as

$$\begin{cases} C_{r_0} = (1\ 0), \\ C_{r_1} = (0\ 1). \end{cases} \tag{5}$$

The received vector with two samples is assumed to be $V_r = (A\ \ 0) + (B\ \ B)$ for the transmitted bit of 0 or $V_r = (0\ \ A) + (B\ \ B)$ for the transmitted bit of 1, where A is each signal sample amplitude, and B is amplitude for time-invariant backgroud light. The demapper calculates the inner product of the received vector V_r and the reference vector C_{r_1} and also calculates the one of the received vector V_r and the reference vector C_{r_0}, then it calculates the difference of these inner products as

$$\begin{aligned}\Gamma_0 &= V_r \cdot C_{r_1}^T - V_r \cdot C_{r_0}^T \\ &= \begin{cases} A & \left(\text{for } V_r = (0 \;\; A) + (B \;\; B)\right), \\ -A & \left(\text{for } V_r = (A \;\; 0) + (B \;\; B)\right). \end{cases}\end{aligned} \tag{6}$$

The differential calculation cancels the interference caused by backgroud lights [7]. Then a demapped bit is obtained as

$$u_r = \begin{cases} 1 & (\text{for } \Gamma \geq 0), \\ 0 & (\text{for } \Gamma < 0). \end{cases} \tag{7}$$

The demapped consecutive r bits are converted to a symbol over GF(2^r) and it forms a received symbol. The received n symbols construct the received vector $Y_r = \left(y_r(0) \;\; y_r(1) \; \ldots \; y_r(n-1)\right)$ over GF(2^r) and it corresponds to the received codeword of RS(n, k) coding. Error correction decoding corrects errors in the received codeword and generates the corrected codeword. And the n-point DFT transforms the corrected codeword to the output vector $X_r = \left(x_r(0) \; x_r(1) \; \ldots \; x_r(n-1)\right)$ over GF(2^r), and the k symbols $x_r(0), x_r(1), \ldots, x_r(k-1)$ correspond to the reconstructed information symbols.

4 Evaluations

We assume that the PIN-PD is used as the PD, then its output signals are disturbed by thermal noises as dominant disturbance. Then the received signals are assumed to be suffered from added Gaussian independent and identically distributed random variables with zero mean and variance σ^2. The mapped signal vector, which is assumed to be either $(A \;\; 0)$ or $(0 \;\; A)$, is contaminated by noises. The signal to noise ratio (SNR) is defined as A^2/σ^2.

When the binary orthogonal signaling is adopted in mapping, the mapped signals are demapped to bits using the demapping scheme 1 or 2, and bit error probability P_{biterr} is obtained as

$$P_{\text{biterr}} = \frac{1}{2}\text{erfc}\left(\sqrt{\frac{A^2}{4\sigma^2}}\right). \tag{8}$$

And each consecutive r bits are converted to a symbol in GF(2^r). Using P_{biterr} in Eq. (8), symbol error probability P_{symerr} is obtained as

$$P_{\text{symerr}} = 1 - (1 - P_{\text{biterr}})^r. \tag{9}$$

And each consecutive n symbols form a symbol vector of length n for $n = 2^r - 1$, then the vector corresponds to a codeword of the non-systematic RS(n, k) code. When n and k are set to $n - k = 2t$ for an integer t greater than 0, the t

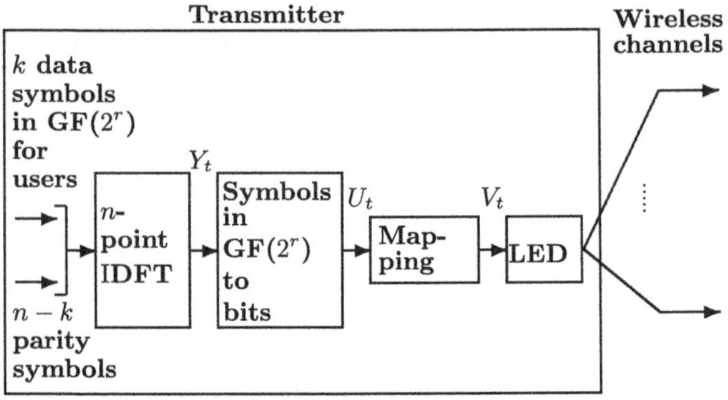

(a) Configuration of transmitter

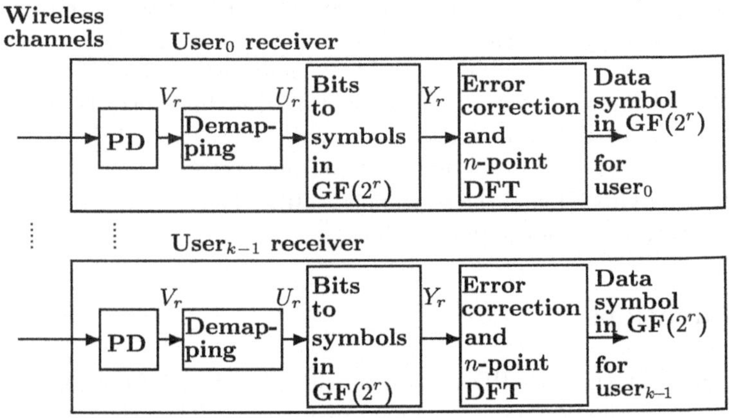

(b) Configuration of receivers

Fig. 1. Downlink system configurations.

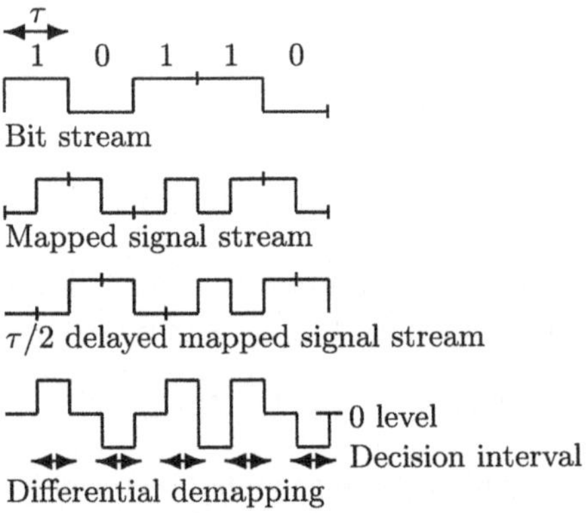

Fig. 2. Demapping scheme 1.

error symbols in the received codeword Y_r are corrected by the error correction decoding.

When there are more than t error symbols in the received codeword, the error correction decoding for the RS(n, k) code cannot correct errors. In such a condition, decoding failure occurs, and its probability P_{decfail} is derived as

$$P_{\text{decfail}} = 1 - \sum_{h=0}^{t} {}_nC_h P_{\text{symerr}}^h (1 - P_{\text{symerr}})^{n-h} \tag{10}$$

The decoded codeword is input to the n-point DFT over GF(2^r) and transformed to a vector $X_r = \left(x_r(0)\ x_r(1)\ \ldots\ x_r(n-1)\right)$. And the k symbols $x_r(0)$, $x_r(1)$, ..., $x_r(k-1)$ correspond to the reconstructed information data symbols. If the decoding failure occurs, the reconstructed symbols are erroneous.

The probability of decoding failure P_{decfail} is obtained by theoretical calculation using Eq. (10) for $r = 8$, $n = 255$, $k = 239$, and $t = 8, 16, 24$, and 32 over GF(2^8). And the results are illustrated in Fig. 3. In this evaluation, the influences of backgroud lights are neglected. Evaluations including backgroud lights require computer simulation and it is future work.

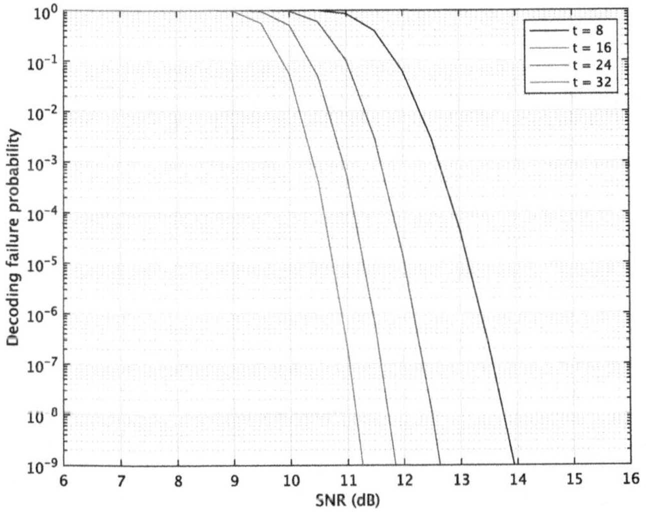

Fig. 3. Probability of decoding failure P_{decfail} of Y_{rl} for $t = 8, 16, 24$ and 32.

5 Conclusion

This study proposed a coded multiplexing scheme for optical wireless communications and showed evaluations of transmission characteristics.

The advantages of the scheme are that the multiplexing procedure includes Reed-Solomon coding for error correction and the demapping procedure includes interference light cancellation. And multiplexing user information data into a multiplexed symbol stream over the finite field contributes to symbol transmission with low peak-to-average power ratio characteristics.

References

1. Khan, L.U.: Visible light communication: applications, architecture, standardization and research challenges. Digit. Commun. Netw. **3**(2), 78–88 (2017)
2. Murai, R., et al.: A novel visible light communication system for enhanced control of autonomous delivery robots in a hospital. In: 2012 IEEE/SICE International Symposium on System Integration (SII), pp. 510–516 (2012)
3. Arfaoui, M.A., et al.: Physical layer security for visible light communication systems - a survey. IEEE Commun. Surv. Tutor. **22**(3), 1887–1908 (2020, Third Quarter)
4. Yamasaki, S., Matsushima, T.K., Ono, K., Tanaka, H.: Variable-length orthogonal codes over finite fields realizing data multiplexing and error correction coding simultaneously. IEICE Trans. Fundam. **E107-A**(3), 373–383 (2024)
5. Blahaut, R.E.: Algebraic Methods for Signal Processing and Communications Coding. Springer, Cham (1992)
6. Chow, C.W., Yeh, C.H., Liu, Y.F., Huang, P.Y.: Mitigation of optical background noise in light-emitting diode (LED) optical wireless communication systems. IEEE Photonics J. **5**(1) (2013)
7. Matsushima, T.K., Yamasaki, S., Ono, K.: Signature codes to remove interference light in synchronous optical code-division multiple access systems. IEICE Trans. Fundam. **E104-A**(11), 1619–1628 (2021)

Body Area Networks and Wearable Systems for Reliable Health Monitoring

Preliminary Study on Adaptive MAC Protocol for Reliable Control in IEEE 802.15.6ma BANs

Kosei Nagai[1](✉), Jaakko Hyry[2], Takumi Kobayashi[2], and Daisuke Anzai[2]

[1] Guraduate School of Engineering, Nagoya Institute of Technology, Gokiso-cho, Showa-ku, Nagoya, Aichi 466-8555, Japan
cmj13119@ict.nitech.ac.jp

[2] Guraduate School of Information, Osaka Metropolitan University, 1-1, Gakuen-cho, Naka-ku, Sakai, Osaka 564-8565, Japan
{jaakko,kobayashi.takumi,d.anzai}@omu.ac.jp

Abstract. Smart biological control support systems that control medical devices based on sensed vital data in a body area network (BAN) have attracted attention. However, the current wireless communication standard IEEE 802.15.6ma does not take stable control of medical devices into consideration, and there is concern that the control system may become unstable. Therefore, in order to achieve stable operation of multiple control systems in a BAN, we propose an adaptive control MAC protocol that derives an upper bound of packet loss probability and based on it, operates dynamically. This protocol increases retransmission opportunities by allocating more timeslots to control systems with high packet error rate (PER), thereby improving the overall stability. In the simulation, the norm-squared mean of the state vector asymptotically approaches zero with adaptive control, resulting in improved stability.

Keywords: BAN · MAC protocol · Control system · Medical devices

1 Introduction

Smart biological control support systems have been proposed that utilize cyber-physical systems and digital twin technologies in body area network (BAN) [1,2] to control medical devices such as gait support robots, myoelectric prosthetic hands, and even vagus nerve stimulators and insulin pumps based on sensed vital data [3,4]. To realize this system, it is essential to design a medium access control (MAC) protocol that enables data transmission to guarantee stable operation of the control target. However, IEEE 802.15.6ma [5], which is currently proposed as a wireless communication standard specifically for BAN, does not

This work was supported in part by JSPS KAKENHI Grant Number JP21H01325 and the MIC/FORWARD # JPMI250830001.

H. Tanaka et al. (Eds.): BodyNets 2025, LNICST 714, pp. 331–339, 2026.
https://doi.org/10.1007/978-3-032-38657-1_27

consider the stable control of medical devices. Furthermore, while similar studies exist addressing signal interference issues when multiple BANs coexist [6] and signal interference between devices due to posture changes [7], the stability of devices based on control theory has not been verified. Consequently, the possibility remains that the control systems of devices could become unstable due to wireless control.

In this study, we examine the conditions for stabilizing multiple control systems in a BAN, and design a MAC protocol whose protocol dynamically changes according to these conditions, in order to achieve stable operation of medical devices in the BAN. The effectiveness of the proposed MAC protocol is verified through computer simulations, and the stability of control in a BAN environment with multiple control systems is also evaluated.

2 Proposal of Adaptive MAC Protocol for Reliable Control

2.1 Principle of Upper Bound on Packet Error Rate for Stable Control

Figure 1 shows a closed-loop control system for the control target G, a discrete-time linear system. State equation of the system uses (1), while (2) shows the signal $\hat{u}(k)$ from the controller. The control input $u(k)$ that through the communication channel is shown by (3), and the state vector $\hat{x}(k)$ that through the communication channel is shown by (4). The probability density function $\theta_1(k)$, $\theta_2(k)$ uses (5) and (6) as follows:

$$x(k+1) = Ax(k) + Bu(k) \tag{1}$$

$$v(k) = Kx(k) \tag{2}$$

$$u(k) = \theta_2(k)\hat{u}(k) \tag{3}$$

$$\hat{x}(k) = \theta_1(k)x(k) \tag{4}$$

$$\Pr\{\theta_1(k) = i\} = \begin{cases} \alpha_1 & i = 0 \\ 1 - \alpha_1 & i = 1 \end{cases} \tag{5}$$

$$\Pr\{\theta_2(k) = i\} = \begin{cases} \alpha_2 & i = 0 \\ 1 - \alpha_2 & i = 1, \end{cases} \tag{6}$$

where $x(k) \in \mathbb{R}^n$ is the state vector, $u(k) \in \mathbb{R}^m$ is the control input, A is the unstable state matrix, B is the input matrix, K is the state feedback gain, α_1 is the packet loss probability for the communication path from the control target to the hub, and α_2 is the packet loss probability for the communication path from the hub to the control target.

In the control system shown in Fig. 1, a necessary and sufficient condition for the existence of a control law such that the closed-loop system is square mean stable is that the packet loss probability α_1, α_2 satisfies the following equation [8]

$$\alpha_1 < \frac{1}{\prod_{|\lambda_i|>1} |\lambda_i|^{2N/N_1}} \tag{7}$$

$$\alpha_2 < \frac{1}{\prod_{|\lambda_i|>1} |\lambda_i|^{2N/N_2}}, \tag{8}$$

where λ_i is the unstable eigenvalues of the state matrix A, N is the cycle length of transmission (number of discrete steps), and N_1 and N_2 are the number of transmission steps within cycle N for the control input and state output, respectively.

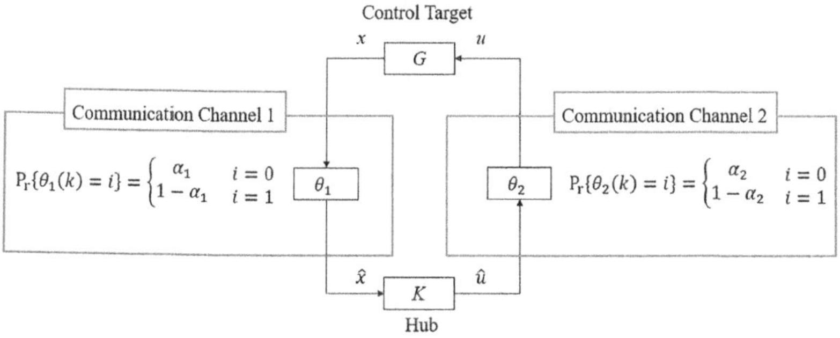

Fig. 1. Closed-loop control system

2.2 Proposed Adaptive MAC Protocol

Figure 2 shows the proposed superframe structure of the adaptive control MAC protocol in this study. This superframe includes a Network Management Period (NMP), a Contention Free Period (CFP), and an Inactive Period (IAP). In CFP, each sensor is allocated a time slot in which it can send packets containing status signals. Figure 3 shows the network topology of the proposed MAC protocol. The hub collects information from sensor nodes in the BAN and sends packets containing control input to each controller. We compare the actual Packet Error Rate (PER) of each control system with the upper bound of the packet loss probability derived by using (7), and propose an adaptive control MAC protocol that allocates more time slots to control systems with low PER characteristics. This increases the retransmission opportunities for control systems with low PER characteristics, thereby achieving stable control of all control systems in the BAN.

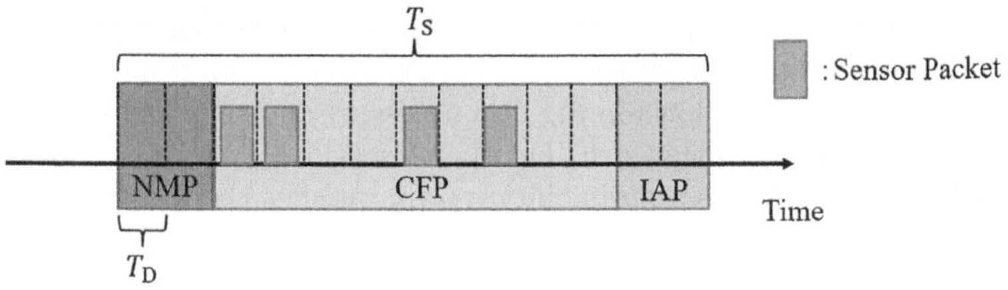

Fig. 2. Superframe structure for proposed MAC protocol

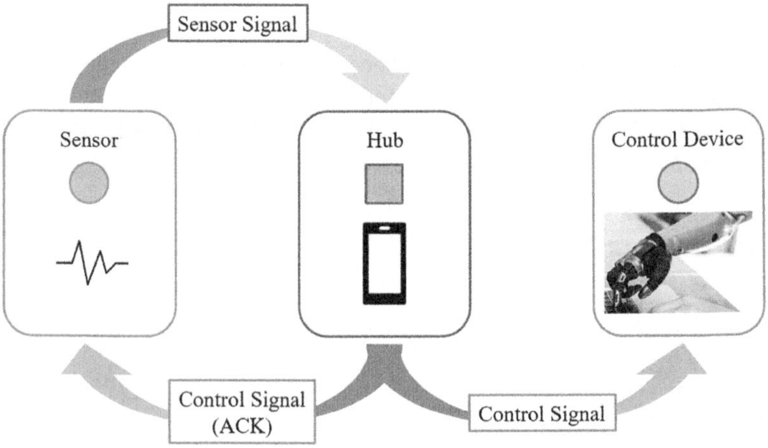

Fig. 3. Network topology of proposed MAC protocol

3 Computer Simulation Environment

This study evaluates the effectiveness of the proposed adaptive control MAC protocol when multiple control systems exist in a BAN. For comparison, we evaluate the effectiveness of adaptive control in improving the stability of the control system, assuming not only the proposed protocol but also the case where the superframe structure is the same but no adaptive control is used.

The parameters set in the computer simulation are shown in Table 1, and the combination of sensors assigned to each control system and the SNR of the communication channels are shown in Table 2. Simulation models 1, 2, and 3 represent the control systems within the BAN, with multiple sensors connected to each control system. In this study, we assume that packet loss occurs only in the communication paths that send signals from the sensors to the hub, and that each control system can always receive control inputs from the hub. The PER of each sensor used for adaptive control is also observable at the hub, and the state matrix A and input matrix B of each control system are also assumed to be known.

To quantitatively evaluate the stability of each control system, we use the expected squared norm of the state vector, $\mathbb{E}\left[\|x(t)\|^2\right]$, where $x(t)$ denotes the system state at time t. This value represents the mean energy of the system state, and a smaller value indicates higher stability. In the simulations, the expectation $\mathbb{E}[\cdot]$ is approximated by the average over N independent runs as

$$\mathbb{E}\left[\|x(t)\|^2\right] \approx \frac{1}{N}\sum_{i=1}^{N} \|x_i(t)\|^2,$$

where $x_i(t)$ is the state vector obtained in the i-th simulation run. The results shown in the figures correspond to this averaged value at each sampling instant. By comparing $\mathbb{E}\left[\|x(t)\|^2\right]$ between the proposed adaptive control MAC protocol and the non-adaptive case, we can quantitatively assess the improvement in the stability of multiple control systems within a BAN.

Table 1. Computer simulation parameters

Communication time	10 s
Superframe length T_S	100 ms
Timeslot length T_D	1 ms
NMP length	5 timeslots
CFP length	90 timeslots
IAP length	5 timeslots
Number of control targets	3
Number of sensors	10
Maximum retransmission	30
Modulation method	BPSK
Sampling rate	100 ms
Packet length	2000 bits
Trials	100

Table 2. Combination of sensors in simulation models

	Sensor index									
	1	2	3	4	5	6	7	8	9	10
SNR	15dB	7dB	7dB	15dB	7dB	15dB	15dB	15dB	15dB	15dB
Simulation model 1	√	√	√		√		√			
Simulation model 2		√	√	√	√					√
Simulation model 3		√	√		√	√			√	

4 Results and Discussion

Figures 4 and 5 show the evaluation results of the norm-squared mean of the state vector of each control system for the MAC protocol without and with adaptive control, respectively. The mean squared error on the vertical axis indicates the deviation from the target value of the sensor associated with each control system. In other words, if this value asymptotically approaches zero, the control system becomes stable; conversely, if this value diverges, the control system becomes unstable. In Fig. 4, the mean squared norm approaches zero for all control systems initially over time. However, it abruptly increases around 3 s, indicating that the control system became unstable without adaptive control. In contrast, Fig. 5 shows that the mean squared norm for all control systems approaches zero over time, achieving nearly zero around 3 s. This confirms that the control system stabilized due to the effect of adaptive control.

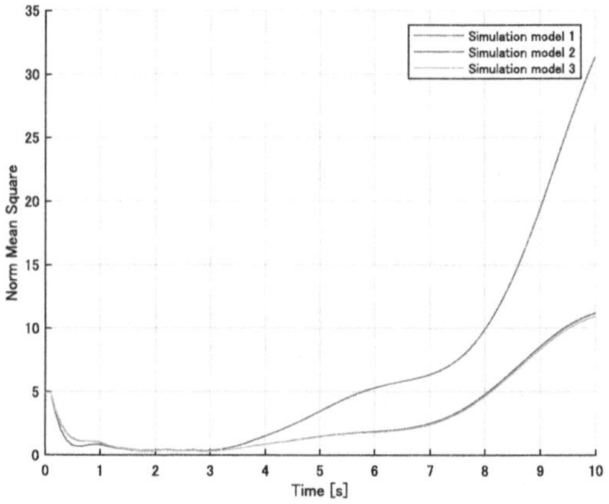

Fig. 4. Simulation result for MAC protocol w/o adaptive control

Tables 3 and 4 show the average of the PER and the upper bound of the packet loss probability for each control system for the MAC protocol without and with adaptive control, respectively. Comparing Table 3 and Table 4 reveals that the average PER and upper bounds of packet loss probability for each sensor show little difference. Despite the lack of difference in average PER and packet loss probability upper bounds, the significant difference in control system stability can be attributed to the difference in packet retransmission opportunities. Without adaptive control, sensors with low SNR characteristics received the same number of allocated time slots as other sensors. Consequently, they could not retransmit packets within their allocated time slots, leading to control being performed with insufficient information and resulting in system instability. In contrast, with adaptive control, sensors with low SNR characteristics could be prioritized for time slot allocation. This allowed them to utilize more retransmission opportunities to send packets, enabling control with sufficient information

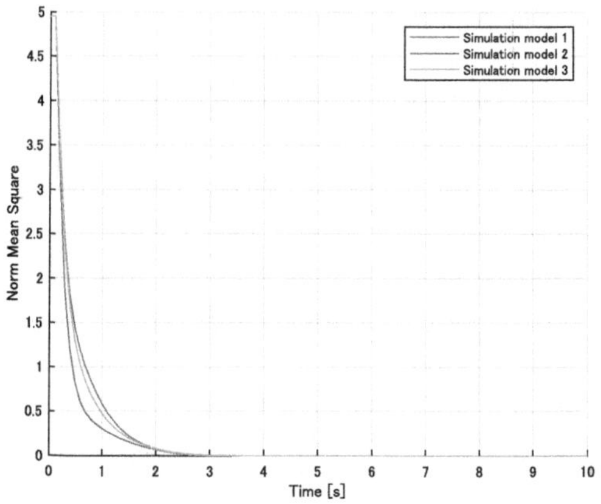

Fig. 5. Simulation result for MAC protocol w/ adaptive control

and resulting in a stable control system. Based on these results, we were able to confirm the effectiveness of the proposed adaptive control method in improving the stability of the control system.

Table 3. Simulation result summary (w/o adaptive control)

	SNR [dB]	Average PER	α_1
Sensor 1	15	$<10^{-4}$	0.611204368
Sensor 2	7	0.9539791	0.611204368
Sensor 3	7	0.9533519	0.611204368
Sensor 4	15	$<10^{-4}$	0.611204368
Sensor 5	7	0.95325487	0.611204368
Sensor 6	15	$<10^{-4}$	0.611204368
Sensor 7	15	$<10^{-4}$	0.611204368
Sensor 8	15	$<10^{-4}$	0.611204368
Sensor 9	15	$<10^{-4}$	0.611204368
Sensor 10	15	$<10^{-4}$	0.611204368

Table 4. Simulation result summary (w/ adaptive control)

	SNR [dB]	Average PER	α_1
Sensor 1	15	$<10^{-4}$	0.611204368
Sensor 2	7	0.95395534	0.611204368
Sensor 3	7	0.95378558	0.611204368
Sensor 4	15	$<10^{-4}$	0.611204368
Sensor 5	7	0.95495739	0.611204368
Sensor 6	15	$<10^{-4}$	0.611204368
Sensor 7	15	$<10^{-4}$	0.611204368
Sensor 8	15	$<10^{-4}$	0.611204368
Sensor 9	15	$<10^{-4}$	0.611204368
Sensor 10	15	$<10^{-4}$	0.611204368

5 Conclusion

In this study, we proposed an adaptive control MAC protocol for stable control of medical devices in a BAN and evaluated its effectiveness. Computer simulation results showed that the stability of the control system can be improved by effectively allocating slots to control systems with low SNR characteristics.

Future studies include the estimation of state and input matrices for each control system, the estimation of PER for each sensor, and the effectiveness of adaptive control in environments where packet loss occurs in the communication path between the hub and each control system.

References

1. Anzai, D.: Introduction to trends of ETSI SmartBAN. In: 2019 URSI-Japan Radio Science Meeting (2019)
2. Hämäläinen, M., et al.: ETSI SmartBAN architecture: the global vision for smart body area networks. IEEE Access **8**, 150611–150625 (2020)
3. Johnson, Z., Saikia, M.J.: Digital twins for healthcare using wearables. Bioengineering **11**(6), 606 (2024)
4. Sun, T., He, X., Li, Z.: Digital twin in healthcare: recent updates and challenges. Digit. Health **9** (2023)
5. IEEE 802.15.6ma Technical Requirements Document [Online]. https://mentor.ieee.org/802.15/dcn/21/15-21-0577-02-006a-technicalrequirements-document.pdf
6. Anzai, D., Inuzuka, R., Kim, M., Hernandez, M., Kohno, R.: Fundamental MAC performance evaluation under multiple IEEE802.15.6ma BAN co-existence. In: 17th IEEE International Symposium on Medical Information and Communication Technology (2023)

7. Mile, A., Okeyo, G., Kibe, A.: Hybrid IEEE 802.15.6 wireless body area networks interference mitigation model for high mobility interference scenarios. Wirel. Eng. Technol. **9**(2) (2018)
8. Ishii, H.: Stabilization under shared communication with message losses and its limitations. In: Proceedings of the 45th IEEE Conference on Decision and Control 4974/4979 (2006)

Performance Evaluation on IEEE 802.15.6ma-Based UWB Ranging in Coexistence Environment

Yuhei Oguri[1(✉)], Jaakko Hyry[2], Takumi Kobayashi[2], and Daisuke Anzai[2]

[1] Graduate School of Engineering, Nagoya Institute of Technology, Gokiso-cho, Showa-ku, Nagoya, Aichi 466-8555, Japan
y.oguri.385@stn.nitech.ac.jp

[2] graduate School of Informatics, Osaka Metropolitan University, 1-1, Gakuen-cho, Naka-ku, Sakai, Osaka 599-8531, Japan
{jaakko,kobayashi.takumi,d.anzai}@omu.ac.jp

Abstract. Ultra-wideband (UWB) has been increasingly integrated into devices such as smartphones and digital keys, where it is expected to be used not only for data transmission but also for high-precision ranging. In particular, the IEEE 802.15.6ma standard for Body Area Network (BAN) considers mutual communication via UWB transmission between Human BAN (HBAN), which are attached to the human body, and Vehicle BAN (VBAN), which are installed in vehicles such as buses. However, as UWB-enabled devices become more widespread, mutual interference among UWB signals may degrade ranging accuracy, highlighting the need for a quantitative evaluation of ranging performance under interference conditions. In this study, we evaluated the ranging accuracy of UWB systems in environments where multiple BANs coexist, using computer simulations that model multipath conditions in a hospital room. Furthermore, to mitigate the effects of interference, we proposed a UWB ranging method that employs M-sequence spreading codes, and verified its effectiveness. Simulation results demonstrate that the use of M-sequences improves ranging accuracy under interference-rich conditions.

Keywords: Ultra-wideband · Ranging · Interference Mitigation

1 Introduction

In recent years, ultra-wideband (UWB) has been increasingly applied to devices such as smartphones and digital keys, leveraging its wide bandwidth to enable high-precision ranging [1]. Among its various applications, the TG6ma for Body Area Network (BAN) has been considering the use of UWB for mutual communication between Human BAN (HBAN), which are worn on the human body,

This work was supported in part by JST [Moonshot R&D][Grant Number JPMJMS2214-06] and the MIC/FORWARD # JPMI250830001.

H. Tanaka et al. (Eds.): BodyNets 2025, LNICST 714, pp. 340–346, 2026.
https://doi.org/10.1007/978-3-032-38657-1_28

and Vehicle BAN (VBAN), which are installed in vehicles [2] [3]. Due to its extremely high distance resolution, UWB is expected to be utilized in a variety of scenarios, such as detecting patient locations in hospitals and enabling keyless entry systems for vehicles. However, as the number of UWB-enabled devices increases, mutual interference between devices becomes a concern, potentially degrading ranging accuracy. Therefore, quantitative evaluation of ranging performance under interference-prone conditions is required. This issue is particularly critical in enclosed spaces such as hospital rooms or vehicle interiors, where the coexistence of multiple BANs leads to complex multipath propagation and signal interference from other devices, making degradation in ranging performance unavoidable. In this study, we evaluate the ranging accuracy of UWB systems under such conditions using computer simulations that replicate a multipath environment in a hospital room. The Time of Arrival (TOA) method is employed for ranging, and the impact of multiple UWB interference sources is analyzed [4] [5]. Additionally, to mitigate the effects of interference, we propose the use of M-sequence spreading codes and quantitatively compare ranging accuracy before and after their application. Through this investigation, we aim to demonstrate the potential for improved ranging performance in interference-rich environments and to provide foundational knowledge for future real-world applications.

2 Principle of Interference Rejection Using M-Sequences

The M-sequence used for interference rejection has the following two characteristics. First, its autocorrelation function exhibits a sharp peak at zero phase difference and remains sufficiently low at all non-zero phase differences. Second, the cross-correlation between different code sequences remains low for all relative phase shifts. Let $a(t)$ and $b(t)$ be two signals that repeat with a common period p, and let τ denote the time shift between them. The cross-correlation function R_{ab} between these signals is defined as follows [6]

$$R_{ab}(\tau) = \frac{1}{p} \int_0^p a(t) \cdot b(t - \tau)\, dt. \tag{1}$$

In this study, interference rejection is achieved by leveraging these two properties. We assumed the communication channel model illustrated in the block diagram in Fig. 1.

3 Simulation Environment

A UWB pulse signal with a bandwidth of 3.1–10.6 GHz is used as the transmitted signal. One transmitter Tx and up to five interference sources In, are employed. The distance between the transmitter Tx and the receiver Rx is fixed at 3 m, while the distance between each interference source In and Rx is randomly selected between 1 m and 6 m using a uniform distribution. Up to six M-sequences (31-bit, BPSK-modulated) are assigned to each signal source. Impulse

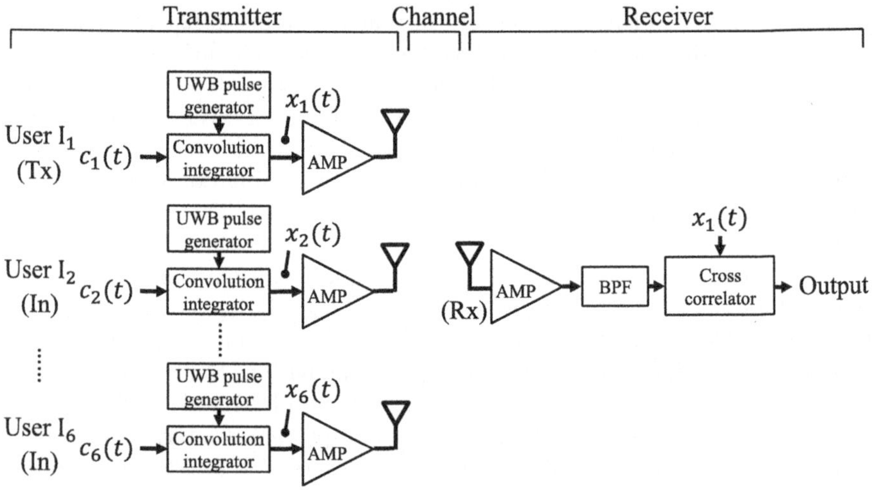

Fig. 1. Block Diagram of UWB Localization Using M-Sequences

trains $c_n(t)$, generated from the M-sequences, are convolved and integrated with the UWB pulse signals. The resulting waveforms, denoted by $x_n(t)$, represent the output signals from each source. Each waveform $x_n(t)$ propagates through the communication channel and is received at the receiver Rx. At the receiver, the signals are cross-correlated with the reference signal $x_1(t)$, which is generated from the M-sequence assigned to the transmitter Tx. This cross-correlation process is intended to extract the signal from Tx, while suppressing the contributions from interference sources In. The resulting waveform is treated as the output of the cross-correlation process. To identify the First Arrival Path (FAP), a thresholding method is applied to the cross-correlated signal [7]. In this method, the threshold is set as a fraction θ of the maximum amplitude of the cross-correlation output, and the first sample exceeding this threshold is identified as the FAP. TOA of this path is then used to estimate the distance between the transmitter and receiver. In this study, three threshold values $\theta = 0.4, 0.7, 1$ are used. The amplitude a_l of the lth path in the power delay profile (PDP) is derived using the path loss model and the following equation:

$$10\log_{10}|a_l|^2 = 10\log_{10}\exp\left(-\frac{\tau_l}{\Gamma}\right), \tag{2}$$

where Γ is the path power decay time constant, and τ_l is the delay time [ns] of the lth path. The arrival time of the lth path is determined by an independent exponential probability density function. The number of reflected paths is modeled as a Poisson-distributed random variable. In this study, $\Gamma = 59.7$ ns, mean arrival time interval $1/\lambda = 1.85$ ns, and mean number of arriving paths $\overline{K} = 38.1$. These parameters were calculated based on empirical data obtained from measurements conducted in an actual hospital room in a previous study. In the measurement setup, UWB signal with a frequency range of 3.0–11.0 GHz

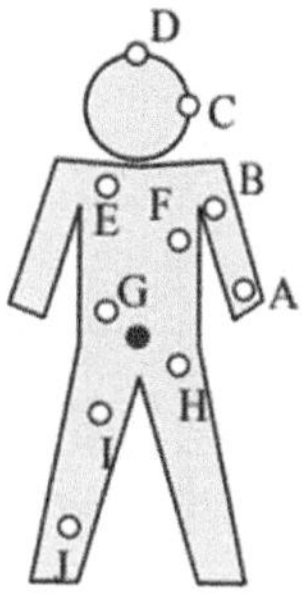

Fig. 2. Measurement setup for the human body [8]

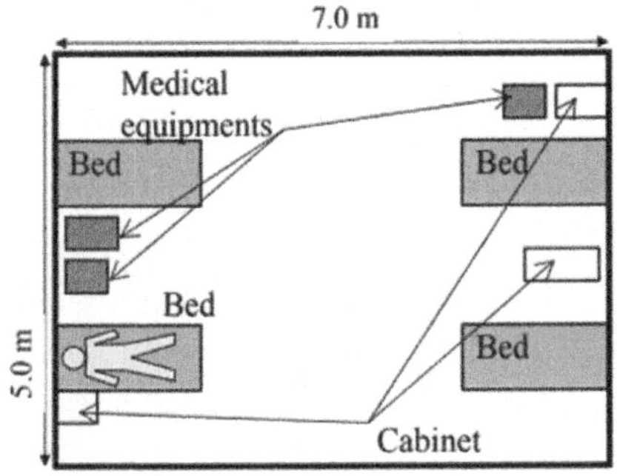

Fig. 3. Layout of the hospital room [8]

was transmitted from the transmitter and received by antennas attached to the surface of the human body. The antenna placement on the human body and the layout of the hospital room during the measurements are illustrated in Figs. 2 and 3 [8].

4 Simulation Results

As an example, Fig. 4 shows the received signal at the receiver Rx when one transmitter Tx and one interference source In are present, with the M-sequence applied. Figure 5 presents the result of cross-correlation between the received signal in Fig. 4 and the waveform $x_1(t)$. In this figure, the blue and red dashed lines indicate the time durations during which the interference signal and the signal from the transmitter Tx are present, respectively. From Fig. 5, it can be observed that the interference signal is significantly attenuated or eliminated, whereas the signal from the transmitter Tx remains clearly visible.
Subsequently, Fig. 6, Fig. 7 show the ranging error in terms of Root Mean Squared Error (RMSE) and success rate of FAP detection in Time of Arrival (TOA) simulation before and after the introduction of M-sequence. The simulation is conducted under the conditions of threshold $\theta = 0.4$ and SNR $= 0$ dB, with 10,000 trials. In Fig. 6, where no M-sequence is applied, both the RMSE and the success rate of FAP detection deteriorate as the number of interference sources increases. In contrast, Fig. 7, which reflects the use of M-sequences, shows that the RMSE and the detection success rate remain relatively stable regardless of the number of interfering signals. This demonstrates the effectiveness of the M-sequence in mitigating the effects of interference on ranging performance. Furthermore, among the three thresholds tested, the threshold $\theta = 0.4$ yielded the best performance. As a result, it is found that the introduction of the M-sequence improve the success rate of FAP detection by up to approximately 60% and reduced the RMSE by up to about 2 m.

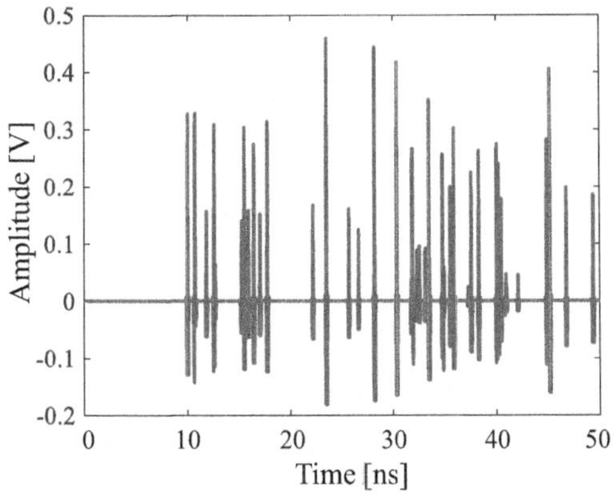

Fig. 4. Received Signal (w/o Additive White Gaussian Noise (AWGN))

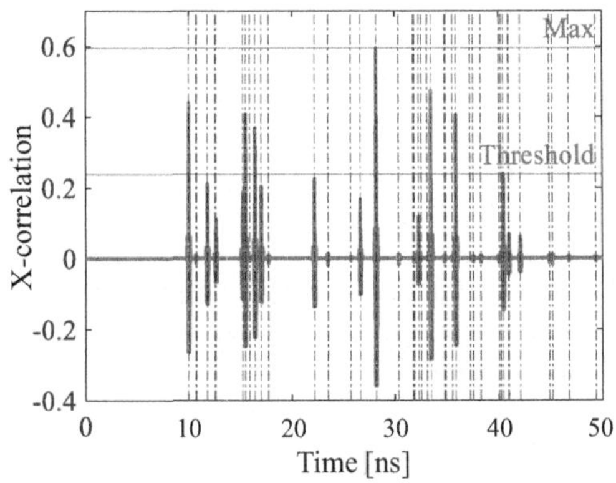

Fig. 5. Cross-Correlated Received Signal

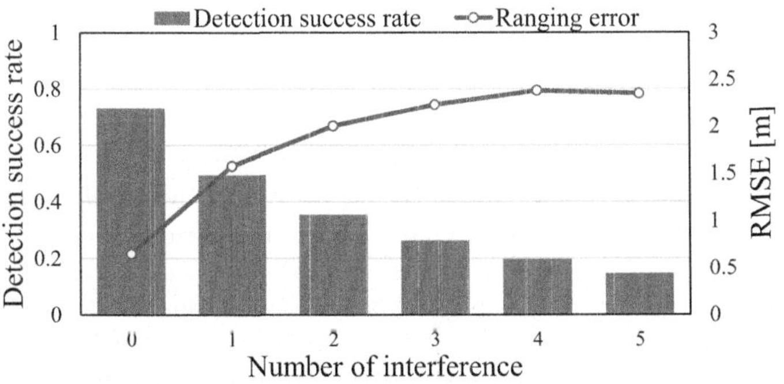

Fig. 6. Decision Rate and RMSE (w/o M-sequence)

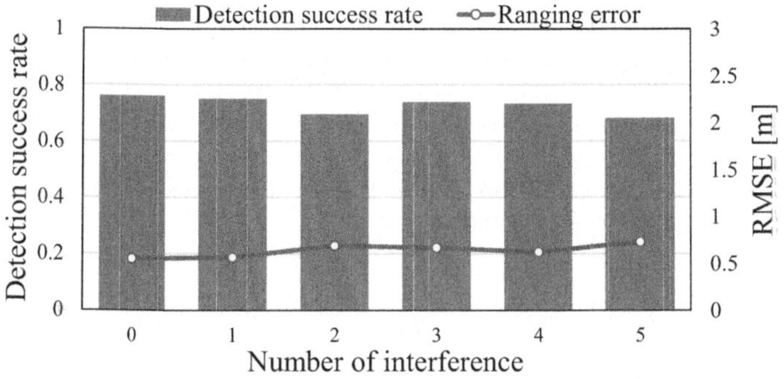

Fig. 7. Decision Rate and RMSE (w/ M-sequence)

5 Conclusions

In this study, we evaluated the change the degradation in UWB ranging accuracy between transmitters and receivers before and after the introduction of M-sequences in a simulated hospital room environment with multiple ultra-wideband BAN interference sources. When the threshold value was set to $\theta = 0.4$, the introduction of M-sequences improved the success rate of FAP detection by up to approximately 60% and reduced the RMSE by up to approximately 2 m. Future work is required to determine the optimal value of the threshold θ.

References

1. Nakagawa, Y., et al.: Development of microwave ultra-wide-band tag location system using stand-alone reader architecture. Panasonic Tech. J. **57**(1), 54–59 (2011)
2. Otto, C., Milemkovic, A., Sanders, C., Jovanov, E.: System architecture of a wireless body area sensor network for ubiquitous health monitoring. J. Mob. Multimed. **1**(4), 307–326 (2006)
3. Hernandez, M., Kohno, R., Kobayashi, T., Anzai, D., Kim, M.: Standardization activities of IEEE P802.15.6ma wireless human and vehicle area networks. In: 2023 IEEE 17th International Symposium on Medical Information and Communication Technology (ISMICT), Lincoln, NE, USA, pp. 01–05 (2023). https://doi.org/10.1109/ISMICT58261.2023.10152145
4. Ning, X., Sha, X., Wu, X.: A TOA estimation method for IR-UWB ranging systems. In: 2010 First International Conference on Pervasive Computing, Signal Processing and Applications, Harbin, China, pp. 684–687 (2010). https://doi.org/10.1109/PCSPA.2010.170
5. Nouali, I.Y., Slimane, Z., Abdelmalek, A.: Change point detection-based TOA estimation in UWB indoor ranging systems. In: 2022 45th International Conference on Telecommunications and Signal Processing (TSP), Prague, Czech Republic, pp. 329–332 (2022). https://doi.org/10.1109/TSP55681.2022.9851238
6. Marubayashi, G., et al.: Spread Spectrum Communication and Its Applications. The Institute of Electronics, Information and Communication Engineers (1998)

7. Guvenc, I., Sahinoglu, Z.: Threshold-based TOA estimation for impulse radio UWB systems. In: 2005 IEEE International Conference on Ultra-Wideband, Zurich, Switzerland, pp. 420–425 (2005). https://doi.org/10.1109/ICU.2005.1570024
8. Takizawa, K., Aoyagi, T., Li, H.-B., Takada, J., Kobayashi, T., Kohno, R.: Path loss and power delay profile channel models for wireless body area networks. In: 2009 IEEE Antennas and Propagation Society International Symposium, North Charleston, SC, USA, pp. 1–4 (2009)

IoT-Based Non-invasive and Non-ionizing Bone Fracture Home-Monitoring System

Matti Hämäläinen[1(✉)], Amher Nazar[2], Juha-Pekka Mäkelä[1], Timo Kumpuniemi[1], Roope Parviainen[3], Juha-Jaakko Sinikumpu[3], and Jari Iinatti[1]

[1] Centre for Wireless Communications, University of Oulu, Oulu, Finland
{matti.hamalainen,juha-pekka.makela,timo.kumpuniemi,jari.iinatti}@oulu.fi
[2] University of Oulu, Oulu, Finland
amher.nazar@student.oulu.fi
[3] Research Unit of Clinical Medicine, University of Oulu and Oulu University Hospital, Oulu, Finland
{roope.parviainen,juha-jaakko.sinikumpu}@oulu.fi

Abstract. Fractures of various bones represent common musculoskeletal injuries requiring clinical intervention. A standard treatment approach involves the realignment of fractured bones followed by immobilization using a cast. This facilitates a proper bone union over time. Throughout the ossification process, alignment is regularly assessed to ensure appropriate healing and to identify any deviations indicative of malunion or other complications. Radiographic imaging, typically using ionizing X-rays, is the primary modality employed for this monitoring. In this paper, we are evaluating the possibility to carry out non-invasive and non-ionizing monitoring using cost-effective Internet of Things (IoT) -based solutions enabling the usage also for patients at their home locations. The proof-of-concept type examination pointed out that the angular displacement could be detected using simple IoT sensor nodes. Avoiding X-rays is a preferable solution as, especially for children and other vulnerable people, the non-ionizing solutions are safer. It is also possible to use IoT -based systems when being outpatient which is one of the keypoints in this paper.

Keywords: accelerometer · angular displacement · sensor

1 Introduction

The children play, run, and climb. Cycling is a popular hobby and electric scooters are very popular today. Also other simple tasks that people do everyday are possible causes for injuries: Falling from a ladder, falling down by a bike, or just slipping on an icy road are incidents that could cause a bone fracture. When falling, typically the forearms, especially wrists, are used first to smooth a drop before hitting the ground. In an unfortunate situation, this may lead to an

H. Tanaka et al. (Eds.): BodyNets 2025, LNICST 714, pp. 347–359, 2026.
https://doi.org/10.1007/978-3-032-38657-1_29

injury, e.g., in the ulna or wrist bones, etc. Not only an forearm or a wrist, but also the bones in a person's legs are prone to break. It is worth to notice that these are examples of illustrative cases encountered by numerous individuals in the society.

There are also other issues which could increase the vulnerability for bone fractures, such as osteoporosis, which can be found among the elderly population. Osteoporosis affects bone structure, making bones more brittle and susceptible to fractures [1]. Additionally, participation in various action sports increases the likelihood of bone fractures. As a result, fractures do not only affect the younger population; elderly individuals are also at greater risk due to the porosity of their bones. Furthermore, fractures can affect individuals across all age groups, particularly those with active lifestyles. The typical management of such trauma involves either surgical intervention and/or casting, depending on the severity of the fracture.

Bone fractures are among the most common injuries worldwide and are recognized as a significant public health issue on a global scale [1]. According to recent data, the global age-standardized incidence rate of fractures was 2,296.2 per 100,000 individuals in 2019. Fractures also contribute substantially to morbidity in the pediatric population. The literature indicates that approximately 27% to 50% of children experience at least one fracture before the age of 18 [2]. Specifically, the incidence of fractures in children under the age of five has been estimated to range between 50 and 100 per 10,000 person-years in European populations [3–5].

The disabling effects of bone fractures extend beyond personal injury; they also have significant societal impacts. Medical treatments and the healing process often result in work absences, unexpected costs, and increased travel requirements for hospital, clinic, or health center. Unfortunately, the need for medical intervention does not end after the initial treatment or surgery. Post-operative evaluations are necessary to assess whether the healing process is proceeding as expected, ensuring that the fractured bone ends are properly rejoined. Currently, *de facto* -standard for follow-up monitoring involves the use of X-ray imaging. While X-rays are effective in monitoring bone healing, they are an ionizing technique and, therefore, are not an ideal method due to the radiation exposure involved. However, they remain a reliable and widely adopted practice for post-fracture monitoring.

During the healing process, misalignment can occur if the angle between the fractured bone segments deviates from the original alignment established during a surgery or casting. Additionally, the relative position of the bone fragments may change. If the deviation exceeds a critical threshold, further surgical intervention may be required. Displacement can occur if, for instance, the reduction in swelling during healing creates an air gap between the limb and the cast, potentially allowing for movement of the bone fragments. Trauma, such as intense impacts to the cast, can also lead to misalignment.

The possible dislocations of the bones, in angular or displacements to any directions, should be rather accurately detected. As pointed out in [6], the acceptable angular change in adults during the healing process in a wrist dorsally (thus, backwards) is 15°. In pediatric cases, greater angular deviations may be tolerated. Depending on the child's age, the tilt angle—defined as the angulation between the healing bone fragments, measured in degrees—can range up to 20–30° [6]. In practice, displacements, or linear spacing in other words, should not happen in our use-case. However, during the study, we considered that movement too, as the experimental results can be utilized in other applications.

The objective of our research was to develop a non-invasive method to monitor the alignment of the fractured bone in real time and without ionizing radioation. A simplified presentation of the environment in this research is depicted in Fig. 1.

Once changes in the alignment of the fracture are detected (i.e., when the predefined threshold is exceeded), an alert can be sent to the patient or communicated to healthcare professionals. Wireless connectivity allows ubiquitous access for medical personnel to remotely monitor the healing process. Following an alert, the patient should visit a hospital for a more thorough examination. In such cases, the use of X-ray imaging is justified and essential. If no changes in the bone position are detected, unnecessary medical visits and X-ray examinations can be avoided.

In this study, we do not focus on any specific bones, as the proposed solution is intended to be generic. However, the forearm bones are used as an example. The ideal solution for healing monitoring is one that is applicable in outpatient settings. Additionally, the monitoring system must be small, durable, and energy-efficient. When attached to the skin, bio-compatibility issues must also be carefully considered [7].

All these motivate us to develop a real-time remote monitoring concept for the observation of the healing process. In this case, real-time means the timeframe within the context of a bone-fracture healing process.

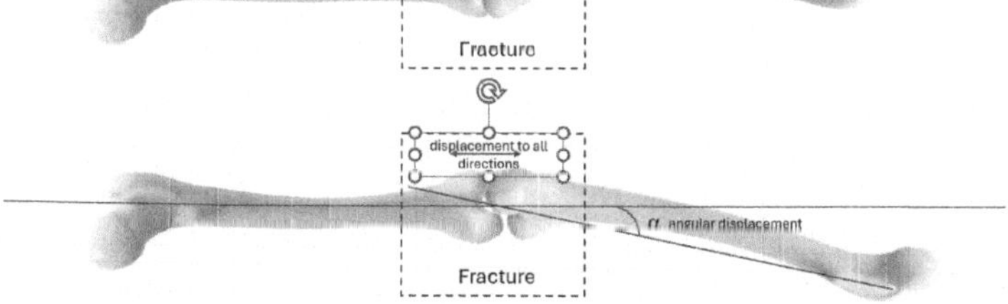

Fig. 1. Parameters to be monitored during the bone ossification.

In the case of all notified changes, either being angular or displacement to any directions, if the ossification process of the bones has not been progressed as expected, a re-evaluation of the trauma by the medical professionals is required.

This paper is structured as follows. In Sect. 2, a short literature review about the methods to study bone fracture healing process is given. In Sect. 3, the Internet of Things (IoT) -based method is proposed. Section 4 describes the experiments that have been carried out and the obtained results are given in Sect. 5. Prospects to continue the started work are discussed in Sect. 6. Finally, Sect. 7 concludes the paper.

2 Related Work

As per today, there are no wearable non-invasive and non-ionizing methods developed for a limb bone fracture healing process monitoring available in the market. However, some preliminary studies how this problem could be solved have been carried out. In [6], two radio frequency (RF) based non-invasive methods have been proposed. The proposed solutions are based on measuring the difference in time-of-flight between the sensor nodes installed both sides of the fracture. Nodes can be located under the cast and on the cast, depending on the solution. The proposed techniques are based on a transmitter-receiver pair (TX-RX pair) and radar approaches.

The TX-RX pair requires several transceiver pairs to be implemented to detect all the angular directions, and the displacement detection is performed using a triangulation to detect possible changes in the relative limb positions. However, it has not been verified yet if this method could provide accuracy being enough for the desired application. In this solution, the sensor nodes need to be attached to the skin, under the cast. However, battery can be located outside or in the cast to make the installation easier and more flexible. Due to the rather short distances/movements need to be detected, high frequencies and high signal bandwidth are needed to fulfill the required detection accuracy. The initial performance could be improved using antenna arrays, but then, the complexity and size of the implementation increases. For high distance resolution, ultra wideband (UWB) signaling is preferred as the achieved delay resolution is inversely proportional to the signal bandwidth [9]. This means that the smaller changes could be detected, the higher should the bandwidth of the probing signal be.

A problem in the radar -based solution would also be related to the short distance the signal propagates. As the radar (at least two are needed to improve the spatial coverage), which could be installed on top of the cast, is only few centimeters away from the bone, the reflected signal receives back the radar very fast. This sets a hard operational requirement for the radar to change its operation mode from transmitter mode to receiver one. Using frequency modulated continuous wave (FMCW) signal, it might be possible to detect a reflected waveform faster, during the transmission time, but the required signal bandwidth still needs to be high [10]. Finally, both of these RF -based techniques require specific focus on antenna design and advanced signal processing to improve their usability in the case of short distances.

Another option presented in the literature is based on commercial bend sensors, as described in [11]. In this case, a flexible bend sensor is attached to a bare skin, the sensor crossing the fracture in both directions. The flex (bend) sensor is detecting the angular changes the possible bone dislocations are causing. As in the previous example, the idea is that the sensor nodes will set an alarm when the predefined threshold value is exceeded. Both of these presented sensing approaches [6] and [11] could be linked to a wireless home network by using an embedded radio transmitter module that enables connectivity. In the implementation, the radio and battery units could be located outside the cast, or within the cast, but the sensor itself should be attached onto the skin. The sensing elements themselves in the bend sensor approach need to be attached to the skin in order to be able to detected the possible angular displacement via the angular alterations between the fractured bones under observation. If the bend sensor is attached to the cast, the small angular changes cannot be detected as the cast is too rigid to move when the bones or tissues underneath are moving.

For example, in [8] and [12], Matlab simulations have been carried out to define how RF based non-invasive monitoring system utilizing machine learning (ML) and artificial intelligence (AI) can be used to improve the healing process monitoring. However, the given solution is not indicating the bone displacement or misalignment, but a healing of tissues by detecting the changes in the tissues' dielectric parameters. Bone fracture itself can be detected by measuring the changes of electromagnetic parameters, such as the dielectric constant and conductivity, as proposed in [13]. The measurements are based on detecting the increased amount of blood, which is then changing the relative permittivity (ϵ_r) of the object. However, an angular information cannot be achieved in this way.

If the monitoring is not targeted for angular change detection but detecting only a displacement/movement, it can be done using simple signal reflection measurements, such as measuring S-parameters S_{11} (a time domain reflectometry measurement), or measuring S-parameters S_{21} and S_{12}, which can be used to indicate a change within the propagation media, thus a fraction in our case [8]. In the measurements, the transmitted signal is passing through the media between the antennas but also reflecting back from any discontinuity, thus a boundary of a bone and a small blood/air gap. Based on this information, the possible fraction can be detected and its location from the antenna can then be calculated. Dielectric parameters of the propagation media have also an impact on the speed of the propagating signal, and thus, on the signal's flight time. This method needs a vector network analyzer, and the measurement installation is prone to noise.

Literature also lists invasive methods to detect bone movements, such as presented in [14]. Here, the ultrasound signal is used in a similar way than the TX-RX pair proposed in [6]. In this approach, the transceivers are implemented in the bones. In this case, the selected uses-cases are dealing with long bones. In the experiments in [15], a strain sensor with a bone plate was implemented to the fractured bone of a rabbit and data was then transferred using Bluetooth Low Energy (BLE) outside of the animal.

3 Proposed IoT -Based Method

Our proposed method is based on the use of cheap IoT nodes to be used to measure nodes' angular positions in the Earth magnetic field. We have selected WT9011DLC-BT50 9-axis accelerometer by WIT Motion [16] for our experiments. The selected IoT node includes accelerometer, gyroscope, angle sensor, inclinometer and magnetometer. In addition, the node provides a radio connectivity for data transfer via BLE. Thus, the sensor node provides all the information necessary to calculate mutual position differences between the two sensors. A node can be connected to computationally more powerful device for data post-processing. The sensor used in the proof-of-concept (PoC) -type study is shown in Fig. 2a. In the experiments the idea was to evaluate whether the sensor placement on both sides of the fracture, installed on the skin, can provide necessary information about the relative angular and location changes of the bones. During the post-processing the difference between the nodes' relative angles were calculated as well as the distance change when the nodes were separated.

The coordinates and the measured parameters are as shown in Fig. 2b. The value scales for yaw and pitch are $z = \pm 180°$ and $x = \pm 180°$, respectively, and for the roll $y = \pm 90°$.

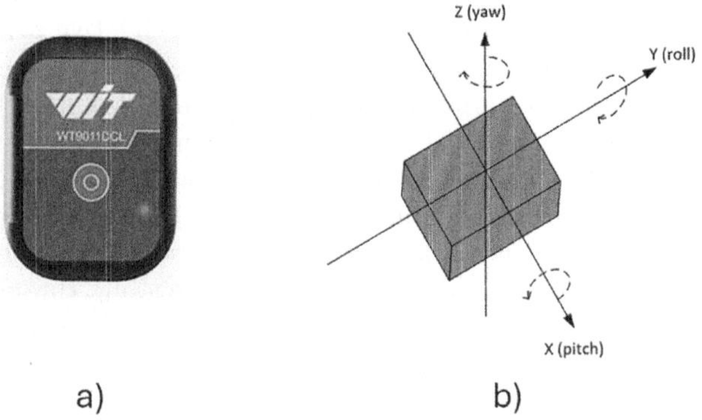

Fig. 2. a) WT9011DCL 9-axis BLE Magnetometer Gyroscope, b) Parameters the sensor provides.

During the data processing, an algorithm to remove gravitational effects were run by subtracting the error vector from the raw angular data provided by the nodes. This is done as

$$\begin{bmatrix} g_x \\ g_y \\ g_z \end{bmatrix} = \begin{bmatrix} -Gsin(x) \\ Gsin(y)cos(x) \\ Gcos(y)cos(x) \end{bmatrix}, \tag{1}$$

where gravity components $\mathbf{g}$ are calculated along the corresponding primary axes and G is the acceleration due to the Earth's gravity field, $G = 9.8\,\mathrm{m/s}$.

Calculation is done in radians. The gravity corrected accelerometer data a_{corr} is then calculated as

$$a_{corr} = \begin{bmatrix} a_x - g_x \\ a_y - g_y \\ a_z - g_z \end{bmatrix} . \tag{2}$$

Thus, the final angular results are showing the relative changes between the sensor nodes without an impact of the Earth's magnetic field.

From the angular data provided by the sensors, rotation matrices around the principal axes (X,Y,Z) can be calculated as [17]

$$R_x = \begin{bmatrix} 1 & 0 & 0 \\ 0 & cos(x) & -sin(x) \\ 0 & sin(x) & cos(x) \end{bmatrix} , \tag{3}$$

$$R_y = \begin{bmatrix} cos(y) & 0 & sin(y) \\ 0 & 1 & 0 \\ -sin(y) & 0 & cos(y) \end{bmatrix} , \tag{4}$$

$$R_z = \begin{bmatrix} cos(z) & -sin(z) & 0 \\ sin(z) & cos(z) & 0 \\ 0 & 0 & 1 \end{bmatrix} , \tag{5}$$

where x, y and z are the angles measured towards the corresponding primary axes X, Y and Z, respectively (Fig. 2b). The sensor orientation in 3D space is calculated as [17]

$$R_i = R_z^i \cdot R_y^i \cdot R_x^i , \tag{6}$$

where i denotes the individual node. In our case, $i \in \{1, 2\}$.

Rotation matrices need to be calculated for both sensor nodes and their relative rotation angle is obtained as [17]

$$R_{rel} = R_1^T R_2 , \tag{7}$$

where the transpose of R_1 (thus R_1^T) reverses the first sensor's orientation and align it with a common reference. Then after, the rotation of the second sensor R_2 relative to the first one, R_{rel}, can be calculated.

Finally, the relative angle Θ between the two sensor nodes are calculated as [17]

$$\Theta = cos^{-1}\left(\frac{trace(R_{rel}) - 1}{2}\right) . \tag{8}$$

As already mentioned, the sensor node WT9011DLC-BT50 [16] contains a BLE 5.0 radio module, which enables a wireless connectivity between the sensor node and a network. Since the node weight is only 9 g, it is suitable for daily use in wearable. However, this research is just a PoC study, and our goal was not to produce a final end-user application, where also the node's dimensions, power consumption, etc. would be optimized. The concrete goal is to evaluate if the proposed approach can be used in the corresponding use-case with the predefined limits.

In addition to the angular change, the dislocation to any directions can be calculated by comparing the relative distances within the primary axes of the nodes between the consecutive samples utilizing the obtained 3D-location information.

4 Experimental Work

The following discussion explains how the PoC experiments were carried out. The idea of this study was to evaluate if the specified IoT -based approach is capable to detect angular and lateral bone displacements and offer the required resolution. For simplicity, in our experiments the sensor nodes were attached to the regular pens, which were mimicking the fractured bone, as shown in Fig. 3. The readings of the angular rule and the angular results reported by the IoT sensors were then compared. This enables easy control of angle between the two pens and measure their relative angles, and then, evaluate the performance of the proposed system. The selected key performance indicators (KPIs) were accuracy and sensitivity to detect dislocation.

Similarly to the angular displacement, the capability of the sensors to detect dislocation changes were studied following the settings shown in Fig. 4. In this test, pens were moved back and forth using different speeds but remaining their relative angle the same ($\alpha = 0°$ as showed in conjunction with the lower bone in Fig. 1). In this case, the measurement was based on the relative velocity between the two nodes. The corresponding relative distance change evaluation was done using the Euclidean norm.

These two relative dislocations are the most interesting parameters to be monitored when the healing of the bone fracture ossification is performed.

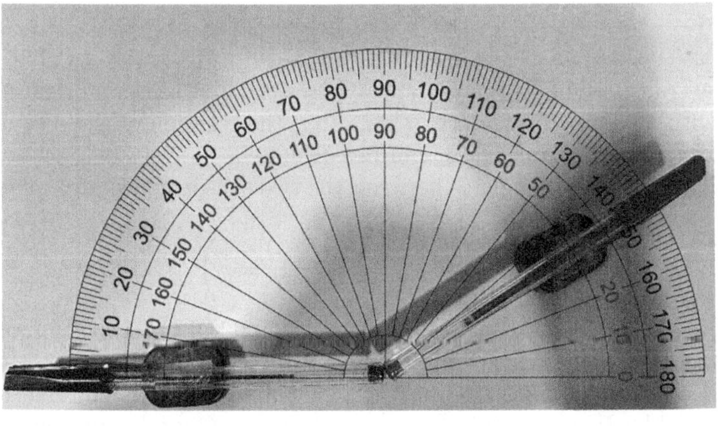

Fig. 3. Nodes installation for angular test measurements.

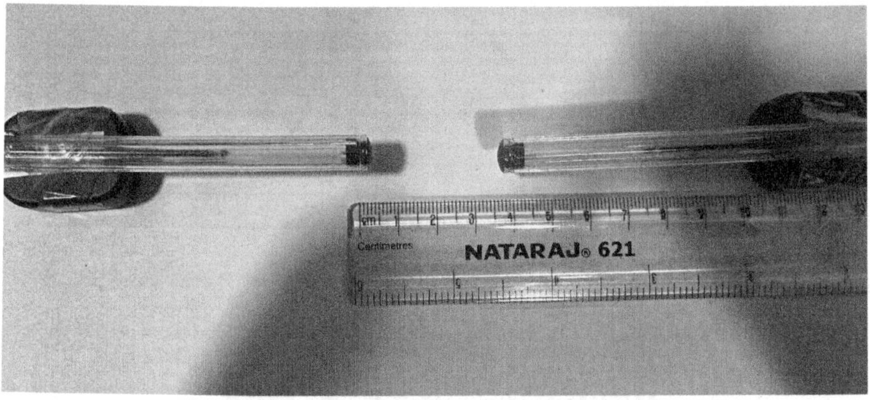

Fig. 4. Measuring displacement.

The sensor nodes were connected to a laptop PC using BLE, which enabled to show the graphical visualization of the results real-time via Matlab application

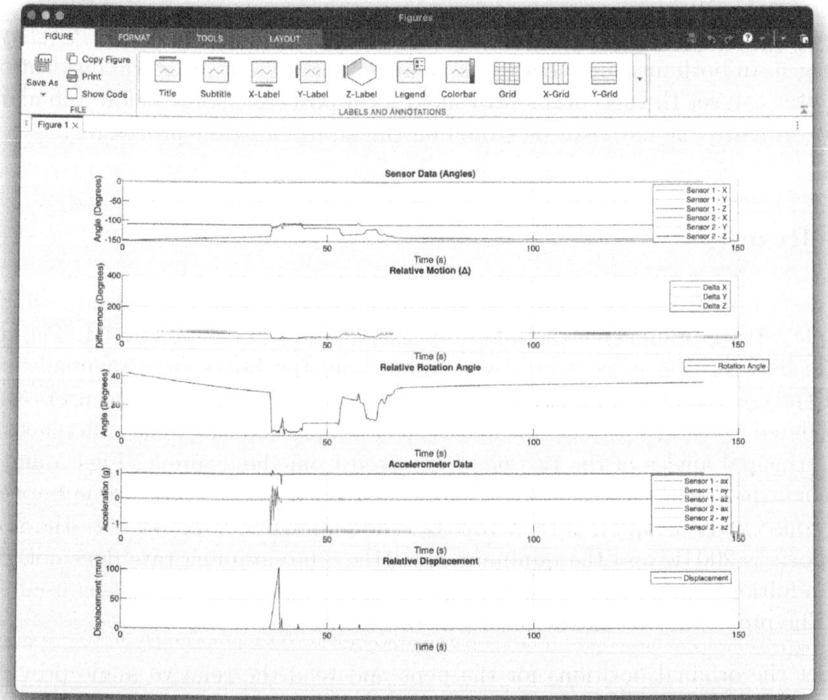

Fig. 5. Real time data.

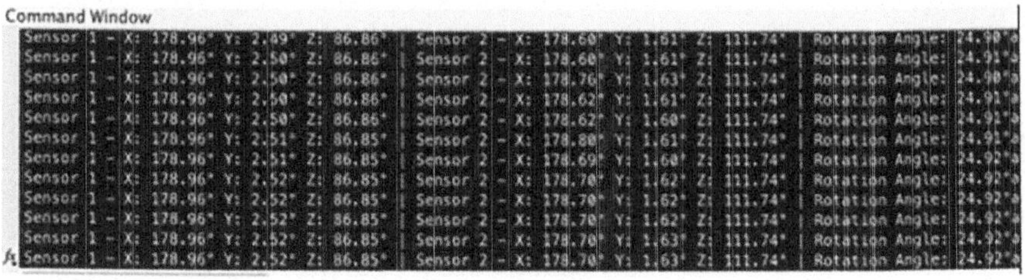

Fig. 6. Captured real time data.

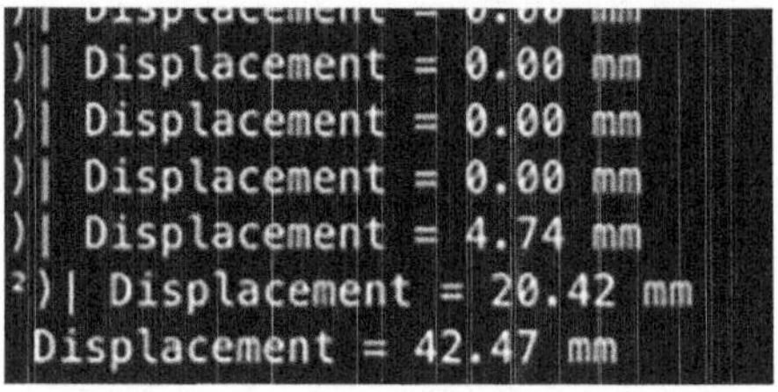

Fig. 7. Captured real data for lateral displacement.

interface, as shown Fig. 5, as well as at the Command Window of the PC shown in Fig. 6. In both measurement cases, being either angular or lateral dislocation, the user can set the acceptable threshold for a posture change before the alarm is set. Finally, the data can be stored on the laptop for post-processing.

5 Results

As described in Sect. 4, the initial performance tests were carried out using a simple settings mimicking the final use-case, as shown in Figs. 3 and 4. The real angle between the pens, which were mimicking the bones, was manually set, and the corresponding relative angle result provided by the WIT sensors were calculated at the PC. The captured real-time data indicates the differences of the principal angles of the two nodes, as seen from the example, Figs. 5 and 6. In our experiments, the sampling frequency, which indicates the time between the consecutive samples, is set to 10 Hz. The maximum sampling rate the node supports is 200 Hz and the minimum is 0.2 Hz. The sampling rate does not give any additional value for our tests so the default value of the node was used.

The procedure to run the tests was the following:

- Set the original positions for the pens and read the relative angle provided by the nodes' data.
- Measure the real angle between the pens.
- Compare the angle value with the one provided by the WIT sensors (from Fig. 6).

- Change the position of the other pen.
- Repeat the procedure.

As shown in Fig. 6, the user interface that is currently in use provides the angular position of the nodes compared to the Earth's magnetic field in the 3D coordinates. Initial tests showed that the WIT sensors are sensitive enough to provide the required angular resolution and sensitivity. Moreover, these tests validated that IoT -based approach could be used to monitor small angular dislocations.

The other purpose of the experiments was to study whether the displacement to any directions could be detected using the same installation. The achieved results are expressed in Fig. 7, where the relative displacement between nodes can be seen. At the beginning, the pens were connected to each other. Then, the pens were separated keeping angle the same. The results after relocating the pens are shown starting from the fourth row in Fig. 7. However, it was observed that the distance measurements require higher forces to be detected and thus the used node is not capable to provide the required information for realistic fractured bone dislocation.

6 Future Work

The work reported in this paper is based on the first PoC type research we carried out using the proposed measurement system. The experiments were carried out to assess whether the proposed method could be used to monitor angular or lateral displacements (to any directions) of the bones during the ossification process. As showed, the angular resolution appears to have high enough accuracy to be used in our medical use-case settings. On the other hand, the velocities caused by the one-way displacement are not high enough to be detected by this approach, but, e.g., in industrial applications, where higher velocities can be achieved, this solution could be applicable.

In the next phase, comparative measurements using a servo motor controlled testbed to automatically change the angle will be carried out using the WIT sensors jointly with the bend sensors used in [11]. The automated measurements will also provide statistically reliable results, as it is possible to carry out longer measurements without the participation of a person.

In addition, the experiments will be done in more realistic settings, thus including artificial tissue material, as well as casting on top of the fractured material. In this case, it is possible to use thicker material, like a wooden bar or even an artificial hand, to mimic human bones. Using the casting increases the realism of the experiment.

Final step could be the clinical tests with volunteers but we are not at that phase, yet. Moreover, testing with humans also requires ethical approval before the experiments could be started.

7 Conclusion

In this paper, we have proposed a non-ionizing and non-invasive IoT -based monitoring system to detect possible changes in the fractured bone ossification process. Currently, a post-monitoring of the healing process is performed by using a regular X-ray control to detect possible misalignment of the fractured bones. Our proposed system, which is based on the use of 9-axis accelerometers, dispenses with the X-rays. Simultaneously, the proposed system enables real-time healing monitoring at home, which is a cost effective way for the post treatment care.

Based on our initial experiments, the used WIT sensor nodes are capable to detect small angular changes between the bones, which might occur during the healing process. However, the measurement technique and the node used is not able to detect dislocations due to the slow changes the bones have when moving one-way away from each others. To enable alarm, the relative movement to any direction between the bone ends needs to be very fast, which is not realistic in our use-case. It should also be noted that the measurement settings were highly simplified and thus, more realistic experiments are required to finally prove the suitability of the proposed concept for bone fracture healing monitoring.

References

1. Wu, A.M.: Global, regional, and national burden of bone fractures in 204 countries and territories, 1990–2019: a systematic analysis from the global burden of disease study 2019. Lancet Healthy Longevity **2**(9), 580–592 (2021). https://doi.org/10.1016/S2666-7568(21)00172-0
2. Jones, I.E., Williams, S.M., Dow, N., Goulding, A.: How many children remain fracture-free during growth? A longitudinal study of children and adolescents participating in the dunedin multidisciplinary health and development study. Osteop. Int. **13**, 990–995 (2002). https://doi.org/10.1007/s001980200137
3. Goulding, A., et al.: First fracture is associated with increased risk of new fractures during growth. J. Pediatr. **146**(2), 286–288 (2005). https://doi.org/10.1016/j.jpeds.2004.09.029
4. Orton, E., Kendrick, D., West, J., Tata, L.J.: Persistence of health inequalities in childhood injury in the UK; a population-based cohort study of children under 5. PLoS One **9**(10) (2014). https://doi.org/10.1371/journal.pone.0111631
5. Mäyränpää, M.K., Mäkitie, O., Kallio, P.E.: Decreasing incidence and changing pattern of childhood fractures: a population-based study. J. Bone Miner. Res. **25**(12), 2752–2759 (2010). https://doi.org/10.1002/jbmr.155
6. Parviainen, R., Kumpuniemi, T., Mäkelä, J.-P., Hämäläinen, M., Sinikumpu, J.-J., Iinatti, J.: Preliminary considerations on non-invasive home-based bone fracture healing monitoring. In: Proceedings of the 14th EAI International Conference on Bio-inspired Information and Communications Technologies. EAI, Okinawa (2023). https://doi.org/10.1007/978-3-031-43135-7_13
7. Food and Drug Administration: Use of International Standard ISO 10993-1, Biological evaluation of medical devices - Part 1: Evaluation and testing within a risk management process. [Docket No. FDA-2013-D-0350], GUI00001811 (2023)

8. Aldelemy, A., et al.: Monitoring bone healing: integrating RF sensing with AI. IEEE Access **13**, 11114–11135 (2025). https://doi.org/10.1109/ACCESS.2024.3524178
9. Lindgren, A., Gong, K.: Measurement of the relative delay between signals propagating in a multipath environment. In: Ocean 1974 - IEEE International Conference on Engineering in the Ocean Environment, pp. 293–298 (1974). https://doi.org/10.1109/OCEANS.1974.1161438
10. Iovescu, C., Rao, S.: The fundamentals of millimeter wave radar sensors. https://www.ti.com/lit/wp/spyy005a/spyy005a.pdf. Accessed 25 July 2025
11. Kumpuniemi, T., Parviainen, R., Mäkelä, J.-P., Hämäläinen, M., Sinikumpu, J.-J., Iinatti, J.: A cost-effective solution for non-invasive home-based bone fracture healing monitoring - preliminary prototype tests. In: Proceedings of the 19th IEEE International Symposium on Medical Information and Communications Systems. IEEE, Florence (2025). https://doi.org/10.1109/ISMICT64722.2025.11059397
12. Siaw, P.O., et al.: Breakthrough in bone healing monitoring: how RF sensing and AI are revolutionising fracture care. In: 2024 IEEE 29th International Workshop on Computer Aided Modeling and Design of Communication Links and Networks (CAMAD). IEEE, Athens (2024). https://doi.org/10.1109/CAMAD62243.2024.10943005
13. Riaz, M., Tiberi, G., Asani, H., Ghavami, M., Dudley, S.: A non-invasive bone fracture monitoring analysis using an UHF antenna. In: 2020 12th International Symposium on Communication Systems, Networks and Digital Signal Processing (CSNDSP). IEEE, Porto (2020). https://doi.org/10.1109/CSNDSP49049.2020.9249570
14. Protopappas, V.C., Baga, D.A., Fotiadis, D.I., Likas, A.C., Papachristos, A.A., Malizos, K.N.: An ultrasound wearable system for the monitoring and acceleration of fracture healing in long bones. IEEE Trans. Biomed. Eng. **52**(9), 1597–1608 (2005). https://doi.org/10.1109/TBME.2005.851507
15. He, Y., Ma, Y., Zhao, Z., Zhang, M.: A biomechanical monitor for bone fracture healing. In: 2023 IEEE Biomedical Circuits and Systems Conference (BioCAS). IEEE, Toronto (2023). https://doi.org/10.1109/BioCAS58349.2023.10388734
16. WITMotion: WT9011DCL 9-axis BLE Magnetometer Gyroscope. https://www.wit-motion.com/BLE/17.html. Accessed 25 July 2025
17. Evans, P.: Rotations and rotation matrices. Biol. Crystallogr. **57**(10), 1355–1359 (2001). https://doi.org/10.1107/S0907444901012410

Research of Detection System for the Heatstroke Which Caused by Wearing Protective-Clothes, Based on Heartbeat Information Using Clothing-Type Wearable Sensors

Kyoko Oe[1(✉)], Hiroyasu Goto[2], and Koji Kuwata[2]

[1] Research Department, Chemical School, Japan Ground Self-Defense Force, Ministry of Defense, 1-40-7 Nisshin, Omiya, Saitama 331-8550, Japan
res-cmlsh@inet.gsdf.mod.go.jp

[2] Department of Nephrology and Endocrinology, National Defense Medical College, 3-2 Namiki, Tokorozawa, Saitama 359-8513, Japan

Abstract. This report is the overview of the research by Chemical School, Japan Ground Self-Defense Force (JGSDF), which analyzed the heartbeat data obtained using wearable sensors. The participants were the member of the Chemical unit of JGSDF, all the participants were male. Training wearing protective-clothes which protects a body from chemical agents in high temperature environment gives a very high heat stress to body. It is very important to have the safety measures for reducing the risk of member's heatstroke. By being exposed to high temperature environment and high humidity in protective-clothes, member's core body temperature rises and it read to dangerous state of body which causes heatstroke. However, even if member's becomes dangerous physical condition, they have to continue working for their duties. It is difficult to avoid onset of serious heatstroke by member's own senses. So, the system which monitors each member's performance and physical condition by administrator is required. Therefore, we try to develop the system that detects signs of heatstroke by real-time monitoring. In this research, I used the clothing-type wearable sensors which combined the small heart rate sensor. We measured heartbeat of members wearing protective-clothes during actual training and attempted to evaluate heat stress. We describe the heatstroke detection system based on heartbeat information which we have challenged.

Keywords: Protective-clothes · Wearable sensors · Heatstroke · Heartbeat

1 Introduction

In CBRN (Chemical, Biological, Radiological and Nuclear) response operations, members must wear protective-clothes and mask to shield themselves from hazardous chemicals while carrying out their duties. Recently temperature of a summer is rising every year. Under such as severe summer environment, training wearing protective-clothes,

H. Tanaka et al. (Eds.): BodyNets 2025, LNICST 714, pp. 360–367, 2026.
https://doi.org/10.1007/978-3-032-38657-1_30

the body undertakes the high physiological burden by heat stress. It is not only reducing performance, but also there is high risk of getting serious heatstroke. Ensuring physical safety is an important issue. We are trying research using every possible approach to prevent severe heatstroke. For example, 1) We have proposed the training protocol of heat acclimation through the original training manual for chemical unit. And we do the blood test before and after the heat acclimation training to evaluate the body's heat acclimation. 2) We adopted the method of sinking body into cold water using ice bath, and investigated the effective methods of pre-cooling and post-cooling to suppress the rise in core body temperature. 3) We are currently working on developing a system that can detect signs of heatstroke by real-time monitoring. These studies help reduce heat stress and support their performance.

2 The Approach to Heatstroke Prevention

2.1 Heat Acclimation Training

The heat acclimation training we proposed is effective even without a special artificial climate chamber. Aiming at wearing protective-clothes in summer, they do endurance exercises like jogging about 1 h wearing a sauna suit or a windbreaker. And moving on to the stage of training using protective-clothes and mask by the end of the rainy season. We had the blood test before and after the heat acclimation training, and investigated the expression rate of Hsp70 (heat shock protein 70) in human peripheral blood mononuclear cells. Figure 1 shows the data of the well-trained and heat-acclimated members, and negative control. The well-trained group's Hsp70 increased significantly rather than negative control group's Hsp70.

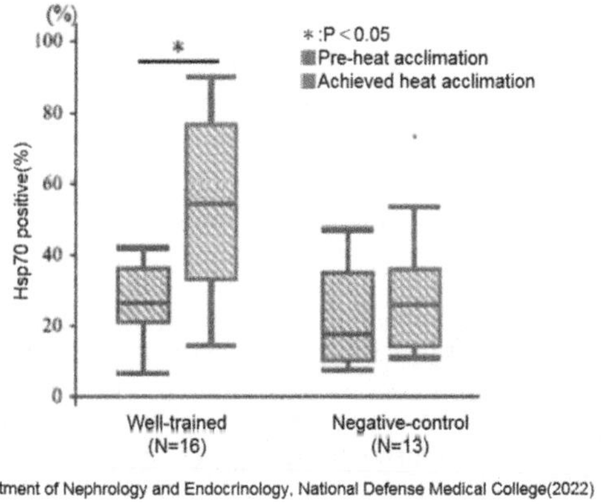

Fig. 1. The expression rate of Hsp70 of well-trained member and negative controls

2.2 Measurement of Vital Data

Rectal core body temperature, which is important data, was measured continuously at one-minute intervals during actual training. After the training, we investigated the feeling of fatigue by VAS (Visual Analogue Scale) and the symptoms of heatstroke by questionnaires. Figure 2a are Results of the rise in core body temperature compared between experienced and inexperienced members. Inexperienced members refer to newcomers who are currently undergoing training and education. At the same training, core body temperature in experienced members were significantly lower than of inexperienced members. Figure 2b shows the results of their feeling of fatigue. Although the inexperienced members were in dangerous body condition, both group's feeling of fatigue were the almost same. From these results, it can be said that to judge only own feeling of fatigue is risky

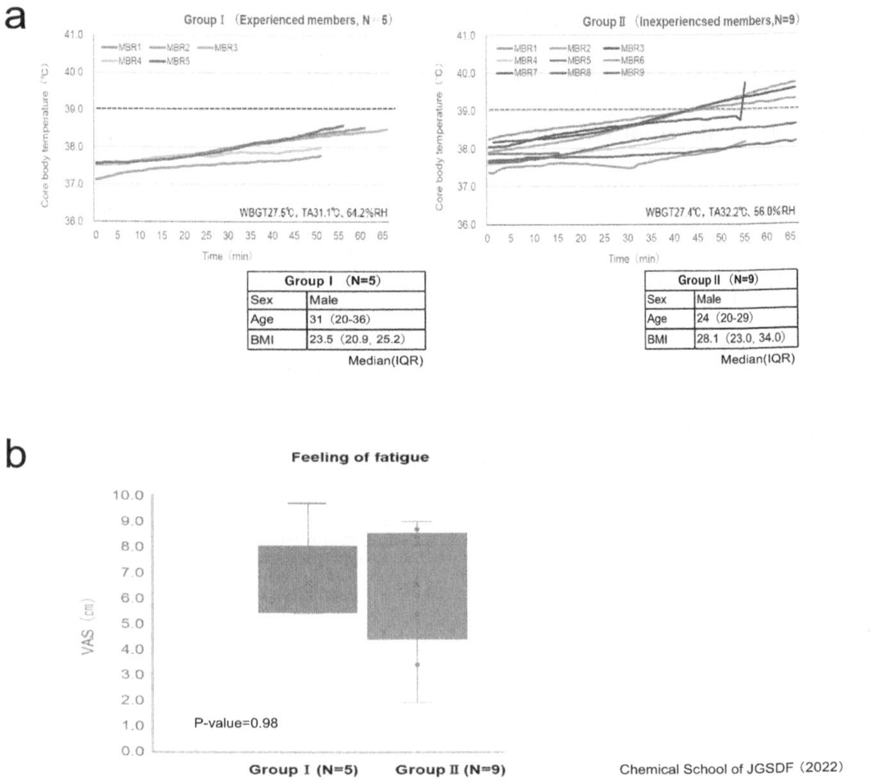

Fig. 2. Comparison between experienced members and inexperienced members. a results of the rise in core body temperature. b results of the feelings of fatigue by VAS

Figure 3 shows the decrease in core body temperature during post-cooling from the peak core body temperature after actual training. Once the core body temperature is over 39.0 °C, it was difficult to bring it down to 38.0 °C. Although the members whose core body temperature was over 39.0 °C, they didn't notice the signs of the onset of heatstroke. So, we investigated for organ damage by the blood test and urinalysis. Table 1 is the result of the blood test and urinalysis after the training. There was slightly organ damage of the members, whose core body temperatures were higher than 39.0 °C, through blood test and urinalysis. Detecting the early signs of heatstroke is one way to prevent severe heatstroke. So, we started research for the development a heatstroke detection system by real-time monitoring.

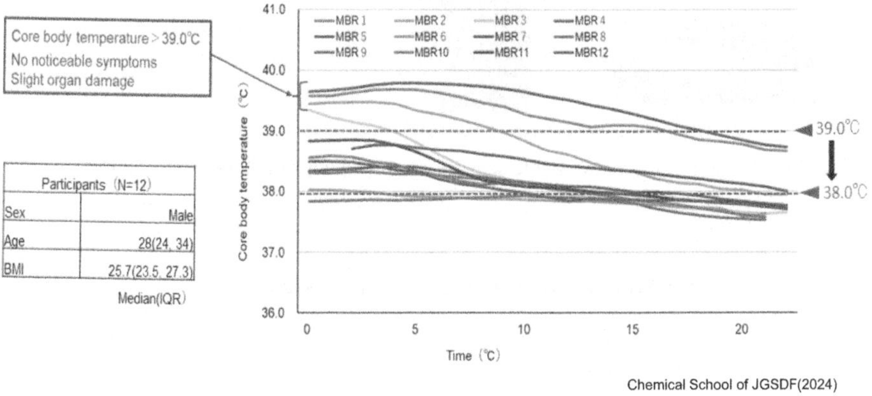

Fig. 3. The decrease in core body temperature during post-cooling from the peak core body temperature after actual training

Table 1. Results of Blood test and urinalysis after actual training.

Blood test	Negative(N=9)	Positive(N=3)	P-value
Age	25 (23-35)	24 (23-30)	0.63
BMI	26.1(22.8, 26.9)	26.2(23.8, 28.7)	0.64
Training Time (min)	85(78-95)	89(88, 96)	0.08
Core body temperature (°C)	38.5(38.2, 38.8)	39.7(39.5, 39.8)	0.01

Urine test(L-FABP)	Negative(N=5)	Positive(N=7)	P-value
Age	25 (23-36)	24 (23-31)	0.61
BMI	23.8 (21.6 26.9)	26.2(25.8, 28.7)	0.33
Training Time (min)	87 (78-92)	86 (78-94)	0.84
Core body temperature (°C)	38.9 (38.2, 39.4)	38.6 (38.3, 39.7)	0.94

Median(IQR)

The left-hand side of Table 1 is the result of blood test for renal function (sCr) and liver damage (AST, ALT, T.bill).
The right-hand side of Table 1 is the result of urinalysis using the test kit that can measures L-FABP (liver fatty acid-binding protein) in urine. We used the L-FABP POC kit (Point-of-Care kit), it is rapid assay kit for heat-induced organ damage.
National Defense Medical Journal separate volume-Vol.72(2025)

3 Practical Research of Heartbeat Measurement Using Clothing-Type Wearable Sensors

3.1 Selection of Wearable Sensors

We selected "COCOMI$_{TM}$ Wear (Toyobo MC Co., Ltd.)"that have electrodes and wiring formed inside the under bust part using the elastic film-shaped conductive material, and combined it with the small heart rate sensor "myBeat, WHS-1 type (Union Tool Co., Ltd.)" to measure heartbeat (Fig. 4). COCOMI$_{TM}$ Wear can be worn under protective-clothes during actual training without any trouble. And we confirmed that a stable heartbeat could be measured.

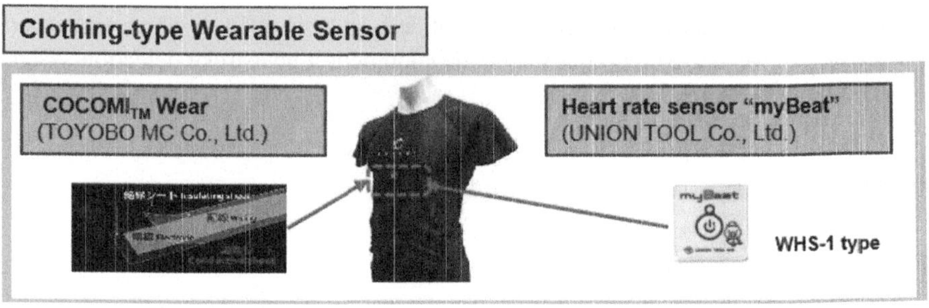

Fig. 4. Clothing-type wearable sensors combined with small heart rate sensor

3.2 Heartbeat Data Measurement Using Wearable Sensors

Heartbeat was measured continuously for three days, including the training day. On the training day, rectal core body temperature was also measured, and blood test and urinalysis were done after the training (Fig. 5).

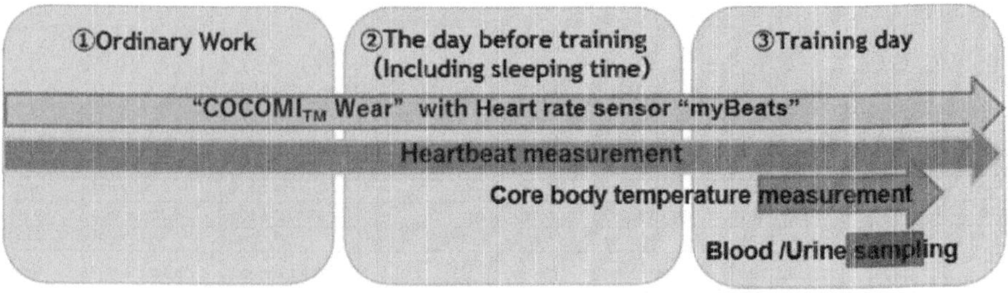

Fig. 5. Vital data measurement flow for three days

3.3 Heartbeat Information Analysis Technology for the Development of a Heatstroke Detection System

To analyze the physiological burden caused by heat stress from the measured heartbeat data, we adopted the analytical method ANAIM$_{TM}$ (Autonomic Nervous Activity Index Map), which is possible to read the mental and physical state. This method utilizes the cardiac cycle RRI (interval between heartbeat peaks obtained from ECG: Electrocardiogram) to express mental and physical state from fluctuations in the autonomous nervous system. Figure 6 is the graph which plotted sympathetic nerve activity index and logarithm of parasympathetic nerve activity index obtained from member's heartbeat data to X-Y axis. The ANAIM$_{TM}$ diagram displays the regression line of the autonomic nerve activity in ordinary life time period, along with the upper and lower regression lines $\pm 3\sigma$. Figure 6 shows the results of the one of member's ANAIM$_{TM}$ diagram which measured during the non-training times. The white line is the regression line obtained from heartbeat data measured ordinary life time period. The green and red lines are $\pm 3\sigma$

of the regression line. In the top graph, the yellow plots indicates the state of break time period, and in the middle graph, the green plots indicates the state of sleeping time period. These represent a relaxed state dominated by the parasympathetic nervous system. In the bottom graph, the light-blue plots indicates after the training time period, the blue plots indicates in the night relax time period, and these also represent a relaxed state.

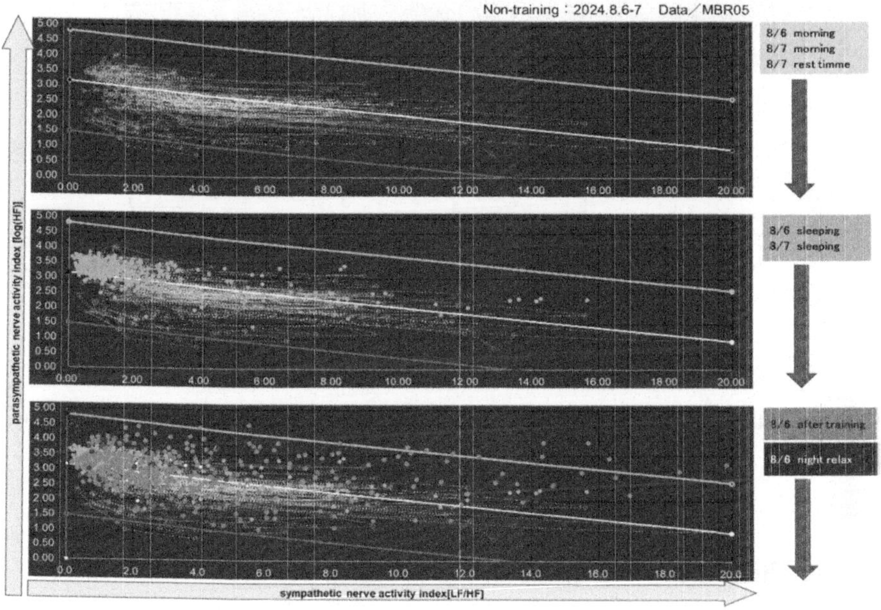

Fig. 6. ANAIM$_{TM}$ diagram of the one of members during non-training time

Figure 7 shows the results of the same member's (in Fig. 6) ANAIM$_{TM}$ diagram and the core body temperature data simultaneously measured during the training times. The red plots in ANAIM$_{TM}$ diagram indicates actual training time period. We can read him mental and physical state from the red plots. That is, he concentrated to training at the early time and he became to in exhaustion damaged state via in anxiety nervous state. In the zone which is indicated by the red plots, the core body temperature begins to rise and it reach to 39.5 °C. The results of the blood test and urinalysis showed that he had slight organ damage.

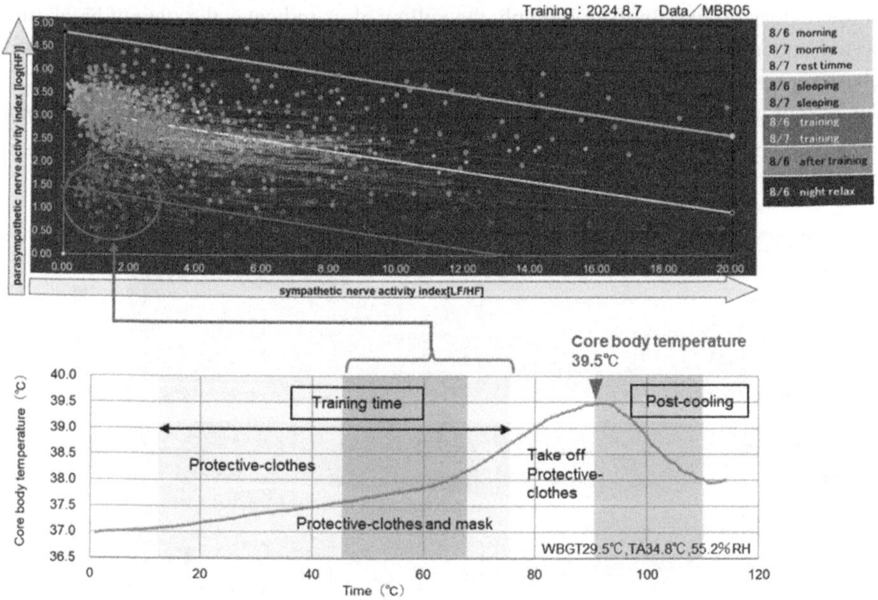

Fig. 7. ANAIM$_{TM}$ diagram and the core body temperature of the one of members during actual-training

4 Conclusion

In CBRN response operations, under the severe summer environment, the members of Chemical unit must wear the protective-clothes and mask for their duties. Therefore the risk of heatstroke is very high. To discover the sign of heatstroke at an early stage is important to prevent serious heatstroke. The technique of analyzing the heartbeat information obtained from the wearable sensors which combined "COCOMI$_{TM}$ Wear" and the small heart rate sensor "myBeat" is one effective method for detecting heatstroke. We are going to continue our research and aim to develop heatstroke detection system by real-time monitoring for them.

Acknowledgement. We would like to deeply thank the members of the Department of Research at Self-Defense Force Central Hospital for their administrative assistance and support for sample collection and laboratory testing. We also thank the members of Chemical unit of JGSDF for cooperation as participants.

References

1. Maeda, S.: Autonomic nerve activity index representation method based on heartbeat information obtained from wearable devices. In: TBIS. 10.3993/tbis (2023)

2. Maeda, S., Toyobo MC Co., Ltd.: How far can mental states be read with wearable devices? In: Monthly Bioindustry. CMC Publishing (2023)
3. Goto, H., Ishikiriyama, T., Oe, K., et al.: Liver fatty acid-binding protein point-of-care testing detects heat-induced organ damage: a pilot study in Japanese male self-defense force personnel. Sci. Rep. **15**, 7197 (2025). https://doi.org/10.1038/s41598-025-91685-7
4. Goto, H., Oe, K., et al.: Natl. Def. Med. J. separate volume 71: 69 (2024)
5. Oe, K., Goto, H., et al.: Natl. Def. Med. J. separate volume 71: 68 (2024)
6. Goto, H., Oe, K., et al.: Natl. Def. Med. J. separate volume 72: 67 (2025)
7. Oe, K., Goto, H et al.: Natl. Def. Med. J. separate volume 72: 67 (2025)

Multi-person Heartbeat Sensing Using Millimeter-Wave Sensor

Tomoyuki Nakasha(✉), Takuya Honma, Katsutoshi Kawai, Tatsuo Toba, and Jun Kuroda

Kyocera Corporation, Yokohama, Kanagawa 220-0012, Japan
tomoyuki.nakasha.ke@kyocera.jp

Abstract. This paper presents a millimeter-wave heartbeat sensing technique that enables simultaneous, non-contact measurement of cardiac activity in multiple individuals. The proposed method addresses key challenges for practical implementation—namely, achieving high-precision measurements and expanding the applicability. In previous studies, chest micro-vibrations induced by heartbeats were accurately extracted using a millimeter-wave sensor, and both heart rate and R–R intervals (RRI) were estimated by analyzing these waveforms. However, this approach was primarily limited to single-person monitoring, restricting its applicability in real-world environments. To overcome this limitation, angular separation processing was applied to the intermediate frequency (IF) signals captured by the sensor. This enabled the system to isolate and extract heartbeat signals corresponding to each individual. The proposed method was validated through five-minute experiments involving two participants, demonstrating high-accuracy estimation of heart rates (maximum error below ±6 bpm for both individuals) and RMSSD—an important index for autonomic nervous system analysis (maximum error below ±6.7 ms). These results highlight the potential of this technique for non-contact, high-precision heartbeat sensing in a wide range of healthcare and safety monitoring scenarios.

Keywords: Millimeter-wave sensing · Multi-person heartbeat sensing · Non-contact monitoring · Vital sign monitoring

1 Introduction

There has been a growing demand for healthcare monitoring systems that utilize vital sensors capable of acquiring respiration and heart rates. This demand is driven by an aging population and increasing health consciousness. While wearable sensors have been widely used for vital sign monitoring, several challenges remain, including the complexity of attachment, discomfort for users, and difficulty in achieving continuous, long-term measurements. To address these issues, millimeter-wave sensing technology—enabling accurate, non-contact, and remote acquisition of physiological information—has garnered significant attention [1,2].

H. Tanaka et al. (Eds.): BodyNets 2025, LNICST 714, pp. 368–379, 2026.
https://doi.org/10.1007/978-3-032-38657-1_31

Millimeter-wave sensing has already been widely adopted in automotive radar systems, particularly for applications such as collision avoidance and vehicle-surround monitoring, owing to its capability to estimate the position and velocity of targets. Beyond these conventional uses, millimeter-wave technology has also demonstrated high sensitivity to subtle vibrations, underscoring its potential for vibration sensing [3]. Notably, it allows for non-contact acquisition of vital signs, such as heart rate and respiration, by detecting minute surface vibrations of the human body. In this study, we propose a method for high-precision estimation of heart rate and R–R intervals (RRI) by sensing body surface vibrations using a millimeter-wave sensor. Furthermore, we introduce a novel approach that incorporates angle-resolved signal processing, enabling simultaneous monitoring of multiple individuals. The effectiveness of the proposed method is experimentally demonstrated and discussed.

2 Heartbeat Analysis for Multiple People Using Millimeter-Wave Sensor

2.1 System Configuration of the Millimeter-Wave Sensor and Heartbeat Analysis Procedure

Figure 1 presents a block diagram of the millimeter-wave heartbeat sensing system. The transmitted signal is generated using a synthesizer, digital-to-analog converter (DAC), local oscillator, and RF amplifier, and is directed toward the subject. The reflected signal from the subject is received by the antenna and downconverted into intermediate-frequency (IF) signals using a mixer. These IF signals are then amplified, digitized, and input to the signal processing unit, where heartbeat estimation is performed.

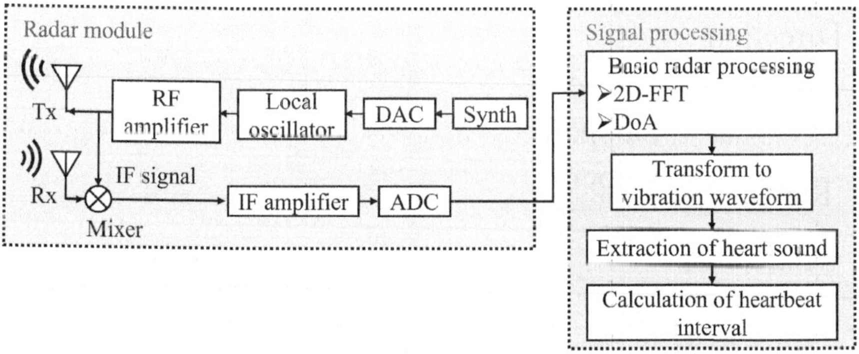

Fig. 1. Block diagram of millimeter-wave heartbeat sensing system.

The signal processing unit comprises several modules: basic radar processing, vibration waveform conversion, extraction of heartbeat-induced chest vibrations, and estimation of heart rate and RRI. In the basic radar processing block, signal processing is applied to the IF signal to extract key information such as distance, relative velocity, and direction. Specifically, by applying a two-dimensional fast Fourier transform (2D-FFT) to the IF signal, both the distance and surface vibration velocity of a person can be extracted. Direction estimation is performed using array signal processing techniques. This process results in the construction of a three-dimensional radar data cube, as shown in Fig. 2, from which direction-based separation and subsequent processing steps are applied to obtain individual chest vibration waveforms. Chest vibration waveforms contain not only heartbeat-induced components but also respiration and body motion artifacts. These non-cardiac components often exhibit large amplitudes and overlapping frequency harmonics, making it difficult to isolate heartbeat signals using simple filtering. To address this challenge, statistical signal processing techniques are employed. As shown in Fig. 3, these techniques enable extraction of the heartbeat-specific vibration peaks from the overall waveform. Heart rate and RRI are then estimated by identifying and analyzing these peaks. The identified peaks correspond to vibrations caused by the closing of heart valves—specifically, the closure of the atrioventricular (AV) valves (associated with the first heart sound, S1) and those caused by the closure of the semilunar valves (corresponding to the second heart sound S2). The time intervals between S1 and S2, and between S2 and S1 exhibit different durations. By analyzing the sequence of peak intervals obtained from the vibration waveform over a certain period, it is possible to estimate whether each peak corresponds to S1 or S2. Consequently, the intervals between the peaks corresponding to S1 can be accurately calculated as RRI.

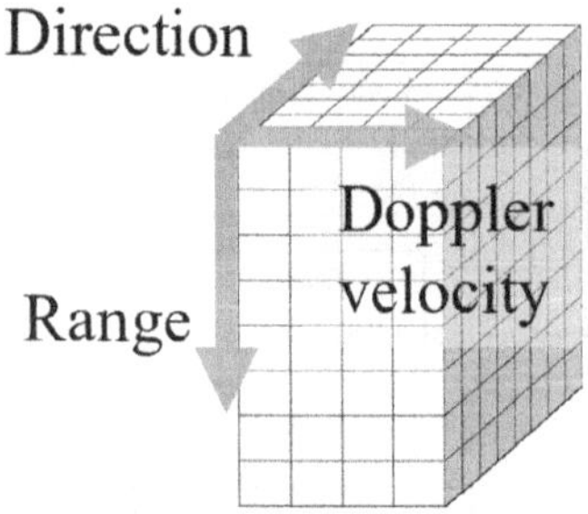

Fig. 2. Radar data cube.

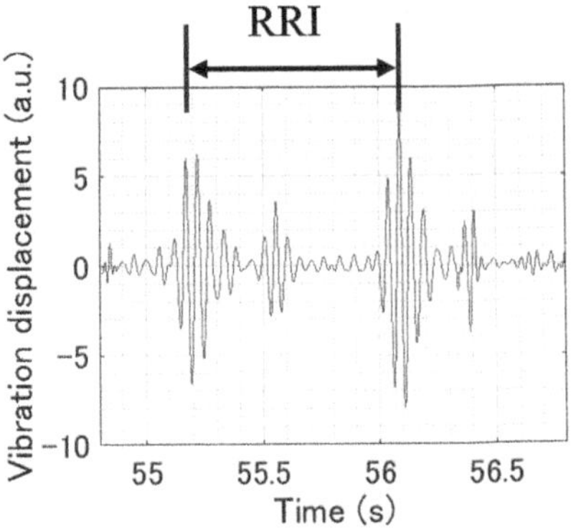

Fig. 3. Heartbeat-induced chest vibration displacement measured by millimeter-wave sensor.

By accurately estimating RRI, heart rate variability (HRV), including the high-frequency (HF) band, can be measured, enabling the analysis of autonomic nervous system activity. In this study, we evaluated the root mean square of successive differences (RMSSD), which is an indicator related to parasympathetic activity and is used, for example, in applications such as driver drowsiness estimation [4]. RMSSD is written as:

$$\mathrm{RMSSD} = \sqrt{\frac{1}{N-1}\sum_{i=1}^{N-1}\left(RR_{i+1} - RR_i\right)^2}, \tag{1}$$

where, N denotes the number of data points, and RR_i represents the ith RRI. The RMSSD was calculated from five-minute RRI data based on the guidelines of the European Society of Cardiology [5].

2.2 Multi-person Analysis Method

Next, the analysis method for multiple individuals is described. This is achieved by applying range separation, angular separation, or a combination of both to the radar data cube, enabling the extraction of chest vibration waveforms for each person. Angular separation is performed using the constrained minimum variance distortionless response (MVDR) method [6]:

$$\hat{w} = R^{-1}C\left(C^H R^{-1} C\right)^{-1} f, \tag{2}$$

where, R denotes the array spatial correlation matrix, C is the constraint matrix that specifies the steering vectors. C^H is the Hermitian (conjugate) transpose of C, and f is the vector containing the desired constraint values. Specifically, as illustrated in Fig. 4, when extracting the chest vibration waveform of person A, a null is formed in the direction of person B to suppress their signal, thereby isolating the signal from person A. Conversely, when extracting the signal from person

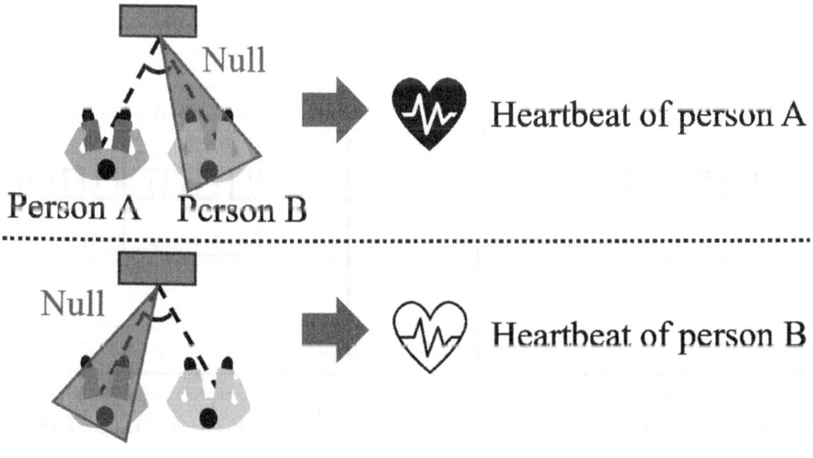

Fig. 4. Analysis method for multiple individuals using angular separation.

B, the process is applied in the opposite direction. By performing such processing in parallel, simultaneous measurement of multiple individuals becomes possible. This approach enables the extraction of chest vibration waveforms for each person, allowing analysis even when multiple people are present at the same time.

2.3 Enhancement of Angular Resolution by Virtual Array Technique

When performing signal suppression using receive null steering, the hardware configuration of the millimeter-wave sensor must be carefully considered. This is because the spatial degrees of freedom for beamforming-based signal suppression—that is, the number of directions in which nulls can be formed—is determined by the number of receiving antennas minus one. In this study, as shown in Fig. 5(a), we assume a hardware configuration comprising two transmitting antennas and four receiving antennas. Therefore, signal suppression is limited to $4 - 1 = 3$ directions. To increase the spatial degrees of freedom, a virtual array is constructed by time-division multiplexing the transmissions from each transmitting antenna [7,8]. The transmitting antennas Tx1 and Tx2 alternately transmit in a time-division manner, and the received signals corresponding to each transmission are captured by the four receiving antennas.

In this case, the spatial channel matrix can be expressed as

$$H = \begin{bmatrix} h_{1,1} \, h_{1,2} \cdots h_{1,4} \\ h_{2,1} \, h_{2,2} \cdots h_{2,4} \end{bmatrix} \in \mathbb{C}^{2\times 4}, \tag{3}$$

where, $h_{m,n}$ denotes the channel response from transmitting antenna m to receiving antenna n. Time-division transmission enables the individual observation of the channel vector for each transmitting antenna, allowing these vectors to be

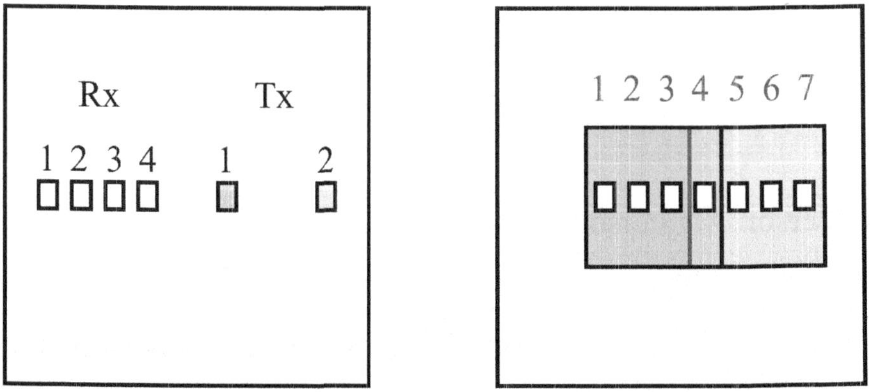

(a) Antenna configuration (b) Formed virtual array

Fig. 5. Antenna configuration of millimeter-wave sensor and formed virtual array.

acquired as separate observation vectors. A virtual array is constructed by considering all possible combinations (i.e., the Cartesian product) of the transmitting and receiving antennas. With two transmitting antennas and four receiving antennas, this results in a maximum of $2 \times 4 = 8$ virtual antenna elements. However, in this study, as shown in Fig. 5(b), due of the specific antenna arrangement, $h_{1,4} = h_{2,1}$. Consequently, the virtual array comprises seven distinct antenna elements.

3 Measurement Using Millimeter-Wave Sensor

3.1 Millimeter-Wave Sensor and Measurement

Experiments were conducted to validate the performance of the proposed method for heartbeat sensing in multiple individuals using the above-described techniques. Table 1 summarizes the specifications of the millimeter-wave sensor. The operating frequency was set to 60–64 GHz, a range commonly used for in-vehicle human detection and occupant monitoring applications. Heartbeat sensing was performed using two transmitting antennas, with a chirp interval of 1 ms. Although this sensor was employed for heartbeat sensing in this study, it is also applicable to remote sensing of various types of vibrations, including human respiration and motion, as well as mechanical vibrations in equipment, infrastructure, and buildings.

Table 1. Specifications of millimeter-wave sensor.

Parameter	Value
Frequency	60–64 GHz
Tx/Rx ant.	3/4 (2 Tx antennas used)
Range resolution	5 cm
Chirp interval	1 ms
Recommend range	0.2–2.0 m (Heartbeat sensing)
Field of view	±50°
Operation temperature	−10–40 °C
Dimension/Weight	64.5 mm × 63 mm × 23.8 mm/94 g

Measurements were conducted using the aforementioned sensor. As a preliminary measure, a single individual was measured while facing the sensor. Subsequently, two-person measurements were conducted.

To facilitate a clear evaluation of sensor performance, the maximum and mean errors of the heart rate compared to the ECG, as well as the error of the RMSSD compared to the ECG, were calculated. The criterion for the maximum heart rate error was set within ±10%, based on commercially available wearable sensors [9]. On the other hand, the criterion for RMSSD error was set within ±10 ms, which is considered practical for applications such as drowsiness estimation inside a vehicle [10]. The accuracy of the measurements with multiple people was evaluated based on these standards.

3.2 Single-Person Measurement

Figure 6 illustrates the setup with a person seated 1.0 m in front of the sensor. Figure 7(a) shows the heartbeat-induced chest vibration waveforms obtained using the millimeter-wave sensor, along with a magnified view. It can be observed that the waveforms accurately capture the heartbeat-induced peaks. Figure 7(b) shows the time courses of heart rate and RRI estimated from these peaks. In the figure, the solid blue line represents the results obtained by the millimeter-wave sensor and the orange dashed line indicates the results from the ECG. It was confirmed that both the heart rate and RRI measured by the millimeter-wave sensor closely matched the ECG results throughout the entire five-minute period. The maximum heart rate error was 4 bpm, and the mean error was 0.0 bpm, well within the target accuracy. The RMSSD error was also 0.0 ms, confirming that favorable results were obtained.

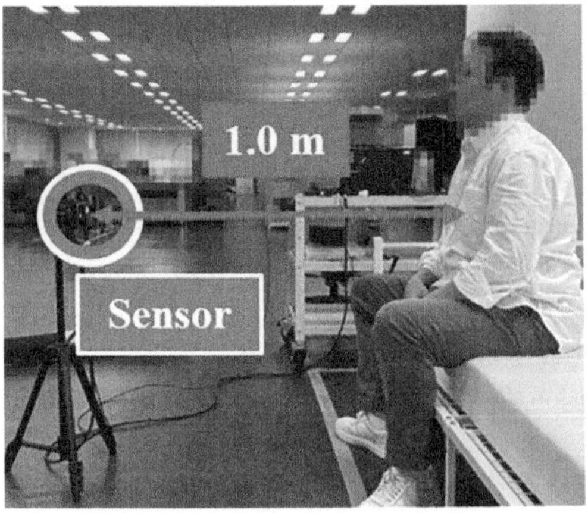

Fig. 6. Single-person measurement scene.

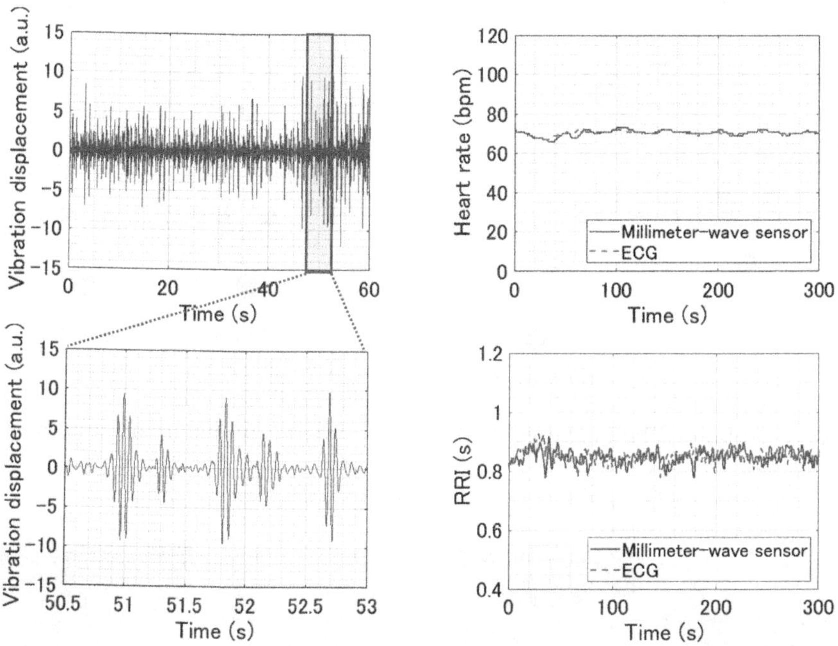

(a) Heartbeat-induced chest vibration displacement (top) and its magnified view (bottom)

(b) Heart rate (top) and RRI (bottom)

Fig. 7. Single-person measurement results.

3.3 Measurement with Two People

Next, the measurements were conducted with two people. As described earlier, two-person arrangement patterns were considered: (1) a non-equidistant configuration, in which people were located at different distances from the sensor, and (2) an equidistant configuration, in which people were at the same distance from the sensor. In the non-equidistant configuration, separation of each individual's chest vibration waveform was achieved using both range and angular separation, based on distance estimates obtained from basic radar processing. In contrast, in the equidistant configuration, range separation could not be applied, and signal separation was performed using only angular separation. Although the equidistant configuration is relatively rare in real-world applications compared to the non-equidistant case, it was included in this study to evaluate the effectiveness of angle-based separation. As illustrated in Figs. 8(a) and 8(b), two arrangement patterns were tested. To ensure reproducibility, these measurements were performed in an anechoic chamber, as shown in Figs. 9(a) and 9(b).

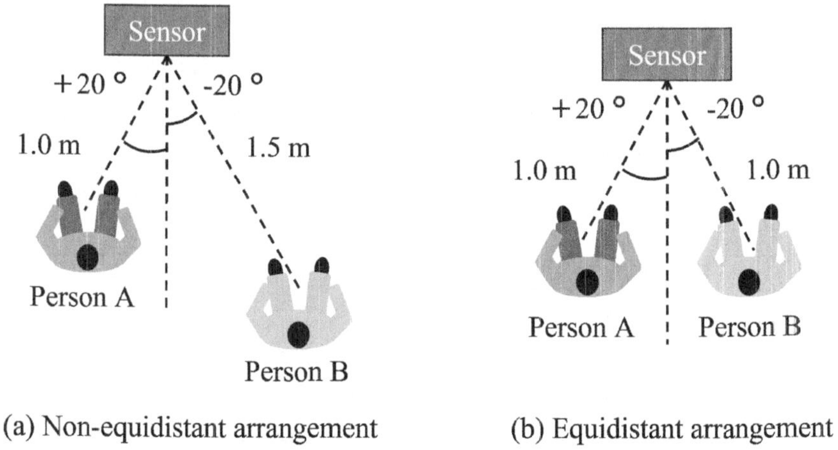

Fig. 8. Arrangements for two-person measurement.

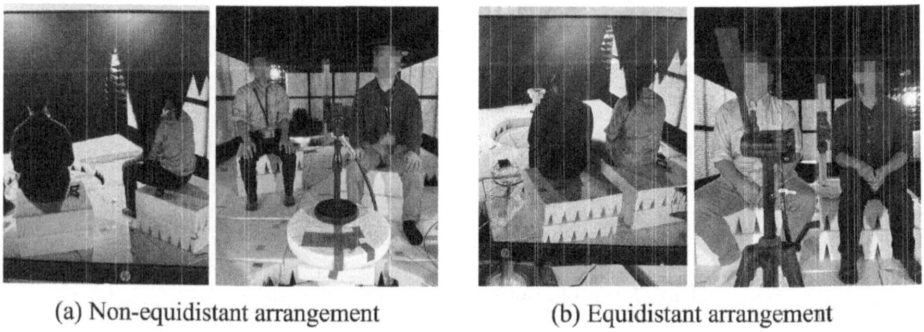

Fig. 9. Measurement scenes with two people.

Figures 10(a) and 10(b) present the heart rate and RRI results for persons A and B in the non-equidistant configuration. The heart rates obtained using the millimeter-wave sensor closely matched the ECG results for both individuals. The maximum and mean heart rate errors were 6 bpm and 1.2 bpm for person A, and 5 bpm and 1.1 bpm for person B, respectively, indicating high agreement with the ECG. For RRI, some discrepancies were observed for person A at the beginning of the measurement, likely due to insufficient extraction of heartbeat-induced vibrations caused by body movement, which could not be completely removed. Nevertheless, the RMSSD error was 1.5 ms for person A and 2.7 ms for person B, both of which meet the target accuracy. These results confirm that when individuals are located at different distances from the sensor, accurate simultaneous measurement is possible through signal separation based on both distance and angular information.

Figures 11(a) and 11(b) show the heart rate and RRI results for persons A and B in the equidistant configuration. As in the previous case, the heart rates

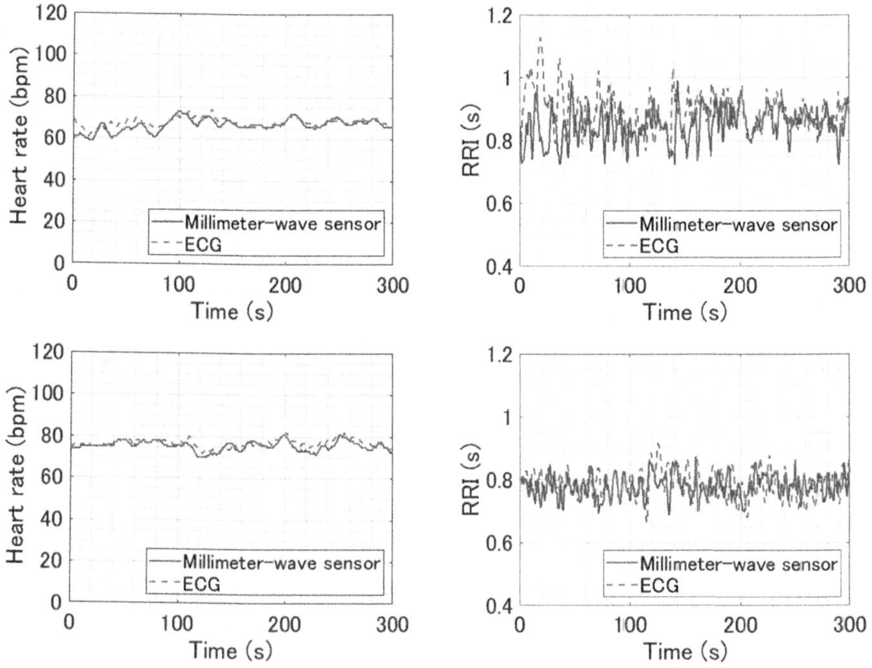

(a) Heart rate of person A (top) and person B (bottom)

(b) RRI of person A (top) and person B (bottom)

Fig. 10. Measurement results in non-equidistant arrangement.

measured by the millimeter-wave sensor for both individuals closely followed the ECG results. The maximum and mean heart rate errors were 6 bpm and 1.6 bpm for person A, and 5 bpm and 1.1 bpm for person B, both satisfying the target accuracy. However, for person A, some irregularities were observed in RRI tracking, resulting in a slightly higher RMSSD error of 6.7 ms. This is attributed to insufficient signal separation in the equidistant configuration compared to the non-equidistant case. Enhancements in angular separation and peak detection processing are planned as part of future work. Nevertheless, the RMSSD errors—6.7 ms for person A and 0.8 ms for person B—still meet the target accuracy. These results confirm that even when individuals are positioned at the same distance from the sensor, it is possible to separate their signals using only angular separation and accurately estimate each person's heartbeats.

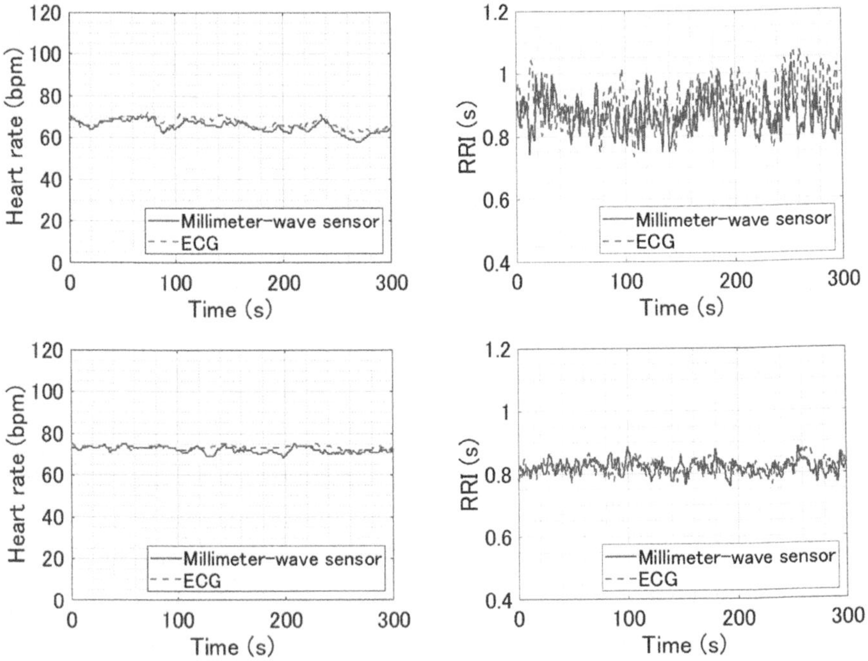

(a) Heart rate of person A (top) and person B (bottom)

(b) RRI of person A (top) and person B (bottom)

Fig. 11. Measurement results in equidistant arrangement.

4 Conclusion

This study investigated heartbeat sensing for multiple individuals using millimeter-wave vital sensing, with the aim of expanding the application scenarios of this technology. By applying statistical signal processing techniques to signals acquired by a millimeter-wave sensor, heartbeat-induced chest vibration waveforms were accurately extracted, enabling reliable heartbeat estimation through waveform analysis. Furthermore, it was demonstrated that simultaneous measurement of two individuals is feasible by separating signals based on angular information and extracting heartbeat data for each person. To validate the proposed method, five-minute experiments were conducted with two participants. The results showed high-accuracy estimation of heart rates (maximum error below ±6 bpm for both participants) and RMSSD, an important index for autonomic nervous system analysis (maximum error below ±6.7 ms). Although some issues were observed in RRI estimation under the equidistant configuration, we plan to address these through enhancements in angular separation and peak detection algorithms. Looking ahead, we aim to further develop this technology for non-contact health monitoring applications, such as patient condition monitoring in hospital wards and nursing facilities, as well as the prevention of sudden infant death syndrome (SIDS) in childcare environments.

References

1. Will, C., et al.: Radar-based heart sound detection. Sci. Rep. **8**(1), 11551 (2018)
2. Ding, Y., Yu, X., Lei, C., Sun, Y., Xu, X., Zhang, J.: A novel real-time human heart rate estimation method for noncontact vital sign radar detection. IEEE Access **8**, 88689–88699 (2020)
3. Kuroda, J., Murakami, Y., Kawaji, S., Sato, M., Yamamoto, K., Sahara, T.: Evaluation of influences of radome on vibration sensing capability of millimeter-wave sensor. In: Proceedings of the IEEE Radar Conference (2022)
4. Suemura, S., Kuroda, J., Toba, T., Ito, T.: Contactless estimation driver drowsiness by using millimeter wave radar and camera. In: 30th ITS World Congress (2024)
5. Task Force of the European Society of Cardiology and the North American Society of Pacing and Electrophysiology. Heart rate variability: standards of measurement, physiological interpretation and clinical use. Circulation **93**(5), 1043–1065 (1996)
6. Capon, J.: High-resolution frequency-wavenumber spectrum analysis. Proc. IEEE (1969)
7. Dohler, M.: Virtual antenna arrays. Ph.D. dissertation, King's College London, University of London (2004)
8. Zhou, C., Gu, Y., Fan, X., Shi, Z., Mao, G., Zhang, Y.: Direction-of-arrival estimation for coprime array via virtual array interpolation. IEEE Trans. Signal Process. **66**(22), 5956–5971 (2018)
9. Nelson, B.W., Allen, N.B.: Accuracy of consumer wearable heart rate measurement during an ecologically valid 24-hour period: intraindividual validation study. JMIR Mhealth Uhealth **7**(3), e10828 (2019)
10. Xu, X., Yu, J., Ma, C., Ren, T., Liu, H., Zhu, Y.: mmECG: monitoring human cardiac cycle in driving environments leveraging millimeter wave. In: Proceedings of IEEE INFOCOM (2022)

Reliable and Interference-Resilient Wireless Networks for Healthcare

Improving Reliability in Hospital WLANs with RL-Based Channel Selection and Contention Window Adaptation

Kousuke Kinoshita(✉) and Kento Takabayashi

Toyo University, 2100 Kujirai, Kawagoe, Saitama 351-8585, Japan
s36C02400059@toyo.jp

Abstract. In recent years, Wireless Local Area Networks (WLANs) have been introduced into hospitals to support various medical applications such as monitoring of vital signs, telemetry, and rapid information sharing among staff. However, unsupervised deployments and the coexistence of heterogeneous devices, for example patient-owned wearables and unmanaged access points, often lead to severe interference and transmission failures. To address these issues, we investigate a scheme that combines channel selection with contention window (CW) adaptation using reinforcement learning (RL). We compare several RL algorithms, such as ε-greedy, Upper Confidence Bound (UCB), and UCB1-Tuned, against conventional CSMA/CA. Computer simulation results show that the proposed learning-based configuration reduces the transmission failure rate. A trade-off is observed in throughput, which decreases in some settings, indicating that further joint optimization of channel choice and CW parameters is required.

Keywords: reinforcement learning · channel selection · contention window · WLAN

1 Introduction

In recent years, Wireless Local Area Networks (WLANs) have been introduced in medical institutions such as hospitals, becoming a core communication infrastructure in their information system. WLAN is used for a wide range of purposes, including medical information systems (such as electronic medical records), internet connectivity, and data transmission for medical devices [1]. For example, by utilizing laptops, tablets, and smartphones as Hospital Information System (HIS) terminals, staff can access and input patient information from anywhere within the hospital, enabling accurate and rapid sharing of patient information among staff members [2].

H. Tanaka et al. (Eds.): BodyNets 2025, LNICST 714, pp. 383–389, 2026.
https://doi.org/10.1007/978-3-032-38657-1_32

While both the 2.4 GHz and 5 GHz bands are being adopted in healthcare facilities, the 2.4 GHz band is classified as an Industrial, Scientific, and Medical (ISM) frequency. It is shared with various devices such as microwave ovens, Bluetooth devices, microwave scalpels, and microwave therapy devices, making it a frequency band prone to radio wave interference. Additionally, communication failures occur due to radio interference from WLAN-enabled diagnostic equipment and medical electrical devices, as well as from mobile phones, wireless-enabled portable game consoles, wireless-enabled IP cameras brought in by patients, and unmanaged WLAN access points [1].

Therefore, to resolve communication failures in hospitals and other medical institutions, we propose a scheme that uses reinforcement learning to select channel selection and the contention window value used in CSMA/CA. We evaluated its performance by computer simulations.

2 Related Technologies

2.1 Reinforcement Learning

Reinforcement learning is a framework in which an agent learns an action policy by interacting with an environment and receiving rewards, without requiring labeled data. The goal is to improve the policy to maximize cumulative rewards [3–5].

Q-Learning
Q-learning is a model-free RL method that estimates the action-value function q(s,a) and updates it from observed rewards and state transitions. By selecting the action with the highest estimated value, the agent can improve its policy without an explicit model of the environment, which enables broad applicability.

ε-Greedy Algorithm
ε-greedy algorithm is an algorithm that determines ε in advance and decides actions based on random numbers and ε. Action a is expressed by the following equation.

$$a(t+1) = \begin{cases} \mathrm{argmax}_{i=1,\ldots,K}\overline{r}_i(t) & \text{probability } 1-\varepsilon \\ \text{random select} & \text{probability } \varepsilon \end{cases} \tag{1}$$

UCB Algorithm
UCB algorithm calculates a value called the UCB score using the following formula and selects the option with the highest calculated UCB score.

$$a(t+1) = \mathrm{argmax}\left(\overline{r_i}(t) + \sqrt{c\frac{\ln n}{n_i}}\right) \tag{2}$$

Here, n_i denotes the number of times the i th channel was selected, and n is the total number of times all channels were selected. Furthermore, $c(>0)$ is a value controlling the degree of exploration. In this study, we employed $c = 2$, known as the UCB1 algorithm, and $c = 1/2$, as proposed in [6–8]. The case with $c = 2$ is referred to as the UCB1 algorithm, and the case with $c = 1/2$ is referred to as the UCB algorithm.

UCB1-Tuned Algorithm

UCB1-Tuned algorithm is an algorithm that adds a variance term to the UCB1 algorithm, expressed by the following equation.

$$a(t+1) = \mathrm{argmax}\left(\overline{r_i}(t) + \sqrt{\frac{\ln n}{n_i}\min\left(\frac{1}{4}, V_i(n_i)\right)}\right) \tag{3}$$

$$V_i(n_i) = (\hat{r}_i(t))^2 + \sqrt{2\frac{\ln n}{n_i}} \tag{4}$$

Here, $(\hat{r}_i(t))^2$ is the variance of $r_i(s)$, $s = 1, \ldots, t-1$.

2.2 CSMA/CA

CSMA/CA (Carrier Sense Multiple Access with Collision Avoidance) is a MAC layer protocol, exemplified by IEEE802.11 WLANs. A terminal wishing to transmit first performs carrier sense on the channel. If the channel is idle, it waits for a fixed period before transmitting. If the channel is occupied, the terminal sets a randomly determined wait time (backoff time) and attempts retransmission afterward. The backoff time is determined based on the contention window (CW).

Backoff time ($T_{backoff}$) is expressed by the following equation.

$$T_{backoff} = \mathrm{rand}[0, CW] \times T_{slot} \tag{5}$$

Here, T_{slot} is one slot. The value of CW is updated as follows when a collision occurs, with the collision count denoted as k:

$$CW_k = \min\left(2^k(CW_{\min}+1) - 1, CW_{\max}\right) \tag{6}$$

Here, $CW_{\min}$ is the minimum contention window and $CW_{\max}$ is the maximum contention window. In IEEE802.11a/g, $CW_{\min} = 15$ and $CW_{\max} = 1023$. Figure 1 shows the mechanism of CSMA/CA used in IEEE802.11.

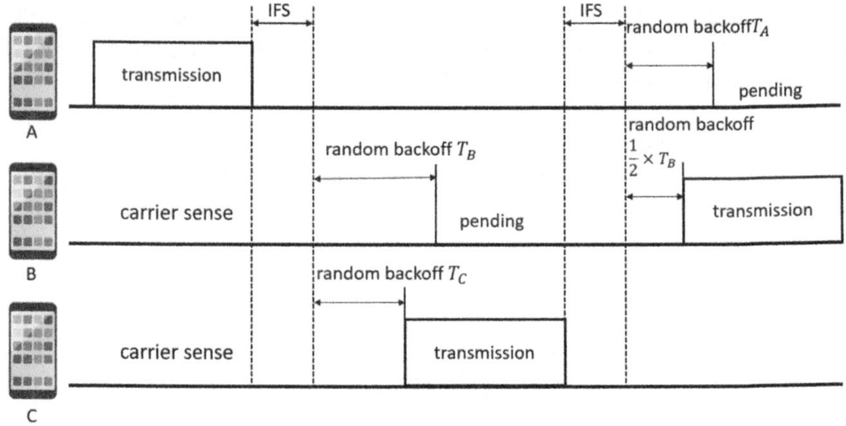

Fig. 1. CSMA/CA mechanism

3 Methodology

We consider a system in which each station selects both the operating channel and the CW according to a learning policy.

3.1 Channel Selection

Channel selection is performed using reinforcement learning. Previous studies demonstrated that reinforcement learning-based channel selection could choose available channels. However, prior research faced the issue of selecting free channels excessively. To resolve this, we calculate a threshold value for the average reward to distribute terminals across multiple channels. We then randomly select channels from those with an average reward above this threshold to avoid excessive concentration. The threshold value V_B for the average reward is calculated using the following formula.

$$V_B = \max(\overline{r_i}(t)) - \alpha \frac{\max(\overline{r_i}(t))}{M} \tag{7}$$

Here, $\max(\overline{r_i}(t))$ denotes the highest average reward value across all channels, M is the transmitted data length, and α is the weighting coefficient, which was set to $\alpha = 0.5$ in this study.

3.2 Contention Window

Contention window selection is performed using reinforcement learning. The value of the contention window was obtained using Eq. (6), but by transforming this into the collision count $a(0 \leq a \leq 6)$ is expressed by the following equation.

$$CW = 2^{4+a} - 1 \tag{8}$$

The value of a is determined using Q-learning. In this study, throughput was calculated and used as the reward. When a collision occurred, the reward was set to -1 regardless of the throughput accordingly.

4 Numerical Results

In this study, the number of channels was set to 5, and the simulation time was 1 s. The number of terminals was increased from 10 to 300 within one episode, and this process was repeated for 100 episodes to perform learning. This was repeated 3000 times, and the average was taken. Channels were assumed to experience noise from some form of communication with the probabilities shown in Table 1. For reinforcement learning, Q-learning was used for contention window selection, while the following algorithms were employed for channel selection: ε-greedy algorithm, UCB algorithm, UCB1 algorithm, and UCB1-Tuned algorithm.

Table 1. Probability of noise due to some form of communication per channel

Channel	Busy Probability[%]
CH1	10
CH2	15
CH3	20
CH4	25
CH5	30

Figure 2 shows the transmission success rate, collision occurrence rate, and transmission failure rate for each algorithm. Figure 3 shows the throughput for each algorithm. Figure 4 shows the rewards per episode for each algorithm.

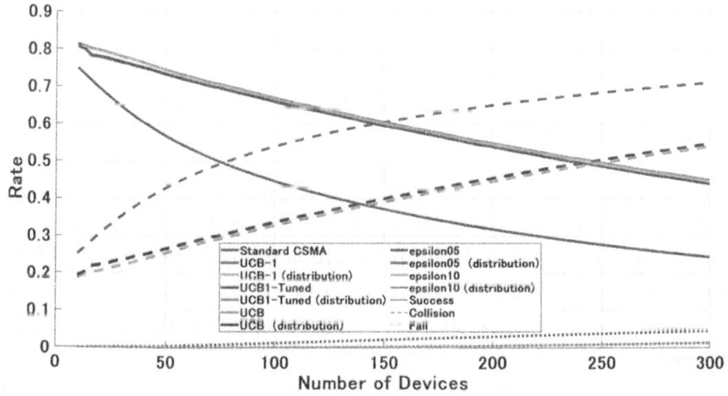

Fig. 2. Transmission success rate, collision occurrence rate, transmission failure rate per algorithm

Figure 2 shows that the transmission success rate increased for all algorithms compared to CSMA/CA, while the collision probability and failure rate decreased.

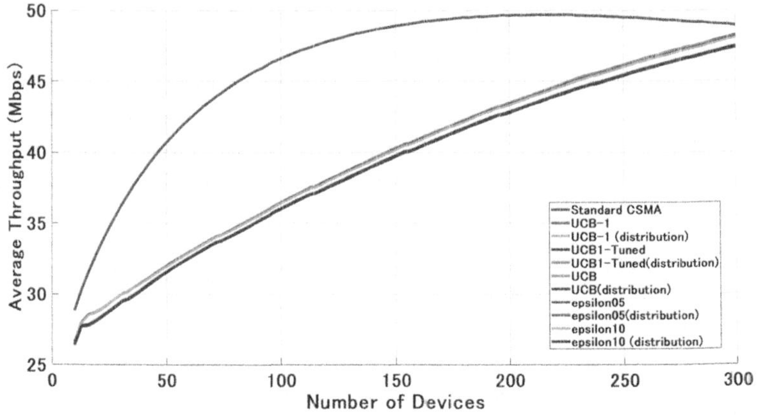

Fig. 3. Throughput of each algorithm

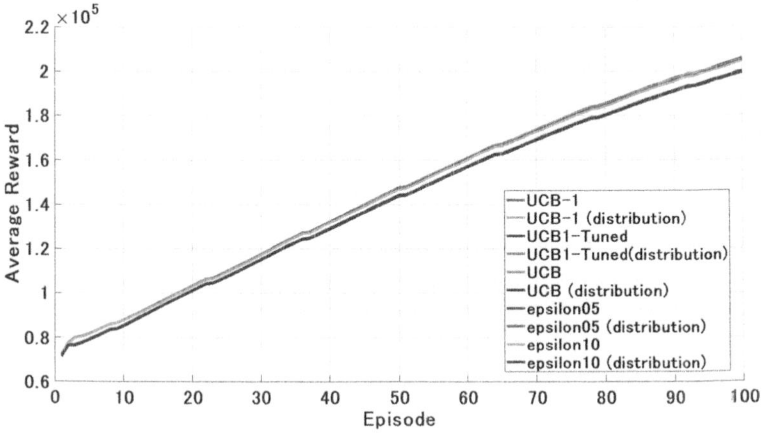

Fig. 4. Reward per episode for each algorithm

On the other hand, Fig. 3 shows that Throughput decreased for all learning algorithms compared with baseline CSMA/CA when the number of terminals was small. As the number of terminals increased, the performance gap between CSMA/CA and the learning-based policies narrowed. The average reward per episode differed across algorithms, reflecting the balance each strategy strikes between exploration and exploitation as shown in Fig. 4.

The proposed framework effectively reduces the transmission failure probability by adapting channel selection and CW values. However, the observed decrease in throughput indicates a trade-off introduced by conservative backoff settings or sub-optimal exploration schedules. This suggests that throughput-oriented reward shaping, joint tuning of CW and data-rate parameters, or multi-objective optimization could further improve performance.

5 Conclusion

We simulated scenarios with the number of terminals ranging from small to large and compared several RL algorithms with CSMA/CA. When channel selection and CW values were learned, the transmission failure probability decreased, but throughput also declined in some regimes.

Future work will focus on maintaining high success rates while improving throughput, for example by refining reward design, considering traffic differentiation, and jointly optimizing MAC and channel choices.

References

1. Radio Environment Council: Guidelines for Safe and Secure Use of Radio Waves in Medical Facilities. Ministry of Internal Affairs and Communications. (in Japanese) (2025)
2. Hanada, E., Kudou, T.: Wireless communication system use in medical hospitals and management of the electromagnetic environment. In: 2024 IEEE Joint International Symposium on Electromagnetic Compatibility, Signal & Power Integrity: EMC Japan / Asia-Pacific International Symposium on Electromagnetic Compatibility (EMC Japan/APEMC Okinawa), Ginowan, Okinawa, Japan (2024)
3. Sutton, R.S., Barto, A.G.: Reinforcement Learning an Introduction, 2nd edn. The MIT Press, Cambridge, Massachusetts, London, England (2018)
4. Sogabe, T.: Introduction to Reinforcement Learning Algorithms. Ohmsha, Tokyo. (in Japanese) (2019)
5. Kuleshov, V., Precup, D.: Algorithms for multi-armed bandit problems. J. Mach. Learn. Res. **1**, 1–48 (2000)
6. Hirano, S., Takabayashi, K., Sakakibara, K.: A study on channel selection method in cognitive radio using UCB algorithm. In: The Institute of Electronics, Information and Communication Engineers General Conference (2022)
7. Dejima, K., Takabayashi, K., Sakakibara, K.: Performance evaluation on channel selection algorithm using reinforcement learning under dynamic channel environment in cognitive radio networks. In: The 74th Joint Conference of the Chugoku Branch of the Electrical and Information Related Societies (2023)
8. Kinoshita, K., Takabayashi, K.: A study on distributed channel selection method for interference avoidance using reinforcement learning. In: The Institute of Electronics, Information and Communication Engineers Society Conference, Saitama, Japan (2024)

Hybrid ARQ with Cyclic-Orthogonal Walsh–Hadamard Spreading for Interference-Robust IEEE 802.15.6ma Based WBANs

Ruon Takahashi(✉) and Kento Takabayashi

Toyo University, 2100 Kujirai, Kawagoe, Saitama 351-8585, Japan
s36c02400093@toyo.jp

Abstract. Wireless body area networks (WBANs) are increasingly deployed in medical and healthcare applications, where stringent reliability and latency are required despite dense device coexistence and unpredictable interference. This paper studies a hybrid automatic repeat request (HARQ) scheme tailored to IEEE 802.15.6ma that integrates forward-error-correction (FEC) with selective retransmissions and applies cyclic-orthogonal Walsh–Hadamard codes (COWHC) as spreading sequences to suppress multiple-access interference (MAI) from asynchronous WBANs. We outline the HARQ procedure, detail the construction and properties of the COWHC set, and evaluate performance by packet-error rate (PER) under additive white Gaussian noise (AWGN) with MAI. The results indicate that, for limited retransmission budgets, HARQ with COWHC yields lower PER than conventional ARQ and maintains orthogonality among concurrently active links, thereby improving reliability without excessive retransmissions.

Keywords: Hybrid ARQ · Hadamard codes · cyclic-orthogonal code sets · WBAN · IEEE802.15.6 ma

1 Introduction

Recent advances in WBAN technology are driving adoption in continuous monitoring, assisted rehabilitation, and other healthcare scenarios [1–6]. However, in practical deployments multiple independent WBANs may operate in proximity with limited coordination, creating asynchronous transmissions that deteriorate link reliability through MAI [7]. Within IEEE 802.15.6ma which is currently being developed as a revision of IEEE 802.15.6, high-QoS packet delivery therefore requires a mechanism that leverages FEC to correct random errors and contains MAI arising from concurrent users [8].

We address these challenges by combining an HARQ mechanism concatenating Reed-Solomon (RS) codes and a LDPC code defined in IEEE 802.15.6ma, where parity information is incrementally provided across retransmissions, with spreading by a cyclic-orthogonal Walsh–Hadamard code set. While FEC mitigates random noise and residual interference, the code design preserves orthogonality among concurrently active sensors, reducing MAI at the de-spread output even under relative delays.

H. Tanaka et al. (Eds.): BodyNets 2025, LNICST 714, pp. 390–397, 2026.
https://doi.org/10.1007/978-3-032-38657-1_33

2 Proposed HARQ Method

Figure 1 schematically illustrates the procedure for the HARQ method considered in this study [8, 9]. First, a CRC is appended to the information bit, which is then encoded using an RS code. Next, the code is encoded using an LDPC code with a coding rate of 1/2. In the initial transmission, only the RS-encoded packet is sent. At the receiver, after decoding the RS code and CRC, it checks for bit errors or packet loss. If any are detected, the receiver temporarily holds the transmitted packet and sends a NACK back to the transmitter. Upon receiving the NACK, the transmitter sends the parity bit sequence generated during the LDPC encoding. The receiver then combines the retained packet with the received parity bit sequence to perform LDPC decoding. This enhances error correction capability before performing error correction.

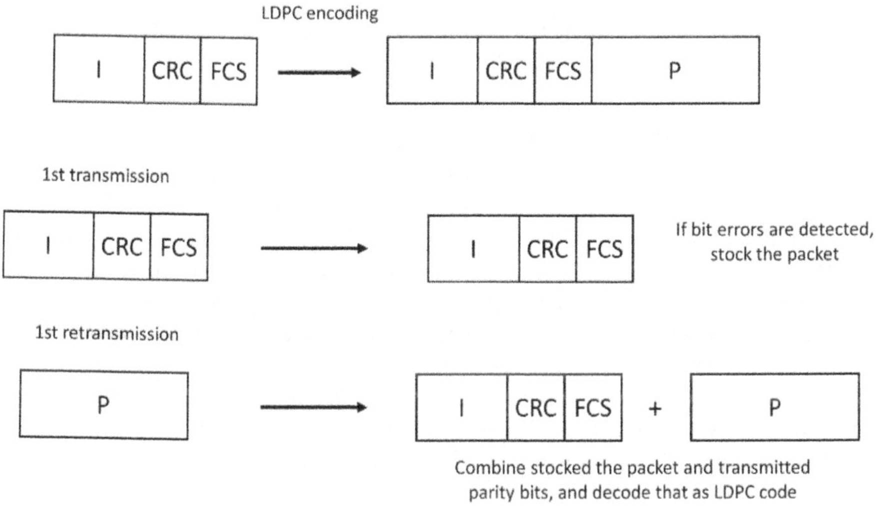

Fig. 1. Proposed HARQ method Overview

3 Cyclic Orthogonal Walsh-Hadamard Codes

Existing Hadamard matrices lose orthogonality when multiple access interference occurs. In this study, the cyclic orthogonal Hadamard codes are used as a spread code to eliminate multiple access interference [10].

3.1 Hadamard Codes

The codes generated from Hadamard matrices H exhibit orthogonality at zero phase. Hadamard codes are $N \times N$ matrices. Starting with the initial condition $H_N = [1]$, higher-dimensional matrices H_N are generated as shown in Eq. (1).

$$H_{2N} = \begin{bmatrix} H_N & H_N \\ H_N & -H_N \end{bmatrix} = H_2 \otimes H_N \tag{1}$$

Using the Hadamard matrix as a spreading code allows signals from other devices to be removed from the received signal, enabling extraction of signals from any desired device. When each row $w_1, w_2, \cdots, w_N$ of the Hadamard matrix is assigned to the transmitted signal $K_1, K_2, \cdots, K_N$ of each user, the received signal y is given by the following Eq. (2).

$$y = K_1 w_1 + K_2 w_2 + \cdots + K_N w_N \tag{2}$$

Here, since the Hadamard matrix is orthogonal at zero phase, multiplying Eq. (2) by w_1 allows us to extract only the signal K_1.

3.2 Cyclic Orthogonal Walsh-Hadamard Codes

The orthogonality of the Hadamard matrix is lost when the codes are phase-shifted. Correlating phase-shifted codes produces nonzero cross-correlation values. When such non-orthogonal codes are used in asynchronous WBAN, multiple access interference (MAI) occurs. Therefore, a set of Cyclic Orthogonal Walsh-Hadamard codes (COWHC) that are mutually orthogonal at all phase shifts $\Phi = 0, 1, \cdots, 2^k - 1$ is used [10]. Each device is assigned a unique code from the COWHC set to eliminate the effects of MAI.

we see that only "some" codes exhibit zero cross-correlation. We are particularly interested in these sets of codes When examined, we can find a unique set of $K = k + 1 = 4$ code from W(8, 3) that have zero cross-correlation in all phases $\Phi = 0, 1, 2, \cdots, 7$ [4]. Here, assuming the codes $w_i (i = 1, \cdots, 8)$ are extracted from the i-th row of W(8, 3), the following code set can be cited as an example of a COWHC.

- $w_1 = (1, 1, 1, 1, 1, 1, 1, 1)$
- $w_2 = (1, -1, 1, -1, 1, -1, 1, -1)$
- $w_3 = (1, 1, -1, -1, 1, 1, -1, -1)$
- $w_5 = (1, 1, 1, 1, -1, -1, -1, -1)$

The COWHC code set selected in this manner can be used for sensor broadcasting in WBANs. While this method limits the maximum number of simultaneously active sensors to $K = k + 1$, it ensures high reliability for all K connections and eliminates collisions.

4 Coexistence Environments Class 3–7

Figure 2 shows the coexistence environment classes assumed. It assumes interference from WBANs and other WBANs using the same IEEE 802.15.6ma standard, as well as interference from systems using other standards. Interference from systems using the same standard is known as interference and can be mitigated as expected interference, but interference from systems using other standards is unexpected.

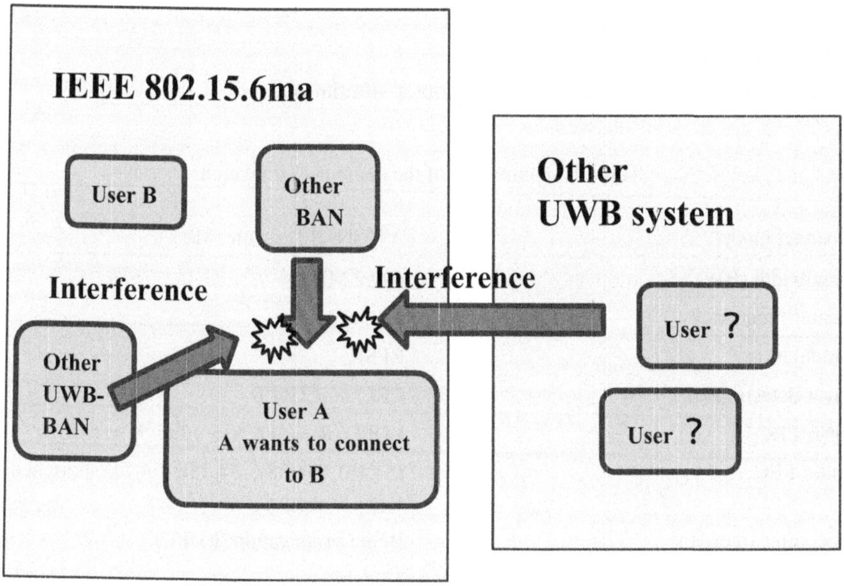

Fig. 2. Coexistence Environments Class 3–7

The assumed bit loss communication channel (Fig. 3) involves consecutive bit loss due to interference with other systems and devices. A maximum of $p_e\%$ of the PSDU length is lost, and the lost length follows a uniform distribution.

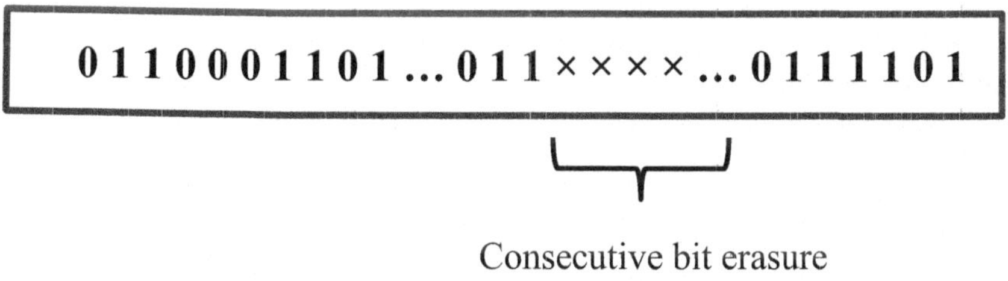

Fig. 3. Bit erasure channel model

For interference from other devices, two types are used: expected devices and unexpected devices. For expected devices, a different row of the COWHC is applied as the spreading code compared to the main device. For unexpected devices, the same COWHC as the main device is applied.

5 Numerical Results

Table 1 shows the parameters of the computer simulation.

Table 1. Parameters of the computer simulation

Channel model	AWGN, Bit erasure, MAI
Bandwidth (BW)	499.2 MHz
Center Frequency	3993.6 MHz
Modulation	BPSK
Error detection code	CRC-16-CCITT
Inner FEC	LDPC (R = 1/2, N = 1296, K = 648)
Outer FEC	(54,46), (54,38), (54,28), (54,14) shortened Reed-Solomon (sRS) Codes
Decoding algorism	Belief propagation (LDPC)
PSDU length (L_{psdu})	1296 bits
Maximum erasure ratio (p_e)	10%
Maximum number of retransmissions (r_{max})	1,4 (LDPC)
ARQ scheme	Stop and wait

Figures 3, 4, 5 and 6 shows the packet error rate versus received SNR when applying a (1296, 648) LDPC code, with the RS code encoding rate set to five levels including no encoding, and with and without COWHC applied, for maximum retransmission counts of 1 and 4. It assumes bit loss of up to 10% of the maximum transmission packet length (648 bits). Figures 3 and 4 show results for a maximum number of retransmissions of 1, while Figs. 5 and 6 show results for a maximum number of retransmissions of 4. For maximum retransmission counts of 1 and 4, the PER reached 1 at all SNRs when COWHC was not applied. This indicates that the error correction codes used alone cannot suppress MAI. Applying COWHC improved the PER compared to not applying it. Furthermore, HARQ achieved a better PER than ARQ. Increasing the maximum retransmission count also improved the PER. These performance evaluation results confirm that applying COWHC sufficiently suppresses MAI (Fig. 7).

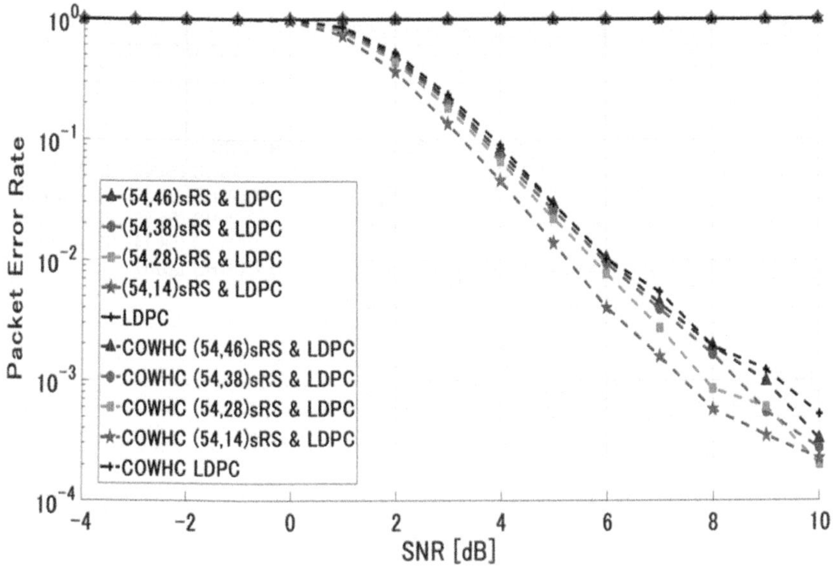

Fig. 4. LDPC ARQ maximum retransmission 1

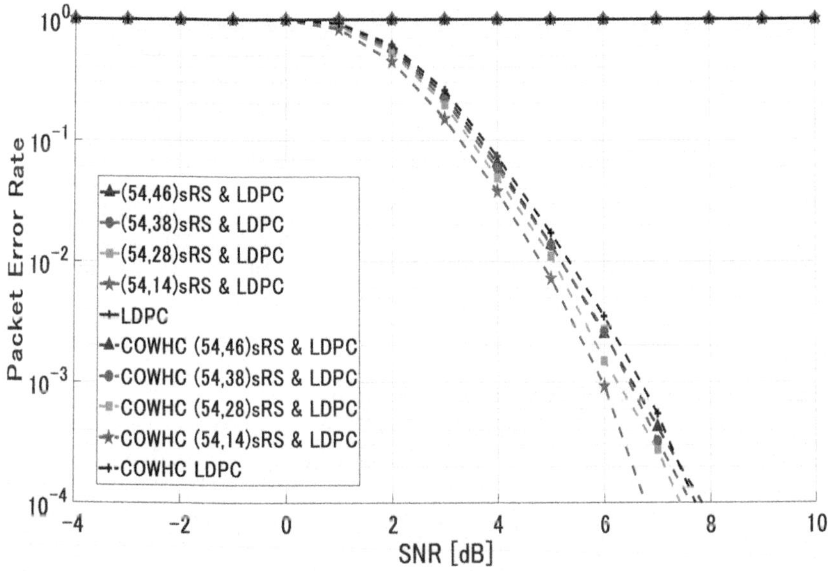

Fig. 5. LDPC HARQ maximum retransmission 1

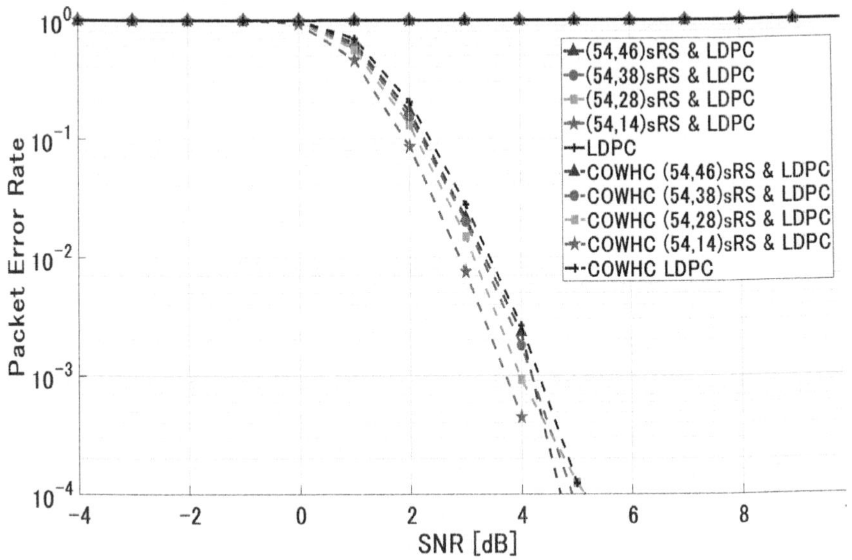

Fig. 6. LDPC ARQ maximum retransmission 4

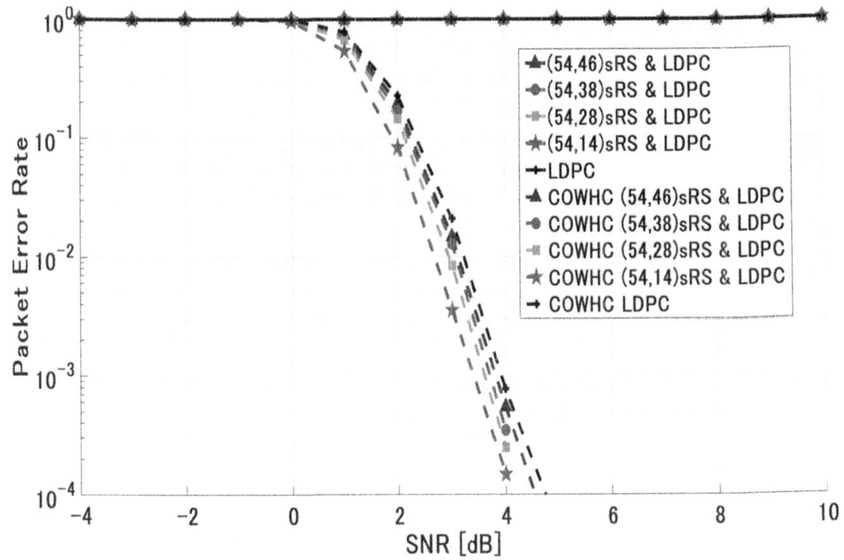

Fig. 7. LDPC HARQ maximum retransmission 4

6 Conclusion

We investigated an HARQ scheme for IEEE 802.15.6ma WBANs that employs COWHC spreading to mitigate MAI from asynchronous coexisting networks. Simulation results showed that combination of COWHC and HARQ improved orthogonality among users and, when combined with incremental redundancy, reduces PER more effectively than ARQ with the same retransmission limit.

Future work includes evaluation under multi-path fading channels and a systematic study of the MAI levels that COWHC can tolerate across activity patterns and timing offsets.

References

1. Alshehri, F., Muhammad, G.: A comprehensive survey of the Internet of Things (IoT) and AI-based smart healthcare. IEEE Access. **9**, 3660–3678 (2021)
2. Dwivedia, R., Mehrotrab, D., Chandrac, S.: Potential of Internet of Medical hings (IoMT) applications in building a smart healthcare system: a systematic review. J. Oral Biol. Craniofacial Res. **12**, 302–318 (2022)
3. Ning, Z., et al.: Mobile edge computing enabled 5g health monitoring for internet of medical things: a decentralized game theoretic approach. IEEE J. Sel. Areas Commun. **39**, 463–478 (2021)
4. Javaid, S., Zeadally, S., Fahim, H., He, B.: Medical sensors and their integration in wireless body area networks for pervasive healthcare delivery: a review. IEEE Sens. J. **22**, 3860–3877 (2022)
5. Selem, E., Fatehy, M., El-Kader, S.M.A.: mobTHE (Mobile Temperature Heterogeneity Energy) aware routing protocol for WBAN IoT health application. IEEE Access. **9**, 18692–18705 (2021)
6. Misra, S., Bishoyi, P.K., Sarkar, S.: I-MAC: In-body sensor MAC in wireless body area networks for healthcare IoT. IEEE Syst. J. **15**, 4413–4420 (2021)
7. Takumi K., Minsoo K., Marco H., Daisuke A., Ryuji K.: Interference mitigation schemes in class 3, 5, 6 and 7 of coexistence in TG6ma. Doc. IEEE802.15-24-0073-07-006a (2025)
8. Kento T., et al.: Hybrid ARQ scheme for high QoS packets in high class of coexistence of IEEE 802.15.6ma. Doc. IEEE P802. 15-23-0576-03-06ma (2024)
9. Ruon, T., Kento, T., Takumi, K., Daisuke, A.: A study on performance evaluation of HARQ scheme in IEEE802.15.6ma standard. In: The Institute of Electronics, Information and Communication Engineers Society Conference 2024, Saitama, Japan (2024)
10. Ali, T., Jamshid, A., Plataniotis, K.N.: Cyclic orthogonal codes in CDMA-based asynchronous wireless body area networks. In: 2012 IEEE International Conference on Acoustics, Speech and Signal Processing (ICASSP), Kyoto, Japan (2012)

Performance Comparison of IEEE802.15.6ma Error Control Scheme with Super Orthogonal Convolutional Code

Kento Takabayashi[1(✉)] and Ryuji Kohno[2,3]

[1] Toyo University, 2100 Kujirai, Kawagoe, Saitama 351-8585, Japan
takabayashi.kento.xp@gmail.com

[2] YRP International Alliance Institute (YRP-IAI), YRP1 Blg., 3-4 HikarinoOka, Yokosuka 239-0847, Kanagawa, Japan
kohno@yrp-iai.jp

[3] Yokohama National University, 79-5 Tokiwadai, Hodogaya-ku, Yokohama 240-8501, Japan

Abstract. With the rapid growth of IoT and healthcare needs, wearable devices and Wireless Body Area Networks (WBANs) have gained attention. IEEE802.15.6, standardized in 2012, and ETSI SmartBAN provided initial frameworks, while the ongoing IEEE802.15.6ma revision aims to create a highly dependable WBAN by introducing UWB high-speed transmission, simplified MAC, multi-WBAN cooperation, hybrid ARQ (HARQ), and so on. This enables applications in medicine, vehicles, and industrial automation. Reliability depends on flexible use of error correcting codes and HARQ, according to coexistence environment level and QoS. By the way, super orthogonal convolutional codes (SOCC) have strong error-correcting capability and compatibility with UWB, making them candidates for adoption in IEEE802.15.6ma. This study evaluates SOCC against existing error control schemes through computer simulations under a coexistence scenario. Numerical results show that HARQ provides high reliability with some delay, while low-rate SOCC achieves strong error correction with real-time performance.

Keywords: WBAN · IEEE802.15.6ma · Error Control Scheme · HARQ · SOCC

1 Introduction

In recent years, with the spread of the Internet of Things (IoT) and increasing health awareness, wearable devices have been attracting attention, which can easily measure an individual's lifestyle and health status, process the measurement data in an integrated manner, and provide meaningful feedback to the user [1–3]. One type of technology supporting the development of the medical and healthcare IoT system is the wireless

H. Tanaka et al. (Eds.): BodyNets 2025, LNICST 714, pp. 398–409, 2026.
https://doi.org/10.1007/978-3-032-38657-1_34

body area network (WBAN), which flexibly connects biosensors placed near the surface of the body [4–6]. Among these, the wireless communication method for WBANs was internationally standardized as IEEE 802.15.6 in February 2012 [7]. In April 2015, the European Telecommunications Standards Institute (ETSI) formulated technical specifications for a Smart Body Area Network (SmartBAN) [8]. In addition, IEEE 802.15.6ma is currently being developed as a revision of IEEE 802.15.6 [9]. IEEE 802.15.6ma is a project to completely revise the 2012 edition of the WBAN standard and is based on the concept of a "Dependable Body Area Network." It aims to expand the network to a highly reliable one that spans people and vehicles by introducing ultra-wideband (UWB) high-speed transmission, simplified MAC, multi-WBAN cooperation, a hybrid ARQ (HARQ), TSN bridging, and more. Once the standardization of IEEE802.15.6ma is complete, it is expected to become widespread as a common platform that achieves "cable-less and high reliability" in fields such as medicine (implant BCI and home monitoring), automobiles (wireless harnesses and in-vehicle sensors), and industrial factory automation (UAV rescue and robot control).

To achieve the high reliability that IEEE802.15.6ma aims at, the method of applying error correction codes and HARQ can be flexibly changed according to the coexistence environment class and the Quality of Service (QoS) of the information being handled [9]. On the other hand, super orthogonal convolutional code (SOCC) is known as an error correcting code that is compatible with UWB, and its adoption as an optional method is being considered in IEEE802.15.6ma [10].

In this research, it is confirmed that SOCC satisfies the requirements of the assumed applications of IEEE802.15.6ma and demonstrate its effectiveness by comparing the performance of SOCC with the error control method of IEEE802.15.6ma in the assumed environment of IEEE802.15.6ma.

2 IEEE802.15.6ma Error Control Scheme

2.1 Coexistence Environment Class

As shown in Table 1, IEEE802.15.6ma has eight coexistence environment classes according to the degree of coexistence with WBANs that have the same or similar standards, other systems that use UWB, and existing systems that use the same frequency band [9]. In particular, when the coexistence environment class is high, such as Class 4 or higher, HARQ is used in addition to error correcting codes as an error control method.

Table 1. Coexistence environment class.

Class	Data type
0	Only one IEEE802.15.6ma WBAN
1	Multiple IEEE802.15.6ma WBANs
2	Multiple IEEE802.15.6 and 15.6ma WBANs
3	Multiple IEEE802.15.6ma WBANs and non-UWB systems
4	Multiple IEEE802.15.6ma WBANs and IEEE802.15.x UWB systems
5	Multiple IEEE802.15.6ma WBANs and non-IEEE802.15.x UWB systems
6	Systems included in Class 4 and 5
7	Systems included in Class 3 to 5

2.2 QoS Levels of Packets Corresponding to User Priority

In IEEE 802.15.6 WBAN systems, various data such as vital signs, skin temperature, blood pressure, ECG, EEG, ECoG, and vehicle controlling commons have different QoS levels corresponding to user priority as shown in Table 2 [7]. Similarly for IEEE802.15.6ma, data packet transmission should be dependable according to QoS levels even in various classes of coexistence environment for dependable WBAN for human and vehicles. Figure 1 shows the concept of channel coding procedure to realize a reliable WBAN system according to QoS in IEEE802.15.6ma. In a low priority QoS case, only a single error correcting code will be applied for a physical layer service data unit (PSDU). On the other hand, an outer and an inner error correcting codes will be serially applied for PSDU in a high priority QoS case. Table 2 shows the concept table of channel coding scheme for IEEE802.15.6ma [9]. As an inner code, IEEE802.15.4ab LDPC ($K = 324, 648, 972, R = 1/2$) or binary convolutional code (BCC) ($K = 7, R = 1/2$) will be selected for the coexistence of IEEE802.15.6ma and IEEE802.15.4ab. As an outer code, shortened Reed-Solomon (RS) codes with $N = 54$ (original code length $N = 63$) will be selected to correct burst errors and erasures due to interference from other WBANs, and the coding rates are changed according to each QoS.

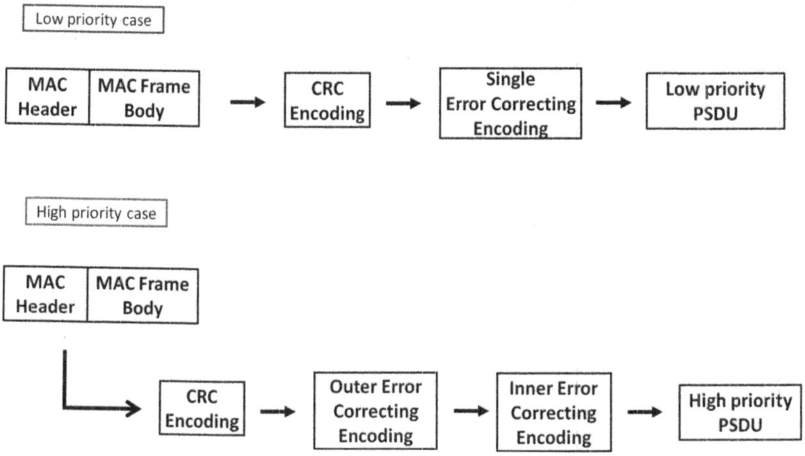

Fig. 1. Concept of channel coding procedure in IEEE802.15.6ma.

Table 2. Concept table of channel coding selection.

User Priority	Inner Code	Outer Code
0	IEEE802.15.4ab LDPC or BCC	No coding
1	IEEE802.15.4ab LDPC or BCC	No coding
2	IEEE802.15.4ab LDPC or BCC	No coding
3	IEEE802.15.4ab LDPC or BCC	No coding
4	IEEE802.15.4ab LDPC or BCC	(54, 46) shortened RS code
5	IEEE802.15.4ab LDPC or BCC	(54, 38) shortened RS code
6	IEEE802.15.4ab LDPC or BCC	(54, 28) shortened RS code
7	IEEE802.15.4ab LDPC or BCC	(54, 14) shortened RS code

2.3 HARQ Scheme in IEEE802.15.6ma

IEEE802.15.6ma considers the half-rate BCC and LDPC as an error correcting code [9]. Hence, a HARQ scheme using those FEC is introduced. Figure 2 summarizes a procedure of the HARQ mechanism in the BCC case. Firstly, the information bit sequence is encoded by the half-rate BCC. An encoded codeword is punctured via the punctured matrices, and codeword 1 and 1' are generated. After that, codeword 1 and 1' are transmitted alternately, and at the receiving side, codeword 1 and 1' are combined to gradually improve the error correction capability. In this HARQ mechanism, the coding rate is decreased to 4/5, 1/2, 1/3, 1/4, and so on.

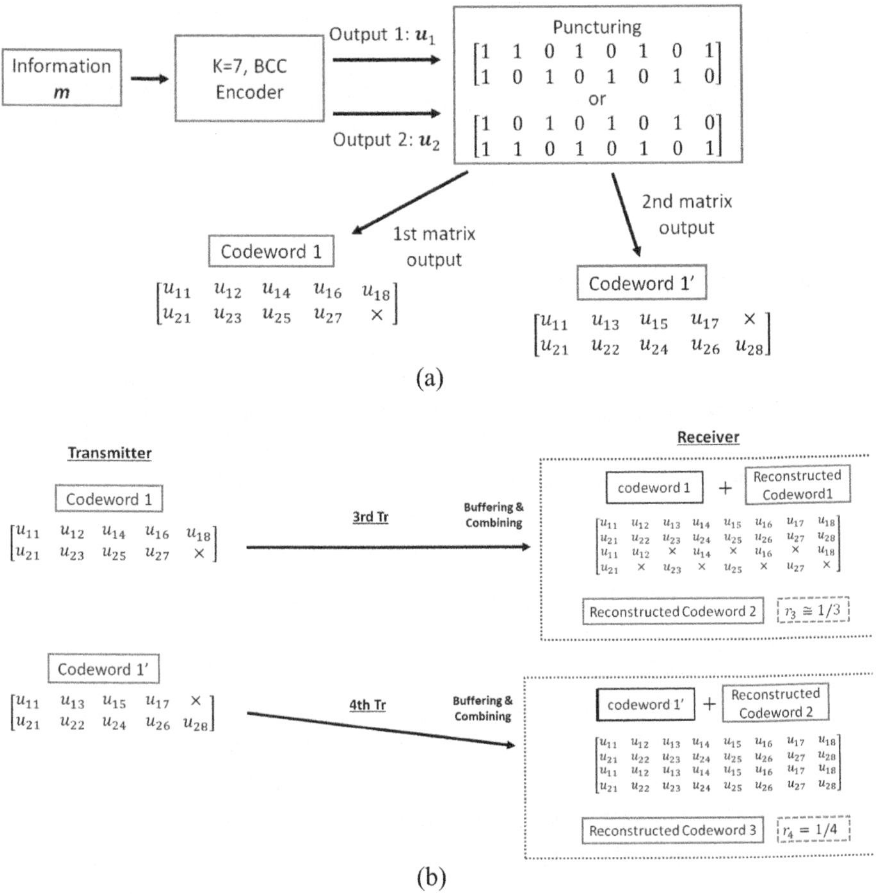

Fig. 2. Procedure of the HARQ mechanism in the BCC case. (a) Generation of codeword 1 and codeword 1' (b) Codeword reconstruction

Figure 3 summarizes a procedure of the HARQ mechanism in the LDPC case. In this case, the mechanism is the same as the HARQ defined in IEEE802.15.6 Std.-2012. First, a CRC is added to the information bit sequence and it is encoded with RS code. Next, this is encoded with an LDPC code with a coding rate of 1/2, and then only the RS-encoded packet is sent in the first transmission. On the receiver side, after RS decoding and CRC decoding, it checks for bit errors or losses, and if any are detected, it temporarily holds the transmitted packet and returns a NACK to the transmitter. After receiving the NACK, the transmitter then transmits the parity bit sequence from the LDPC encoding, and the receiver combines the held packet with the received parity bit sequence to perform LDPC decoding, improving its error correction capability and then correcting errors.

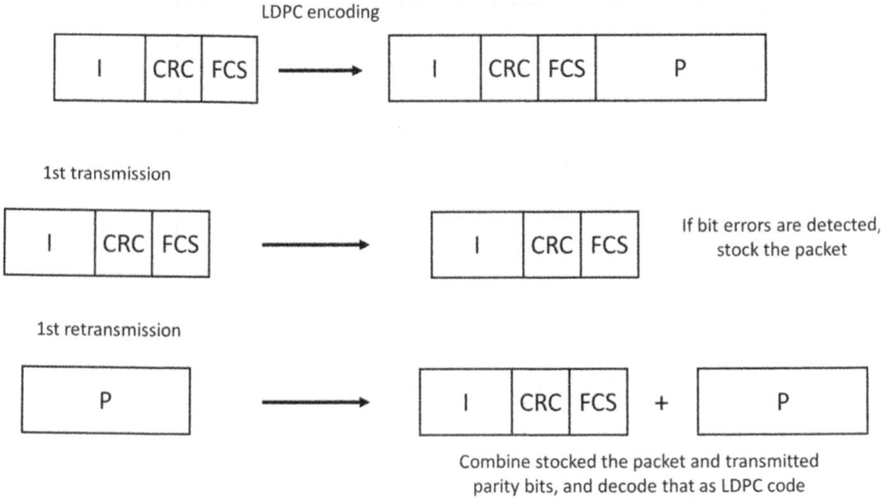

Fig. 3. Procedure of the HARQ mechanism in the LDPC case.

3 Super Orthogonal Convolutional Code

It is possible to design an error-correcting SOCC with a very low coding rate, resulting in this type of code having very strong error-correcting capabilities. SOCCs have attracted attention as error correction codes for code division multiple access (CDMA) using the spread spectrum [10]. Therefore, SOCCs are compatible with the UWB, as they have a very wide bandwidth. The encoder of an SOCC is shown in Fig. 4. The SOCC encoder consists of $K - 1$ shift registers and a block orthogonal encoder with a Hadamard matrix of order 2^{K-2}. Here, K represents the constraint length. The encoder maps the bits stored in the shift registers up to $K - 2$ th to the Hadamard sequence with a sequence length of 2^{K-2}. Then, the SOCC symbols are generated by applying an exclusive-OR to the output of the Hadamard sequences, the input bit and the $K - 1$ th stored bit. The coding rate R_{SOCC} of an SOCC is $2^{-(K-2)}$. Viterbi decoding can be used to decode SOCCs as well as general convolutional codes.

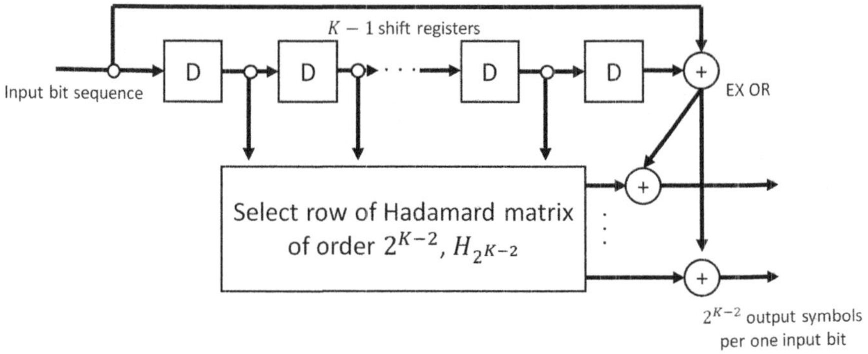

Fig. 4. SOCC encoder configuration.

4 Numerical Results

This section compares the performance of the IEEE802.15.6ma error control method and SOCC in the assumed environment of IEEE802.15.6ma by computer simulation. Table 3 lists the parameters for computer simulation. This computer simulation assumes bit erasure channel, which simulates asynchronous interference from other systems assuming coexistence environment classes 3 to 7. It is assumed that consecutive bit erasures of up to p_e% of the length of PSDU L_{PSDU} occur as shown in Fig. 5. p_e is uniformly distributed in the interval 0 to p_e. In addition, the IEEE model CM3 was selected as the channel model. This channel model is used when assuming communication in a wearable WBAN (Human WBAN: HBAN) [9, 11].

Table 3. Simulation parameters.

Parameter	Details
Channel model	IEEE model CM3, Bit erasure channel
Bandwidth (BW)	499.2 MHz
Center Frequency	3993.6 MHz
Modulation	BPSK
Error detection code	CRC-16-CCITT
Inner FEC	IEEE802.15.4ab BCC, LDPC (R = 1/2), SOCC (R = 1/2, 1/4, 1/8, 1/16)
Outer FEC	(54,46), (54,38), (54,28), (54,14) shortened Reed-Solomon (sRS) Codes
Slot length	0.886 ms
PSDU data rate	125 Mbps
PSDU length (L_{PSDU})	1296 bits

(continued)

Table 3. (*continued*)

Parameter	Details
Maximum erasure ratio (p_e)	0.3
Max number of transmission	0 (SOCC), 3 (ARQ and HARQ)
ARQ scheme	Stop and wait

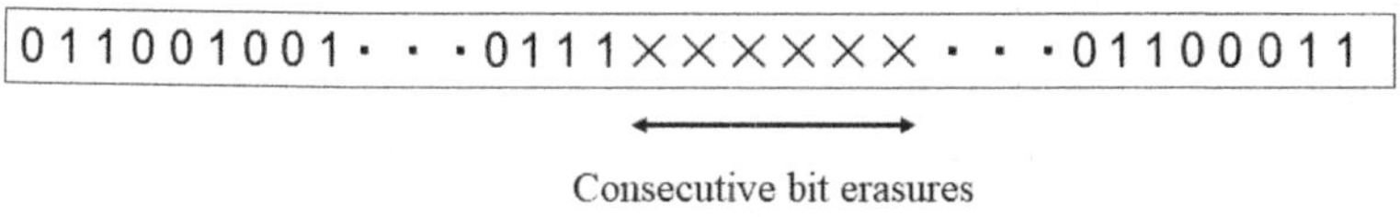

Fig. 5. Example of consecutive bit erasures.

Figures 6, 7 and 8 show packet error ratio, PSDU throughput and average delay performances of each scheme as a function of E_b/N_0 respectively. In the cases of LDPC and BCC, the PER of HARQ has better improved compared with ARQ and HARQ. In particular, when we look at the case of BCC, the difference was very large. This is because HARQ using BCC can improve error correction capability with each retransmission. When considering concatenated coding with RS codes, the best performance was obtained in combination with the (54, 46) sRS code in comparison of E_b/N_0. This means that although a combination with a low-coding-rate RS code provides high error correction capability, it is not energy efficient. Regarding the comparison in Fig. 6(c), BCC and half-rate SOCC could not achieve a PER of 10^{-2}. On the other hand, LDPC and low-rate SOCCs could achieve that. Especially low-rate SOCC cases whose coding rates were 1/4, 1/8 and 1/16 were much better than BCC and LDPC in low E_b/N_0 areas without retransmission.

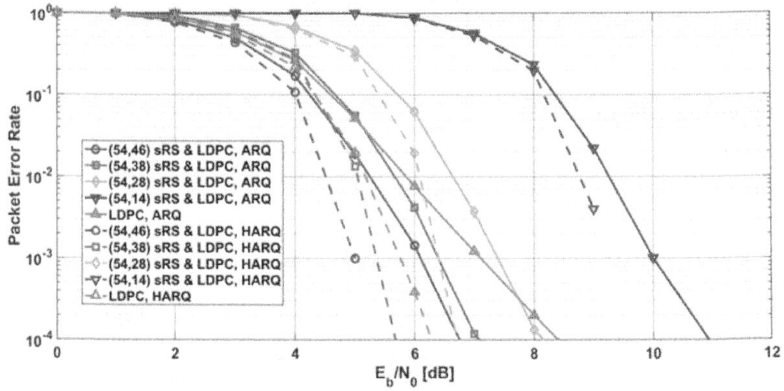

(a)

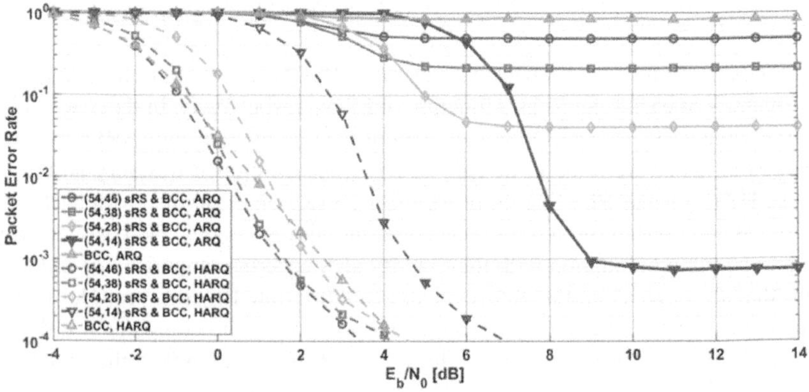

(b)

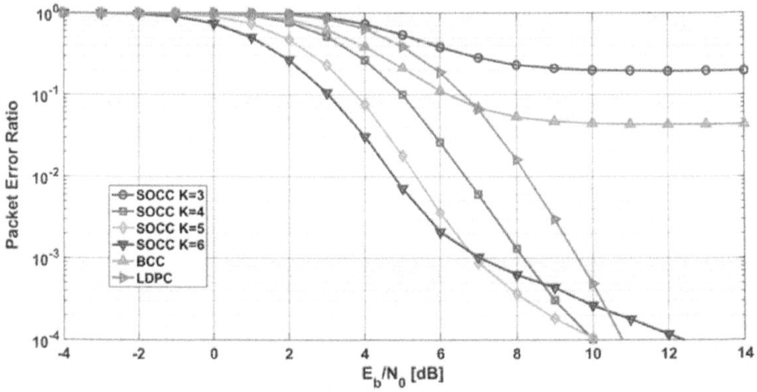

(c)

Fig. 6. Packet error ratio of each scheme as a function of E_b/N_0. (a) LDPC case (b) BCC case (c) SOCC case

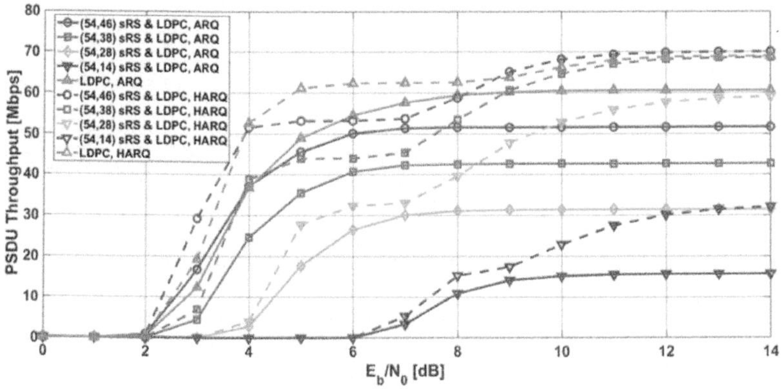

(a)

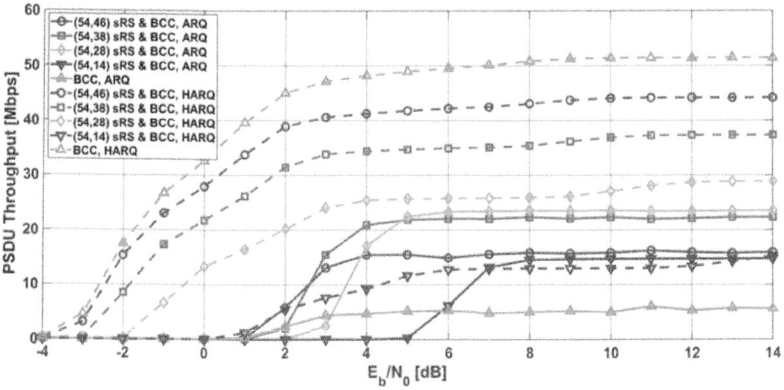

(b)

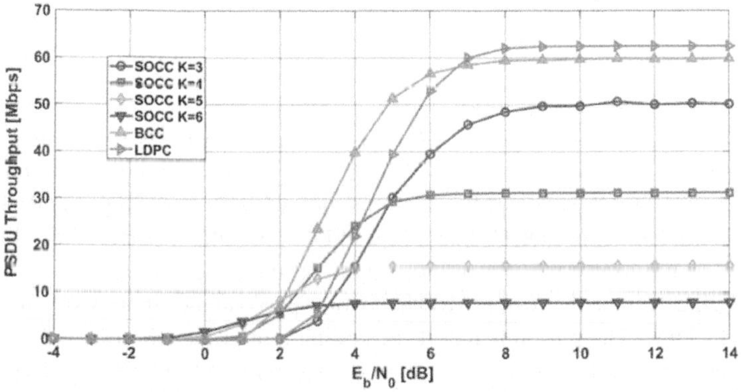

(c)

Fig. 7. PSDU throughput of each scheme as a function of E_b/N_0. (a) LDPC case (b) BCC case (c) SOCC case

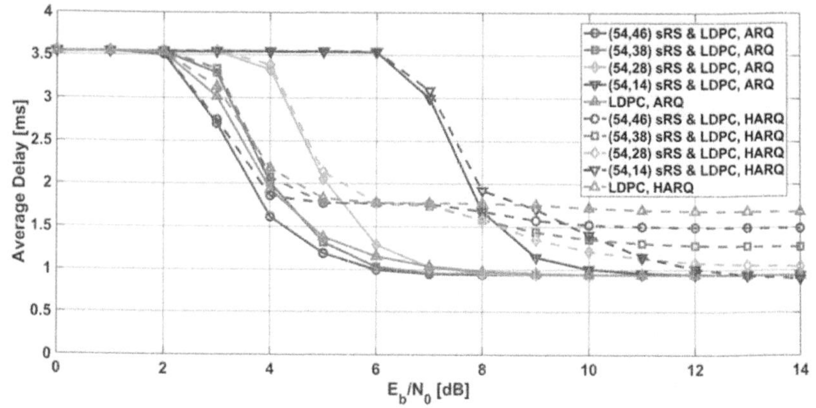

(a)

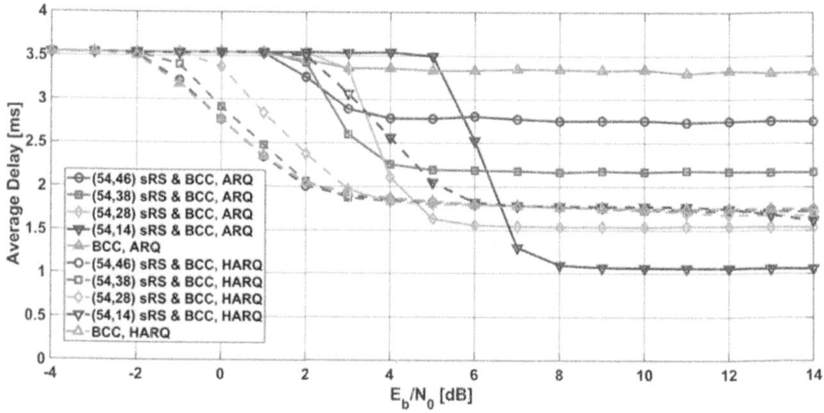

(b)

Fig. 8. Average delay of each scheme as a function of E_b/N_0. (a) LDPC case (b) BCC case

Next, the PSDU throughput of HARQ was also better than that of ARQ in both cases of LDPC and BCC, especially high E_b/N_0 areas. By adjusting the coding rate, it was possible to reach 30 Mbps except for a combination with a low-coding-rate RS code. On the other hand, Low-rate SOCCs had a less PSDU throughput performance than other cases. However at least 7.8 Mbps or more could be stably achieved.

Finally, the average delay of HARQ had worse performance than ARQ, in particular the case of LDPC. The reason is that if the coding rate of the RS code was high or RS code was not used, at least one retransmission was required in the case of HARQ. On the other hand, the average delay of HARQ had basically better performance in the BCC case, especially low E_b/N_0 areas. In the high E_b/N_0 region, the average delay was longer than that of simple ARQ with a low RS code due to one retransmission. However, it still maintained a low delay of several ms or less. For comparison in SOCC, the delay is constant at one slot time, approximately 1 ms since no retransmissions are performed.

5 Conclusion

This study has evaluated performances of HARQ and SOCC when applying an on-body to on-body channel model based on the scenario assumed in IEEE802.15.6ma. In this condition, HARQ has been significantly superior in terms of PER and PSDU throughput, and HARQ also maintained a low average delay. Then, low-rate SOCCs have had better PER performances but a less PSDU throughput than other schemes. However, at least about 8 Mbps or more could be stably achieved. In other words, HARQ is suitable for cases where a certain degree of delay is acceptable and very high reliability is required. On the other hand, in cases where real-time performance and a certain degree of high reliability are required, SOCC with a low coding rate can be said to be more suitable.

As for the future work, the effectiveness will be demonstrated through evaluation assuming other specific scenarios, for example a vehicle WBAN case.

References

1. Alshehri, F., Muhammad, G.: A comprehensive survey of the Internet of Things (IoT) and AI-based smart healthcare. IEEE Access. **9**, 3660–3678 (2021)
2. Dwivedia, R., Mehrotrab, D., Chandrac, S.: Potential of Internet of Medical hings (IoMT) applications in building a smart healthcare system: a systematic review. J. Oral Biol. Craniofacial Res. **12**, 302–318 (2022)
3. Ning, Z., et al.: Mobile edge computing enabled 5G health monitoring for internet of medical things: a decentralized game theoretic approach. IEEE J. Sel. Areas. Commun. **39**, 463–478 (2021)
4. Javaid, S., Zeadally, S., Fahim, H., He, B.: Medical sensors and their integration in wireless body area networks for pervasive healthcare delivery: a review. IEEE Sens. J. **22**, 3860–3877 (2022)
5. Selem, E., Fatehy, M., El-Kader, S.M.A.: mobTHE (Mobile Temperature Heterogeneity Energy) aware routing protocol for WBAN IoT health application. IEEE Access. **9**, 18692–18705 (2021)
6. Misra, S., Bishoyi, P.K., Sarkar, S.: I-MAC: In-body sensor MAC in wireless body area networks for healthcare IoT. IEEE Syst. J. **15**, 4413–4420 (2021)
7. IEEE Standard for Information Technology: Telecommunications and information exchange between systems—local and metropolitan area networks; specific requirements. In: Part 15.6: Wireless Medium Access Control (MAC) and Physical Layer (PHY) Specifications for Wireless Personal Area Networks (WPANs) Used in or 12 around a Body (2012)
8. ETSI. Smart Body Area Network (SmartBAN); technical report on smart coordinator for SmartBAN networks. ETSI TR 103 944 V1.1.1 (2023)
9. Kohno, R.: Overview of activity of IEEE802.15 TG15.6ma for revision of IEEE802.15.6-2012 wireless BAN with enhanced dependability. In: IEEE 802 Plenary, Madrid, Spain (2025)
10. Takabayashi, K., Tanaka, H., Sakakibara, K.: Performance evaluation of an on-body wireless body network based on an ultra-wideband physical layer under a dynamic channel model. Electronics. **11**(21), 3491 (2022)
11. Yazdandoost, K.Y., Sayrafi-an-Pour, K.: Channel model for Body Area Network (BAN). In: IEEE P802.15Working Group for Wireless Personal Area Networks(WPANs). IEEE P802.15-08-0780-10-0006 (2009)

Coordinator-to-Coordinator(C2C) Communication and Ranging for Coexisting Multiple UWB-BANs

Ryuji Kohno[1(✉)], Takumi Kobayashi[2], and Chika Sugimoto[3]

[1] Yokohama National University, YRP International Alliance Institute, Yokosuka, Kanagawa 239-0847, Japan
kohno@yrp-iai.jp

[2] Osaka Metropolitan University & YRP International Alliance Institute, Osaka 536-0025, Japan
kobayashi.takumi@omu.ac.jp

[3] Yokohama National University, Yokohama, Kanagawa 240-8501, Japan
sugimoto-chika-zb@ynu.ac.jp

Abstract. This paper describes proposed core technologies in physical (PHY) and Medica-Access-Control (MAC) layers to recognize dynamic environment of coexisting multiple Ultra-Wide Band (UWB) wireless Body Area Network (BAN) into a new revision standard IEEE802.15.6ma for dependable BAN. Since an individual BAN is used to be independently operated in practical use cases, recognition of overlaid communication coverage ranges and contentions among packets due to geographical overlay of coexisting BANs are important. We have proposed schemes of communication and ranging between coordinators or hubs of neighboring multiple BANs in the revision standard IEEE802.15.6ma to perform stable synchronization and avoid contention among coexisting multiple UWB-BANs. This paper describes coordinator-to-coordinator (C2C) communication and ranging schemes in PHY and successive procedure in MAC in IEEE802.15.6ma. Their system performance of these cross-layer technologies is investigated in typical channel and environmental models.

Keywords: UWB · BAN · coexistence · C2C · IEEE802.15.6ma

1 Introduction

A wireless body area network (BAN) originated for wearable and implant vital sensors and actuators in a human body for medical healthcare of which original standard IEEE802.15.6 was established in 2012 [1]. BAN has been applied for remote medicine such as detecting COVID-19 and care of elderly people etc. These decays, demand of BAN uses has been expanding for animals, robotics, vehicles etc. while a large marketing size of automotive use makes BAN more successful in commercial. After 10 years passed of the standard establishment, amendment and revision of IEEE802.15.6

H. Tanaka et al. (Eds.): BodyNets 2025, LNICST 714, pp. 410–425, 2026.
https://doi.org/10.1007/978-3-032-38657-1_35

were required and task group of the revision TG15.6ma started for wireless BAN with enhanced dependability to wireless sensing and controlling human and vehicle body area networks (HBAN and VBAN) for medical healthcare and automotive uses in 2022 [2–4]. In particular, HBAN based on Ultra-Wide Band (UWB) radio for Brain-Machine-Interface (BMI) requires highly dependable and high speed transmission of electrocorticogram (ECoG) together with electroencephalogram (EEG) and other vital data for machine learning and remote robotic control [5]. VBAN makes a new market in automotive industry such as digital keys, wireless harness, etc. Moreover, a new applications in mixed human and vehicle uses such as avoiding elderly driver's traffic accidents etc. The revision standard IEEE802.15.6ma should satisfy requirement to manage interference and contention among overlaid BANs in PHY and MAC. The more BANs use, the more contention and inference cause performance degradation. The revision of physical (PHY) and media access control (MAC) has focuses on resolving these problems in coexistence of BANs [6]. This paper focuses on the proposed and involved coordinator-to-coordinator(C2C) communication and ranging schemes in a presence of coexisting multiple BANs in IEEE802.15.6ma. Typical system performance is illustrated in typical coexistence models. The following chapters describe first major features of the new revision standard IEEE802.15.6ma shortly. Coexistence assurance scenario including C2C communication and ranging is described. Typical system performance analysis is investigated according to the number and geographical distribution of multiple BANs.

2 Dependable WBAN Standard IEEE802.15.6ma

Shortly core technologies in PHY/MAC layers and progress of the revision standard IEEE802.15.6ma to achieve enhanced dependability will be summarized.

2.1 Main Features of the Revision Standard of Dependable BAN; IEEE802.15.6ma

IEEE802.15.6ma is a revision standard IEEE802.15.6–2012, so basically backward compatibility is ensured. However, it focuses on impulse radio type of UWB in PHY layer while IEEE802.15.6–2012 covers narrow band and human body communication (HBC) modulation. More additional channel and environmental models, error-control of channel codes and hybrid ARQ have been applied for combination of newly defined classes of coexistence and QoS priority levels of user packets in HBAN and VBAN.

(1) Channel and Environmental Models: To design dependable PHY layer of technologies in human and vehicle bodies, various channel propagation and environment with undesired and interfering signals have been modeled. The part of human body is listed in Table 1 while vehicle part can be referred in [7].
(2) Coexistence Classes: IEEE802.15.6ma classifies various coexisting networks in Table 2. Primarily it is designed to ensure dependability of Class 1 of only same new standard multiple BANs which are overlaid in communication range in partial and full.

Table 1. Channel Models of IEEE802.15.6ma

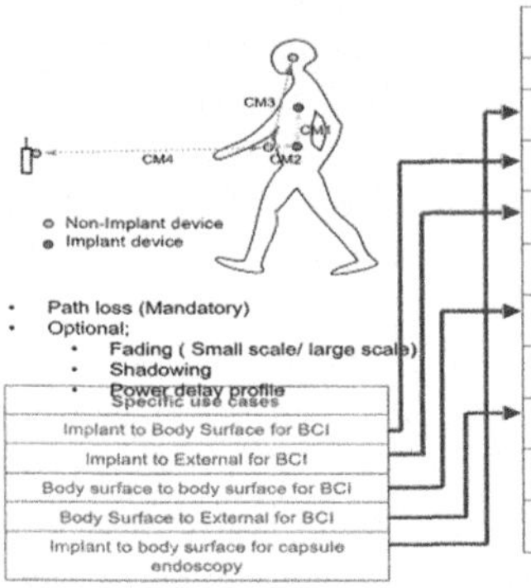

Scenario	Description	Frequency Band	Channel Model
S2	Implant to Body Surface	402-405 MHz.	CM2
S2.1	Implant (upper body) to Body Surface	3.1-10.6 GHz UWB	CM2.1
S2.2	Implant (head) to Body Surface	3.1-10.6 GHz UWB	CM2.2
S3	Implant to External	402-405 MHz, 3.1-10.6 GHz UWB	CM2
S4	Body Surface to Body Surface (LOS)	400, 600, 900 MHz 2.4, 3.1-10.6 GHz	CM3
S4.1	Body Surface to Body Surface (LOS)	3.1-10.6 GHz CM4.1	CM4.1
S5	Body Surface to Body Surface (NLOS)	400, 600, 900 MHz 2.4, 3.1-10.6 GHz	CM3
S6	Body Surface to External (LOS)	900 MHz 2.4, 3.1-10.6 GHz	CM4
S6.1	Body Surface (head) to External (LOS)	3.1-10.6 GHz	CM6.1
S7	Body Surface to External (NLOS)	900 MHz 2.4, 3.1-10.6 GHz	CM4

Table 2. Classes of Coexistence

Coexistence environment class	15.6ma BAN	15.6-2012	Non-UWB (Wi-Fi, unlicensed 5G)	IEEE Stds 802.15 UWB (15.4, 15.8)	Non-IEEE Std 802.15 UWB (ETSI)	Note
0	—	—	—	—	—	A single BAN
1	✓	—	—	—	—	Multiple BANs
2	✓	✓	—	—	—	
3	✓	—	✓	—	—	Non-UWB systems
4	✓	—	—	✓	—	Multiple UWB systems
5	✓	—	—	—	✓	
6	✓	—	—	✓	✓	
7	✓	✓	✓	✓	✓	Multiple: BANs, non-UWB and UWB systems

(3) QoS Levels or Priority Order of User Packets: Under primitive channel capacity or Shannon bound, priority order of user data packets corresponding to required QoS levels has been defined in Table 3 in a sense that the higher QoS of packets should be the higher priority of packets to be protected against channel errors and interference while the lower to be sacrificed under the constrain capacity bound.

Table 3. Priority and QoS Levels of User Packets

Priority	User priority	Traffic designation	Frame type
Lowest	0	Background (BK)	Data
	1	Best effort (BE)	Data
	2	Excellent effort (EE)	Data
	3	Video (VI)	Data
	4	Voice (VO)	Data
	5	Medical data or network control	Data or management
	6	High-priority medical data or network control	Data or management
Highest	7	Emergency or medical implant event report	Data

2.2 Progress of the Revision Standard IEEE802.15.6ma

After Interest Group(IG) of dependable wireless started in 2014, Project Authorization Request(PAR) and Criteria for Standards Development(CSD) of amendment and revision of Study Group(SG) for Dependable BAN were approved in WG802.15 in 2021 and TG15.6ma started in 2022, and TG15.6ma summarized necessary documents such as Channel Model Document(CMD) [7] and Technical Requirement Document(TRD) [8] in covering use cases. Timeline of TG15.6ma is shown in Fig. 1. The first Letter Ballot (LB) of draft P802.15.6ma_D03 was successfully completed in Oct. 2024, comments resolution was proceeded in Nov. 2024. The first for D04, second for D05, and third recirculation for D06 were completed in Feb., April, June 2025, respectively. WG15 approved unconditional approval for Standard Association (SA) Ballot in July and then LAN/MAN Standard Committee (LMSC) approved to start SA Ballot in August 2025. Figure 1 shows an expected timeline.

3 Core Technologies for Coexistence of Multiple BANs

To enhance dependability in BAN, novel technologies have been investigated in PHY and MAC layers [9].

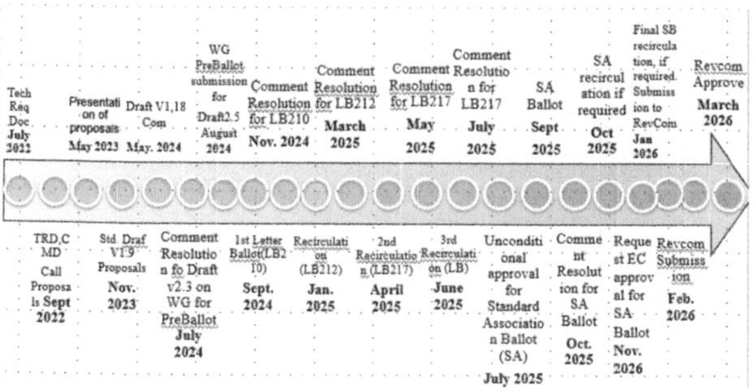

Fig. 1. Expected timeline of IEEE802.15.6ma Standard

3.1 Physical Layer of Technologies

(1) Core Technologies in PHY layer to satisfy technical requirement for enhanced dependability.
   i) In feedback loop for remote monitoring sensors or radars and feedback controlling actuators, real-time cognition of varying condition on site and adaptive reconfiguration in messy, small, and dense areas are requested to guarantee worst performance with permissible delay and errors.
   ii) Within a permissible limited feedback delay, propagation paths connecting between nodes and coordinator should be found to keep connectivity by diversity, channel switching etc.

Table 4. FEC and Hybrid ARQ for 64 Combinations of 8 QoS Levels and 8 Classes of Coexistence

Coexistence Class	0	1	2	3	4	5	6	7
QoS Level								
0	LDPC/BCC	LDPC/BCC	LDPC/BCC	LDPC/RS	LDPC/RS	LDPC/BCC	LDPC/RS	LDPC/RS
1	LDPC/BCC	LDPC/BCC	LDPC/BCC	LDPC/RS	LDPC/RS	LDPC/BCC	LDPC/RS	LDPC/RS
2	LDPC/BCC	LDPC/BCC	LDPC/BCC	LDPS/RS	LDPS/RS	LDPC/BCC	LDPS/RS	LDPS/RS
3	LDPS/BCC	LDPS/BCC	LDPS/BCC	LDPS/RS	LDPS/RS	LDPS/BCC	LDPS/RS	LDPS/RS
4	LDPC/RS	LDPC/RS	CFP/HARQ	LDPC/RS	LDPC/RS	LDPS/BCC	LDPC/RS	LDPC/RS
5	LDPC/RS	LDPC/RS	CFP/HARQ	CFP/HARQ	CFP/HARQ	LDPC/RS	CFP/HARQ	CFP/HARQ
6	LDPS/RS	LDPS/RS	CFP/HARQ	CFP/HARQ	CFP/HARQ	LDPS/RS	CFP/HARQ	CFP/HARQ
7	LDPS/RS	LDPS/RS	CFP/HARQ	CFP/HARQ	CFP/HARQ	LDPS/RS	CFP/HARQ	CFP/HARQ

iii) For such a dynamic environment and QoS requirement changing situation, sophisticated PHY technologies are requested to guarantee minimum requirement of performance.

(2) Error Control: Channel Coding and Hybrid ARQ

Forward Error Correction(FEC) by channel coding, Automatic Repeat reQuest(ARQ), and their hybrid have been investigated to satisfy technical requirement in various channel model, QoS levels of user packets, and classes of coexistence considering compatibility with IEEE802.15.6-2012 and another UWB PAN IEEE802.15.4ab, etc. Table 4 shows its summary in draft P802.15.6ma_D06 [2]. LDPC/BCC and LDPC/RS mean concatinated codes with LDPC as inner code, Binary Convolutional Code(BCC) and Reed-Solomon(RS) code as outer code. CFP/HARQ means packets in Contention Free Period(CFP) are protected with Hybrid ARQ(HARQ).

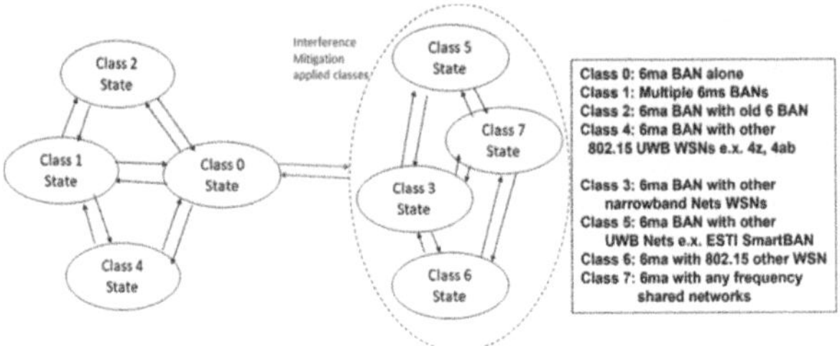

Fig. 2. Diagram of state transitions for coexistence class environments

(3) Interference Mitigation Technologies

Interference mitigation technologies in time and space domains in PHY layer [10] can result in classes 0,1,2 from classes 3,4,5,6 shown in Fig. 2. to satisfy technical requirement for enhanced dependability in the focused use cases. Then interference in classes 1 and 2 may be resolved by protocol to avoid contention of packets in MAC layer [10, 11].

3.2 MAC Layer of Technologies for Coexistence

(1) Hybrid Protocol of Contention Free and Contention Access

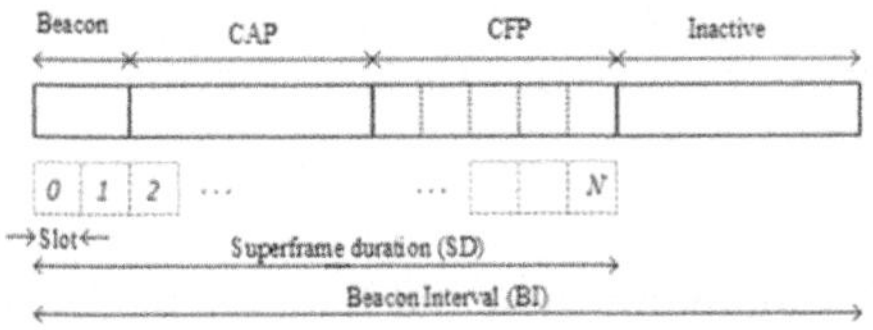

Fig. 3. Superframe Structure with Contention Access Period (CAP) and Contention Free Period (CFP) in IEEE802.15.6 and 6ma

In feedback loop for Hybrid Protocol of Contention Free and Contention Access One of uniqueness in MAC of IEEE802.6 and 6ma is hybrid between contention free and contention access protocols in Fig. 3.

(2) Control and Data Channels

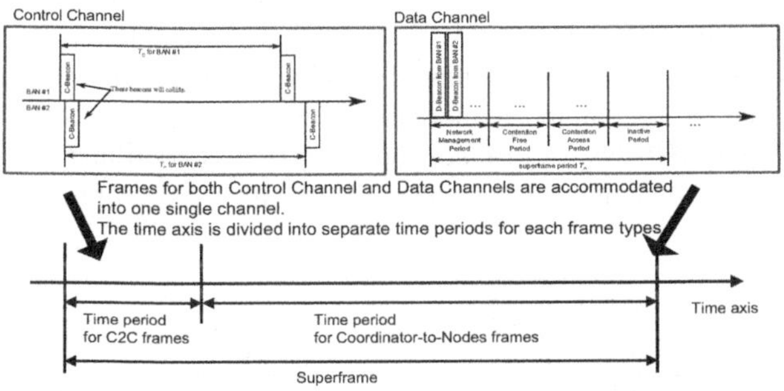

Fig. 4. Control and Data Channels in two or one UWB frequency bands

A new concept of control and data channels has been applied for enhanced dependability in IEEE802.15.6ma. If UWB device supports more than two UWB frequency bands, control channel is used to manage beacon detection, synchronization, and coordinator-to-coordinator(C2C) communication and ranging among coexisting multiple BANs etc. while data channel is used to transmit data packets. On a case of only one UWB band available, control and data channels in separate in time periods in Fig. 4.

4 Coordinator-to-Coordinator (C2C) Communication and Ranging

The revision IEEE802.15.6ma proposes new coexistence mechanisms in MAC and PHY. Control and data channels (CDC) with UWB bands defined to enhance dependability in classified coexistence by controlling access to avoid contention in MAC. The detail coexistence mechanism has been described in MAC function of the draft and coexistence assurance document [9, 12].

4.1 Necessity of C2C Communication and Ranging in Coexisting Multiple BANs

C2C ranging and communication is performed through a link between BAN Coordinators, separate from links between a BAN Coordinator and BAN Nodes in each BAN in case of coexisting multiple BANs, i.e. Classes 1 and 2 of coexisting classes.

To avoid complexity, it would be preferable to use the same PHY as the link between a BAN Coordinator and BAN Nodes. Interference and collisions in dense situations can be taken care. Links between coordinators can be utilized to control channel access between 2 or more BANs to reduce collisions and interference, especially in situations where BANs are densely located. C2C ranging can be performed to identify situation of geographically distribution of possible coexisting multiple BANs in dynamic motion. Various use cases should be taken care such as Fig. 6(a), (b) and more. Figure 6(b) shows a case of vehicle BAN(VBAN) and human BAN(HBAN)s inside the vehicle ($n > 5$). For a van or a bus that can accommodate more than five people, its VBAN should be able to accommodate more HBANs for instance, up to 15 HBAN coordinators. The coverage area of the VBAN should also be considered along with the size of the vehicle.

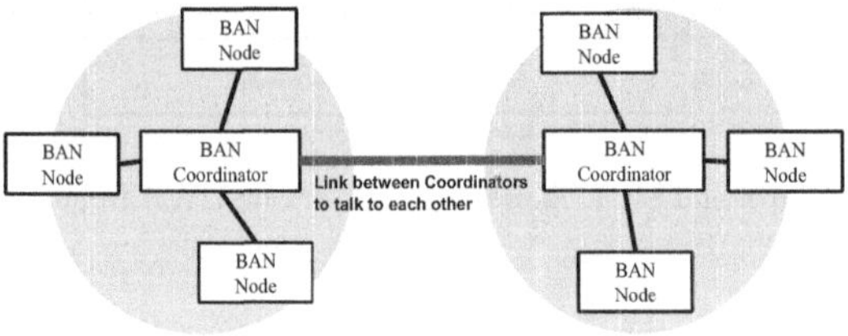

Fig. 5. Coordinator-to-Coordinator(C2C) Communication between Neighboring Two BANs

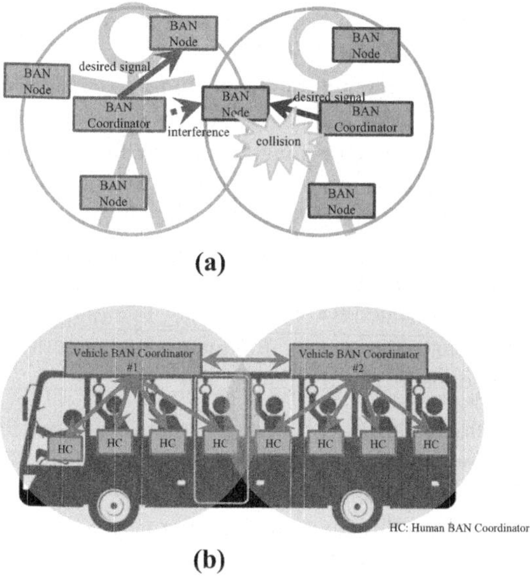

Fig. 6. (a) Use Case of Two HBANs of Covering Ranges Overlapped. (b) Use Case of Coexisting and Communicating Multiple HBANs and VBAN

4.2 Procedure of C2C Communication and Ranging in Coexisting Multiple BANs

The revision supports BANs operating with high reliability in dense environments coexisting with intra-interference and inter-interference due to other wireless systems in the same frequency band. Figure 2 shows state transition among several classes of coexistence environment defined in Table 2. In Fig. 2, the state transition probabilities are approximated in consecutive super-frames. Furthermore, the duration of the CAP and CFP are determined by the type of QoS associated with every super-frame, or group frame and available resources to avoid congestion.

As shown in Fig. 2, coexistence environment classes 0, 1, 2, and 4 perform enhanced dependability. During clear channel assessment (CCA) and beacon periods, a BAN coordinator may analyze the type of synchronization preamble detected from a 15.6ma, 15.6, or 15.4 system. These classes are relatively easy to detect as those involve 15.6ma, 15.6, or 15.4 radios, where all the specification in PHY and MAC such as type of beacons, super-frame structure, MAC frame and functions are known, and compatible. MAC function of the revision can detect overlaid coexisting legacy and new BANs and IEEE802.15.4 UWB WSNs by the known specification of PHY and MAC. Particularly class 1 of multiple new BANs coexistence can use with new schemes such as.

- Control and data channels in UWB bands defined to enhance dependability in classified coexistence by controlling access to avoid contention in MAC.
- Coordinator-to-coordinator (C2C) negotiation among coexisting multiple BANs to identify the number of full and partial overlaid BANs and to synchronize a group of overlaid BANs. Basically an individual BAN is operated independently. If covering ranges of two BANs are overlaid, then desired and interfering packets will cause

contention as shown in Fig. 7. C2C communication can manage which packet should be taken care by individual coordinators.
- C2C ranging among coexisting multiple BANs to monitor and identify transition of coexisting status. Another core technology for coexistence in IEEE802.15.6ma is Coordinator-to-Coordinator(C2C) communication and ranging in Fig. 5. In control channel, coordinators of coexisting BANs should communicate one another to synchronize clocks, determine group BAN coordinator which is a leader of coordinators of coexisting BANs, and identify geographical layout of the BANs by C2C ranging based on UWB TDOA or TOA which is much precise rather than RSSI. In fact, C2C ranging between co-located BANs is quite key to monitor dynamic motion such as approaching closer and leaving out. Ranging between co-located BANs can be performed as the same manner as IEEE802.15.4z [13].

Coexistence environment classes 3, 5, 6, and 7 where every specification may not be known. Coordinators of new BANs may detect unknown coexisting systems overlapped frequency bands with a new BAN and suppress or cancel interference from other radios with digital filters and antenna directivity in time, frequency, and space domains. Then class 3,5, and 6 may result in classes 0, 1, 2, and 4.

5 Performance Evaluation for MAC of UWB-BAN in Cases if Geographical Distribution of Multiple BANs

To confirm basic performance of MAC in UWB-BAN draft of IEEE802.15.6ma, computer simulation results with updated decision rule and layout is presented in cases of random geographical distribution of multiple coexisting BANs.

5.1 Simulation Models

In simple analysis of packet errors, all packets which have contentions are counted as packet errors [14]. However, even if packets have contentions, some packets can be correctly received according to signal-to-interference and noise ratio (SINR). In this analysis, packet errors may be counted more carefully considering SINR in case of contention [15].

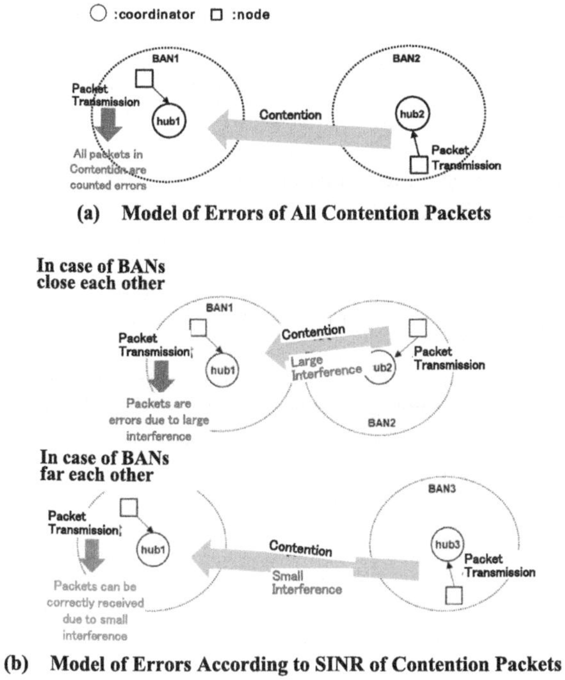

Fig. 7. Models of Packet Errors in Cases of Contentions among Co-located BANs

Number of BANs can be more flexibly changeable. Diameter of the circle can be flexibly changeable. Random geographical distribution is assumed according to the flowing manner. Although simple analysis assumes a layout of BANs pentagon, in this packet error analysis, a layout of BANs is randomly distributed in a circle.

A BAN location (x, y) can be calculated in case of circle with diameter d (Fig. 8 and Table 5).

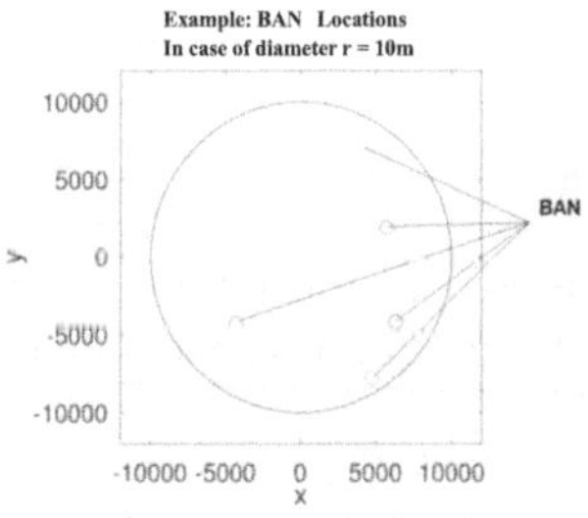

Fig. 8. Model of Geographical Distribution of BANs

$$\begin{cases} x = r \sin\theta \\ y = r \cos\theta \end{cases} 0 \le \theta \le 2\pi, 0 \le r \le d$$

- r and Θ can be calculated uniform random numbers in (0,1).
- BAN location can be derived

$$\begin{cases} \theta = 2\pi u \\ r = \sqrt{d^2 v} \end{cases}$$

Table 5. Simulation Specification

Diameter of circle inside which BANs are distributed	1.0, 2.5, 5.0, 7.5, 10
Number of Asynchronous BANS	0, 1, 2, 3, 4
Number of Simulation Trials	100

T_S	4 ms	Number of BANs	5
T_D	40 μs	Number of Nodes (/BAN)	5
Number of superframes	250	Maximum number of retransmission (CFP) times	5
Number of NMP slots	5	Maximum number of retransmission (CAP) times	5
Number of CFP slots	60	Maximum number of random waiting slots (CAP)	10
Number of CAP slots	30	Normal packet (CFP)	Poisson distribution
Number of IAP slots	5	Normal packet (CAP)	Poisson distribution
Gap	0 ~ 499	Packet length	2000 bit
Tx power	-10 dBm		

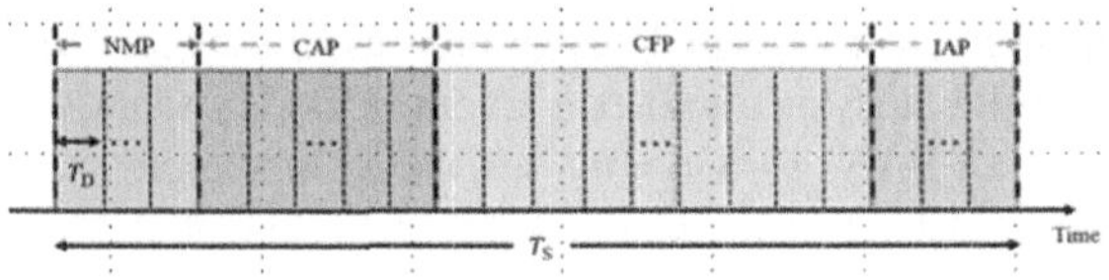

where assumed that layout of BANs was reset every simulation trial, Asynchronous BANs are randomly selected in each simulation trial.

5.2 MAC Simulation Results

Throughput versus Packet appearance probability λ or offered traffic load in cases of different no. of coexisting BANs and covering geographical range.

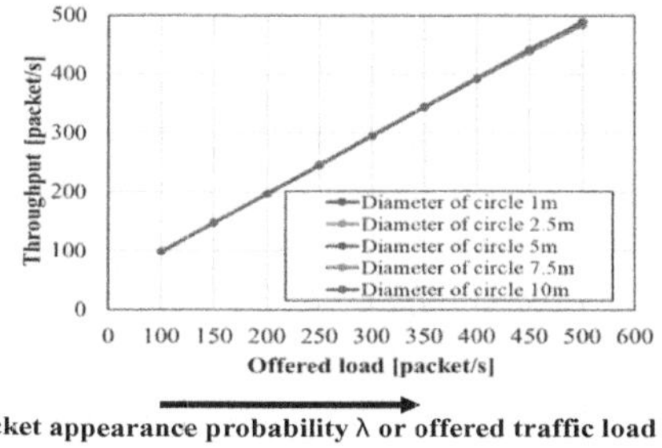

(a) No. of Asynchronous BANs = 0

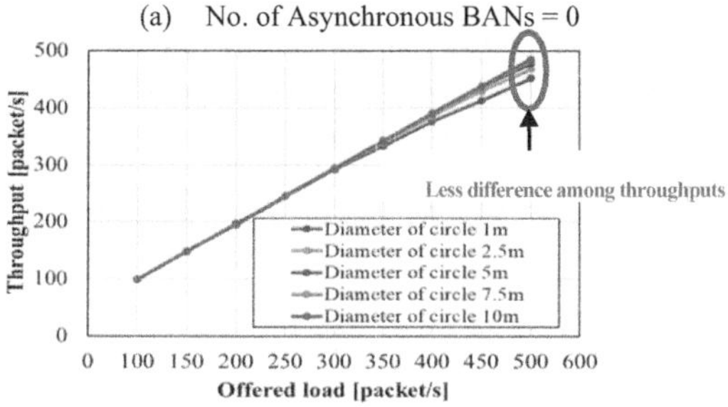

(b) No. of Asynchronous BANs = 1

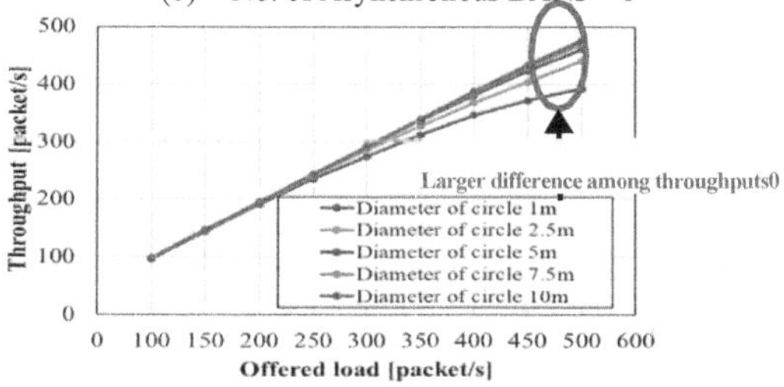

(c) No. of Asynchronous BANs = 4

Fig. 9. Throughput According to Offered Loads or Packet Appearance Probability λ in No. of Coexisting BANs

Figure 9 shows larger variance of throughput according to packet appearance probability λ or offered traffic load in case of the larger number of asynchronous BANs. It is noted that the larger packet traffic or offered load, the larger throughput in case of less than 5 m in diameter, but a minor difference of throughout in case of more than 5 m in diameter.

5.3 MAC Simulation Results in Case of the Number of Asynchronous BANs According to Distance

Although in above simulation, assumed that number of asynchronous BANs are fixed, then the fixed number of asynchronous BANs are randomized in geographical distribution. In practical implementation, according to distance among BANs, the number of asynchronous BANs may change.

Throughput versus Packet appearance probability λ or offered traffic load in cases of different no. of coexisting BANs and covering geographical range are shown in Fig. 10.

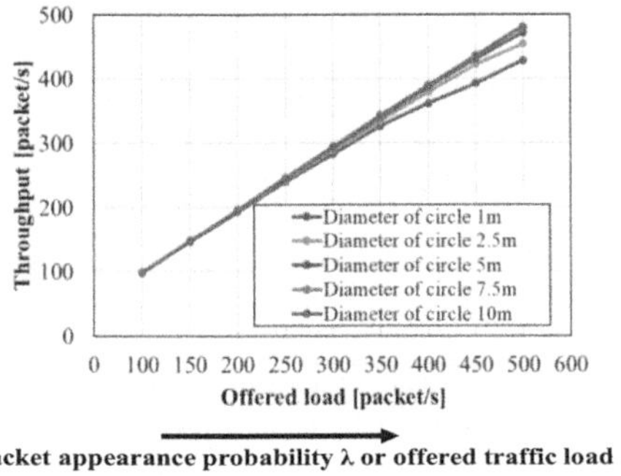

(a) Case of asynchronous BANs at random No. of Asynchronous BANs = 2

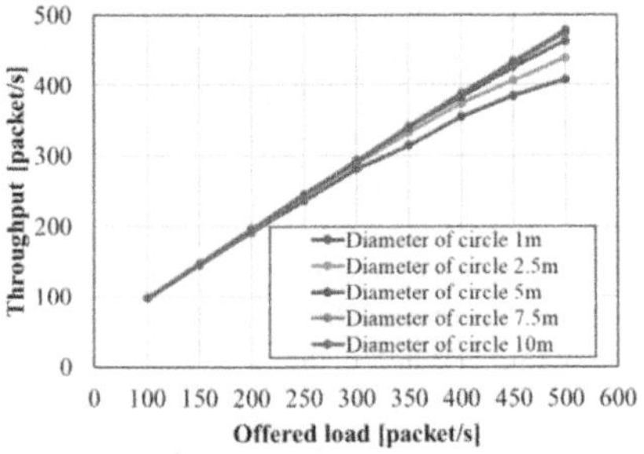

(b) Case of asynchronous BANs at random No. of Asynchronous BANs = 3

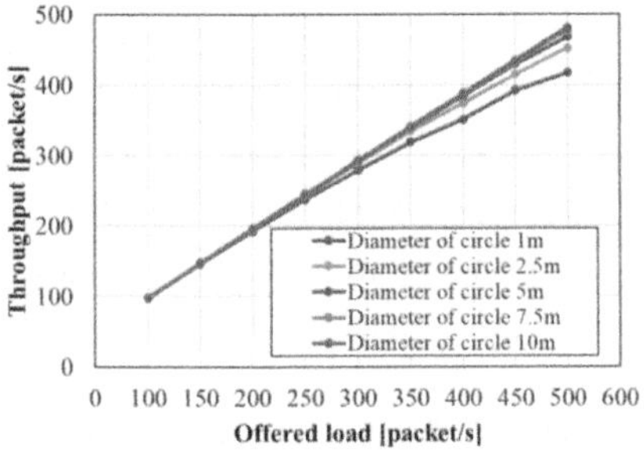

(c) Case of asynchronous BANs according to distance

Fig. 10. Throughput versus Packet appearance probability λ or offered traffic load in cases of different no. of coexisting BANs and covering geographical range.

In the specification of this simulation, the number of asynchronous BANs is set randomly from 1 to 4. Therefore, the result of this simulation is the average of the result in five and it is intermediate to the result in the case where the number of asynchronous BANs is 2 and 3. Simulations are performed in cases of different decision rule of packet error rate and geographical distribution of coexisting BANs. The simulation confirms that throughput is quite dependent on the number of asynchronous BANs. In case of coexisting BANs closer than 5 m, throughput may significantly degraded as increase of asynchronous BANs. However, in case of BANs far than 5 m, throughput is a little different even different number of asynchronous BANs,

These simulations confirm that if a group BAN coordinator can control the number of asynchronized coexisting BANs less than 5 within covering range of 5 m in diameter, then packet error rate can be under controlled and result in permissible throughput in a certain range of packet traffic or offered load. The covering range 5 m is dependent on transmission power of each BAN.

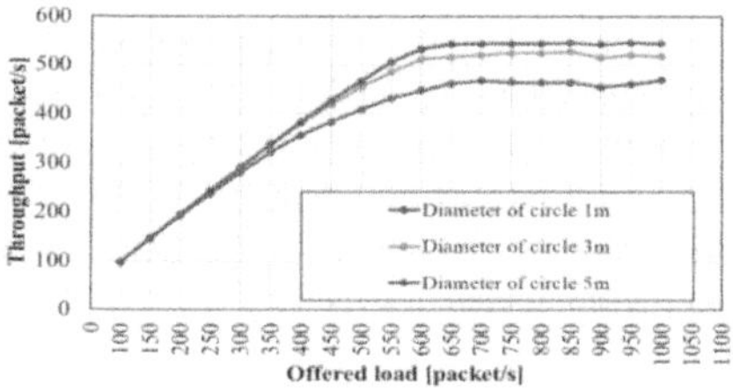

(a) Transmission Power = -10dBm

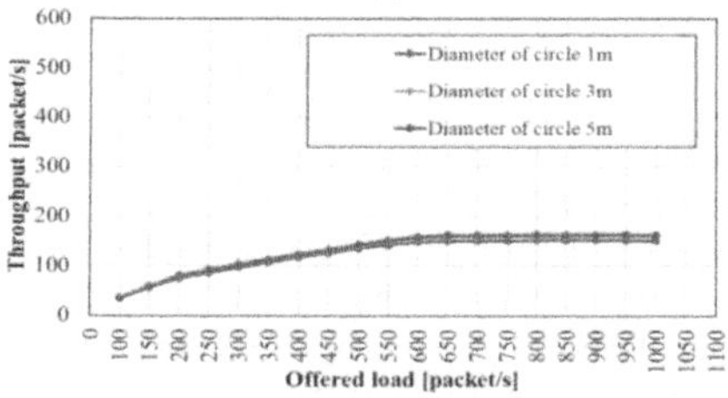

(b) Transmission Power = -45dBm

Fig. 11. Throughput According to Transmission Power

5.4 MAC Simulation Results in Case of the Number of Asynchronous BANs According to Transmission Power

Although Figs. 9 and 10 show throughputs in case of TX power = -10 dBm, Fig. 11 shows throughput according to TX power. It is noted that variance of throughput in case of larger diameter decreases as TX power decreases. There's is few differences among diameters 1, 3 and 5 m in case TX power > -40 dB.

This simulation is meaningful in the sense that the new standard MAC of IEEE802.15,6ma is robust against uncontrollable coexisting BANs,

6 Concluding Remark

This paper has described main features of the revision of IEEE802.15.6-2012, i.e. IEEE802.15.6ma for HBAN and VBAN with enhanced dependability. To ensure dependability or stable management or synchronization of inter-coordinators of coexisting multiple BANs. Through activities of IEEE802.15.6ma, various novel technologies to enhance dependability in PHY and MAC layers have been presented such as error-controlling schemes cognitively switched in state transition among classes of coexistence, space-time interference mitigation in PHY, C2C ranging and communication for classes 1 and 2 of coexisting multiple BANs, and modes 1 and 2 of control and data channels of frequency bands and time slots in MAC. Particularly this paper described principle of C2C communication and ranging and performance evaluation of MAC based on these C2C communication and ranging. It is confirmed that MAC and PHY of IEEE802.15.6ma can ensure dependability even in various cases of coexistence. The authors encourage more people to attend professional engineers meetings for making standards where more opportunities to get hints for research and develop of novel technologies for practical demands as well as theoretical interests.

Acknowledgement. This paper is a part of results of the Commissioned Research of the National Institute of Information and Communications Technology (NICT), Japan under a grant for the development and application of an implantable device for BMIs using high-speed wireless data transfer and big data analyses of neural information. Grant No. JPJ012368C22801. Moreover, This work is partially funded by Academy of Finland via 6G Flagship (grant 318927), by the European Union's Horizon2020 program under

References

1. IEEE Std 802.15.6TM-2012
2. P802.15.6ma Draft P802.15.6ma-D06
3. Kohno, R.: Overview of activity of IEEE802.15 TG15.6ma for revision of IEEE802.15.6–2012 wireless BAN with enhanced dependability. Doc. IEEE802.15-25-0033-04-06m 2025
4. Kohno, R.: Upcoming a new standard of wireless BAN with multimodal AI for business innovation in medical healthcare, automotive, and their crossover fields. keynote speech. The 5th International Conference on Intelligent Medicine and Health (ICIMH2024) Harbin, China (2024)
5. Kohno, R., Kobayashi, T., Sugimoto, C., Kinjo, Y., Hämäläinen, M., Iinatti, J.: Medical healthcare network platform and big data analysis based on integrated ICT and data science with regulatory science. IEICE Trans. Com. **E102-B**(6), 1078–1087 (2019)
6. Kohno, R.: Comprehensive research and business of universal platform with BAN/cloud/AI for medical healthcare and other SDGs. In: The 11th International Conference on Computer and Communications Management. Keynote Speech, Nagoya, Japan (2023)
7. Kobayashi, T., Sayrafian, K., Anzai, D., Hernandez, M., Kohno, R.: TG6ma channel model document for enhanced dependability. Doc. IEEE 802.15-22-0519-09-06ma (2024)
8. Hernandez, M., Kohno, R., Kobayashi, T., Kim, M.: Technical requrement document. Doc. IEEE802.15-22-0577-06-006ma (2022)
9. Kohno, R.: TG15.6ma Coexistence assessment document. Doc.IEEE802.15-24-0348-06-006a, Walshawa, Poland (2025)
10. Kobayashi, T., Kim, M., Hernandez, M., Kohno, R.: Interference mittigation schemes in class 3, 5, 6, and 7 of coexisitence in TG6ma. Doc. IEEE802.15-24-0073-10-006a, Madrid, Spain (2025)
11. Ogawa, S., Goto, T., Kobayashi, T., Sugimoto, C., Kohno, R.: MAC protocol with interference mitigation using negotiation among coordinators in multiple wireless body area networks. In: 14th EAI International Conference on Body Area Networks(BodyNets2019). Florence, Italy (2019)
12. Kohno, R., Kim, M., Kobayashi, T., Hernandez1a, M.: Coordinator-to-coordinator(C2C) ranging and communication for multiple BAN coexistence. Doc. IEEE802.15-24-0642-00-006a, Vancouver, Canada (2024)

13. IEEE Std 802.15.4z CAD: https://mentor.ieee.org/802.15/dcn/18/15-18-0523-06-004z-coexistence-document-15-4z.docx
14. Anzai, D., Nagai, K., Kobayashi, T., Hernandez, M., Kohno, R.: Selection of suitable preamble sequence sets in UWB wireless communications in the presence of multiple coexisting VBANs. Doc. IEEE802.15-25-0246-07-006a, Vancouver, Canada (2024)
15. Kohno, R.: Simulation results of performance evaluation for MAC of UWB-BAN draft of IEEE802.15,6ma in cases of random geographical distribution of multiple coexisting BANs. Doc. IEEE802.15-24-0602-00-006a, Vancouver, Canada (2024)

Human-Centric Sensing, Haptics, and Data Standardization

Objective Evaluation of the Fabric Handle ~Sensitivity (Kansei) Design of Textile Materials~

Mari Inoue(✉)

Kobe University, 3-11 Tsurukabuto, Nada-ku, Kobe City, Hyogo 657-8501, Japan
inouema@kobe-u.ac.jp

Abstract. Comfort in clothing can be understood through three elements: the fabric's handle (the tactile and visual impression of woven or knitted materials), ease of movement (perceived through the pressure of the clothing), and thermal sensation (understood through the thermal properties of the fabric such as insulation, air resistance, and thermal conductivity). Traditionally, these sensory elements have been evaluated subjectively, but recent advancements have made it possible to assess them scientifically. This study organizes the components that constitute clothing comfort, with a particular focus on objective evaluation methods for fabric handle. Specifically, it introduces the Kawabata Evaluation System (KES) for measuring physical properties and presents case studies on how handle quantification is applied in the field of smart textiles. Objective evaluation of fabric handle enables clothing design that aligns with users' sensory preferences, serving as a key to integrating comfort, functionality, and aesthetic value. In the development of future smart textiles, handle assessment is expected to play a vital role as a bridge between sensory design and scientific analysis.

Keywords: Fabric handle · Objective evaluation · Smart textile

1 Introduction

Fibers have a thin and elongated shape, with molecular chains oriented along the fiber axis, resulting in increased strength. For textile fibers, both the elastic modulus and strength in the fiber axis direction can be about 5 to 10 times greater than in isotropic conditions, while the specific gravity remains almost unchanged, maintaining a value of approximately 1 to 1.3, making it suitable for lightweight and strong clothing materials. These thin fibers are gathered to form yarn, which is then woven or knitted into fabric, becoming the material for clothing. The fabric is shaped into a three-dimensional form to create garments that wrap around the human body. As clothing materials, fabrics not only need to encompass the body but also must deform with body movements. The elongation properties of fabrics are nonlinear, easily deforming with slight changes while showing considerable stiffness under large deformations. Furthermore, since fabrics frequently come into contact with the skin, they must possess a softness that does not

H. Tanaka et al. (Eds.): BodyNets 2025, LNICST 714, pp. 429–437, 2026.
https://doi.org/10.1007/978-3-032-38657-1_36

harm the skin. These properties of fabric are influenced by the thickness, shape, and physical properties of the fibers, as well as the structural design of the yarn and fabric. Additionally, various fibers should be blended to create excellent properties and enhance the quality/price ratio. Although fibers are rigid materials, their collective structure, which contains a lot of internal space, allows for easy deformation and provides a softness that conforms to the body. The performance of clothing materials is critically dependent on their compatibility with humans. Clothing materials are expected to match human sensibilities, being comfortable, beautiful, and endearing.

Research has been conducted to objectively derive sensory elements such as warmth, coldness, itchiness when touched, smoothness, and fluffiness of fabrics from their material properties. As shown in Fig. 1 [1], comfort in wearing clothes is captured by three elements: handle (the feeling received from the fabric's touch and appearance), ease of movement (perceived by the fabric pressure), and thermal sensation (captured from the thermal properties of the fabric such as insulation, air resistance, and thermal conductivity). In particular, the research on quantifying the 'handle' of fabric from its physical properties was established by Professor Sueo Kawabata of Kyoto University and Professor Masako Niwa of Nara Women's University in the 1970s to 1980s [2]. Based on this measurement method, physical properties of fabrics such as tensile, bending, shearing, compression, and friction properties are measured and correlated with human subjective evaluations to quantify comfort related to the tactile experience. This method has been applied not only to clothing [3–6] but also to various products such as automotive seats, steering wheels, non-woven masks, sanitary products [7–9] and so on. This research will explain the objective evaluation of 'handle' and introduce examples of applying this system to smart textiles equipped with wearable devices.

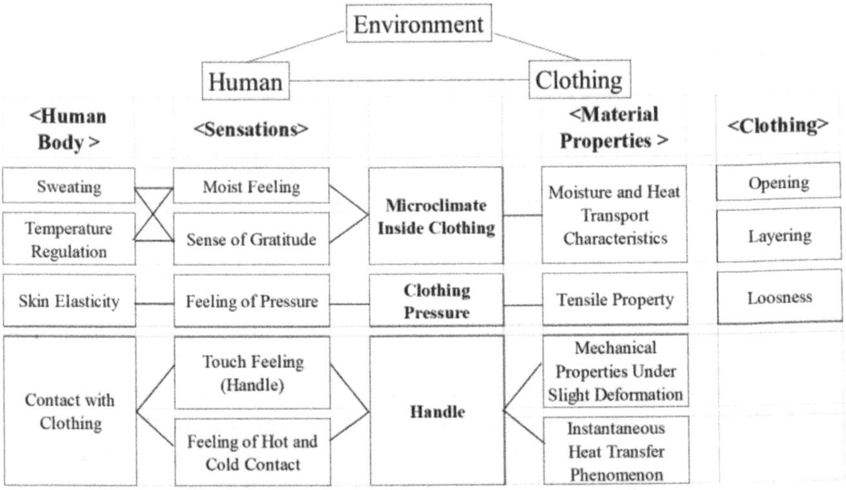

Fig. 1. The main factor of clothing comfort [1]

2 Development of Fabric Handle and Objective Evaluation System as a Total Hand Evaluation

The fabric used for clothing is a material that interacts with human sensibilities. The evaluation of fabric begins with touching it by hand, followed by advanced data processing in the brain. This involves the accumulation of past experiences. It is not evaluated solely on instinctive physiological responses. Since data collection is primarily based on the tactile sensation, it is thought that the detection mechanism is a function of the nerve endings; however, the information obtained from many detection mechanisms is immediately sent to brain processing, leading to conclusions through several processes such as sensory reorganization, primary synthesis, and secondary synthesis. The properties of materials that humans perceive have been vaguely expressed with the term 'handle' because the details of the fabric's evaluation are not clear. However, to elucidate the material performance regarding how humans feel comfortable with fabrics and their connection to human sensibility, there is a strong desire to externalize the judgment process and criteria to recreate an objective evaluation method. In 1932, Pierce proposed that it might be possible to measure the mechanical properties of fabrics. The strong demand for such assessments in clothing fabrics is likely due to the fact that the essential quality of the fabric is determined by its 'pleasant handle,' which fundamentally questions its compatibility with humans. In the 1970s, Kawabata developed an objective evaluation method with the cooperation of skilled professional evaluators, put it into practical use, and later expanded its application in the industry along with the accumulation of databases. Below, I will summarize and explain this objective evaluation method and its development.

2.1 Primary Hand and Total Hand

Good handle means that the fabric has properties that are desirable to humans, and this judgment is basically made by touching the fabric with one's hands. The judgment process of an expert judge is as follows.

First stage of judgment: Based on the feel of the fabric, the character of the fabric is summarized by several textural expressions. These expressions are summarized into three values (KOSHI, NUMERI, FUKURAMI). These are named Primary Hand Values. Table 1 shows these handles.

Second stage of judgment: Next, the combination of the strength and weakness of each primary hand is used to determine whether the handle is good or bad in terms of quality. This final evaluation of "goodness" is called the total handle, or Total Hand.

2.2 Numerical Expression of Handle

Each Primary Hand has its own strength and weakness, for example, "*KOSHI*". Total Hand Value, which expresses the degree of goodness, also expresses the degree of goodness, i.e., strength and weakness. The numerical expression of the degree of strength and weakness is named Hand Value and Total Hand Value, respectively, and the HV of the Primary Hand is expressed as a numerical value ranging from 10 to 1 from strong to

Table 1. Definition of the primary hands [2].

Handle		Definition
(Japanese)	(English)	
KOSHI	Stiffness	A feeling related with bending stiffness. Springy property promotes this feeling. The fabric having compact weaving density and woven by springy and elastic yarn makes this feeling strong.
NUMERI	Smoothness	A mixed feeling come from smooth, limber and soft feeling. The fabric woven from cashmere fiber gives this feeling strongly.
FUKURAMI	Fullness & softness	A feeling come from bulky, rich and well formed feeling. Springy property in compression and thickness accompanied with warm feeling are closely related with this feeling.

good, and the Total Hand as a numerical value ranging from 5 to 1 from good to bad, as shown in Table 2.

Table 2. Total Hand Value [2].

THV	Evaluation
5	excellent
4	good
3	average
2	below average
1	poor
0	out of use

2.3 Development of Objective Evaluation Equations

The response that a person receives when touching a fabric with his/her hands is related to the mechanical qualities and surface properties of the fabric. Thermal response is also a factor, but it may be included in the item when the fabric is used in direct contact with the skin, as in the case of underwear. Figure 2 is a conceptual diagram of converting the subjective judgment process into an objective method, using the mechanical quantity-handle value conversion equation, via the Primary Hand Value and Total Hand Value.

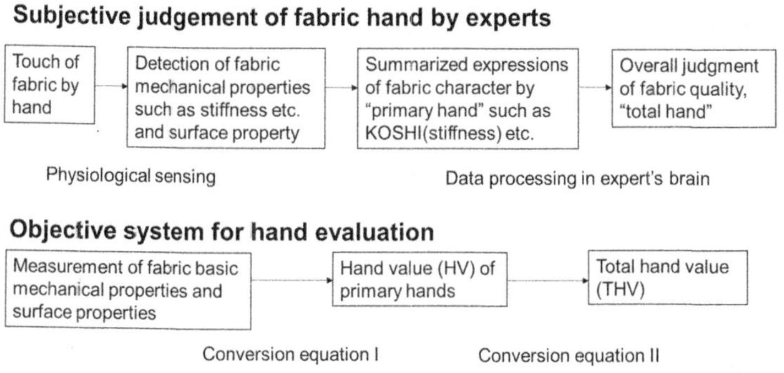

Fig. 2. The relationship between subjective evaluation and objective evaluation

Around 1970, Kawabata developed [2] and put into practical use an objective evaluation method with the cooperation of expert judges, and later, as the database was accumulated, its application was extended to the textile industrial world. The objective evaluation method and its development are summarized below.

In the conversion Eqs. (1) and (2), the dynamic quantities are converted into three or five Primary Hand Values (HV_i) by the constant coefficient group C_{ij}, which are then transformed into a linear equation including the quadratic terms of the HV values, and *THV* is derived by the coefficient group C_i. However, the dynamical quantity parameter *Xi* is the value obtained by normalizing each of the 16 dynamical characteristics X_i (i = 1 to 16) by the mean and standard deviation of the population. The above judgment process is an estimated simulation of the human judgment process in judging handle and consists of two steps.

$$HV_i = C_{i0} + \sum_{j=1}^{16} C_{ij} \frac{X_j - \overline{X}_j}{\sigma_j} \quad (1)$$

$$THV = C_{00} + \sum_{i=1}^{3} C_{i1} \cdot \frac{Y_i - M_{i1}}{\sigma_{i1}} + C_{i2} \cdot \frac{Y_i^2 - M_{i2}}{\sigma_{i2}} \quad (2)$$

C_{ij} in these equations were determined by multivariate regression analysis using the average of the results of about 250 samples subjectively judged by several skilled persons under the criteria. However, the block residual method for each characteristic was used to calculate the Primary Hand. For each block of each mechanical characteristic, we regressed the subjective values against the subjective values and selected the block with the highest accuracy. The regression equation is added to the first regression equation at the beginning, and the regression equations are connected in the same way. The accuracy of the discriminant equation was checked by using a new sample different from the one used to create the regression equation.

The above mathematical modeling by multiple regression is not a new method, but two important points when applying such a method are (1) the preparation of reliable subjective judgment data and (2) the setting of characteristic parameters related to sensitivity and its high measurement accuracy. Human and familiar properties generally have nonlinear dynamic properties. Such nonlinear properties need to be measured precisely within the deformation range where handle is relevant, generally in the low load range. The measurement of such nonlinear behavior in the low load range requires a new measurement system based on a concept different from that of conventional strength tests. In developing an objective system, Kawabata developed the Kawabata Evaluation System (KES) to measure 16 property values (Table 3) derived from tensile, bending, shear, compressive, and surface properties of fabrics. This system, called KES, along with the handle transformation equation, became widely used in textile research.

3 Experiment

The following is an example of the application of the handle objective evaluation method described above to smart textiles.

Table 3. Measurement Properties [2].

Blocked Properties	Symbols	Characteristic value
Tensile	*LT*	Linearity
	WT	Tensile energy
	RT	Resilience
Bending	*B*	Bending rigidity
	2HB	Histeresis
Shearing	*G*	Shear stiffness
	2HG	Histeresis at $\phi = 0.5°$
	2HG5	Histeresis at $\phi = 5°$
Compression	*LC*	Linearity
	WC	Compressional energy
	RC	Resilience
Surface	*MIU*	Coefficient of friction
	MMD	Mean deviation of *MIU*
	SMD	Geometrical roughness
Weight & Thickness	*W*	Weight per unit area
	T	Thickness at 0.5 gf/cm^2

3.1 Samples

A total of five samples (T1 – T5) were used: three garments with wearable devices (all samples are sleeveless upper garment knit underwear) and two commercial sleeveless upper garment knit underwear for comparison.

The fiber composition of the samples is shown in Table 4. For the sample with the device, measurements were conducted separately for the "sensor part," and "fabric part.

Table 4 Samples.

<table>
<tr><th></th><th>For use</th><th>Composed fiber</th></tr>
<tr><td>T1</td><td rowspan="3">Wearable shirts</td><td rowspan="4">Polyester</td></tr>
<tr><td>T2</td></tr>
<tr><td>T3</td></tr>
<tr><td>T4</td><td rowspan="2">T shirts</td></tr>
<tr><td>T5</td><td>Cotton</td></tr>
</table>

3.2 Wearing Experiment

The subjects were five male university students. The protocol for the wearing experiment consisted of 10 min of rest after wearing, 10 min of running at 6 km/h, and 10 min of rest. Subjective evaluations were conducted immediately after wearing the garments, before running, during running, after running, and after resting. The subjective evaluation items were “hard to soft,” “rough to not rough,” “uncomfortable to good fit on the skin,” and “unfavorable to favorable” for each of the above sample areas. All were rated on a 7-point scale from -3 to $+3$, including 0, with the latter side as positive.

3.3 Measurement of Physical Properties and Application to Handle Objective Evaluation Equation

Samples were cut from each section of each specimen, and tensile (EMT, LT, WT, RT), bending (B, 2HB), shear (G, 2HG, 2HG5), compressive (LC, RC, WC), and surface (MIU, MMD, SMD) properties were measured using KES (Katotech, Inc.). The maximum load was set at 50 N/m for tensile properties, and for the hard samples that could not be measured under those conditions, measurements were made under the following conditions: initial load of 300 N/m or 100 N/m for shear properties, maximum shear angle of $\pm 2°$, and maximum curvature of $\pm 1.0\ \text{cm}^{-1}$ for flexural properties.

Basic handle values (*KOSHI, NUMERI, FUKURAMI*) and total handle value (*THV*) were calculated using the existing handle objective evaluation Eq. [2].

4 Results and Discussion

First, samples T4 and T5 feel drier than samples T1 through T3 with terminals, and are rated as soft, not rough, good fit feeling. The likability was highly rated at 1 or more, compared to -1.5 to -0.5 for T1 to T3. Correlation coefficients were calculated for each subjective evaluation item of the sensor part and the desirability, and high correlations were obtained for all items.

T4 and T5 were rated more desirable than T1, T2, and T3. The least favorable rating was obtained during exercise for all samples. The measured results of mechanical and surface properties of the fabric part and the sensor part of each sample are shown in Figs. 3 and 4: T1, T2, and T3 have higher values in bending (B, 2HB) and shear (G,

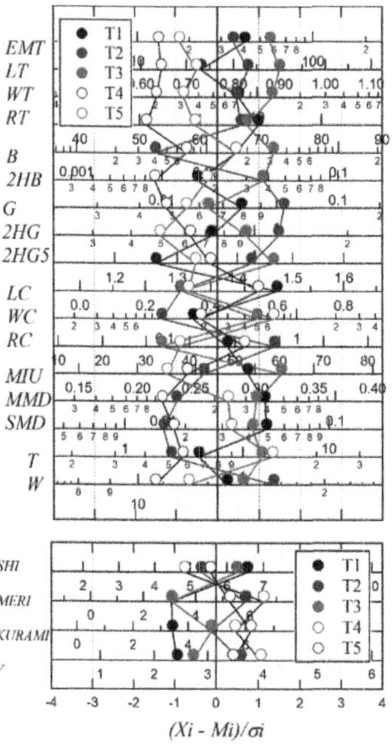

Fig. 3. Physical Properties and Objective Handle of T1 – T5 (Fabrics Parts)

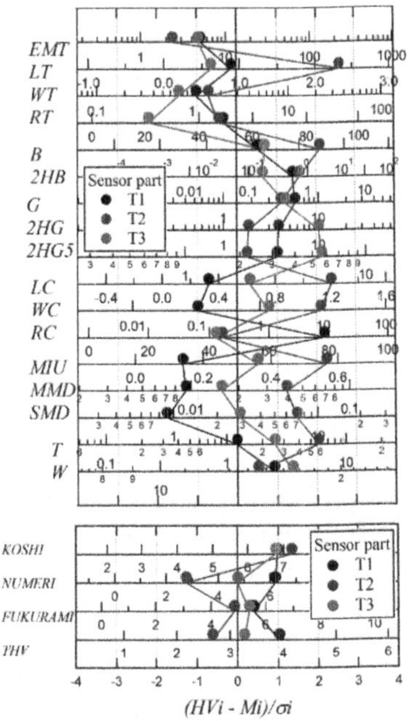

Fig. 4. Physical Properties and Objective Handle of T1 –T3 (Sensor Parts)

2HG, 2HG5) properties than T4 and T5. Strong correlations were obtained for these properties and each subjective evaluation item. From these results, it is clear that the samples T1 to T3 with wearable devices have larger bending and shear properties than T4 and T5, and are not very comfortable to wear.

When basic handle values and overall handle values were calculated using existing handle objective evaluation equations, a strong correlation of 0.80 or more was found between softness and *KOSHI* values, and a correlation of 0.83 was also found between softness and desirability. Therefore, the hardness of the sensor part of the garment with wearable device may have been a factor in the unfavorable evaluation.

5 Conclusions

This study introduces an objective evaluation system for fabric handle established around 1980, and shows an example of application of this system to smart textiles with wearable devices. Experimental results showed that the presence or absence of the wearable device affected the coldness, stiffness, roughness, discomfort, difficulty in stretching, stiffness, and tightness of the garment, and that there was a correlation between the presence and absence of the wearable device and desirability. In addition, it was found that the wearable device increases the bending and shear properties, which is a factor that causes the fabric to be evaluated as undesirable because it has a stiff handle. As described above, it is clear that the objective evaluation system for fabric handle can be applied to the wearability of smart textiles.

KES is a technical system that deals with the engineering problem of mapping sensory information to physical values (which can be put on electrical signals) in tactile sensation.

Clothing is "the smallest portable environment". Among food, clothing, and housing, clothing is the only activity that humans engage in, and it adds color to our lives. When considering textile products as applications of smart textiles, it is essential to view clothing life from a global perspective, connecting it to environmental, social, and economic factors, and to build a sustainable future.

Acknowledgement. This research was supported by JSPS KAKENHI Grant Numbers 22H00950 and 23 K22221. I gratefully acknowledge the financial support provided under the category of Grant-in-Aid for Scientific Research (B), funded by the Japan Society for the Promotion of Science (JSPS). I also extend our sincere thanks to all collaborators and institutions involved in this project for their valuable contributions and insights.

References

1. Harada, T.: Main factors affecting wear comfort on the field tests. Sen'i Kikai Gakkaishi (J. Text. Mach. Soc. Jpn.). **36**(4), P212–P217 (1983)
2. Kawabata, S.: The Standardization and Analysis of Hand Evaluation, 2nd edn. The Textile Machinery Society of Japan (1980)
3. Peirce, F.T.: The "handle" of cloth as a measurable quantity. J. Text. Inst. **21**, T377–T416 (1930)
4. Sakaguchi, H., Niwa, M., Kawabata, S.: J. Text. Mach. Soc. Jpn. **31**, T43 (1986)
5. Sakaguchi, H., Niwa, M., Kawabata, S.: J. Soc. Fiber Sci. Technol., Jpn. **45**, 214 (1989)
6. Sukigara, S., Fujimoto, T., Niwa, M.: Sensorial comfort/discomfort of lingerie based on hand assessment and objective evaluation. Sen-I gakkaishi. **49**(6), 294–305 (1993)
7. Mari, I., Matsumoto, M., Nakagawa, K., Ando, H.: Proc. of the 27th textile research symposium. pp. 127 (2008)
8. Niwa, M., Inoue, M., Kawabata, S.: Objective evaluation of the handle of blankets. Text. Res. J. **71**(8), 701–710 (2001)
9. Inoue, M., Maeda, M., Tagami, E., Imamura, Y., Miyazawa, K.: A study on wearing comfort of pants type diapers for elderly people. J. Jpn. Res. Assoc. Text. End-Uses. **51**, 327–332 (2010)

Design and Demonstration of a Standardized Container Structure for Sensor Data Distribution

Takumi Seike[1(✉)], Masato Yoshimi[1,2], Takahiro Ito[2], and Hirokazu Tanaka[2]

[1] TIS Inc., TOYOSU BAYSIDE CROSS TOWER, Koto-ku, Tokyo 135-0061, Japan
{seike.takumi.999,yoshimi.masato}@tis.co.jp

[2] Graduate School of Information Sciences, Hiroshima City University, Hiroshima 731-3194, Japan
{ito-t,hitanaka}@hiroshima-cu.ac.jp

Abstract. The sharing and utilization of data obtained from diverse sensors are becoming increasingly important as foundational technologies supporting next-generation systems such as wearable devices and the metaverse. However, many existing data distribution methods rely on proprietary implementations and implicit assumptions, posing challenges in terms of reproducibility, sustainable operation, and flexible interoperability across heterogeneous systems. To ensure interoperability in the distribution of data with varying formats and types, standardized data formats are essential. This study proposes a framework in which the structure and semantics of information are separated from the raw data by decoupling the data body from its formalization method. We materialized this concept into a concrete data structure. The result has been reflected in IEC 63430, an international standard aiming to enhance data distribution, and is expected to serve as an interface for future data exchange. This paper details the design principles and structural features of the proposed format, presents the results of a prototype implementation, and discusses future perspectives.

Keywords: Sensor data · Data interoperability · Information reconstruction · IEC 63430 · Data format · IoT standardization

1 Introduction

1.1 Information, Data, and Their Distributability

According to ISO/IEC 2382 [1], "information is knowledge concerning objects such as facts, events, things, processes, or ideas, including concepts, that has a specific meaning within a given context." In addition, the same standard defines "data" as a representation of information that is formalized in a manner suitable for communication, interpretation, or processing, and that can be reinterpreted as information. This relationship is illustrated in ISO/IEC 2382 as shown in

H. Tanaka et al. (Eds.): BodyNets 2025, LNICST 714, pp. 438–445, 2026.
https://doi.org/10.1007/978-3-032-38657-1_37

Fig. 1. In other words, the distributability of information refers to the property whereby formalized data can be transmitted to others and interpreted by the receiver as the original information.

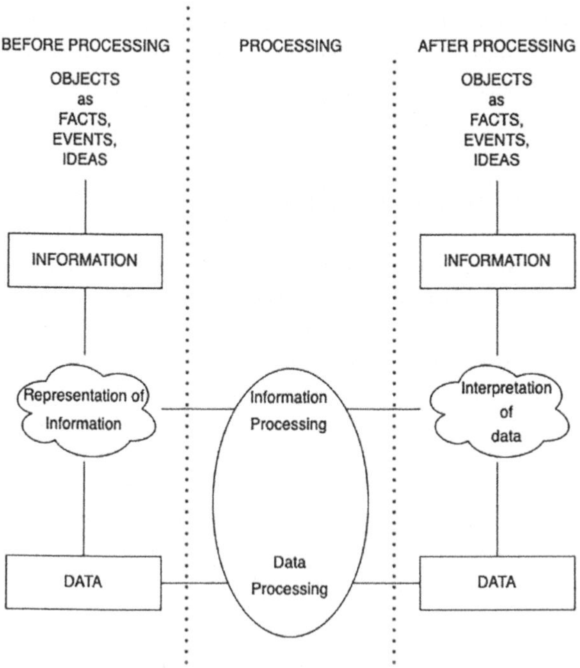

Fig. 1. ISO/IEC 2382 Interrelationships between information and data

When information is transformed into data and distributed, it is sometimes necessary to know the rules—i.e., the formalization method—used to convert the information into data in order to reconstruct the original information from the data. In some cases, such as with predefined data formats (e.g., IP packets or encoded images), it is sufficient if all parties involved in the distribution are aware of the format in advance. However, in the case of sensor-generated data, the information does not necessarily follow any predefined data format.

1.2 Diversification of Data and Related Challenges

To enable the distribution of information, both the sender and the receiver must share an agreement—i.e., a formalization method—for converting between data and information.

In domains such as audio and video, well-known formalization methods exist. In such cases, the information distribution process can rely on explicitly indicated formats or implicit assumptions. For example, formats such as MP3 or

H.264 allow the receiving party to automatically recognize and process the formalization method, enabling the reconstruction of information without requiring explicit agreements. On the other hand, data generated by IoT sensors [2] and wearable devices is highly diverse in terms of the types of information it represents, and each may use its own unique formalization method. In such scenarios, there is often no mechanism for referencing standard formalization methods, nor is there an implicit shared understanding. This creates a challenge in that there is no common foundation to ensure correct interpretation of data as meaningful information.

2 Clarification of the Challenges

At present, standardized formalization methods have not been sufficiently established for the wide variety of information types. As the types of information being converted into data are expected to continue increasing, it is not realistic to define a separate formalization method for each one. Even if such methods could be defined, interoperability cannot be ensured unless they are widely adopted and commonly used among multiple vendors. Consequently, data distributability would remain limited.

To address this challenge, it is necessary not to predefine formalization methods for all types of information, but instead to establish a mechanism that allows the formalization method itself—or clues that lead to it—to be transmitted and shared along with the data during distribution.

3 Standardization of Data Format via IEC 63430

By resolving these challenges, data distributability can be significantly improved, and the development cost of information systems that handle diverse types of data can be reduced.

Against this background, we have designed a data structure in which a header is attached to an arbitrary payload, enabling the corresponding formalization method to be obtained. In this paper, we refer to this data structure as a *container* (Fig. 2).

Information about the data structure and formalization method is stored as schema metadata in a file. The schema is referenced in order to interpret the information from the payload data. This concept forms the core idea of the data format that has been internationally standardized as IEC 63430 [3].

3.1 Header Format and Schema Retrieval Mechanism

A unique identifier is assigned to each schema. The header of a container stores the schema identifier, which is used to interpret the information contained in the payload of that container. Information systems that handle containers retrieve the corresponding schema using the identifier embedded in the header. When

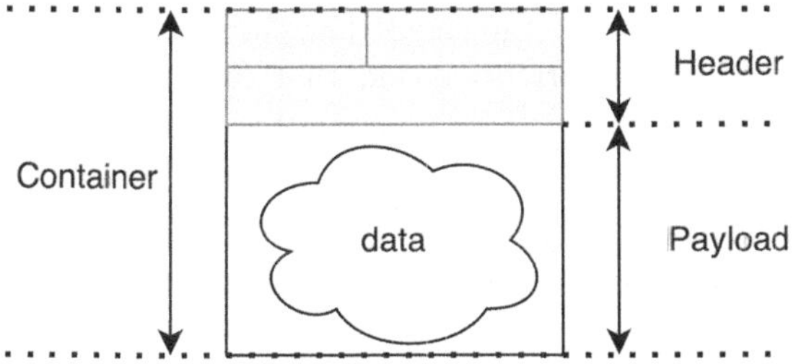

Fig. 2. Data structure of the container

retrieving schema information, the system refers to a schema repository. The schema repository serves to provide schema information in response to schema retrieval requests from the information system. This mechanism enables flexible and dynamic interpretation of data without requiring the payload to conform to a predefined data format.

3.2 Container Generation Method

A container is a structure in which a header is attached to an arbitrary payload. This header includes the following three essential elements:

- **Preamble**
  Indicates the start of the header and also serves to describe optional settings associated with the container.
- **Container Size**
  Specifies the total length of the container (header + payload). This information allows the system to detect and extract individual containers from a continuous stream of data.
- **Schema Identifier**
  Indicates the schema information that should be referenced to interpret the payload data as information. The identifier is assigned at the time of schema registration in the schema repository and is used consistently across the scope in which the container is distributed.

3.3 Operational Validation

To verify the effectiveness of the proposed approach, we conducted a validation to confirm that it is possible to distribute information while separating the data body (payload) from its formalization method (schema information). Specifically, we used sensor data collected from a smartphone to continuously transmit containers and confirmed that the receiver could reference the schema information to correctly interpret and visualize the data.

On the receiving side, we confirmed that the data was successfully reconstructed into meaningful information and that its content was visually accessible through graph rendering, thereby validating the feasibility of information distribution.

The validation was carried out according to the following steps:

1. **Creation of Schema Information and Registration in the Schema Repository**
   Create schema information that describes the structure of the sensor data, and register it in the schema repository.
2. **Generation and Transmission of Containers**
   Continuously generate and transmit containers from a smartphone, attaching a header that includes the previously created schema identifier.
3. **Reception, Interpretation, and Visualization Based on Schema Information**
   Retrieve the appropriate schema information from the schema repository on the receiving side, and reconstruct the payload into meaningful information. By visualizing the result as a graph, we confirmed that the content could be accessed visually. This indicates that the data was correctly interpreted and successfully conveyed to the receiver as meaningful information.

3.4 Creation of Schema Information and Registration in the Schema Repository

Sensor data is acquired from the gyroscope on a smartphone, and this data is used to construct the payload. The schema information corresponding to this data is created based on two sources: the output of the gyroscope and the current timestamp.

Table 1. Schema information

Field Name	Type	Offset	Length
timestamp	int	0	8
x	float	8	8
y	float	16	8
z	float	24	8
alpha	float	32	8
beta	float	40	8
gamma	float	48	8

Table 1 shows the schema information, where each row corresponds to a single data element. Each element includes a field name, data type, offset, and length.

This schema consists of a timestamp representing the current time (an 8-byte integer) and values obtained from a gyroscope sensor. The schema comprises the following seven elements:

- `timestamp`: An 8-byte integer value representing the current timestamp.
- `x, y, z`: Three-axis angular data representing the orientation of the device (yaw, roll, pitch).
- `alpha, beta, gamma`: Three-axis values representing the device's acceleration.

The six elements related to orientation and acceleration are all recorded as 8-byte double-precision floating-point values.

This schema information is registered in the schema repository and can be referenced using the schema identifier specified in the container header. Based on this identifier, the information system retrieves the corresponding schema and interprets the payload within the container.

3.5 Transmission Using Containers

Next, containers are created using the acquired sensor data. The creation of a container is performed according to the following steps:

1. **Preamble Selection**
   Select a preamble to indicate the start of the container and append container type and optional information.
2. **Size Calculation**
   Calculate the total size of the container by adding the header length to the payload length.
3. **Assignment of Schema Identifier**
   Write the schema identifier, which corresponds to the previously registered schema information, into the header.
4. **Payload Assembly**
   Combine the timestamp and six sensor values (`x`, `y`, `z`, `alpha`, `beta`, `gamma`) in binary format to form the payload.
5. **Container Construction**
   Concatenate the header and payload to complete the container.

The generated containers are continuously transmitted at approximately 20 units per second. This enables stable data distribution while maintaining real-time characteristics.

3.6 Reception, Interpretation, and Visualization Based on Schema Information

On the receiving side, the schema identifier is first extracted from the container header, and the corresponding schema information is retrieved from the schema repository based on this identifier. Following the retrieved schema information, each data element (`timestamp`, `x`, `y`, `z`, `alpha`, `beta`, `gamma`) is extracted from the payload and interpreted. To verify that the data has been correctly reconstructed, the extracted information is visualized in graph form (Fig. 3).

The above figure shows the data extracted from the container, stored in a database, and visualized as graphs. The two graphs represent the following:

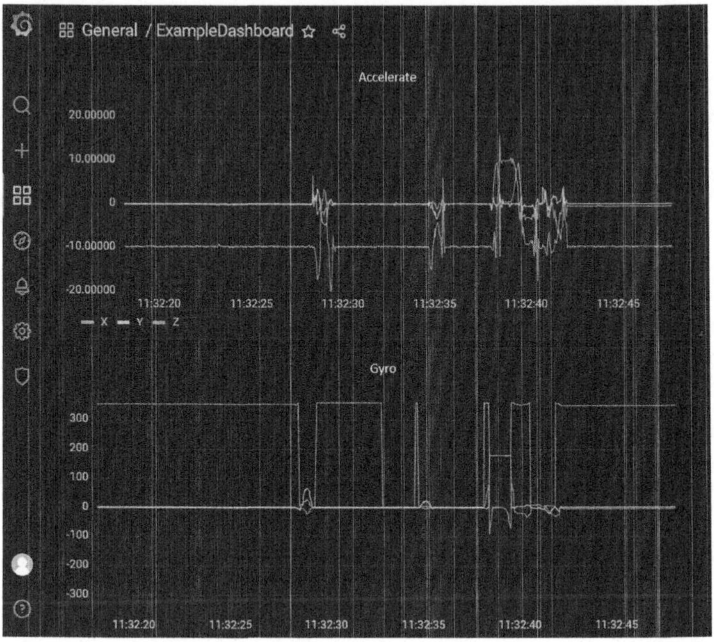

Fig. 3. Visualized graph

- Upper graph: Time-series changes in three-axis acceleration (`alpha`, `beta`, `gamma`).
- Lower graph: Time-series changes in three-axis orientation (`x`, `y`, `z`: yaw, roll, pitch).

The graphs are configured to update in real time, and synchronized changes corresponding to variations in the smartphone's orientation and acceleration were observed. These results verify that the interpretation based on the schema information was correctly performed and that information distribution using the container functioned properly. However, several challenges remain to be addressed for broader practical applications.

4 Conclusion

In this study, we designed and implemented a mechanism that separates the data body from its formalization method (schema information), allowing the formalization method and its interpretation cues to be transmitted and shared independently of the data body. The validation confirmed that the proposed approach enables information distribution at the container level and dynamic data interpretation based on the schema.

5 Challenges

Future challenges and perspectives are discussed below.

5.1 Schema Repository and Schema Information Management

In this validation, the schema repository was constructed within a single environment. For future deployment, the following issues need to be addressed:

- Mechanisms for ensuring consistency and sharing schema information across multiple schema repositories.
- Interoperability when schema information is managed independently by different vendors or communities.
- The necessity of standardizing the uniqueness and assignment rules for schema identifiers.

5.2 Future Prospects

In this validation, we focused on schema information for primitive sensor data. In real-world applications, further developments may include:

- Supporting cases where existing formalization methods (e.g., JSON, MPEG, etc.) are directly used as the payload.
- Schema design for structured data and information containing semantic annotations.
- Establishing a common data interpretation platform across heterogeneous devices and industry domains.

In the future, we aim to verify the flexible applicability of schema-enhanced container formats to these unexplored use cases and continue our research with an emphasis on interoperability and scalability.

References

1. International Organization for Standardization and International Electrotechnical Commission: ISO/IEC 2382: Information technology – Vocabulary. ISO/IEC, Geneva, Switzerland (2015)
2. Lin, J., Yu, W., Zhang, N., Yang, X., Zhang, H., Zhao, W.: A survey on Internet of Things: architecture, enabling technologies, security and privacy, and applications. IEEE Internet Things J. **4**(5), 1125–1142 (2017)
3. International Electrotechnical Commission: IEC 63430: Data container format for wearable sensor. IEC, Geneva, Switzerland (2025)

Standardization and Concept of Heterogeneous Media Data Stream Alignment

Masahiro Ide[1,2](✉) and Masato Yoshimi[1,3]

[1] TIS Inc., Tokyo, Japan
{ide.masahiro,yoshimi.masato}@tis.co.jp
[2] Tokyo City University, Yokohama, Kanagawa, Japan
[3] Hiroshima City University, Hiroshima, Japan

Abstract. The convergence of the physical and digital worlds has accelerated the emergence of services that integrate heterogeneous media data, extending beyond conventional video and audio to include sensor signals, and haptic interactions. However, existing international standards remain largely focused on traditional multimedia such as video and audio. This gap has resulted in fragmented implementations, limited interoperability, and difficulties in reusing data across applications. To address these challenges, IEC TC100/TA18 has initiated Technical Report (TR) on Heterogeneous Media Data Stream Alignment. This paper reports on the objectives and progress of this effort. Specifically, it introduces representative combinations of heterogeneous media, presents a conceptual three-layer framework (input, process, output) for alignment, and discusses the applicability of wearable sensor standards. Finally, the paper outlines the ongoing standardization process and the roadmap.

Keywords: Multimedia service · Standardization · Virtual Reality

1 Introduction

Driven by advances in digital technologies, new multimedia services have emerged that combine not only conventional video and audio but also sensor signals and haptic data (Fig. 1). While standards exist for combining conventional media data (e.g., video, audio) into "multimedia data", currently there is no standard covering these emerging media data. As a result, each service independently implements its own approach, leading to issues such as limited interoperability, reusability, scalability and data silos.

To address these challenges, IEC TC100/TA18 has initiated Technical Report (TR) IEC TR 63669 on the alignment of heterogeneous media data streams. The purpose of this activity is to establish a standardized framework that integrates diverse media types beyond conventional video and audio. Specifically, the TR introduces realignment combinations of heterogeneous media, proposes a conceptual three-layer model (input, process, output) for alignment, and identifies candidate items for standardization based on the analysis of relevant technologies and standards.

H. Tanaka et al. (Eds.): BodyNets 2025, LNICST 714, pp. 446–453, 2026.
https://doi.org/10.1007/978-3-032-38657-1_38

This paper reports on the objectives and progress of IEC TR 63669. It introduces representative service examples and challenges that combine heterogeneous media, presents the conceptual three-layer alignment framework, and highlights the applicability of existing wearable sensor standards—specifically SmartBAN (IEC 63203-801-1 [1], IEC 63203-801-2 [2]) and IEC 63430 [3] — as practical foundations for realizing the conceptual framework. Finally, it outlines the ongoing standardization process and provides a roadmap from Technical Report (TR) to International Standard (IS).

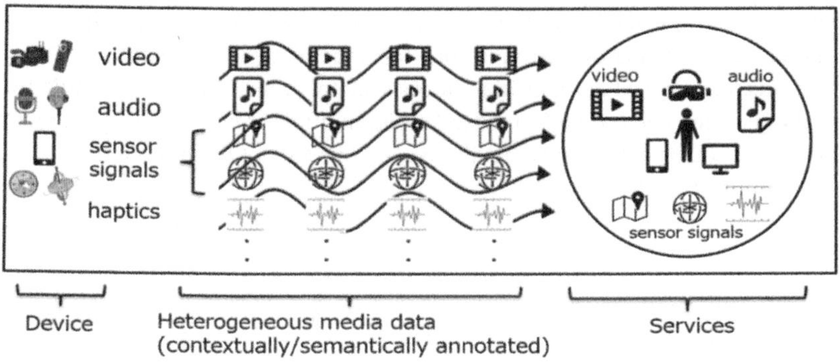

Fig. 1. Abstraction of services by heterogeneous media Data

2 Examples and Challenges

This section introduces representative examples of services that integrate heterogeneous media data (Fig. 2) and discusses the specific challenges they face in the absence of standardized alignment mechanisms.

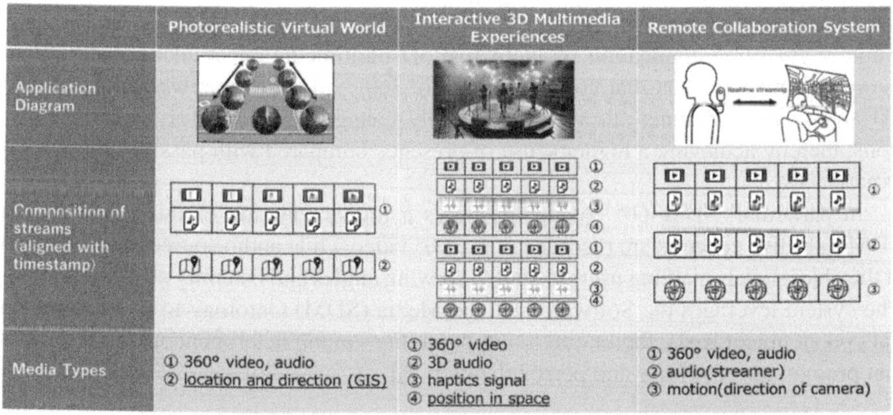

Fig. 2. Examples of services combining heterogeneous media data

2.1 Photorealistic Virtual World

A typical example of heterogeneous media integration is the construction of photorealistic virtual worlds by combining 360° video with geospatial information captured at the time of recording. Each video frame is associated with location data through computational or manual processes, enabling the creation of an interactive virtual environment (Fig. 3). Applications such as MovieMap [4] and 360RVW [5] have demonstrated the feasibility of this approach, supporting experiences such as virtual city exploration and cultural heritage tours. Compared with traditional 3D-CG modeling, which requires significant resources, this method offers a more scalable and cost-efficient solution. However, the lack of a standardized framework for integrating geospatial data with video streams leads to increased implementation costs and poor interoperability. Furthermore, these datasets often need to be re-indexed along multiple axes, such as time, location, or semantic attributes, which existing ad-hoc systems cannot flexibly support.

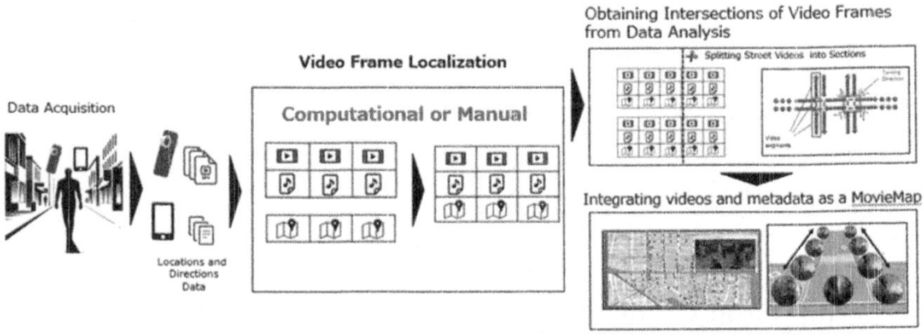

Fig. 3. Process of creating a MovieMap database

2.2 Interactive 3D Multimedia Experiences

Another emerging application is interactive 3D multimedia experiences, exemplified by virtual music events that combine multiple 360° video streams with object-based 3D audio. Such systems allow users to freely change viewpoints or listening positions, thereby achieving a higher sense of presence compared with passive audiovisual experiences.

In particular, SDM360^2 [6] demonstrates a implementation of this approach. In SDM360^2, live concerts are recorded with 360° video while audio sources are managed at the object level, enabling users to switch viewing angles and listening positions at will. The system leverages the Software Defined Media (SDM) Ontology to manage media data on an object basis, facilitating interoperability among heterogeneous data sources and promoting reusability and personalization [6].

Some implementations additionally incorporate haptic feedback, as in the case of Tactile TV [7], which delivers vibration signals synchronized with video and audio. These approaches highlight the growing demand for immersive and multimodal interaction. At the same time, aligning multiple audiovisual datasets across both temporal and spatial dimensions remains technically difficult, and the absence of standardized schema or formats results in application-specific implementations that are costly and difficult to reuse.

2.3 Remote Collaboration System

A further representative case is the remote collaboration system, which integrates real-time streams of video, audio, and sensor data such as orientation or motion to support immersive cooperative experiences. T-Leap [8], for example, provides stabilized 360° video by combining gyroscopic data with live recordings, enabling remote guided tours with reduced motion discomfort (Fig. 4). Remote work guidance systems employ 3D cameras or motion sensors to capture an instructor's gestures and line of sight, overlaying them on workers' displays for intuitive instruction. VR meeting platforms such as Horizon Workrooms [9] extend this concept by synchronizing avatars, voice communication, and interactive tools in shared virtual spaces. These systems demonstrate the potential of heterogeneous media integration for real-time collaboration, yet they also expose critical challenges. Synchronization across heterogeneous streams is difficult to achieve consistently, latency requirements are strict, and no widely adopted standards exist for the integration of sensor data with audiovisual channels.

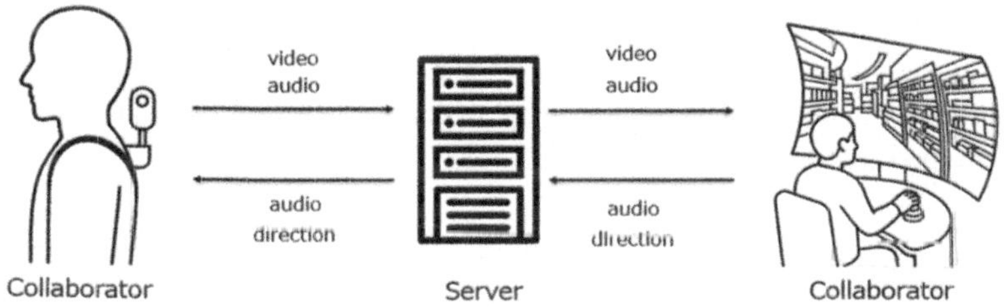

Fig. 4. Architecture of the T-Leap system

3 Conceptual Framework for Alignment

The service examples introduced in the previous section highlight a common challenge: there is no standardized framework for combining heterogeneous media data streams. Each application or product currently implements its own ad-hoc solution, which leads to interoperability problems, limited reusability, scalability concerns, and fragmented data silos. To address these issues, IEC TR 63669 conceptualizes the alignment of heterogeneous media data streams as a three-layer process (Fig. 5).

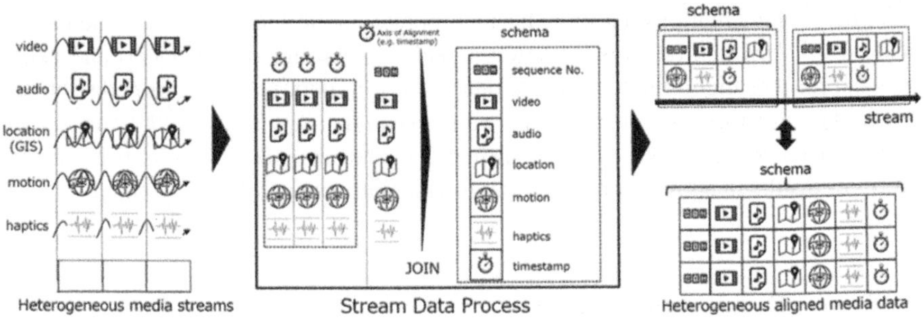

Fig. 5. Concept of alignment of heterogeneous media data streams

3.1 Input Layer

The input layer receives heterogeneous media data streams, including video, audio, sensor signals, and static media such as images or 3D models. While streams often include ordering information (timestamps, sequence numbers), static media may not. Therefore, flexible mechanisms are required to associate such data with sequential streams when necessary. Potential standardization items at this layer include data formats and protocols.

3.2 Process Layer

The process layer aligns incoming data streams using sequence information such as time codes, sequence numbers, or coordinates. Metadata is attached and integrated through schema representations that describe relationships across streams. This enables the bundled management of heterogeneous data as a coherent set. Candidate items for standardization at this layer include alignment methods and schema definition/representation.

3.3 Output Layer

The output layer delivers aligned multimedia data in forms suitable for end-user applications. It allows for conversion into different stream formats and supports query-based re-indexing along different axes, such as time or space (Fig. 6). For real-time use cases, such as remote collaboration, methods for delay evaluation are also necessary. Standardization topics here include data formats, protocols, and evaluation methods.

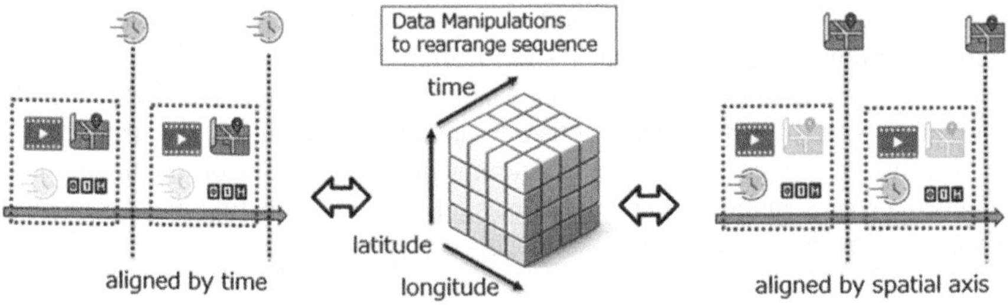

Fig. 6. Flexible alignment of multimedia streams

4 Applicability of Wearable Sensor Standards

The conceptual framework introduced in Sect. 3 describes the alignment of heterogeneous media data streams through three layers: input, process, and output. To realize this framework in practical applications, existing wearable sensor standards can serve as a foundation for interoperability and consistency.

SmartBAN (IEC 63203-801-1 [1], IEC 63203-801-2 [2]) provides mechanisms for time synchronization and data collection across multiple wearable devices. This capability contributes to the input and process layers by ensuring that heterogeneous data streams can be captured and synchronized with high temporal accuracy.

IEC 63430 (Data container format for wearable sensor) [3] defines a standardized structure for storing and transmitting sensor information. It supports the input and output layers by providing interoperability and enabling consistent handling of data originating from diverse devices and systems.

These standards do not function in isolation but rather complement each other in realizing the conceptual framework. SmartBAN contributes to synchronization across input and process layers, while IEC 63430 ensures interoperability and reusability at the input and output layers. Together, they provide the basis for implementing heterogeneous media alignment, establishing a path toward scalable and interoperable virtual-society services.

5 Standardization Activities and Process

The development of IEC TR 63669 is part of ongoing standardization activities in IEC TC100/TA18. The project was initiated in 2024 with the objective of clarifying use cases and concepts for heterogeneous media data stream alignment, and it represents the first step toward establishing a future International Standard (IS).

The initial draft of the Technical Report was circulated in early 2025, followed by discussions in the project team (PT) under TC100/TA18. Feedback from national committees and experts is being incorporated to refine the scope, terminology, and conceptual framework. Subsequent milestones include the committee draft (CD) circulation and consensus building toward final publication.

Looking ahead, the standardization process is expected to follow the conventional IEC pathway: from Preliminary Work Item (PWI) to Technical Report (TR), and subsequently to New Proposal (NP) and International Standard (IS). This staged approach enables the community to first consolidate requirements and conceptual models, and then to move toward detailed technical specifications.

By documenting representative use cases, the conceptual alignment framework, and identified gaps, IEC TR 63669 serves as a foundation for future standardization work. The outcome of this effort will guide subsequent specifications on alignment methods, schema representations, and data formats, ultimately supporting interoperable and scalable multimedia services across heterogeneous environments.

6 Conclusion and Future Work

This paper presented the objectives and progress of IEC TR 63669 on heterogeneous media data stream alignment. We discussed representative service examples that integrate diverse media types, introduced a conceptual three-layer framework for alignment, and highlights the applicability of existing wearable sensor standards—specifically SmartBAN (IEC 63203-801-1 [1], IEC 63203-801-2 [2]) and IEC 63430 [3] —as practical foundations for realizing the conceptual framework.

IEC TR 63669 provides an important foundation for bridging the gap between fragmented implementations and interoperable multimedia systems. By formalizing alignment methods, schema definitions, and data formats, it aims to ensure that heterogeneous media—such as video, audio, sensor signals, and haptic interactions—can be combined in a consistent and reusable manner across applications.

Future work will include proof-of-concept implementations, interoperability testing, and closer collaboration with industry stakeholders to validate the proposed framework in real-world environments. These activities will further support the transition from Technical Report to International Standard and strengthen the role of heterogeneous media alignment in enabling scalable and reliable multimedia services in the emerging virtual society.

References

1. IEC 63203-801-1. Wearable electronic devices and technologies – part 801-1: basic test methods for the external operating environment – method for testing the performance of wearable systems in relevant scenarios – section 1. IEC TC124 (2021)
2. IEC 63203-801-2. Wearable electronic devices and technologies – part 801-2: basic test methods for the external operating environment – method for testing the performance of wearable systems in relevant scenarios – section 2. IEC TC124 (2021)
3. IEC 63430. Data container format for wearable sensor. IEC TC100/TA18 (2024)
4. Sugimoto, N., Ebine, Y., Aizawa, K.: Building movie map – a tool for exploring in a city – and its evaluations. In: Proc. ACM Multimedia (2020)
5. Takenawa, M., Sugimoto, N., Wöhler, L., Ikehata, S., Aizawa, K.: 360RVW: Fusing real 360° videos and interactive virtual worlds. In: Proc. ACM Multimedia (2023)
6. NTT InterCommunication Center (ICC): Tactile TV. https://www.ntticc.or.jp/en/archive/works/tactile-tv/. Accessed 18 Aug 2025
7. Atarashi, R., Sone, T., Komohara, Y., et al.: The software defined media ontology for music events (SDM3602). In: Proc. SAAM '18 (2018)

8. Manabe, M., Uriu, D., Funatsu, T., et al.: Exploring in the city with your personal guide: design and user study of T-leap, a telepresence system. In: Proc. 19th Int. Conf. Mobile and Ubiquitous Multimedia (MUM), pp. 96–106. ACM (2020)
9. Meta Platforms, Inc.: Horizon workrooms. https://www.meta.com/workrooms/. Accessed 18 Aug 2025

A Consideration for Standardization of Haptics Technology

Kazuhiro Murakami(✉)

Meiji University, 1-1, Kanda Surugadai, Chiyoda-Ku, Tokyo 101-8301, Japan
kaz_murakami_pdx@meiji.ac.jp

Abstract. Alongside vision and hearing, haptic technology is an essential component forming the basis of current virtual reality and metaverse experiences. However, this technology remains in its developmental stages. Unlike other sensory technologies, it involves numerous receptors throughout the human body, leading to the existence of diverse individual technologies across various categories and fields. By creating a flexible, standards-based framework for haptics that includes a broad-ranging haptics stimulus descriptor enabling systematic overall understanding, classification, and grouping of these diverse technologies, categories, and fields, along with the relevant terminology and definitions, we believe it is possible to achieve appropriate and smooth technological progress while maintaining quality, without hindering the advancement of this technology.

This paper introduces the progress of standardization and the development of the environment within International standard IEC TC100. It specifically details "Haptics stimuli descriptors," one of its components, which was standardized as an IEC technical specification in June of this year. Furthermore, it outlines the significance and challenges of future haptics standardization, along with potential solutions.

Keywords: Haptics technology · Haptics stimuli descriptors · International standard

1 Progress and Background of Haptics Standardization Within International Standard IEC TC100 TA18

Haptic transmission technology is one of the sensory transmission technologies that has become crucial, alongside visual and auditory technologies, for building current virtual reality and metaverse environments. However, compared to visual and auditory technologies, haptic transmission technology is still in its infancy. Additionally, since the entire human body, including the brain, acts as a receptor, haptic technology encompasses a wide variety of categories and fields.

As shown in Fig. 1, International standard IEC TC100 TA18 therefore compiled a technical report examining the overall landscape of haptics technology, its use cases, and potential standardization items. Based on this report, the group standardized technical

H. Tanaka et al. (Eds.): BodyNets 2025, LNICST 714, pp. 454–460, 2026.
https://doi.org/10.1007/978-3-032-38657-1_39

specifications for descriptors that enable the logical classification and grouping of diverse haptic technologies. Furthermore, the group created an international standard for the terminology and definitions used in haptics technology, which lays the groundwork for the smooth and appropriate standardization of diverse haptics technologies. Below, we describe the specific contents of this work, as well as the challenges encountered while advancing the standardization of various haptics technologies.

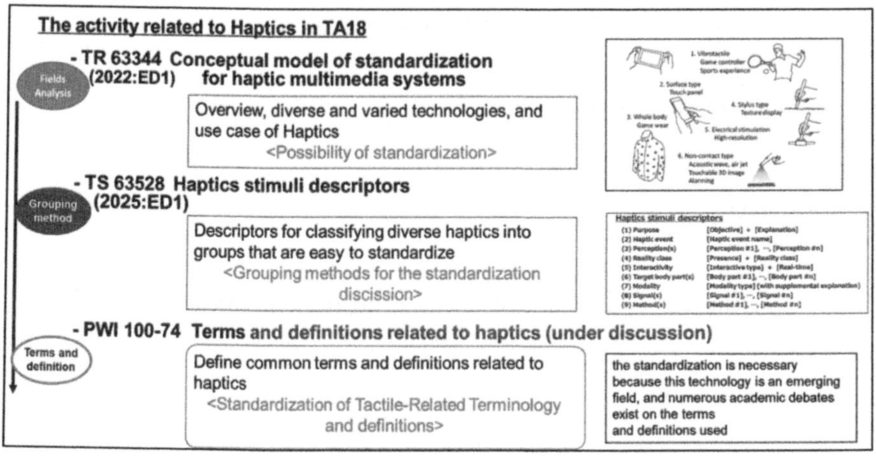

Fig. 1. The groundwork for advancing the standardization of various haptic technologies within International standard IEC TC100 TA18

2 Haptic Stimulus Descriptors

2.1 Outline

The overall picture of haptics technology, its use cases, and candidate items for standardization (reality level, interaction mode, data format and network topology, and device characteristics) were compiled in technical report IEC TR 63344:2022 ED1. Based on these, the technical specification IEC TS 63528:2025 ED1 Haptics stimuli descriptors were standardized as the next step. This technical specification enables the classification and grouping of haptic stimuli by descriptors such as purpose, effect, target receptor, target location, and reality class. It consists of nine items (twelve items including sub-items). To avoid restricting the diverse and evolving haptic technologies and to facilitate documentation even for technologies still under research, (1) Mandatory (must be described), (2) Optional (preferably described), and (3) Conditional (described if currently available) are categized in description. (Refer to Fig. 2)

This facilitates flexible expression of the parameters and characteristics of various haptic stimuli, enables easy classification and grouping of related stimulus sets, and establishes an environment conducive to appropriate standardization discussions within these groups.

Here, we briefly explain these haptic stimulus descriptors and illustrate their parameters and characteristics using several examples.

Haptics stimuli descriptors

(1) Purpose	[Objective] + [Explanation]	<Mandatory>
(2) Haptic event	[Haptic event name]	<Mandatory>
(3) Perception(s)	[Perception #1], ···, [Perception #n]	<Mandatory>
(4) Reality class	[Presence] + [Reality class]	<Mandatory>
(5) Interactivity	[Interactive type] + [Real-time]	<Optional>
(6) Target body part(s)	[Body part #1], ···, [Body part #n]	<Optional>
(7) Modality	[Modality type] (with supplemental explanation)	<Conditional>
(8) Signal(s)	[Signal #1], ···, [Signal #n]	<Conditional>
(9) Method(s)	[Method #1], ···, [Method #n]	<Conditional>

Fig. 2. Haptics stimuli descriptors

2.2 Contents of the Descriptors

Purpose

<Definition>

[Objective] - [Explanation]

Objective: How to use about the target haptics.

Explanation: Brief description including scene and scenario of the use and what effect it has on humans.

<Information level>

Mandatory

Haptic event

<Definition>

[Haptic event]

Haptic event: Specific haptic sensation recognized by human brain through their own touch or passively received by their bodies together with sensory information that humans have experienced and stored up to now.

<Information level>

Mandatory

Perception(s)

<Definition>

[Perception #1], ··· [Perception #n]

Perceive by intrinsic cutaneous sensory organs and by mechanoreceptors including tendon-, muscle-, and semi-circular canal-related sensors (Pressure, vibration, hardness, softness, warmth, cold, coarseness, pain, friction, weight, acceleration, balance, and etc.).

*Multiple perceptions can be described

<Information level>

Mandatory

Reality class

<Definition>

[Existence] - [Reality class]

Existence: Indicates whether it exists in reality (Physical) or in the imagination never existed before now (Imaginary)

Reality Class:	Class A:	Stimuli are reproduced.
	Class B:	The stimulus is different from the actual stimulus, but humans cannot perceive the difference
	Class C:	A mere stimulus, using with an under standing that

<Information level>

Mandatory

Interactivity

<Definition>

[Relational] - [Real-time]

Relational: What user actions will be responded to

D: Dynamic I: Interactive N: Non-interactive

Real-time: Is control/playback real-time or preset

R：Realtime P: Preset

<Information level>

Optional

Target body part(s)

<Definition>

[Body part #1], ··· [Body parts #n]

Human body part(s) to which Haptics is presented;
toes/ feet/ lower limbs/ hips/ torso/ neck/ head/ shoulders/ arms/ elbows/ fore-arms/ wrist /hand/ five fingers (little finger, ring finger, middle finger, index finger, thumb)/ eye/ nose/ face/ upper lip/ lower lip/ teeth/ gums /jaws /tongue /larynx /abdominal cavity/ back/ genital organs (Based on the body part reproduction chart (homunculus) of the human primary somatosensory system)

*no distinction between left and right

<Information level>

Optional

Modality

<Definition>

[Combination of senses] - [Supplementary explanation]

Combination of senses:

A: haptics and visual B: haptics and auditory

C: haptics, visual, and auditory D: haptics only

Supplementary explanation:

Effects of vision and touch on the sense of touch

<Information level>

Optional

Signal(s)

<Definition>

[Signal #1], ··· [Signal #n]

A piece of data that provides specific information about how a human sensory element is stimulated. Relevant signal data, if possible, may be described as descriptors.

<Information level>

Conditional

Method(s)

<Definition>

[Method #1], ··· [Method #n]

Means of how to achieve haptics. A piece of data that provides specific information about how a human sensory element is stimulated.
Relevant signal data, if possible, may be described as descriptors.

<Information level>

Conditional

2.3 Examples of Haptics Descriptors Table

If a particular haptic event can be represented by a table listing all the descriptors according to the definitions of these descriptors, it would be possible to give a concise and clear description of the various aspects and characteristics of the event. If a table such as the example below Figs. 3 and 4 of haptics descriptors table were presented, it would allow the various haptic events to be classified and understood at a glance.

Descriptors		Contents
Purpose	Objective	button sensation on CID
	Explanation	reproduce realistic button sensation on the flat panel CID in the vehicle explanation
Haptic event		button click sensation
Perception(s)		vibration perception, pressure perception
Reality class	Presence	Physical presence
	Reality class	class B
Interactivity	Interactivity type	D (Dynamic) or I (Interactive)
	Real-time	R (Real-time)
Target body part(s)		5 fingers
Modality	Modality type	C (haptics, visual, and auditory)
	(Explanation)	N/A
Signal(s)		vibration wave-form, frequency, displacement/acceleration, attenuation rate, pressure sense, the delay between reaching the pressure threshold and starting vibration for click sensation
Method(s)		Using vibration

Fig. 3. Haptics button sensation on CID in vehicles description example according to haptics stimuli descriptors

Descriptors		Contents
Purpose	Objective	Mid air sensation
	Explanation	When you touch or move the object that is projected in the air, it reproduces the tactile feedback. (ex. rain, breeze, a sense of certainty)
Haptic event		Mid air sensation
Perception(s)		vibration perception
Reality class	Presence	physical presence
	Reality class	class B
Interactivity	Interactivity type	D (Dynamic) or I (Interactive)
	Real-time	R (Real-time)
Target body part(s)		5 fingers, palm
Modality	Modality type	C (haptics, visual, and auditory)
	(Explanation)	If availabe
Signal(s)		vibration wave-form, frequency, strength of Irradiation
Method(s)		ultrasonic waves with several method (ex. array forming)

Fig. 4. Haptics sensation in the air description example according to haptics stimuli descriptors

3 The Significance and Challenges of Advancing Haptics Standardization

3.1 The Significance of Standardization

As mentioned earlier, haptics is an evolving technology, and each step forward in its development is expected to yield greater effects and results through integration with other technologies. However, releasing products or technologies at a level where users cannot recognize their immature state risks diminishing the overall perception and value of haptics. To prevent this, it is essential to accurately assess the maturity level of each haptic technology and demonstrate products or technologies with effects currently acceptable within those prerequisites.

Therefore, appropriate standardization, aligned with the maturity level of haptics, must progress in a more concrete manner.

For instance, vibrational warnings require users to learn that the vibration signifies a warning or to recognize it as distinct from ordinary vibrations.

However, if the vibrational stimulus is that humans have previously experienced and memorized, no learning or familiarization is necessary. Humans can instantly perceive what warning is being signaled and its urgency level. (If the characteristic vibration felt when a large lorry suddenly approaches from behind while driving could be faithfully reproduced, instinctive recognition, understanding, and avoidance decisions regarding the warning would be possible. Furthermore, if the pressure and haptics sensations felt on the finger when pressing a button could be reproduced, the tactile feel of a button could be recreated on a flat, buttonless panel. This would allow the confirmation sensation of having pressed and selected the button to be felt instantly and without doubt.)

3.2 Efficacy of Descriptors

The necessity of this learning and mastery can be determined by the distinction in the aforementioned descriptors' reality levels: Class A (complete reproduction), B (stimuli differing from reality but indistinguishable to humans), and C (mere stimuli where the subject is pre-informed of what they represent).

For other descriptors, similar distinctions can be made clearer through discussions within haptic stimuli that allow for such grouping.

3.3 Challenge

It is becoming apparent that standardization efforts are currently being pursued in a fragmented manner by individual organizations rooted in specific fields or product groups. It is considered that a more effective approach to standardization would be to consolidate activities within an organization that has examined the overall picture of haptics, defined descriptors for stimuli, and prepared terminology and definitions to represent them. Alternatively, standardization efforts could proceed in the same direction by referencing such an organization.

References

1. IEC TC100 TA18: IEC TR63344:2022 ED1. Conceptual model of standardization for haptic multimedia systems
2. IEC TC100 TA18: IEC TR63528:2025 ED1. Haptics stimuli descriptors

Multi-function Integrated Reliable and Unconscious Virtual Vital-Sign Sensor (MIRUWS) and Its Service

Shigenobu Minami[1(✉)], Masafumi Tamura[1], Toshio Ikeda[1], Takuji Suzuki[1], Hirokazu Tanaka[2], Kaisei Ishihara[3], Kazuhiro Sumitomo[3], Akikatsu Kamiya[4], and Keisuke Shima[4]

[1] MIRUWS Co. Ltd., Sapporo, Japan
minami@miruws.com
[2] Hiroshima City University, Hiroshima, Japan
[3] Tohoku Medical and Pharmaceutical University, Sendai, Japan
[4] Yokohama National University, Yokohama, Japan

Abstract. This paper describes a novel cyber-physical system (CPS) called MIRUWS (Multi-function Integrated Reliable and Unconscious Virtual Vital Sensor), which can continuously, precisely and concurrently estimate wellness data comprising emotion, vital and life data. Several types of physical domain sensor can be implemented in various parts of the body, such as the human body or a car body. The virtual sensor is realized by combining physical sensors and software analysis on an edge device and cloud server, respectively. As the performance of the virtual sensor is determined by the performance of both the physical sensors and the software analysis, it is necessary to define the virtual sensor as a single entity. This paper presents the combined performance of the virtual sensor in the form of the sleep stage and sleep apnea syndrome and blood stream pressure estimation performance of MIRUWS. In addition to the above features, MIRUWS offers highly secure personal health record (PHR) and privacy control functions. Since wellness data is highly sensitive, we believe that secure storage and privacy control are essential for a wide variety of wellness data applications. This paper demonstrates that MIRUWS is a novel cyber-based wellness sensor with secure storage and privacy control functionalities.

Keywords: PHR · PDS · SAS · Sleep Stage · Emotion · Stress · Blood Pressure

1 Introduction

These days, wellness has become a very important keyword. Since a medically healthy life does not always equate to a happy and fulfilling life, wellness has been recognized as an indicator of a good life. There are many indicators that can be used to measure wellness, such as emotion, vitality, and lifestyle. Recent wearable sensors, such as smart watches or wristbands, are being developed to visualize these indicators. However, currently, none of these sensors can provide precise emotion, vital, and lifestyle estimations

H. Tanaka et al. (Eds.): BodyNets 2025, LNICST 714, pp. 461–469, 2026.
https://doi.org/10.1007/978-3-032-38657-1_40

continuously and simultaneously with a small body and at a low cost. This is because attaining these requirements requires a lot of computing resources. Although the combination of physical sensors and smartphone applications is usually adopted to overcome this implementation problem, using AI processing for precise wellness data estimation, such as emotions, requires a lot of computing resources. Additionally, it is difficult to implement quickly and maintain applications for rapidly changing operating systems and new types of products. Considering these issues, we decided to develop a cyber-physical system with a virtual vital signs sensor called MIRUWS. It is composed of a small, simple, and low-cost physical sensor and advanced intelligent signal processing in the cloud.

2 Concept of MIRUWS

As shown in Fig. 1, the MIRUWS concept is based on the idea of a virtual vital sign sensor, which is independent of the implementation. Implementation changes gradually but drastically over time. This is because progress in technology, especially LSI technologies, will allow complex algorithms, such as AI algorithms currently implemented in high-performance servers, to be included in edge devices, such as wristbands.

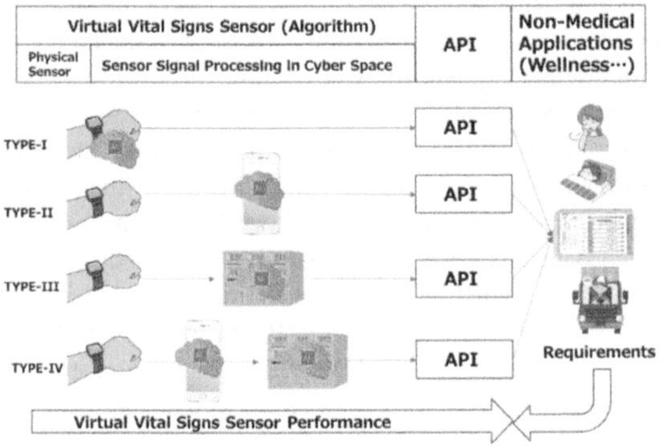

Fig. 1. Virtual Vital Signs Sensor configurations

(a) **TYPE I:** All complex sensor signal processing, such as AI, is implemented in a wearable sensor device. Since the device, such as a wristband, should be as small and low-power as possible, we have to wait for very low-power AI chips to be developed.
(b) **TYPE II:** Currently, most virtual vital sign sensors are implemented in this configuration. Due to progress in smartphone technology, it has become possible to include AI processing. Some high-performance smartphones can estimate wellness data, such as stress levels and sleep patterns. However,
(c) **TYPE III:** Some wearable sensors connect directly to a server without the need for a smartphone. Although a mobile network is needed via a SIM card, users can easily use the sensors without handling a smartphone.

(d) **TYPE IV:** This approach allows for flexible allocation of processing. The smartphone can be used as a gateway or for AI processing together with AI learning on the server.

2.1 MIRUWS M3

The multi-function, integrated, reliable, wearable virtual vital sensor (MIRUWS) maps the algorithms in cyberspace is converted into a Type III or Type VI physical setup. The current generation of MIRUWS [1] is the M3, and its configuration is shown in Fig. 2. Original vital sign signals, such as electrocardiograms (ECGs), pulse, and acceleration waves, are obtained by a body area network (BAN) and analyzed using sophisticated signal processing to determine sleep status, sleep apnea syndrome (SAS), stress, emotions, blood stream pressure, vascular resistance, and blood flow velocity. It should be noted that all these analyses use only pulse, ECG, and body motion data.

All processing outputs are combined with subjective user information obtained via questionnaire to estimate the risk of sleep disorders, SAS, hypertension, frailty, heat stroke, etc.

Even though the outputs of the MIRUWS are emotional, vital, and life data used for nonmedical applications, data security and privacy are still very important functionalities. MIRUWS includes unique security and privacy protection technologies. A Personal Health Record (PHR) is also a mandatory function, even for nonmedical applications. With PHR functionality, the application can utilize the history of nonmedical data, such as wellness data.

MIRUWS has a variety of output options, including web APIs, CSV files, and printable PDF files. The MIRUWS IoT container contains privacy control information and will be used to transfer data to third parties under a data protection policy. Currently, this container format is unique to MIRUWS. However, once the IoT container with privacy control is standardized, we can send the container to any data user who adopts the new IoT container standard (MIRUWS M4 ~).

In addition to the above features, the MIRUWS M3 offers unique functionalities, including risk analysis advice and recommendations utilizing sleep status, SAS risk, stress level, emotional status, vascular resistance, blood flow velocity, and blood stream pressure. These functions are carried out automatically based on a doctor's guidance.

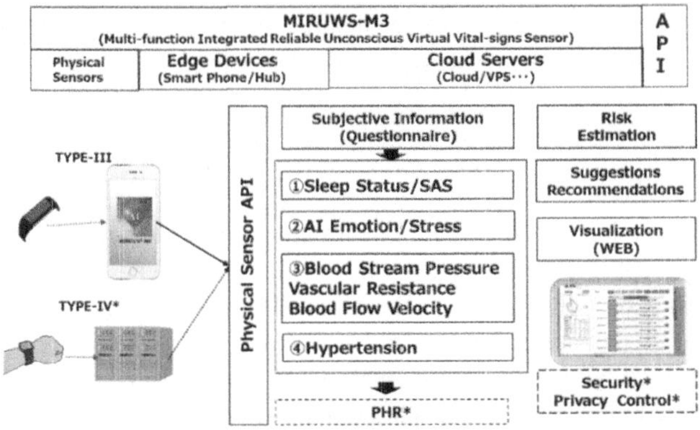

Fig. 2. MIRUWS M3 Configuration (* MIRUWS M4)

3 MIRUWS WEEAK for Sleep

Since our goal is to promote wellness for everyone, we would like to make our cutting-edge technologies available to seniors and children who do not have smartphones, as well as to those who are not very familiar with IT. The unique "MIRUWS WEEAK" service is already available to everyone, including those who are not tech-savvy. The first of these services is "MIRUWS WEEAK for Sleep", which targets those suffering from sleep disorders or SAS. Since some people are too busy to identify the reasons for their poor health, we have reduced the time required for sleep disorder and SAS risk estimation to one week. Usually, a medical diagnosis of SAS requires an overnight polysomnography (PSG) test. However, even with this medical method, it is difficult to attain a correct risk estimation in cases of day-to-day condition changes, such as stressful and relaxing days. We have therefore decided on a one-week measurement period to make SAS screening as easy as possible. Precise medical testing is then carried out on those screened as high-risk candidates. In this approach, screening accuracy is paramount. According to our clinical trial involving 50 subjects at risk of SAS, the sensitivity was 91% and the specificity 85% for subjects with a mid-high apnea-hypopnea index (AHI).

The service outline is shown in Fig. 3. Test results can be viewed in paper form or on a web page, as shown in Fig. 4, and a detailed report of a specific day can also be obtained, as shown in Fig. 5. As shown in Fig. 4, stress, emotions and the number of steps are depicted alongside sleep disorders and SAS risk. This is because these indexes may strongly affect sleep disorders and SAS risk, as can be seen in Fig. 5, where we observed stress and tension increase during SAS events.

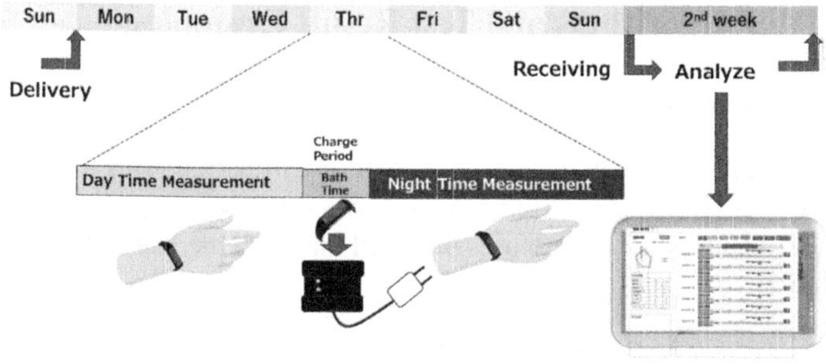

Fig. 3. MIRUWS WEEAK for Sleep Outline

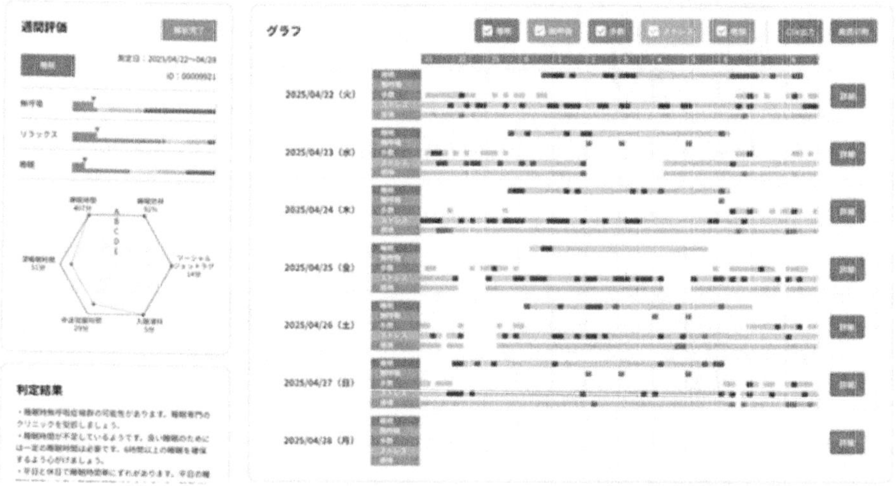

Fig. 4. Web Page for Visualization

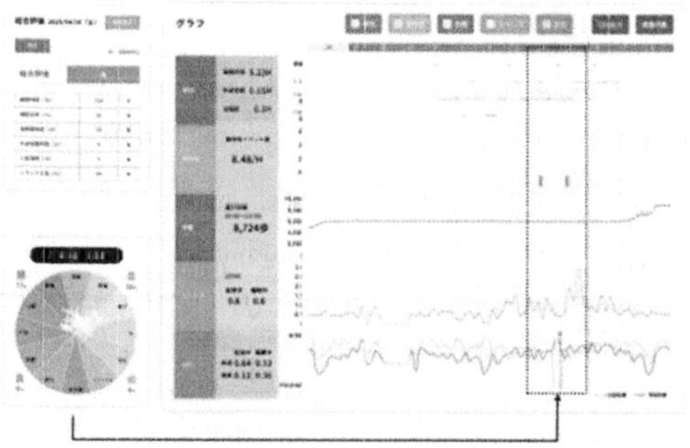

Fig. 5. Detail Page for Selected Day

4 MIRUWS Algorithms and Test Result Examples

4.1 Emotion Estimation by Knowledge Distillation (KD)

Teacher AI is used to attain high-precision emotion estimation using simple pulse data. A model that was learned using brain waves, sweating, subjective test results, etc., is applied. The student model, which uses only PPI input via the KD method [2], is shown in Figs. 6 and 7.

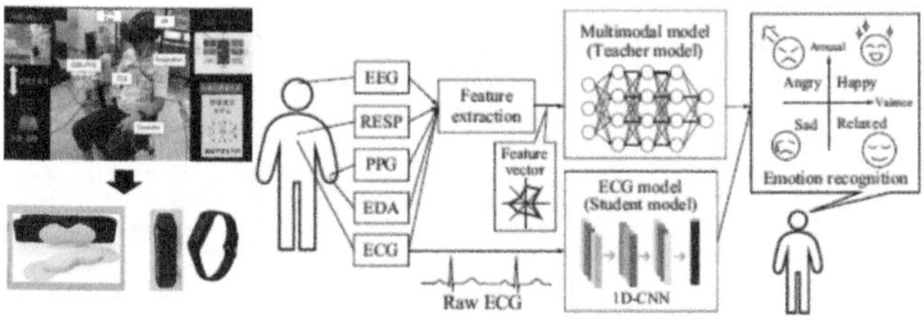

Fig. 6. Knowledge Distillation method applied for the Emotion Estimation

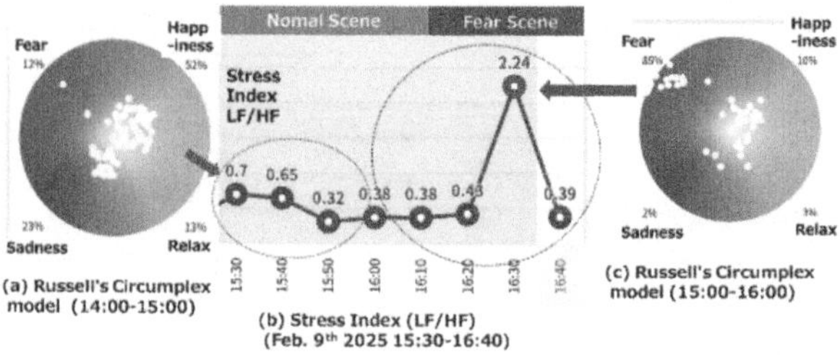

Fig. 7. Emotion Estimation Example with Stress Index during Drama Viewing

Stress index is obtained using traditional LF/HF autonomic balance estimation. As seen in Fig. 8, we can observe emotion change from 12% fear emotion index in normal scene to 85% fear index in fear scene in a suspense drama. It is also observed rapid increase of LF/HF index at the fear scene.

4.2 Blood Stream Pressure Change (BPSC) Estimation

Instead of cuff type blood pressure monitor, characteristics of blood stream and blood vessels are measured by precisely analyzing pulse wave. BSPC which indicates hypertension risk is obtained by using machine learning [3] as shown in Fig. 8.

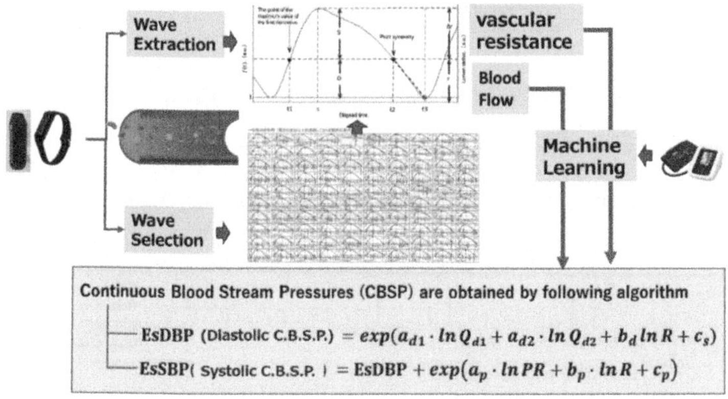

Fig. 8. C.B.S.P. Algorithm Outline

C.B.S.P estimation results for day and night times are shown in bellow. A seen here, C.B.S.P increases are observed in early morning (night) and fear scene in drama viewing (day) (Fig. 9).

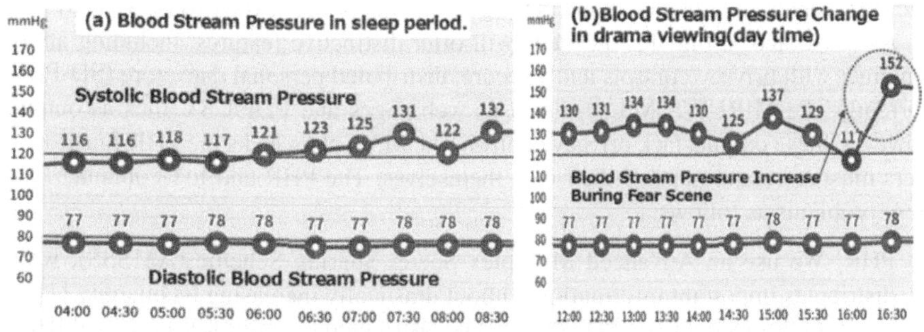

Fig. 9. BSPC estimation results example for suspense drama and sleep

4.3 Sleep Quality and SAS Risk Estimation

By analyzing PPI, sleep quality and SAS risk are estimated. Clinical trial tests are carried out for 50 sleep apnea suspected patients, comparing polysomnography(PSG) results. As for sleep stage, around 73% match is attained by comparing PSG results. As for SAS risk, sensitivity = 0.91 and specificity = 0.87 are measured comparing AHI obtained by PSG (Fig. 4) by using five nights data (Figs. 10 and 11),

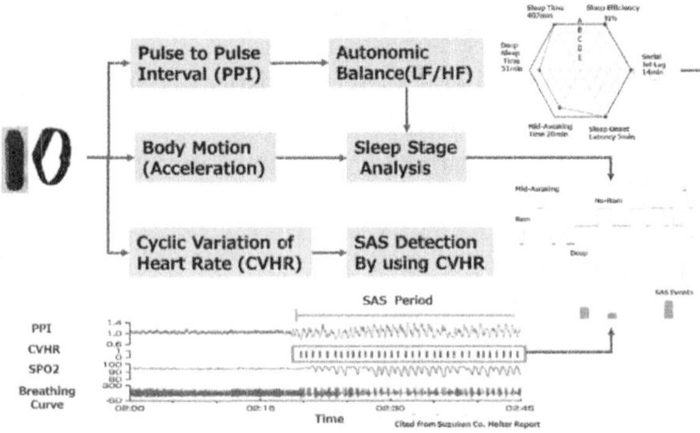

Fig. 10. Sleep-Disorder and SAS Risks Estimation Algorithm

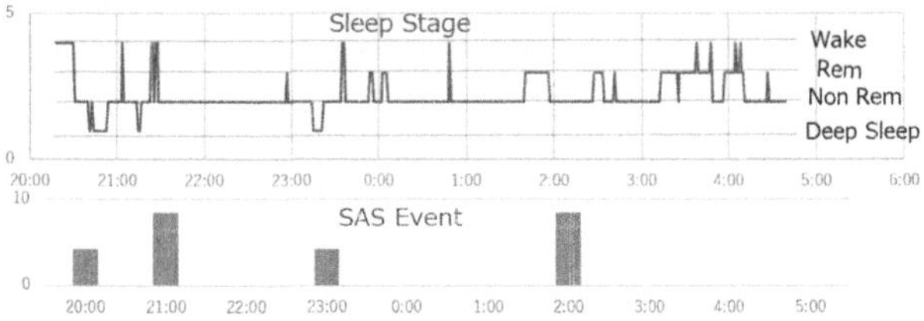

Fig. 11. SAS Risk Estimation Result Example

5 Privacy and Security Protection (Under Development)

The PHR function will be included in the 2025 model of the next MIRUWS M4 system.

As illustrated in Fig. 12, the PHR will offer distinctive features, including an IoT container with privacy controls and a secure, distributed personal data store (SD-PDS). Currently, the MIRUWS M3 system uses web pages and PDF/CSV files as outputs. However, these outputs lack privacy control. The M3 system lacks the PHR function, so users must store and manage their data themselves. The PHR and IoT container solve these problems as follows:

(1) PHR: We use an Advanced Multiplex Secret Sharing Scheme (AMSSS), which distributes important information without drastically increasing its quantity [4].

With this technology, PDS data can be distributed to multiple servers in different locations, such as Hokkaido, Tokyo, and Osaka. Even if one of the servers goes down due to an earthquake, the remaining servers can still produce the original data.

(2) IoT Container: In order to implement a variety of privacy control policies ranging from general consent to GDPR-based, service-specific consent, we use the recently standardized IoT container. As shown in Fig. 12, a service provider or data user offers information to the owner. Once the owner agrees to the offer, a service definition table based on the offer is created and included in the IoT container.

Because the container format is end-to-end compliant, we are proceeding with international standardization activities to incorporate privacy policies into IoT containers.

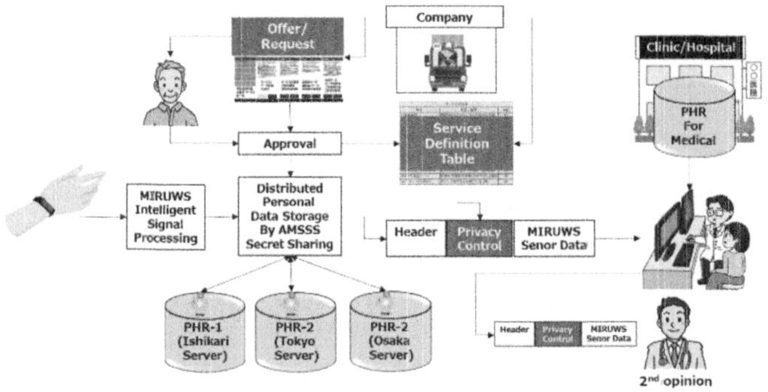

Fig. 12. PHR and IoT Container Functions in MIRUWS M4

6 Conclusions and Acknowledgement

Thanks to the collaboration of academia, industry, engineering, and medicine, the efficient and successful development of the MIRUWS M3 service was possible. Our future plans for M4 and MX (future models) include incorporating new virtual sensor functions, such as heat stroke, frailty, and dementia risks, while maintaining a simple, user-friendly interface. We are also planning to propose our privacy protection method as an international standard to promote the global exchange of personal sensor data while maintaining privacy. To achieve this goal, we are promoting open collaboration on research and development within consortiums.

We would like to thank Professor Katsutoshi Tanaka of Kitasato University for his advice on sleep disorders, sleep apnea syndrome, and lifestyle improvement. We would also like to thank Dr. Toshiya Osanai of Hokkaido University Hospital for conducting clinical trials on neurosurgery recovery monitoring. Our thanks also go to Prof. Masao Yamasawa of the Research and Development Initiative at Chuo University and Mr. Kunihiko Yoshimitsu of Nova Shield Co. Ltd., for AMSSS implementation.

Finally, we would like to thank the following organizations for supports: the Northern Advancement Center for Science and Technology, the Hokkaido SME Comprehensive Support Center, the City of Sapporo, and the Hokkaido Prefecture.

References

1. Minami, S., et. al.: A multi-function integrated virtual vital-signs sensor: MIRUWS. EMBC 2025 Poster Session Wed. 299
2. Nishihara, T., et.al.: Drivers' affect recognition system utilizing multimodal bio signals. The Proc. of JSME annual Conference on Robotics and Mechatronics (2021) (Japanese)
3. Sumitomo, K., et.al.: A cuffless blood pressure monitoring using machine leaning. The 48th Annual Scientific Meeting of the Japanese Society of Hypertension, abstract collection (2024) (Japanese)
4. Yamasawa, M., et.al.: Performance evaluation for secret sharing implementation methods. The 41th Symposium on Cryptography and information Security, Proc. SCIS2024, 3F-4 (Japanese)

Author Index

H. Tanaka et al. (Eds.): BodyNets 2025, LNICST 714, pp. 471–472, 2026.
https://doi.org/10.1007/978-3-032-38657-1

The manufacturer's authorised representative in the EU is Springer Nature Customer Service Centre GmbH, Europaplatz 3, 69115 Heidelberg, Germany. If you have any concerns regarding our products, please contact ProductSafety@springernature.com

Printed and bound by CPI Group (UK) Ltd, Croydon, CR0 4YY
13/10/2026
02232357-0020